Anesthesia for Ambulatory Surgery

Anesthesia for Ambulatory Surgery SECOND EDITION

EDITED BY

Bernard V. Wetchler, M.D.

Director, Department of Anesthesiology
Medical Director, Ambulatory SurgiCare
The Methodist Medical Center of Illinois
Clinical Professor and Chief, Division of Anesthesia
University of Illinois
College of Medicine at Peoria
Peoria, Illinois

WITH 21 CONTRIBUTORS

J. B. Lippincott Company
PHILADELPHIA   NEW YORK   ST. LOUIS
LONDON   SYDNEY   TOKYO

Acquisitions Editor: Nancy Mullins
Coordinator: Lori J. Bainbridge
Production: Editorial Services of New England, Inc.
Compositor: Compset, Inc.
Printer/Binder: R. R. Donnelly & Sons Co.

6   5   4   3   2   1

**Library of Congress Cataloging-in-
Publication Data**
  Main entry under title:
Anesthesia for ambulatory surgery / edited by
  Bernard V. Wetchler ; with 21 contributors—
  2nd ed.
      p.   cm.
  Includes bibliographical references.
  Includes index.
  ISBN 0-397-51038-1
    1. Anesthesia.   2. Surgery, Outpatient.
  I. Wetchler, Bernard V.
  [DNLM: 1. Ambulatory
Surgery.   2. Anesthesia.   WO 192 A579]
  RD82.A677   1990
  617.9'6—dc20
  DNLM/DLC
  for Library of Congress   90-6558
                                                CIP

To Jorie

always understanding

always supportive

always interested

Contributors

■ ■

Jeffrey L. Apfelbaum, M.D.
Associate Professor, Department of Anesthesia and Critical Care, University of Chicago Pritzker School of Medicine, Director, Outpatient Surgery, University of Chicago, Chicago, Illinois

Jeffrey L. Apfelbaum, M.D., graduated from Northwestern University Medical School and completed his residency and fellowship at the Hospital of the University of Pennsylvania, with specialty training in ambulatory anesthesia and operating room management. Since 1988, Dr. Apfelbaum has been the Director of Outpatient Surgery and the Director of the Preoperative Anesthesia Evaluation Clinic at the University of Chicago Hospital. He has contributed extensively to the field of ambulatory anesthesia through his efforts in both research and teaching. He currently serves on the Board of Directors of the Society for Ambulatory Anesthesia and is an officer in that organization. Dr. Apfelbaum's interests include professional sports, gourmet dining, and photography, which he enthusiastically shares with his wife Carol and son Sean.

Benjamin G. Covino, Ph.D., M.D.
Chairman, Department of Anesthesia, Brigham and Women's Hospital; Professor of Anaesthesia, Harvard Medical School, Boston, Massachusetts

Benjamin G. Covino obtained his Ph.D. degree in Physiology from Boston University. He began his professional career as a cardiac physiologist with particular interest in the field of cardiac arrhythmias related to hypothermia. He received his M.D. degree from the University of Buffalo and took his anesthesia training at the Massachusetts General Hospital. He has been Chairman of Anesthesia at the Brigham and Women's Hospital since 1979. For the past 20 years, he has been active from a research and clinical point of view in the field of regional and local anesthesia, and he is particularly interested in the role of regional anesthesia in ambulatory surgery. When he gets the chance, he enjoys skiing and tennis.

Anne Frey Dean, R.N., B.S.N.
President, Continuing Resources, Inc., Deland, Florida

Anne Dean received her nursing degrees from San Antonio College and the University of Texas Health Science Center. She was instrumental in planning, equipping, and staffing the Outpatient Surgery Center at Southwest Texas Methodist Hospital and served as its director. Ms. Dean has consulted on over 150 projects, has spoken at many national and international meetings on the subject of ambulatory surgery, and has authored several articles and two books, *Designing and Managing an Ambulatory Surgery Program* and *All Systems Go.* She is a member of the American Academy of Medical Administrators and the American Nurses Association and is a past president of her local AORN chapter. A former art major, Ms. Dean spends her spare time redoing a 100-year-old Victorian estate. She enjoys fishing, hiking, reading, and music of all kinds.

Burton S. Epstein, M.D.
Seymour Alpert Professor and Chairman, Department of Anesthesiology, The George Washington University School of Medicine and Health Sciences, Washington, D.C.

Burton S. Epstein graduated from the George Washington University School of Medicine and completed a residency in anesthesiology at the Hospital of the University of Pennsylvania. He joined the faculty of George Washington University Medical Center in 1964 and was present during the time their ambulatory surgery unit opened in 1966. He has written and spoken extensively on the subject of ambulatory surgery. He lectured on outpatient anesthesia at the ASA refresher course in 1972 and his first article on the subject was published in 1973. He served as Chairman of the Department of Anesthesiology at the Children's Hospital National Medical Center, Washington, D.C., from 1974 through 1983. He is an avid tennis player. He and wife Diane have two sons, Steve, who is a psychiatrist, and Jerry, who is a practicing attorney.

William A. Flexner, Dr.P.H.
Chief Executive Officer, Option Technologies, Inc., Mendota Heights, Minnesota

William A. Flexner is moving from his fourth through his fifth and into his sixth career. As a consultant, he is winding down the extensive traveling and client work that he has done for the past 10 years in the health care industry, where he focused on assisting health service organizations to adapt and change to a market-driven orientation. As an entrepreneur, he is stimulating the growth of his new firm that develops tools, techniques, and technologies to help improve business meetings. Option Technologies' first product OptionFinder has already received national awards as an opinion-gathering and feedback software for use in meetings and is enjoying rapidly growing sales both in the United States and around the world. As a teacher, Dr. Flexner is looking forward to creating a series of courses for either undergraduate or graduate education that will focus on the development of critical thinking skills. To get things started, the beginning week of each course will focus on the physiologic, historical, sociologic, aerodynamic, anthropologic, animal husbandry, and business aspects of the Frisbee.

A. Beth Frost
President, Somebody Really Good, Inc., Port Washington, Wisconsin

A. Beth Frost has served as Associate Administrator of Business Development of Milwaukee Medical Clinic, a 100-physician multispecialty group practice, and as Executive Director of North Shore Surgical Center, also located in Milwaukee. She also held the post of Vice-President of Marketing of a 1500-bed multihospital system. Ms. Frost formed her company, Somebody Really Good, Inc., a business development, marketing, and speaking and training firm, in 1988. She has educated health care personnel from the front line on through the executive suite on marketing and quality service. Ms. Frost is also an amateur actress and has performed annually in summer stock musical comedies. She and her husband Robert are the parents of 16-year-old twin sons.

Barbara Gold, M.D.
Assistant Professor of Anesthesia, University of California Medical Center, San Francisco, California

Born and raised in San Francisco, Barbara Gold received her M.D. degree from Stanford University. She then completed residencies in Internal Medicine and Anesthesia at the Hospital of the University of Pennsylvania. She recently joined the anesthesia faculty at the University of California, San Francisco, and has been active in their Ambulatory Surgery Center. Her research interests include developing patient selection criteria for ambulatory surgery and responses of medically compromised patients to outpatient surgery. Dr. Gold is married and has two children.

James Lewis Griffith, J.D.
Griffith & Burr, P.C., Philadelphia, Pennsylvania

James Lewis Griffith received his J.D. degree in 1965 from Villanova University School of Law. He has been a very active lecturer and teacher in law and medicine at several universities and has presented on a variety of subjects, including ambulatory surgery, at many national programs. He serves as an editorial consultant to *Same Day Surgery*, *Hospital Infection Control*, *Peer Review*, and *Medical Economics*. His entire professional practice has featured a combination of defending hospitals and physicians. He is a member of the Pennsylvania Supreme Court Committee on Jury Trial Instructions. Mr. Griffith's other interests include sailing, canoeing, and travel.

Raafat S. Hannallah, M.D.
Professor of Anesthesiology and Pediatrics, The George Washington University School of Medicine and Health Sciences; Vice-Chairman, Department of Anesthesia, Children's National Medical Center, Washington, D.C.

Raafat S. Hannallah was born in Egypt and graduated in Medicine from Cairo University in 1966. Following his anesthesia training at McGill University in Montreal, he remained on the faculty at the Montreal Children's Hospital and helped develop its modern hospital-based day surgery unit. He is currently the director of the residency training program in pediatric anesthesia at Children's National Medical Center, where he is actively involved in the day-to-day functions of its busy ambulatory surgery unit. His particular interests include anesthesia induction in children, regional anesthesia, and management of airway problems, and he has lectured extensively on these subjects. He is interested in classical music, traveling, and gourmet dining.

John A. Henderson, M.A.
President, SMG Marketing Group, Inc., Chicago, Illinois

John A. Henderson, Australian born, obtained his degree from the University of Stockholm, Sweden, and the University of Grenoble, France. He began his professional career as a Professor of Economics at universities in both France and Sweden. Upon his arrival in the United States, he worked as the Director of Marketing at the American Hospital Association before founding SMG Marketing Group, Inc., an international consulting and marketing services company in 1977. Mr. Henderson has written extensively on ambulatory surgery in *Modern Healthcare, Health Industry Today, FASA Update,* and *Same Day Surgery.* He has spoken at many national meetings, including those of the American Association of Outpatient Surgeons, the Federated Ambulatory Surgery Association, and the Society for Ambulatory Anesthesia. His interests include extensive overseas travel, and he is fortunate to spend his summers in Greece every year. The introductory chapter on ambulatory surgery was written during his vacation at his London house in a beautiful rose garden he tends while staying there.

Surinder K. Kallar, M.D.
Professor of Anesthesiology, Director of Ambulatory Anesthesia, Medical College of Virginia, Virginia Commonwealth University, Richmond, Virginia

Surinder K. Kallar was born in Punjab, India, and graduated from Rohtak Medical College, India. Following her anesthesia training in England, she joined the residency program in anesthesia at the Medical College of Virginia. Upon completion of her training, she joined the faculty of the Department of Anesthesiology in 1975. She has been Director of Ambulatory Anesthesia since 1981. Her interest in teaching and in ambulatory anesthesia led her to organize the first meeting on ambulatory anesthesia in Williamsburg, Virginia, in 1983, where national authorities in ambulatory anesthesia met. This meeting later led to formation of the Society for Ambulatory Anesthesia. Dr. Kallar is a past president of the Society for Ambulatory Anesthesia and has written and spoken extensively on the subject of ambulatory anesthesia. Her research experience includes clinical studies on the newer shorter-acting intravenous agents. Dr. Kallar's hobbies include aerobics, travel, photography, and music.

Deborah S. Kitz, Ph.D.
Executive Director, Abington Surgical Center, Willow Grove, Pennsylvania

Deborah S. Kitz, Ph.D., is Executive Director of the Abington Surgical Center, a freestanding facility located in Willow Grove, Pennsylvania. She is also Senior Fellow at the Leonard Davis Institute of Health Economics, Lecturer in the Department of Anesthesia, and Research Associate in the Section on General Medicine, all at the University of Pennsylvania. Dr. Kitz attended Trinity College in Hartford, Connecticut, and received her bachelor's and doctorate degrees from the University of Pennsylvania. Previously, she was co-director of the Center for Research in Day Surgery at the University of Pennsylvania and Director of Governors and Chapter Activities for the American College of Physicians. Her research interests include clinical cost-benefit and cost-effectiveness analysis, clinical-economic issues related to ambulatory surgery, and the impact of reimbursement schemes on decision-making of institutional administrators. Dr. Kitz enjoys musical theater, bicycling, rowing, and (easy) home renovation projects.

Leslie K. Leider, M.H.A.
President, Leider Planning Associates, Minneapolis, Minnesota

Leslie K. Leider received his masters degree in Hospital and Health Care Administration from St. Louis University. Prior to starting his firm in 1987, he was a health care consultant with Ernst & Whinney and Robert Douglass Associates, Inc., and Assistant Vice President at St. Mary's Hospital in Minneapolis. He is a member of the American College of Healthcare Executives, was an associate of the American Association of Healthcare Consultants, was a faculty member of the University of Minnesota Hospital Administration Program (Independent Study Program), and has served on the faculty of the American Hospital Association's seminar, "Ambulatory Surgery: Implementing and Managing a Successful Hospital Program," since 1982. When he is not consulting and parenting his two children, he can usually be found enjoying the theater, windsurfing during the short Minneapolis summers, and cross-country and downhill skiing during the long winters.

Peter M. Mannix, M.H.A.
Associate Vice President of Strategic Planning, Mercy Health Services, Farmington Hills, Michigan

Peter M. Mannix directs Mercy Health Services' strategic plan development encompassing the parent company and its five major subsidiary organizations. Prior to joining MHS, Mr. Mannix was Director of Facility Development of Health Management Services, Syracuse, New York, and was a hospital consultant with Robert Douglass Associates, Inc., Minneapolis, Minnesota, and Herman Smith Associates, Hinsdale, Illinois. His project experience focused on the development of long-range plans, certificate of need, and building consultations. A number of these studies are specifically related to ambulatory surgery programs. For five years, he was a faculty member of the widely successful American Hospital Association seminar, "Ambulatory Surgery: Implementing and Managing a Successful Hospital Program." When not jogging, he can be found backpacking, having recently completed his second Alaskan adventure.

Slade H. McLaughlin, J.D.
Griffith & Burr, P.C., Philadelphia, Pennsylvania

Slade H. McLaughlin was born in Philadelphia, graduated from Ursinus College, and received his J.D. degree from Villanova University in 1982. His professional practice involves the defense of medical practitioners in malpractice cases. His other interests include scuba diving, long-distance running, and rafting.

Herbert E. Natof, M.D.
Founder and Past Medical Director, Northwest Surgicare (Medical Care International), Arlington Heights, Illinois

Herbert E. Natof was born, raised, and educated in Illinois, graduating from the University of Illinois College of Medicine in 1954 and completing his residency in anesthesiology at the University of Illinois Research and Education Hospitals in 1957. While visiting the Phoenix Surgicenter in 1971, he met Wallace Reed, and from that moment on became deeply involved in the ambulatory surgery concept. He was one of the founders of Northwest Surgicare, the fourth freestanding ambulatory surgery center in the United States. He has served on the Board of Directors of the Federated Ambulatory Surgery Association, as a representative of the AMA to the Professional and Technical Advisory Board for Ambulatory Care of the Joint Commission, on the ASA Committee on Ambulatory Surgical Care, and as a surveyor for the Accreditation Association for Ambulatory Health Care. He enjoys swimming, long walks, and suffering with the Chicago Cubs. His secret ambition is to publish a novel, and he is currently working on his second.

Cynthia Alexander Nkana, M.D.
Associate Medical Director, Methodist Ambulatory SurgiCare, The Methodist Medical Center of Illinois, Peoria, Illinois

Cynthia Alexander Nkana has fond memories of her childhood and early adult life in Evansville, Indiana. Her undergraduate studies were completed at Indiana State University. When she graduated from the Medical College of Wisconsin in 1979, 10% of her class went into anesthesia residency programs. Amidst the unspoiled beauty of West Virginia she took her anesthesia training at West Virginia University. She returned to the midwest to begin her anesthesia practice at The Methodist Medical Center of Illinois in Peoria. Following her exposure to its active ambulatory surgery center, she quickly realized the importance of the anesthesiologist in maintaining the efficiency of the facility and also in providing for patient safety. She currently finds working in ambulatory surgery one of the most interesting and exciting areas of her practice. Her mosts precious moments are spent with her husband and three children, who are due a "thank you" for relinquishing some of their family time so that she could contribute to this book. She relaxes at the piano, playing the music of Mozart and Schubert.

Fredrick K. Orkin, M.D., M.B.A.

Associate Medical Director, UCSF Surgery Center; Associate Professor of Anesthesia, University of California (San Francisco) Medical Center, San Francisco, California

Quite by accident, Fredrick K. Orkin discovered the wisdom of Francis Weld Peabody, who decades before modern medicine noted that new physicians "are too 'scientific' and do not know how to take care of the patients" and emphasized that "the secret of the care of the patient is in caring for the patient" (*JAMA* 88:877–882, 1927). An interest in returning care to the overall patient underlies Dr. Orkin's enthusiasm for ambulatory surgical care, as well as his other professional interests. A graduate of the Wharton School's Health Care Management Program, he has studied manpower and physician payment issues relating to quality of care. He is also the Chairman of the American Society of Anesthesiologists' Committee on Manpower and is editor of the sourcebook *Complications in Anesthesiology*. He is married and has two teenagers.

Beverly K. Philip, M.D.

Director, Day Surgery Unit, Brigham and Women's Hospital; Assistant Professor of Anaesthesia, Harvard Medical School, Boston, Massachusetts

Beverly Khnie Philip received her M.D. degree from Upstate Medical Center, State University of New York, and her anesthesia training at the Peter Bent Brigham Hospital, Boston, Massachusetts. Dr. Philip organized the Day Surgery Unit at the Brigham and Women's Hospital, Boston, in 1980 and remains its director. She teaches the practice of ambulatory anesthesia, showing that excellent care yields patients' appreciation. Dr. Philip has spoken to national and regional audiences on how to establish a hospital-based program and on tailoring anesthesia to fit the special needs of ambulatory surgery. She has a particular interest in ambulatory regional anesthesia and has spoken and published on that subject. Dr. Philip is married and has two sons. She is a scuba diver with experience in underwater archeology and in marine-life collection. She is also an avid dancer and skier and is a Senior Member of the National Ski Patrol.

Bernard V. Wetchler, M.D.

Director, Department of Anesthesiology, Medical Director, Ambulatory SurgiCare, The Methodist Medical Center of Illinois; Clinical Professor and Chief, Division of Anesthesia, University of Illinois College of Medicine at Peoria, Peoria, Illinois

Born and raised in New York City, Dr. Wetchler graduated from New York Medical College and completed his anesthesia training at the Flower and Fifth Avenue Hospitals. Since moving to Peoria, Illinois, in 1955, he has juggled a private practice with his administrative and teaching duties. He has written and spoken extensively on the subject of ambulatory surgery anesthesia, is Chairman of the ASA Committee on Ambulatory Surgical Care, is ASA representative to the JCAHO Accreditation Program for Ambulatory Healthcare Professional Technical and Advisory Committee, is Vice Chairman, Executive Committee, World Federation of Societies of Anaesthesiologists, and was the first president of the Society for Ambulatory Anesthesia (SAMBA). Dr. Wetchler is a jogger (whose pace has slowed since the first edition of this book was published in 1985) who likes travel and pasta.

Harry C. Wong, M.D.
Professor of Anesthesiology, University of Utah School of Medicine, Salt Lake City, Utah

Born of immigrant Chinese parents in Beloit, Wisconsin, Dr. Wong was the fifth of seven children. He received his M.D. in 1958 from the University of Wisconsin in Madison, where he also completed his anesthesiology residency. Since 1961, he has lived in Salt Lake City, Utah, and has been in the private practice of anesthesiology. Dr. Wong joined with two other anesthesiologists, Drs. John Adair and Wallace Ring, to found the Salt Lake Surgical Center in 1976. He has been a frequent speaker and contributor to the literature about ambulatory surgery care and computer applications; he is President of the Society for Ambulatory Anesthesia (SAMBA), was Chairman of the ASA Committee on Ambulatory Surgical Care, represented the ASA on the JCAHO Ambulatory Healthcare Professional and Technical Advisory Committee, having served as its Chairman, and has served on the Board of the Federated Ambulatory Surgery Association and the Board of the Accreditation Association for Ambulatory Health Care. Dr. Wong has commented on his "good fortune to have a lovely wife, Jean Nagahiro Wong, and four children." His leisure time is devoted to tennis, photography, and travel.

Preface

■ ■

The 20th century should be viewed as the time when ambulatory surgery became viable, when it slowly came into acceptance, when we realized that hospitalization was not the only method of providing quality care, and when within its last decade we will see the number of ambulatory surgical procedures with which anesthesiologists are involved exceeding the number of inpatient procedures. We no longer try to determine why this has happened; physicians and the public now accept ambulatory surgery readily. Ambulatory surgical care has proven itself to be cost-effective, safe, and convenient to the patient, the patient's family, and the physician.

With the development and use of short-acting anesthetic and analgesic agents, anesthesia has played a major role in the growth of ambulatory surgery. The future success of any ambulatory surgery program depends on anesthesiologists' participation and the quality of anesthesia provided. To maintain a position of continued involvement and leadership, anesthesiologists must understand how we arrived where we are today and what our role will be tomorrow in managing the ambulatory surgery patient.

Initially, with improvement and change in anesthetic and surgical techniques, the ambulatory setting became a realistic choice for many procedures. Today, largely because of a thrust toward cost containment, ambulatory surgery is being substituted for inpatient surgery in ever-increasing numbers. Practicing anesthesiologists are quickly realizing the special needs of ambulatory surgery patients and the special problems that exist in managing such patients.

Whereas originally ambulatory surgery meant short procedures on ASA physical status 1 or 2 patients, we are currently seeing more physical status 3 patients, more geriatric patients, and because of improved surgical techniques and instrumentation, a continually expanding list of acceptable procedures. As we view the future, less complicated procedures will be performed in physicians' offices, while more complicated surgeries will shift to the ambulatory setting. Add to this innovative methods of postoperative care (*i.e.*, medical motels, home health care nursing, freestanding surgical recovery centers), and there is little doubt that the increasing complexity of procedures performed in an ambulatory setting will continue during the 1990s.

As we are faced with external pressures from government, industry, and third-party payors to perform more significant surgical procedures on patients who are no longer only physical status 1 or 2, we must, as physicians, make our position known that where a surgical procedure is performed is still a medical decision and not one dependent only on reimbursement. Third-party payors will continue to send us their asthmatics, their obese patients, and their diabetics, but they must allow us the right to evaluate each patient individually, as well as the right to exercise sound medical judgment before the patient is considered acceptable for an ambulatory surgical procedure.

What are the challenges to the future growth of ambulatory surgery? What are the challenges anesthesiologists may face as this subspecialty of anesthesia continues to grow? *Anesthesia for Ambulatory Surgery* was written to provide anesthesiologists with the information needed to understand and meet the challenges.

Many different people helped make this book a reality; I now have the opportunity to acknowledge their help. I wish to thank the individual authors for the excellent quality of their contributions to this volume and hope that you, the reader, find our efforts worthwhile; the members of my department who understood the importance of what I was doing and who allowed me the time to complete this book; and my secretaries, Pam Blayney and Carolyn Pierce, to whom I owe a special thank you—and so do all of you who read this book.

Bernard V. Wetchler, M.D.

Contents

■ ■

xvii

Anesthesia for
Ambulatory Surgery

Ambulatory Surgery: Past, Present, and Future

1

JOHN A. HENDERSON

INTRODUCTION
Surgery in Transition
Hospitals and physicians are seeing dramatic shifts in the surgical market from the inpatient to the outpatient setting. Forces causing the shift in surgeries include changes in reimbursement, physician practice patterns, consumer awareness, cost containment, and technology. These many simultaneous changes are having an important impact on the way health care is delivered.

The series of events that gave impetus to the growth of ambulatory surgery started with the beginning of the 20th century. As the chronology of ambulatory surgery reveals, the rate of change continues to accelerate. The following list points out some of the many events that have led us to this point.

1909: Nicoll first documented the practice of outpatient surgery when he presented to the British Medical Association the results of 8988 operations on outpatients performed at the Glasgow Royal Hospital for Sick Children between the years 1899 and 1909.[1]

1916: Waters opened the Down-Town Anesthesia Clinic in Sioux City, Iowa, for minor surgery and dental cases. His was the prototype of the modern freestanding center. In 1916 he stated, "When the war is over, I trust many of you may develop down-town minor surgery and dental clinics of much larger scope."[2]

1937: Hertzfeld reported on more than 1000 outpatient pediatric hernia repairs performed with the use of general anesthesia.[3]

1959: Webb and Graves reported their experiences with ambulatory surgery.[4]

1962: A formal ambulatory surgical program was initiated at the University of California at Los Angeles.

1966: George Washington University opened its ambulatory surgical facility.

1968: The Dudley Street Ambulatory Surgical Center opened in Providence, Rhode Island. Lacking support from the state health department, which considered it to be no more than a physician's office, and finding no support from third-party insurance carriers, the Dudley Street facility could not maintain itself financially.

1970: The Phoenix Surgicenter (a freestanding facility) opened in Phoenix, Arizona. Ralph Waters' message had been heard. A plaque in its lobby proclaims, "Dedicated to the principle that high-quality outpatient surgical care can be provided in a caring, personal environment, in a freestanding ambulatory facility at a lower cost than other alternatives."

1974: The Society for Advancement of Freestanding Ambulatory Surgery Centers (FASC) was established. It is now known as the Federated Ambulatory Surgery Association (FASA).

1978: The Society for Office Based Surgery was founded. It is now known as the American Society of Outpatient Surgeons (ASOS).

1983: Porterfield and Franklin advocated office outpatient surgery. Of 18,000 procedures, 5038 were performed with the use of general anesthesia.[5]

1984: The Society for Ambulatory Anesthesia (SAMBA) was organized. Outpatient anesthesia was becoming recognized as a specialty.

1987: Hospital-affiliated ambulatory surgery accounted for 9.8 million operations performed within a hospital setting (approximately 45%).

1988: Nine-hundred and eighty-four freestanding outpatient surgery centers performed 1,702,397 surgical operations.

1989: There were 984 Medicare-participating freestanding ambulatory surgery centers in the United States.

In the past, patients preferred hospitalization as long as Medicare, Medicaid, or their group health insurance benefits covered the costs. Most insurance plans covered inpatient rather than outpatient procedures. In the 1980s, however, this unilateral decision making by physicians began to change in accordance with a greater awareness of choices by educated health care consumers. Many procedures previously performed on an inpatient surgery basis, especially elective procedures, were shifted to outpatient settings. In the last few years, patients have been receptive to ambulatory surgery and have accepted that it can be performed away from the inpatient hospital setting.

Hospitals responded to the market by opening and expanding ambulatory surgery facilities and continued to capture the majority of the outpatient business. However, with the increase in the number of physicians performing office-based surgery and ambulatory surgery centers, hospitals have begun to lose a portion of their business. Whereas physicians used to influence their patients to have surgery in the hospitals where they preferred to practice, patients are now reviewing all their options and are turning to ambulatory surgery provided in many different settings.

Competitive and marketplace forces and the relaxation of legislation concerning ambulatory surgery have opened a new market to entrepreneurial physicians. Physicians are forming group practices, performing office-based surgery, and opening freestanding surgery centers resulting in direct competition with hospitals. As new technology lowers the risk for ambulatory surgical procedures, more physicians will move to the ambulatory arena. Those inpatient cases which remain in the hospital will be the more intensive procedures requiring longer-term recovery and overnight stays.

It is evident that surgery delivery patterns are changing rapidly. This is resulting in changes in how health care is delivered, how patients are receiving their health care, and which physician they select for surgical care.

The Shift to Ambulatory Care Services

It is clear that government legislation affecting health care delivery has been significant. It is also becoming increasingly evident that other factors will continue to affect inpatient utilization and, in particular, inpatient surgical utilization.

Cost control has been the primary driver of new developments in the health care industry, particularly in the area of ambulatory health care. Pressure from employers, the government, consumers, and third-party payors to reduce the cost of service delivery have fueled much of the growth in this area.

Some of the most significant growth in ambulatory health facility utilization has occurred not only in surgical utilization, but also in diagnostic services, such as x-ray procedures, laboratory tests, physical therapy, cardiopulmonary tests, and other treatments. Since many of these procedures have historically been performed on an inpatient basis, these shifts in utilization indicate changing health care delivery patterns.

The fact that the hospital is the most important player in ambulatory surgery delivery should not be lost. However, the surgical pie is being further fragmented as more procedures move away from the hospital to other outpatient sites. This shift in surgery delivery patterns being experienced in the United States parallels that of other Western countries where day surgery and clinic-based (physician's office) surgery are common practice.

This shift in total ambulatory surgical activity is clearly demonstrated in Table 1-1. With hospitals controlling nearly 90% of the ambulatory surgery in 1984 compared to a little over 70% in 1990, it is clear that the emerging surgical markets of the 1980s have played an important role in shaping the direction of ambulatory surgery.

Economic Issues and Considerations

The fundamental attractiveness of ambulatory surgery is its ability to provide surgical services at lower cost than inpatient surgery. Employer groups, the government, and other third-party payors view this as a preferable alternative to inpatient hospital care. They encourage and often offer incentives to consumers

TABLE 1-1. Percent Shift in Ambulatory Surgical Activity

	1984	1988	1990*
Physician's office-based	4.5	7.0	8.6
Surgery center-based	6.9	15.7	19.4
Hospital outpatient-based	88.6	77.3	71.9
TOTAL	100.0%	100.0%	100.0%

*Projection
SOURCE: SMG Marketing Group, Inc., Chicago, Ill., February 1989.

(physicians and patients) to utilize ambulatory surgery. Consumers, on the other hand, are attracted not only by the lower cost, but also by the convenience, quality of care, and personal attention.

Much of the cost advantage is believed to come from specialization, which allows efficient use of personnel and facilities and permits tight scheduling of surgical cases. The elimination of ancillary services (e.g., cafeteria, laundry, and so on), lack of 24-hour staffing, and limited laboratory or x-ray services also have contributed to the lower cost per patient. An important cost-containing feature of ambulatory surgery is the elimination of what many view as unnecessary pretesting (laboratory, ECG, x-ray).

Factors Affecting the Growth of Ambulatory Surgery
While the health care industry is fighting to cope with changing financial incentives and technological advances, growth in ambulatory surgery and, in particular, freestanding surgery centers will result in further shifts in delivery. Hospitals have always had an important role in ambulatory surgery. Freestanding surgery centers, on the other hand, as relatively new entrants, have grown and positioned themselves as strong competitors to hospital-based care. In addition, office-based surgery is becoming an increasingly important alternative for ambulatory surgery. Ambulatory surgery will continue to play an important role in the health care system in the 1990s for the following reasons:

1. *Physician involvement.* Physicians have been challenged during the eighties by managed health care programs playing a greater role in health care delivery. This has restricted physician involvement in many aspects of health care delivery. As a result, many physicians, seeing their influence diminished, are seeking to be involved in alternate delivery sites and their administration. In addition, physicians are narrowing their medical specializations as they develop market niches to practice. The emergence of "super-specialties" concentrating in a limited number of procedures is evolving. Much of the new technology in surgery requires specialized training to utilize equipment for many surgical operations.

2. *Technological advancements.* Technological advances in surgical procedures are changing the scope of freestanding ambulatory surgery centers. Each year

more procedures can be done on an ambulatory basis. It has been estimated that today over 60% of all surgeries can be performed on an ambulatory basis. Rapid changes in medical technology, such as lasers, anesthesiology, and endoscopy, have influenced the mix of procedures performed at surgery centers. Over half of all surgery centers have already incorporated laser technology. Cataract surgery, previously conducted on an inpatient basis, is now being conducted almost exclusively on an outpatient basis for both Medicare and non-Medicare patients.

Computers, biogenetics, and new pharmaceuticals reduce body tissue damage and decrease the recovery time for patients. Site-specific ("magic bullets") pharmaceuticals are also reducing recovery times, postponing the need for surgery or, in some cases, making surgery unnecessary.

3. *Medical reimbursement.* Significant changes in Medicare reimbursement have increased the number of approved procedures that can be conducted in an ambulatory setting. The list of approved procedures for surgery centers was expanded in April of 1987 to incorporate over 200 procedures and 1600 surgical codes. This will undoubtedly increase the use of ambulatory surgery.

The result of legislative changes allowing Medicare reimbursement for certain procedures at surgery centers has, for example, seen the number of ophthalmologic operations increase sixfold, now exceeding the number of gynecologic operations. In addition, when outpatient ambulatory visit groups (AVGs are the outpatient equivalent of inpatient diagnosis-related groups; DRGs) come into effect, they are likely to increase the number of procedures. Financial pressures from third-party payors and others have encouraged consumers to have surgery conducted on an outpatient basis.

Ambulatory surgical fees are increasing so rapidly that costs are, in many cases, only 10% less than inpatient surgical costs. Surgeons and hospitals apparently are making up for lost income opportunities caused by the government's prospective payment system for Medicare inpatient procedures and its continuing freeze on physicians' fees.

4. *Consumer awareness.* Consumer awareness and acceptance of ambulatory surgery has increased significantly throughout the 1980s. Consumers are changing their pattern of health care consumption. Patients are more hesitant to be hospitalized for borderline problems and are more inclined to use ambulatory care services and physician offices.

Few problems have been experienced in the quality of care delivered (both within the facility and postoperatively) in the ambulatory surgery setting. Surgery centers, for example, have personnel trained and equipped to handle emergencies that may arise and have associations with local hospitals to handle serious complications should they arise. Since consumers are the ultimate users of hospital services, any change in their utilization patterns has a direct effect on procedures and where consumers will turn for their care.

5. *Integration into the health care system.* Freestanding surgery centers are being integrated into the health care delivery system. Many surgery centers have de-

veloped contractual arrangements with managed care plans, nursing homes, and other alternate providers. This will undoubtedly increase the acceptance of these facilities in the future. Managed or directed care programs give patients financial incentives to use physicians and hospitals as conservatively as possible. It has been a primary program of the managed care plans to contain costs and eliminate many expensive inpatient procedures.

As of 1988, almost 58% of surgery centers contracted with health maintenance organizations (HMOs) and 52% contracted with preferred provider organizations (PPOs). Considering that both freestanding ambulatory surgery centers and preferred provider organizations are relative newcomers to the health delivery system, the degree of penetration is especially significant.

6. *Personal insurance and employer coverage.* Major employers are attempting to hold down health care costs through reduced employee health care benefits, such as reduction in first dollar coverage, greater copayments and deductibles, and usage of alternative delivery systems. There is significant pressure among employers to cut health care benefits. Many corporations are now requiring their employees to pay more of their personal and medical coverage. This will encourage greater use of ambulatory surgery to maintain health care expenditures.

THE SETTINGS OF AMBULATORY SURGERY

The first edition of this book (1985) divided ambulatory surgery facilities into hospital-affiliated (integrated, separated, and satellite) and freestanding (entrepreneurial ownership). Office-based surgery also was included. Within a short period of time, we have noted an increased participation of hospitals in the freestanding arena, an increase in the number of freestanding centers owned and managed by hospital corporate chains, and an increase in the number of physician's office-based surgery suites. In this edition, ambulatory surgery settings are divided into

> **Hospital:**
> Integrated
> Separated
> **Freestanding:**
> Hospital-affiliated
> Independent
> Hospital corporate chain
> **Physician's office-based surgery**

Ambulatory surgery is performed in all these settings. (The advantages and disadvantages of hospital and freestanding facilities are discussed in the section on facility planning in Chapter 10.) Within the hospital setting, ambulatory surgery is categorized into integrated within the hospital operating suite, separated from the hospital operating suite, or as a freestanding (satellite) facility located away from the hospital campus.

The freestanding label is also given to a surgery center when it is distinct and independent from the hospital campus. This facility can maintain its autonomy but can be affiliated with the hospital. These facilities are usually owned and managed by physicians, by a for-profit subsidiary of a hospital, or by a multifacility health care corporation.

The hospital-integrated facility results when a hospital establishes a formal ambulatory surgery program by incorporating outpatient services into an already existing inpatient surgery program. The separated facility is constructed specifically for ambulatory surgery and is located within the hospital or on the hospital grounds. In many cases the facility may be connected to the hospital by a tunnel or bridge. There are also partially integrated systems where a common operating room or postanesthesia care unit (PACU) is used by both inpatients and outpatients, but other facilities (*i.e.*, waiting room, holding, and so on) are separate.

A freestanding hospital-affiliated facility is owned by a hospital and is located at a distance from the hospital. This is, in fact, a freestanding surgery center operated by the hospital to provide surgery availability for their physicians. Physician's office-based surgery is performed in a physician's office where there is an established surgical suite.

THE HOSPITAL SETTING: INTEGRATED, SEPARATED, AND FREESTANDING

With the advent of diagnosis-related groups (DRGs) and the requirement that many procedures be performed on an outpatient basis to be reimbursed, hospital-based ambulatory surgery increased significantly during the 1980s (Figure 1-1). Inpatient surgery, on the other hand, has experienced a decline.

Hospitals have turned away from their mainstay of inpatient surgery to ambulatory surgery. Although the hospital is still where most ambulatory surgery is performed, many of the traditionally inpatient cases have become ambulatory

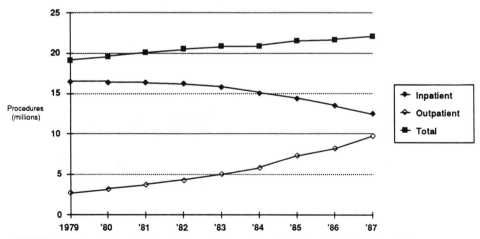

FIGURE 1-1. Hospital setting inpatient and outpatient. (American Hospital Association, 1988.)

TABLE 1-2. Hospital-Based Surgical Activity, 1983–1986

	No. of Operations		Percent Share	
	1983	1986	1983	1986
Hospital inpatient	16,047	13,068	76.1	59.7
Hospital outpatient	5,033	8,823	23.9	40.3
TOTAL	21,080	21,891	100.0	100.0

SOURCE: American Hospital Association, Chicago, Ill., 1983, 1986.

cases. If it were not for the pressures of third-party payors and the growing threat of surgery centers, it is unlikely that ambulatory surgery would have experienced such growth in the hospital environment.

It should be noted that ambulatory surgery has grown more in the hospital-based environment than in other market segments. Hospitals have responded to the competition of non-hospital-based surgery settings with aggressive marketing programs and the expansion of their own hospital-based ambulatory surgery facilities (Table 1-2). In 1980, less than 15% of hospitals had ambulatory surgery programs. Today, virtually all acute care hospitals have ambulatory surgery suites (Figure 1-2).

Hospitals are also competing by establishing their own freestanding (satellite) facilities and also by affiliating with freestanding surgery centers. Hospital affiliations with freestanding surgery centers have tended to be beneficial to both parties. Hospitals provide the surgery centers with the necessary volume to become profitable, while the surgery centers help hospitals to contain ambulatory

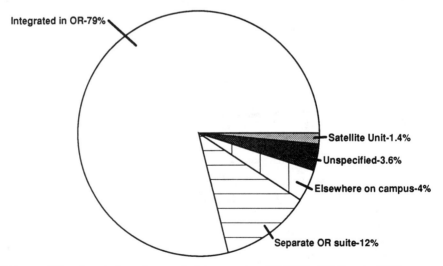

FIGURE 1-2. When hospitals perform ambulatory surgery. (SOURCE: AHA Survey, 1987.)

surgery costs. Many new centers entered joint ventures with hospitals for financial and political assistance, as well as for a management partner. The number of hospital affiliations is growing and is expected to have a greater influence in the market as more hospitals shift services to surgery centers because of financial pressures. Hospitals, however, are continuing to lose ambulatory surgery market share as a result of the rapid growth in freestanding surgery centers and physician's office-based surgery.

By the year 1993, hospitals are expected to perform equal numbers of inpatient and outpatient surgeries. The outpatient market will overtake the inpatient market at a point slightly above 12.5 million procedures per year. As more surgical procedures shift to outpatient settings, the surgical intensity of inpatient procedures will increase.

The number of hospital-affiliated freestanding (satellite) facilities continues to grow, although at a conservative pace. Hospitals continue to recognize that placing these facilities "on campus" is more efficient for both physicians and the hospital. Hospitals appear to be responding to competition by developing freestanding facilities in specific market areas.

FREESTANDING AMBULATORY SURGERY
The Evolution of Freestanding Surgery Centers

Freestanding ambulatory surgery centers, commonly known as surgicenters or same-day-surgery centers, have grown in scope and size since their inception in 1970. Non-hospital-owned surgery centers were perceived as a bridge between the physician's office and the hospital. As technological advances made more surgical procedures possible in the ambulatory setting, surgery centers flourished. Physicians felt that they could offer better service at lower costs without jeopardizing their patients' safety. Surgeons could direct their patients to ambulatory surgery facilities or to their own offices.

George Washington University, in Washington D.C., and the University of California, in Los Angeles, opened the first ambulatory surgery departments during the 1960s to alleviate shortages of staffed beds. Prior to that time, minor outpatient surgery was only occasionally conducted in physicians' offices.

The concept of building an ambulatory surgery facility separate from the hospital was first introduced in 1969 by Dr. Charles Hill in Providence, Rhode Island. Although his attempt was unsuccessful owing to a lack of both interest and financial backing, the idea of a freestanding facility remained alive.

In 1970, Drs. Wallace A. Reed and John L. Ford (anesthesiologists) opened their Surgicenter in Phoenix, Arizona. Since 1970, this center has been a model for many of the more than 1000 surgery centers currently in operation in the United States.

The American Medical Association endorsed the use of surgery centers in 1971. However, the number of such centers did not begin to increase significantly until 1975. Even more rapid growth was triggered in 1981 by the American College of Surgeons' approval of the concept of ambulatory surgery. During that year, the number of new centers doubled. Throughout the 1980s, surgery centers have continued to proliferate as acceptance has grown, the number of procedures considered acceptable for these facilities has grown, and reimbursement has improved.

Surgery centers developed as an alternative to hospital care and traditional medical service delivery. Use of the term *freestanding ambulatory surgery center* refers to both location and range of services. These facilities may be located in specially designed, single-unit buildings or in office complexes. They may be restricted to one surgical specialty (e.g., ophthalmology, oral surgery, or plastic surgery) or may provide multiple specialty services.

In some states, centers are not licensed and are considered to function as doctors' offices. In other states, these centers fall under a clinical or institutional classification. Under this classification, they are licensed and must receive (where applicable) local health systems agency (HSA) and state certificate of need (CON) approval before opening.

Profile of Freestanding Surgery Centers Today

As of January 1989, 984 freestanding ambulatory surgery centers had been established. These 984 centers have a total of 2769 surgical suites and performed 1,702,397 surgical operations in 1988. A summary of national data for 1986, 1987, and 1988 is provided in Table 1-3. It is apparent in this table that surgery centers are not only opening at a rapid rate but are experiencing increased volume as well.

Many surgery centers have evolved into highly specialized facilities by offering procedures that utilize sophisticated technology. Although the initial cost of this technology is high, the volume of cases quickly lowers the cost per case, allowing these centers to capture a local market niche. In addition, the newer technologies may increase patient safety while reducing the duration of surgery and making for an easier postoperative recovery.

Surgery Center Ownership

The overwhelming dominance of independently owned surgery centers has been maintained throughout the 1980s. In 1988, independent ownership of ambulatory facilities already open accounted for 78.0% of the market, while the share of hospital-owned centers declined to 7.5% (Figure 1-3). For the fourth consecutive

TABLE 1-3. Summary of Freestanding Ambulatory Surgery Centers

	1986	1987	Percent Change	1988	Percent Change
Number of ambulatory surgery centers	633	853	34.8%	984	15.3%
Total operating suites	1,930	2,414	25.1%	2,769	14.7%
Total surgical operations	1,100,240	1,476,236	34.2%	1,702,397	15.3%

SOURCE: SMG Marketing Group, Inc., Chicago, Ill., June 1989.

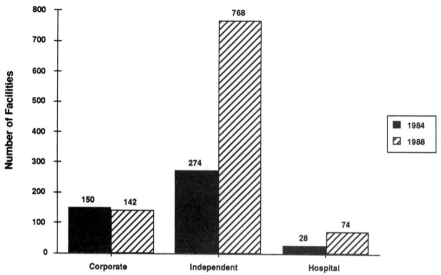

FIGURE 1-3. Freestanding facilities by ownership, facilities open for one year or more.
SOURCE: SMG Marketing Group, Inc., June 1989.

year the corporate chain-owned facilities saw their market share fall. Independents can be expected to maintain their position as corporations close unprofitable facilities and hospitals continue their conservative opening of facilities.

The strong growth of independently owned facilities began in 1984 when they surpassed the development of corporate and hospital-owned centers. Many physician groups and medical clinics saw the opportunity to generate additional revenue by adding ambulatory surgery services. In the past three years, independent freestanding ambulatory surgery centers have gained greater attention and have dominated industry growth.

Multifacility Corporate Chains

Multifacility corporations currently operate 14.5% of the freestanding ambulatory surgery centers. This is a significant drop from 1985, when this same group represented 25% of all facilities. It had been expected that the multifacility corporate chains would grow faster than the other market segments; however, the reverse is occurring. Surgeries in corporate facilities are decreasing as a percentage of the market. The independent sector of the market has grown faster and is taking a greater share (Table 1-4).

Multifacility corporations are finally beginning to recover from their attempts to rapidly develop and purchase existing centers in the early 1980s. Increasing operating income, divestiture of unprofitable centers, and the reduction of development and overhead costs have combined to bring the corporations into profitability. The multifacility corporations are heavily involved in marketing to both physicians and patients. Patient advertising presents a treatment package as an identifiable product and emphasizes the convenience and safety of ambulatory surgery.

TABLE 1-4. Market Share Analysis by Percent of Surgeries, 1985–1988

Ownership (Freestanding Facility)	Percent of Surgeries					
	1986	Percent Change, 1985–1986	1987	Percent Change, 1986–1987	1988	Percent Change, 1987–1988
Corporate	22.7%	−7.1%	19.6%	−1.4%	21.2%	0.8%
Independent	65.7%	3.9%	67.9%	−0.5%	67.8%	−0.2%
Hospital	11.6%	2.2%	12.5%	0.8%	11.0%	−1.2%
TOTAL	100.0%		100.0%		100.0%	

SOURCE: SMG Marketing Group, Inc., Chicago, Ill., June 1989.

Physician marketing, however, is vital to the corporate market. Corporations target physicians through referrals and financial incentives. Referrals come through direct advertising to patients, who in turn draw their physicians to the surgery center to perform the procedures. This is only one method that allows centers to work with physicians to market their practices, to generate new patients, and to establish physician loyalty.

Many of the chains have offered physicians equity, which gives the physician an incentive to perform procedures in the surgery center. This financial arrangement allows the physician to participate in the success of the surgery center. Only recently has this approach been implemented by some of the multifacility corporations, although it remains to be seen how effective this will be to the success of the centers. One limitation to this financial arrangement is possible restrictions placed on Medicare reimbursement through the Ethics in Patient Referrals Act. This bill may disallow payment for patients referred to a facility in which the referring physician has a financial interest. (The term *financial interest* has a variety of definitions and will vary depending on contractual and financial arrangements.)

Most of the chains, believing that their biggest competition is the hospital, are forming joint ventures with hospitals. This arrangement has proven to be mutually beneficial. Hospitals can draw patients through their physician infrastructure, and the surgery centers provide economical care for their patients. Corporations are also beginning to form relationships and joint ventures with HMOs, PPOs, and employer and business coalitions along with physician groups.

Surgery Center Utilization Averages

Utilization in ambulatory surgery centers has been gradually increasing as many of the centers have established strong physician referral patterns and set up a position in the surgical care delivery market. All types of freestanding surgery centers performed an average of 1670 surgeries annually in 1988 in 2.7 operating rooms with an average of 670 procedures conducted per operating room. This is an average of 3.0 surgeries per day per operating room. Corporate-owned facilities have the highest number of operating rooms per facility with 3.5 and perform

TABLE 1-5. 1988 Freestanding Facility Utilization Averages*

	Corporate	Independent	Hospital	Total
Operating room per facility	3.5	2.2	3.2	2.7
Surgical operations per facility	2455	1456	2391	1670
Surgical operations per operating room	711	648	750	670

*Data based on facilities open one year or more.
SOURCE: SMG Marketing Group, Inc., Chicago, Ill., June 1989.

the largest volume of surgeries per facility. Hospital-owned centers perform the most surgeries per operating room (Table 1-5).

Utilization characteristics by facility ownership (open one year or more) increased in 1988 over the two prior years for all ownership categories except hospital-owned. Independently operated facilities experienced the greatest growth in number of facilities and surgical procedures in 1988.

The smaller facilities continue to increase their utilization as they become recognized specialty centers in their local markets. Ophthalmologists, plastic surgeons, and gynecologists dominate the single-specialty surgery centers and have higher than average facility utilization. In some markets, these centers advertise aggressively to achieve name recognition and draw patients away from hospitals.

It is expected that as centers become better accepted and physician referral patterns become established, a dramatic increase will occur in the middle range of 1000 to 2999 annual surgeries. This tendency is beginning to appear in independent and corporate centers open for two to three years and has contributed to the increased utilization in this type of surgery center. Since over a third of all existing centers have opened in the past four years, increases in total surgical volume will continue over the next few years.

The volume of patients at a surgery center is controlled by the available operating rooms. Currently, there is an average of 2.7 operating rooms per facility in the United States. However, most new facilities are being constructed with 4 operating suites. Break-even in these centers is estimated at 3 surgeries per day per operating room. With a current average of 3.0 operating rooms per facility, break-even is reached with 2340 surgeries over a 5-day, 52-week year. It takes approximately three years to reach this level of operation to attain profitability.

As the surgery center concept becomes better accepted by both physicians and the community they serve, it is expected the centers will reach profitability. The main objective of the surgery center industry will be to improve center utilization.

Surgery Center Procedures

The majority of surgical procedures conducted on an ambulatory basis are usually performed on patients who are healthy and do not exhibit any symptoms that might lead to complications during surgery. There are, however, an increas-

TABLE 1-6. Specialty Surgical Procedures Performed at Freestanding Centers, 1987–1988*

Surgical Procedure	Percent Performed†	
	1987	1988
Ophthalmology	27.2%	27.5%
Gynecology	20.4%	19.4%
Otorhinolaryngology	10.8%	10.3%
Orthopedic	10.2%	9.6%
General surgery	9.1%	8.5%
Plastic	8.9%	8.0%
Podiatry	4.9%	4.6%
Urology	3.8%	3.8%
Gastroenterology	NA	2.5%
Dental	1.8%	1.8%
Pain block	NA	0.8%
Neurology	NA	0.4%
Other	2.7%	2.8%
TOTAL	100.0%	100.0%

*Ninety-eight percent of open surgery centers provided the detailed procedure data used here.
†*Percent performed* means percentage of total surgery center operations.

ing number of American Society of Anesthesiologists' physical status 3 and 4 patients entering into the surgery center environment.

The average procedure lasts less than 2 hours, with the patient usually having surgery in the morning and departing by midafternoon. Most ambulatory surgery has been performed on patients under 65 years of age. However, as new surgical techniques allow older patients to undergo surgery with less trauma, Medicare patients are currently utilizing and are expected to utilize ambulatory surgical facilities with greater frequency.

One example of Medicare beneficiary utilization of ambulatory centers is cataract surgery. Several years ago this surgery would have required extensive hospitalization. Today, ambulatory surgery can be performed. Ophthalmology has seen its market share increase from approximately 8% of all procedures in 1984 to over 27% in 1988 (Table 1-6). This 300% increase can be directly related to Medicare's acceptance and reimbursement of cataract surgery performed on an ambulatory basis.

Although freestanding surgery facilities offer a wide range of surgical services, ophthalmology is the most common (27.5% of all procedures), with gynecology the second most common type performed (19.4%). These gynecologic services include therapeutic abortions, tubal sterilizations, and dilatation and curettage procedures (D&C). Following gynecologic procedures are otorhinolaryngology (ENT, 10.3%) and orthopedic surgery (9.6%). Although ENT procedures have always been strongly represented in the ambulatory surgery setting, the growth of orthopedic surgery reflects a new trend. Specialization is another trend in surgery centers. This is exemplified by the growth of single-specialty surgery centers, with ophthalmologic and women's centers in the forefront.

It should be noted that urologic procedures continue to increase their overall share, more than doubling the percentage from 1985. Urologic disorders represent an area of continued growth for ambulatory surgical services. Most women's centers can handle problems of incontinence and infertility at the same facility.

The averages for all procedures performed in surgery centers in 1987 and 1988 conceal wide regional variations caused by differences in regulatory climate and popularity of specific surgeries performed on an ambulatory basis.

PHYSICIAN'S OFFICE-BASED SURGERY

Historically, the surgeon's office has always been a setting for minor surgery. However, as the mid-1980s approached, surgeons performed fewer office procedures because of the following reasons[6]:

1. The availability of organized ambulatory surgery programs in hospitals and freestanding surgery centers;
2. The fear of malpractice suits;
3. Savings on cost of equipment and related supplies; and
4. The reluctance of insurance companies to pay facility fees for procedures done in the office.

As the pendulum continues its swing toward cost containment, one would expect to see more of the minor procedures, particularly those done under local anesthesia, being performed in physicians' offices. In addition, reimbursement incentives are being offered to physicians if they perform surgery in an office setting.

Of importance to anesthesiologists is the number of surgical procedures being performed in office settings under general anesthesia. Many surgeons would like to do more but have not been able to obtain anesthesiologists' coverage. Office-based surgery was pioneered by oral surgeons and plastic surgeons; this has now spread to other specialties, including otolaryngology, ophthalmology, gynecology, and orthopedics.

Hospitals and independent freestanding surgery centers are wary of this trend and the effect it may have on eroding some of their patient base. With the growth of group practices and their multispecialty clinics, it is anticipated that groups will pursue even more ambulatory surgery in the office setting. The number of surgeries in physicians' offices has increased significantly over the past decade, with approximately 842,000 procedures performed in 1988 (Figure 1-4).

The original purpose of the Society for Office-Based Surgery (founded in 1978) was to create a national awareness of the benefits and cost savings of ambulatory surgery, to set standards for quality of care, and to provide an educational forum and information base. With an expanded purpose that now includes liaison with insurance companies and participation in accreditation processes to ensure

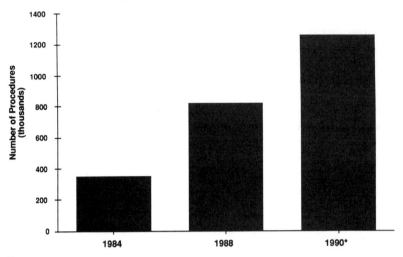

*Projection

FIGURE 1-4. Physician's office-based surgery. (SMG Marketing Group, Inc., February 1989.)

quality of care, the society changed its name in 1986 to the American Society of Outpatient Surgeons (ASOS).

As new reimbursement requirements by third-party payors have influenced the growth of ambulatory surgery as a whole, they also have had a significant influence on the growth of surgery performed in physicians' offices. Even though reimbursement for equipment needs, supplies, and staff to perform surgery in the office is more the exception than the rule, more physicians are electing to perform office-based surgery because they can schedule more cases, better control their own time, control costs, and control staffing. An office surgical suite gives the physician a greater sense of autonomy, which some physicians view as a return to the traditional practice of medicine.

A 1985 study by the House Subcommittee on Health and Long-Term Care found the physician's office to be the least costly location for patients to have ambulatory surgery, hospital-integrated ambulatory facilities being the most expensive. This is principally due to less overhead in the physician's office. Physicians, however, are dissatisfied with reimbursement from third-party payors because many do not provide payment beyond the physician's fee (no reimbursement for facility costs).

The study also revealed some marked differences in certain procedure costs depending on the setting. For example, cataract surgery performed in a physician's office or a surgery center was found to cost half the amount of similar surgery in a hospital's integrated ambulatory department. Significant savings can be achieved by performing certain surgeries in an outpatient setting instead of in an inpatient setting, and in many cases, complete reimbursement of specified procedures may hinge on surgery being performed exclusively in an ambulatory setting. Otherwise, to receive reimbursement as an inpatient, there must be adequate documentation in the judgment of the third-party payor.

Although facility reimbursement is not included in all third-party payor procedures, a number of Blue Cross Blue Shield plans offer reimbursement incentives for such procedures. Examples in effect in 1986 include the following: In North Carolina, there is a maximum reimbursement of $100 to cover the cost of equipment and supplies for any one of 88 office-based procedures. In New York and Arizona, surgeons receive 20% to 25% above the usual and customary fees for designated procedures performed in their offices. In Illinois, a special program provides an additional allowance of $50 for the cost of supplies for any of 14 procedures performed in-office. There are concerns when physicians receive bonus reimbursements for shifting procedures to an office setting. The medical community must be certain that the quality of care and patient safety are never sacrificed in an attempt to increase revenue.[7]

With these reimbursement changes, equipment sophistication, and competition from surgery centers, physicians are performing more in-office surgeries. This office may either be a solo practice, a partnership, or a group arrangement, but one that is distinct from a freestanding surgery center.

Physicians should weigh many factors when contemplating an office-based surgical suite. There is no doubt that the facility will be convenient (to both physician and patient), would be less intimidating to a patient than a hospital setting, and has the potential for attracting new patients. Will adequate reimbursement be received to compensate for the incurred costs of special equipment (both surgical and anesthesia), staff, supplies, pharmaceuticals, and general overhead? Additional factors include litigation risk, expense to the patient (if insurance will not pay for office surgery), and the importance of obtaining accreditation. Physicians who perform in-office surgery can choose to have their office operating rooms inspected and accredited, but they are currently not required to do so.

For the purpose of accreditation (where anesthesia is administered), ASOS has established three levels of care (Table 1-7). Porterfield and Franklin have been strong advocates of level 3 office-based surgery: "Our experiences constitute 16 years of office outpatient surgery procedures. Over this time we have performed 13,000 procedures under local anesthesia with or without sedation and 5038 procedures under general anesthesia. There is a significant cost saving in these outpatient procedures."[5] They continue:

> ... if general anesthesia is to be used in an outpatient [office] facility, the services of a trained, competent and compassionate anesthesiologist should be enlisted. This person must be delegated the responsibility for final selection of patients, including a veto power over the surgeons' selection. Only in this manner can a safe and effective environment exist for the benefit of the patients.

Their conclusion is that the availability of general anesthesia for surgery in the office facility offers the following advantages:

1. Patient satisfaction
2. A broadening of the scope of procedures performed in the office facility

TABLE 1-7. Equipment and Anesthesia Levels

Anesthesia Capability	Examples of Appropriate Operation	Equipment Needed	1989 Probable Costs
Level 1: Local anesthesia	Myringotomy and tubes (13 years or older) Bartholin cyst Skin excisions/local flaps I&D abscess	(Essentially a treatment room) Blood pressure device Crash cart/Defibrillator Ambu bag Endotracheal equipment O_2 tank Appropriate lighting Cautery OR chair Autoclave Portable suction	$15,000–$20,000
Level 2: Monitored anesthesia care (MAC)	Septoplasty Septorhinoplasty Cystoscopy Rhytidectomy Blepharoplasty Breast biopsy D&C Laparoscopy (open) Minilap tubal	*Add:* Anesthesia machine ECG monitor Pulse oximeter Alarm system Gurney Auxiliary power supply Continuous noninvasive blood pressure unit	$35,000–$50,000
Level 3: MAC plus general anesthesia	Herniorrhaphy Vaginal tubal ligation Hand surgery (nonjoint replacement) Closed laparoscopy Cosmetic surgery (unlimited)	*Add:* End-tidal CO_2 monitor Central O_2 and suction	$75,000–$120,000

NOTE: For room size and other requirements, see *AAHC Accreditation Handbook*, 1989 Edition, Chapter 8: Facilities and Environment (National Fire Protection Association, Inc., Quincy, Mass.) as well as *1983 Life Safety Code*; also refer to your own applicable state and local codes.
(SOURCE: American Society of Outpatient Surgeons, San Diego, 1989.)

3. Cost savings to the patient or insurance carrier
4. Convenience to the surgeon

The disadvantages are:

1. Increased startup cost of the office facility
2. Increased responsibility for the surgeon and office staff

As the surgical caseload moves from inpatient facilities to outpatient facilities to physicians' offices, anesthesia practice patterns may have to change in order for anesthesiologists to maintain a share of the available caseload. Before providing anesthesia coverage for an office-based surgical procedure, the prudent anesthesiologist should check the equipment provided, its preventive maintenance program, and whether the office has been accredited to perform surgery. This issue is discussed in Chapter 2.

INNOVATIVE POSTOPERATIVE CARE
To meet tomorrow's challenges, to increase our capability of performing more significant surgical procedures on an ambulatory basis, we are seeing an increasing number of different postoperative health care services, referred to as *after-care services:*

Hospital hotels
Outpatient observation
Freestanding medical motels
Home health care nursing
Freestanding recovery centers

Hospital Hotels
By the conclusion of the 1980s, almost 50% of all surgical procedures performed in hospitals were done on an ambulatory basis. As a result, hospitals consolidated under-utilized beds into one floor or area and developed guest services. Carolyn Jacoby, a Boston attorney, in an article that appeared in *Hospital Risk Management* (August 1986), said, "The riskiest part of bed and breakfast programs is drawing the line between guest and patient." Patients and their families equate space within the hospital as the hospital; however, there is a general feeling that a well-managed program need not be a liability burden.

If your ambulatory surgery unit or department manages a large number of elderly patients or you are a referral center that has patients traveling more than one hour to access care, then a hospital hotel (or medical motel as described later on in this section) could enhance your program's growth. Ambulatory surgery patients, patients undergoing endoscopic procedures or cancer treatments, and elderly cataract patients who live alone are all an absolute market for a hospital hotel.[8]

Outpatient Observation

Following implementation of the Medicare DRG program of prospective payment, it became evident to many institutions that changes had to be made in evaluating patients prior to admission. Some type of extended outpatient evaluation period became the answer to Medicare admission denials. The concept of evaluating patients on an outpatient basis for a longer period of time before a decision of disposition was made has given rise to observation areas or rooms for ambulatory surgery patients requiring additional observation before discharge. Ambulatory surgery patients going into observation beds for less than 24 hours following admittance to the ambulatory facility can be considered as nonhospitalized patients for the purposes of reimbursement by Medicare and other third-party payors. The addition of observation beds allows for patients to receive needed care for short (6 to 8 hours) or extended periods of time (up to 24 hours), have them still be considered as ambulatory patients, and not tie up valuable space in the postanesthesia care unit. Fees for observation units are usually prorated on length of stay; however, fees for maximum length of stay (less than 24 hours) are less than one-day room rates for inpatients.

Outpatient observation areas offer patients continuity of care with maximum payment from third-party payors, decrease health care costs by charging hourly for care received, and offer an added service to physicians for observation of any patient who needs additional time for evaluation before discharge to home or possible admission into the hospital.[9] Surgical short-stay units offer a viable alternative to hospital guest service facilities when managing the ambulatory surgery patient.[10]

Freestanding Medical Motels

Usually, a nonmedical facility, the freestanding medical model offers the ambulatory surgery patient a comfortable, inexpensive, and convenient place to recuperate while being cared for by family or friends. Home health care nurses may provide transitional care. This type of facility allows surgeons to perform more complex procedures on patients who do not require around-the-clock hospital care but who may need some additional attention from a home health agency nurse. Hospitals have entered into partnership arrangements to reserve a certain number of rooms on a yearly basis. A medical motel also can provide a place to stay and other services for patient's families. The majority of motel staffs have no medical qualifications, but personnel usually are trained in cardiopulmonary resuscitation.[11]

Home Health Care Nursing

By utilizing home health care nursing services, ambulatory facilities have the capability of expanding the complexity of procedures performed. By utilizing this service, Texas Outpatient Surgicare has been able to perform vaginal hysterectomies and major ligament repairs on an ambulatory basis.* For example, a patient has a vaginal hysterectomy at 8 A.M. and following surgery remains in the facility

*Battaglia C, personal communication, 1989.

until 5 P.M. At that time, if a decision is made to transfer to home care, the patient is then transported home in an ambulance with a registered nurse in attendance. The registered nurse has availability of intravenous fluids, narcotics, and antibiotics. Registered nurses (8-hour shifts) remain in attendance for 48 hours. The surgeon makes no home visits but maintains telephone contact.

Freestanding Recovery Centers

The Surgical Recovery Center which opened in Phoenix, Arizona, in 1979 originally catered to plastic surgery patients. It now takes care of a wide variety of surgery patients who are transferred directly from a hospital's PACU, from freestanding ambulatory surgery centers, from physicians' offices, and occasionally from hospitals on the first or second postoperative day for further nursing care. The caliber of nursing care is comparable to that of a hospital PACU; surgeons visit on the evening of surgery or the next morning to check on their patients and write appropriate orders (including discharge orders).

The California legislature passed a bill that allows 12 facilities (freestanding, hospital, skilled nursing facility) to add or utilize up to 20 beds for recovery of surgical patients. Patients may occupy these beds for up to three days following their surgical procedure. This demonstration project is to be evaluated three years after final implementation. The purpose behind the bill was to evaluate whether freestanding surgery centers could perform inpatient-type surgical procedures and provide postoperative care more economically than hospitals without compromising either care or safety. It is estimated that 30% of all surgeries currently performed in California on an inpatient basis could be transferred to ambulatory surgery care utilizing this innovative recovery concept.

If the concept of postoperative recovery care works in California, other states are certain to institute similar legislation or permit licensing of such facilities.[12] Whichever of the preceding innovative approaches is utilized, a 30% to 60% saving is projected over traditional hospitalization. If *ambulatory surgery* was the buzzword of the 1970s and 1980s, *after-care services* may become the buzzword of the 1990s.

REIMBURSEMENT ISSUES

Both third-party insurers and Medicare have expanded their reimbursement policies to include surgery performed in an ambulatory setting, particularly in physician's offices. Almost all group health policies now cover same-day surgery. In addition, the Health Care Financing Administration (HCFA) has devised specific reimbursement rates for ambulatory surgery. As of 1987, HCFA increased the list of covered procedures from 100 to 200 and reimbursable surgical codes from 400 to 1600. Reimbursement rates apply to surgery performed in all types of ambulatory facilities (physicians' offices, surgery centers, and hospitals) but are an incentive to perform surgical procedures outside a hospital location.

Prior to 1985, reimbursement to hospitals for ambulatory surgery was considerably greater than to non-hospital-based freestanding centers. Since 1985, there has been an equalizing of the rate, with reimbursement (1989) being the same for designated procedures in hospital departments and freestanding centers. The Health Care Financing Administration has finalized its recommendations on how Congress should extend prospective payment to ambulatory surgical procedures (ambulatory visit group or AVG). Further recommendations are due in the early 1990s.

Medicare reimbursement for physicians' fees in a surgery center is 100%, while in physicians' offices it is only 80%. This creates a disincentive for physicians to perform surgery on Medicare patients in their office. HCFA's reasoning for this discrepancy is that physicians' offices do not have the added expense of a peer-review organization (PRO) review of office procedures, budgets, and objectives. PRO review is a federal requirement for surgery centers, but at present, not for physicians' offices. The direct result of the expansion of covered services and the increase in reimbursement is the increased use of freestanding facilities as less expensive alternatives to traditional inpatient hospital care.

MEDICARE AND STATE CERTIFICATION

Approximately 90% of freestanding surgery centers were certified by Medicare, and nearly 80% were certified by their respective state governments as of December of 1988. It can be assumed that certification is an important factor for these facilities, especially with the importance of both Medicare and Medicaid reimbursement for procedures conducted on an ambulatory basis. As was noted earlier, the expansion of the number of procedures covered by Medicare has increased the importance of facility certification. There is no doubt that the number of certified facilities will continue to grow in the future.

The majority of centers not certified are independently owned facilities. This suggests that independent facilities are less likely to serve Medicare/Medicaid patients. Overall, most centers that are certified meet both federal and state standards.

At this time, physicians offering surgery in their offices do not fall under state or federal health facility licensing requirements. There are efforts to change this with the continuing growth of physicians' office-based surgery.

GROWTH FORECAST FOR AMBULATORY SURGERY
Historical Analysis

The growth in ambulatory surgery has covered all delivery settings. Hospitals have seen their volume increase from 5 million surgeries in 1983 to over 10 million by 1989. Surgery centers performed nearly 2 million procedures, with office-based surgery exceeding 1 million procedures in 1989. The major challenge facing hospitals is the loss of surgical patients to the non-hospital-based ambulatory surgery suites. This has forced hospitals to move rapidly to confront the reality of the changing demands of the marketplace.

Physicians' office-based surgery, on the other hand, has always been in existence. It was not considered a threat to hospitals because the types of procedures historically undertaken were minor and relatively uncomplicated. However, over the past several years physicians performing office surgery have been aggressively pursuing new technology that allows them to conduct more complicated procedures that were traditionally performed in hospitals and more recently have been done in ambulatory surgery centers.

As a result, even though both hospitals and surgery centers conduct the majority of the procedures, it is likely that more physicians will set up office-based surgical suites utilizing the new technology and reimbursement to enhance their revenue stream. It should be noted that there still exists an incentive for physicians to conduct surgery in hospitals or surgery centers since reimbursement is greater. Physicians do not receive reimbursements for facility costs in their own facilities from Medicare, Medicaid, and many third-party insurers.

Ambulatory Surgery Projections into the 1990s

There are now over 800 surgical procedures not requiring overnight hospitalization that can be performed in ambulatory surgery facilities. Estimates of the number of surgeries that can be conducted on an outpatient basis have ranged from 50% to 60%, the most recent projection being that greater than 60% of all procedures will be conducted on an ambulatory surgery basis by 1995. Revised Medicare reimbursement formulas, new technological developments, and a growing demand for outpatient procedures will stimulate growth opportunities for ambulatory surgery.

Hospital Projections Through 1995

The complex nature of the health care industry and the numerous influencing factors in the delivery system deserve special consideration when making projections. Given the following caveats, the SMG Marketing Group has attempted to project the growth of surgical operations in the U.S. hospital markets through 1995.

1. Changes in governmental regulations and reimbursement to hospitals and other health facilities
2. Changes in methods of health care delivery that can affect a hospital's position in the market
3. Changes in medical and surgical techniques that can allow many medical services traditionally undertaken in a hospital to be moved to off-site health facilities

SMG Marketing Group has determined that surgical operations will continue to rise to 29.5 million total cases in 1995 (Table 1-8). It is expected that an increasing number of surgical cases will be handled on an ambulatory basis (Figure 1-5).

Changes in reimbursement by Medicare/Medicaid and third-party insurers will accelerate the movement of cases to an outpatient basis. SMG Marketing Group projects that almost 65% will be done in that way by 1995. Changes in technology, although unpredictable, are expected to lower the cost and availability of health care while increasing the intensity of the average case within the community hospital.

TABLE 1-8. Surgery Projections (in millions), 1988–1995

Year	Total Surgeries	Ambulatory Surgeries	Percent Ambulatory
1988	24.8	11.8	47.6%
1990	26.8	14.1	52.6%
1992	27.9	16.5	59.1%
1995	29.5	18.5	62.7%

SOURCE: SMG Marketing Group, Inc., Chicago, Ill., June 1989.

Office-Based Surgery Growth

The growth of surgery in physicians' offices will depend primarily on the following factors:

> Equipment costs
> Third-party reimbursement
> State and federal regulation
> Liability insurance

If reimbursement rates change to include facility costs, then physicians will be more inclined to use their offices. If, on the other hand, physicians continue to receive the same reimbursement as in the surgery center, they will probably perform surgery on patients in that setting.

State certification criteria may constrain the growth of physicians' office-based surgery in some regions of the country where there are stringent requirements for surgery performed outside the hospital. In addition, the proposed AVG reimbursement system and the overall level of Medicare reimbursement may place

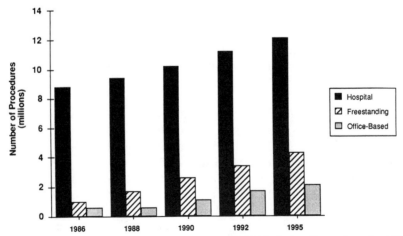

FIGURE 1-5. Growth projections, ambulatory surgery. (SMG Marketing Group, Inc., June 1989.)

limitations on physicians' willingness to participate in this program, thus restricting their patients' use.

Physicians must maintain their cost advantage while increasing their credibility with the public as providers of safe, high-quality surgery in their offices. Continued growth also will hinge on the ability of physicians to meet the following criteria:

> To deliver high-quality care
> To establish internal peer-review procedures for quality assurance and utilization
> To gain accreditation from a national association
> To obtain adequate reimbursement
> To have a substantial enough patient base to support expenses

Consumer acceptance of surgery in physicians' offices also will contribute to this growth. In addition, further technological advances also will mean that new and more complicated procedures may be undertaken in this setting.

Limitations to Growth

The growth projected for ambulatory surgery into the 1990s can be affected by many factors that can potentially change the freestanding surgery center market. These factors include the following:

1. The response of hospitals to the establishment of surgicenters in their service areas could become stronger as they use their political and marketing clout to defend their mainstay business of surgeries. However, as centers become better established, hospitals that are politically stronger may influence legislation limiting their growth. In addition, the hospitals themselves will establish ambulatory surgery programs in direct competition with the freestanding centers.

2. Changes in medical technologies could increase the number of procedures conducted in surgicenters.

3. Legislative changes could encourage the use of ambulatory surgery in both the hospital and freestanding settings. The regulatory and legislative climate could become more restrictive as centers proliferate and affect the traditional hospital environment.

4. Cost-containment efforts could change the current use patterns of outpatient facilities beyond what has been taken into account in these projections.

5. The degree of physician specialization could allow many more types of surgery centers through the advancement of surgical technologies.

6. Potential restrictions could be placed on Medicare reimbursement to surgery centers through the Ethics in Patient Referrals Act. This bill would affect payment

for patients referred to a facility in which the referring physician has a financial interest.

New Developments

New develoments in ambulatory surgery should continue to fuel increased growth. Technology, legislative changes, and increased consumer awareness of health care costs should continue to influence the market over the next several years.

Increased usage of the YAG, argon, and CO_2 lasers in surgery has moved many procedures that were exclusively inpatient to an ambulatory setting. For example, advances in uterine surgery for the control of dysfunctional bleeding could eliminate invasive hysterectomies, allowing over 200,000 inpatient surgical procedures to be performed on an outpatient basis each year. Similar advances in ophthalmology may markedly affect the number of invasive procedures for the treatment of glaucoma and cataracts.

Third-party insurance companies are following the federal government's lead by requiring the use of ambulatory surgery (hospital or freestanding) for more procedures. Many of these insurance companies are using financial pressure (higher percentage reimbursement for ambulatory procedures) to encourage physicians and patients to utilize ambulatory centers except in high-risk situations.

Surgery centers expect heightened awareness of their services as patients, in conjunction with their own physicians, make decisions based on cost, service, and convenience of care provided. As copayments and deductibles increase, consumers are taking a more active role in selecting their health care providers.

The net effect of changes in ambulatory surgery has divided the health care industry into the hospital market that manages high-intensity surgical procedures as well as ambulatory procedures and an alternate-care market that promotes ambulatory surgical procedures.

REFERENCES

1. Nicoll JH: The surgery of infancy. Br Med J 2: 753, 1909
2. Waters RM: The down-town anesthesia clinic. Am J. Surg [Suppl] 33: 71, 1919
3. Herzfeld G: Hernia in infancy. Am J Surg 39: 422, 1938
4. Webb E, Graves H: Anesthesia for the Ambulant Patient. Philadelphia, JB Lippincott, 1966
5. Porterfield HW, Franklin LT: The use of general anesthesia in the office surgery facility. Clin Plast Surg 10: 292, 1983
6. O'Donovan TR, O'Donovan PG: The future is now. In Wetchler BV (ed): Anesthesia for Ambulatory Surgery (pp 1–32). Philadelphia, JB Lippincott, 1985
7. Office-based surgery is target of some insurer incentive plans. Same-Day Surgery 10(12): 159, 1986
8. The patient can stay overnight, visit the doctor the next day and then go home. Same-Day Surgery 10(8): 95, 1986
9. Kaye J: Observation: The health care link for continuity of care. Nursing Management 19(8): 62, 1988
10. Holland C, Cox L, Johnston R: Medical short stay: A viable alternative. Nursing Management 19(8): 38, 1988

11. Patient hotels are a new twist in same-day surgery arena. Same-Day Surgery 10(8): 93, 1986
12. Postoperative recovery centers give same day surgery facilities way to expand caseload. Same-Day Surgery 12(1): 6, 1988

SUGGESTED READINGS

Cotton P: Ambulatory Care DRGs Looming as Analysts "Bundle" Services. Medical World News, May 8, 1989

Davis JE: The Major Ambulatory Surgical Center and How It Is Developed. Surg Clin North Am 67: 671, 1987

Henderson J: Freestanding Outpatient Surgery Centers: A Market in Transition. Health Industry Today, August 1986

Henderson J: Physician Office-Based Surgery: Significant Growth Opportunity. Health Industry Today, August 1987

Henderson J: Freestanding Centers Gaining on Surgical Suites. Modern Healthcare, June 3, 1988

Henderson J: Surgery Center Growth Continues with Integration into the Health Delivery System. FASA Update, July–August 1989

Mapple M: Same Day Surgery Centers: Landmines or Goldmines? Journal of Post Anesthesia Nursing 2–4: 262, 1987

Shannon K: Ambulatory surgery (Special Section). Hospitals 59: 1985

Webb E, Graves H: Anesthesia for the Ambulant Patient. Philadelphia, JB Lippincott, 1966

Wong HC: What Could Wreck the Same-Day Surgery Movement. Medical Economics for Surgeons, December 1985

Legal Implications

2

■ ■

JAMES LEWIS GRIFFITH, SLADE H. McLAUGHLIN

In any discussion today of anesthesia and the risks of anesthesia, there must be consideration of the legal climate that prevails in this country. There is a tremendous preoccupation in this country with the legal risks associated with the practice of medicine, and particularly with a specialty such as anesthesiology that deals with control of the basic cardiopulmonary functions of the body during surgical procedures and control of sensations through the use of topical, local, or regional anesthetic blocks. The purpose of this chapter is not to give specific legal advice, but rather to suggest an approach in terms of risk management to prevent, to the extent possible, litigation.

Obviously, any specific case has its own particular facts and circumstances. In addition, the laws in various states also may be materially different. It should be understood that each case must be considered on its own merits and that specific legal advice should be sought each time it is necessary. It also should be understood that the discussion in this chapter is not intended to state what the law is, but rather to provide a standard that may, in fact, be higher than the minimal requirements developed through case law to date. It is hoped that if all participants adhere to these elevated standards, the risk of harm to patients and, accordingly, the risk of legal involvement on the part of anesthesiologists and ambulatory care centers will be materially reduced.

GENERAL CONSIDERATIONS
Terms
Ambulatory care centers are diverse in their nature and function. Each may have its own merits, safety considerations, and risks. Generally, throughout this chap-

ter, recognition has been given to two principal types of ambulatory care centers: the hospital unit and the freestanding unit. Within the category of the *hospital unit*, there are two subcategories: *integrated* and *separated*. Unless specifically stated otherwise, a reference to a hospital unit is meant to include both subcategories, and the material presented is meant to apply to both these units. The term *freestanding unit* includes the following subcategories: (1) *satellite* (both hospital-owned and joint venture) (hospital/physician), (2) *independent*, and (3) *corporate chain*. The term *freestanding unit* refers to an independent freestanding ambulatory center and does not include the hospital unit or any of its subcategories. The terms *ambulatory surgery center*, *ambulatory center*, and *center* have been used interchangeably throughout this chapter and are intended to include both hospital and freestanding units. The term *office-based surgery* (or office surgery) refers to any procedure performed in a physician's office setting.

Corporate Negligence

Since the last edition of this book was published, an additional theory of legal liability has emerged from several court decisions. Previously, a center was liable primarily only on a vicarious basis; that is, liability was imposed because of the negligence of an agent, servant, or employee. No longer can a center defend itself on the ground that Dr. X, who was negligent, was an independent contractor. Now, under the theory of corporate negligence, a center is deemed to be the provider of all care delivered at the center regardless of the identity or contractual status of the actual perpetrator of the negligent act and will be held jointly liable with the negligent actor for any harm to a patient. A center is now viewed similarly to a hospital as the responsible party for all that occurs on its premises.

This change in legal focus clearly mandates a renewed interest by centers in all aspects of peer review and quality assurance. More important, it is now the center that must police strict adherence to its guidelines and policies. The credentialing standards and the responsibility to carry out all aspects of a peer-review program must be viewed as the legal responsibility of a center, and if the failure to perform any aspect of its mandate results in patient harm, a case of direct corporate negligence may result.

The purpose and focus of this chapter is to provide suggestions to both individual health care providers and to the administration of all centers as to what they must insist on for their own legal protection and financial security. If your name (*i.e.*, hospital, corporate entity, physician) is on the sign in front of the building, you and your staff must take charge and govern accordingly. Adverse public awareness caused by one recalcitrant, noncompliant surgeon or anesthesiologist can cost a center its reputation, its referrals, and even pose a threat to its financial security. In practical terms, if a center is held liable under a theory of direct corporate negligence, it can be expected to pay the full amount of a patient's verdict, and if the person (physician, nurse, or whomever) who actually caused the harm is not insured or is inadequately insured, the center is left with no adequate financial source from which to recoup its payment of the patient's verdict. The center is now cast in the role of the enforcer or "policeman" of all professional services performed on its premises. To view the role of the center otherwise is naive, irresponsible, and potentially financially disastrous.

Surgeon Selection

A center must be careful to choose surgeons who strive to provide first-rate surgical services under maximum safety conditions. Today, ambulatory surgery centers are held to the same standard of care as hospitals (see *JCAHO Accreditation Manual for Hospitals*, 1990 Hospital-Sponsored Ambulatory Care Services). Since virtually all hospitals have established criteria to assess the propriety of allowing a particular surgeon to practice at their facilities, it is essential that all ambulatory surgery centers develop and adopt standards as to the qualifications that a surgeon must meet and as to minimum safety guidelines that he or she must follow in using the center's facilities.

The standards developed by the Accreditation Association for Ambulatory Health Care (AAAHC)* provide that surgical procedures should be

> ... performed only by health care practitioners who are licensed to perform such procedures within the state in which the organization is located and who have been granted privileges to perform those procedures by the governing body of the organization, upon the recommendation of qualified medical personnel and after medical review of the practitioner's documented education, training, experience, and current competence.

Consideration should be given to the appointment of a surgical director of the center. In the *JCAHO Accreditation Manual for Hospitals* (1990), Standard SA.1.3, Surgical and Anesthesia Services, states

> Each organized department/service providing surgical services is directed by a member(s) of the medical staff with appropriate clinical and *administrative* experience relevant to the types of services provided.

A careful review of SA.1.3.2.1–1.3.3.5 is a good starting point in outlining the duties to be carried out by such a director. See also SA.1.4 with respect to the director of the anesthesia service.

Clearly, any ambulatory treatment center that allows a surgeon to practice at its facility without a prior review of his or her education, training, experience, and current competence is leaving itself open to the possibility of being jointly (equally) liable for any negligence committed by that surgeon. To prevent this risk, an ambulatory center should perform an initial screening of all surgeon applicants using guidelines and standards substantially similar to those employed by established hospitals. In a hospital ambulatory care unit, the problem is simplified by the fact that privileges in the unit are ordinarily limited to surgeons who have been reviewed and granted privileges by the hospital to operate in the inpatient unit. With respect to freestanding units, no surgeon should be permitted to do any procedure that he or she does not have privileges to do in

---

*Copies of these standards may be obtained by writing directly to the Accreditation Association for Ambulatory Health Care, Inc., 9933 Lawler Ave., Skokie, IL 60077-3702, or calling (708) 676-9610. In addition, the Joint Commission on Accreditation of Healthcare Organizations publishes an *Accreditation Manual for Ambulatory Health Care* that applies to freestanding facilities only. This manual can be obtained by writing to JCAHO, One Renaissance Blvd., Oakbrook Terrace, IL 60181, or calling (708) 916-5600.

an inpatient operating suite. The issue of how the practitioner who does not have hospital privileges is accorded ambulatory privileges is addressed later in this chapter in the section "Legal Commentary: 20 Questions" (Question 10). Unqualified or underqualified applicants should be denied privileges at the facility. Additionally, peer review on a regular basis, as well as thorough investigation and evaluation of any maloccurrences, is required to ensure the continued competence of the surgeons practicing at the facility. Institution of the aforementioned procedures will unquestionably reduce the number of lawsuits against the center and will ensure that the facility's patients receive an appropriate level of medical care.

Under no circumstances should a freestanding unit be turned into a "retreat" for surgeons who are unable to obtain surgical privileges at other institutions. It is advisable to select only surgeons with demonstrated competence whose judgment and ability are respected and who currently have privileges at other reputable institutions.

A final word of caution is in order. Once standards and guidelines are established, they *must* be enforced. Otherwise they can be used as a basis of liability against the center by a skillful plaintiff's attorney in a malpractice action. (See pages 75–76.) For example, an ambulatory center may establish guidelines requiring that certain preoperative diagnostic studies be performed on patients. If a surgeon fails to order these tests and a complication and injury occur as a result of the surgeon's failure to order the diagnostic tests, the center may be held jointly liable with the surgeon for failing to enforce the medical standards it has established. Clearly, this type of vicarious liability can be prevented with a modicum of effort by enforcing the standards and regulations established by the facility.

Procedure Selection

The range of treatment that may be provided in an ambulatory surgery setting is quite wide and often encompasses procedures as simple as the removal of a mole and as extensive as breast reconstruction. The complexity of the procedures attempted at an ambulatory surgery center should be circumscribed by the type of unit (*i.e.,* hospital-affiliated unit or independent freestanding ambulatory surgery unit).

The hospital-affiliated unit is usually connected to or in physical proximity with a hospital. Such hospital-affiliated centers have the advantage of easy access to many of the hospital's ancillary services and facilities, such as pathology and radiology. In addition, the hospital can provide the convenience of timely consultation with specialists in the event of an emergency. The hospital setting provides an extra margin of safety that may not be available at some freestanding units. For this reason, a greater range and complexity of procedures may be authorized in a hospital-affiliated unit than might be appropriate at a non-hospital-affiliated unit.

The primary consideration of a freestanding ambulatory surgery unit in determining what procedures it will permit is the availability of extensive and in-depth emergency care for sudden and unexpected maloccurrences. Surgeons at these freestanding facilities must not be allowed to become too ambitious in the procedures they undertake. Any operation that poses a substantial threat to a patient's life is best performed on an inpatient basis.

Some reasonable judgment must be made as to what types of procedures the freestanding surgery unit should handle. This determination should be made only after considering the adequacy of the unit's facilities, the qualifications of its personnel, and the proximity of the center to the nearest hospital. The experience of other centers also may be taken into consideration, assuming the units are comparable to the facility in question.

Patient Selection

Patient selection is a shared responsibility of the ambulatory center and the physicians who practice there. The center should develop general rules and guidelines to ensure that there is some uniformity of decision-making with regard to patient selection and to ensure further that patients who are not proper candidates for ambulatory surgery are identified. Patient selection should be made with a number of considerations in mind.

First, the capabilities of the facility should never be overestimated. A patient who is scheduled to undergo an extremely difficult and intricate operation that poses a significant risk of complications is not a proper candidate for outpatient treatment. This patient should be hospitalized so that all the hospital's extensive resources may be brought to bear on the patient's problem if an emergency does develop. Treatment of a patient in a setting that is neither equipped nor staffed to handle untoward events is medically inappropriate and an invitation to legal disaster.

Second, physicians must be attuned to the needs and wants of their patients. For example, the hypercritical patient who is obviously unhappy and apprehensive that his or her procedure is being performed in an outpatient clinic should be admitted to an inpatient facility instead. This patient is a lawsuit waiting to happen. Ambulatory surgical procedures should be attempted only on patients who, after appropriate explanation, have no objection to undergoing same-day surgery that will involve recovery in a home environment.

The final, and perhaps most important, consideration in determining whether a patient is an acceptable candidate for ambulatory surgery is whether that person's past medical history or present state of health would place him or her at an unreasonable degree of risk by performance of the procedure in an outpatient setting. Evaluation of every patient should include a careful and detailed history, with particular emphasis on prior surgical experience and problems. For example, patients with a history of massive bleeding during surgery or patients who have previously experienced a severe reaction to anesthesia are poor candidates for ambulatory surgical care. Any medical history or physical examination that raises the possibility that the facility may be confronted with a sudden, catastrophic emergency or prolonged postoperative recovery excludes consideration of ambulatory surgery. It is foolish to proceed in an outpatient setting under such circumstances, since it is then likely the physician will be sued for undertaking the procedure in a facility that is ill-equipped to handle a complication that might have been anticipated.

Where there is any indication from past medical history, present state of health, or otherwise that a patient is at risk of developing a complication the surgical center may not be able to handle as efficiently as a hospital, the procedure should be performed in an inpatient setting. Again, it must be stressed that a physician will be able to isolate patients with a predisposition to the development of complications only if appropriate preoperative diagnostic procedures are performed and careful present and past medical histories are obtained.

ANESTHESIA MANAGEMENT OF THE AMBULATORY PATIENT

The anesthesia management of a particular patient is the responsibility of the director of anesthesia services and the person who administers the anesthetic agent. If the person who administers the anesthetic is a nurse-anesthetist, ultimate responsibility for his or her acts or omissions also may rest on the surgeon, the anesthesiologist, the director of anesthesia services, or the ambulatory center that employs the nurse-anesthetist. It is therefore imperative that there be strict adherence to the rules and regulations not only of the ambulatory surgery center but also of the various licensing, regulatory, or reviewing agencies. See pages 49 to 52 for a more detailed discussion of agency standards and guidelines.

Some of the guidelines that have been published are discussed later in this section, but a word of caution is necessary at the outset. Strict adherence to the standards established by an industry or profession may be essential to proving that one acted in accordance with accepted standards of care. However, this alone is not a guarantee that one will avoid legal difficulties. No profession or industry can ever isolate itself from legal liability simply by adopting a standard of care and then proving that it followed that standard. Standards are often the real issues on trial. The courts have repeatedly stated that in each case it is for the jury to determine whether a standard followed by a physician was inadequate or unsafe. The physician is always responsible for treating the patient in the safest possible manner and in the event of an emergency or other misadventure must act quickly and appropriately to protect the patient.

Hospital Units

Hospital-affiliated ambulatory surgery units are required to have published regulations that pertain to most situations and procedures. There must be a departmental chain of command and formalized supervision. These and other similar procedures are specifically required by the *Accreditation Manual for Hospitals*, a publication issued by the Joint Commission on Accreditation of Healthcare Organizations (JCAHO), formerly the Joint Commission on Accreditation of Hospitals (JCAH).* The materials promulgated by the JCAHO are published as "standards." Each standard is followed by an "interpretation" section that further defines the scope of required action implicit in the standard.

If a hospital unit has submitted to a JCAHO survey and is accredited, it is

*This publication, which applies only to hospitals and hospital-affiliated ambulatory units, may be obtained by writing to the Joint Commission on Accreditation of Healthcare Organizations, One Renaissance Blvd., Oakbrook Terrace, IL 60181, or calling (708) 916-5600.

understood that the unit has agreed to comply with the JCAHO standards. The patients are deemed to be, in effect, the beneficiaries of these standards to the extent that they pertain to patient safety during the administration of anesthesia.

ACCREDITATION STANDARDS ON TRIAL

The following is an abbreviated, hypothetical version of a case involving patient injury in a hospital relating to problems with the anesthesia apparatus. It is a synposis of what any experienced malpractice trial lawyer has heard on more than a few occasions, and it illustrates the accreditations trap.

Q: Doctor, is your hospital accredited by the JCAHO?

A: Yes.

Q: Are you familiar with the accreditation process?

A: Yes.

Q: Have you received the JCAHO standards for accreditation as they relate to anesthesia services?

A: Yes. [If the answer is "No," the witness becomes vulnerable for not having ever read what is supposed to be an applicable standard in the hospital.]

Q: Does your hospital have regulations for anesthesia safety?

A(1): Yes. [At this point, the witness can be examined as to whether there was compliance with the hospital's own regulations or about the inadequacy of those regulations.]

A(2): No. [The witness is then vulnerable because, under a number of the standards, the director is responsible for developing such regulations.]

Q: Does your department have a program for continuing education?

A: No. [Another violation of JCAHO standards.]

Q: In this specific case, what inspection of the apparatus that was to be used did you carry out?

A: None. I assumed it was working properly, since it had been used the day before without problems.

Q: Doctor, was there a written regulation in your hospital that required you to inspect all the equipment before it was used?

A: No. [A violation of JCAHO standards.]

Q: Doctor, if there has been such a regulation, would you have complied with it?

A: Yes. [Now the failure to comply with the standard may be argued as the cause of the injury if such a preprocedure check would have found the defect or leak in the delivery system.]

Q: After the incident in the operating room, were there any specific problems that this patient had?

A: Yes. We were concerned that the patient might have an increase in secretions, and it was very important that the patient be suctioned at frequent intervals.

Q: How frequently did you intend to do so?

A: At least once every half hour and more frequently if necessary.

Q: What specific instructions did you give to the recovery room personnel?

A: None. They are well trained. [A violation of JCAHO requirements.]

Q: Well, Doctor, were the personnel in the recovery room informed of the event in the OR?

A: Not by me.

Q: By anyone?

A: I do not know.

Q: Well then, how were the recovery room personnel supposed to know about this specific problem?

A: I do not know.

Q: Why didn't you tell them?

A: I was getting ready to do another case.

Q: Do you know that the patient became obstructed in the recovery room, became cyanotic, and as a result, suffered cerebral anoxia, resulting in brain damage?

A: I know that now.

Q: If the recovery room personnel had been told by you of the particular problem you encountered during the procedure and had been in-

Continued

structed by you to aspirate as frequently as you had previously indicated, would that not have significantly reduced the risk of airway obstruction?

A: Yes.

Q: And this brain death injury could have been prevented if you had given such instructions and they had been carried out?

A: I suppose so. [At this point, get out the checkbook.]

Q: By the way, Doctor, where in the anesthesia record does it describe the fact that the patient's drop in oxygen saturation was caused by the leak you found in the delivery system?

A: It is not written there. [A violation of JCAHO standards and a basis for arguing fraudulent concealment of the problem to prevent a lawsuit.]

It is important for a facility to be accredited, but accreditation is not an honor—it is an ongoing responsibility to comply with the very standards that you agreed would govern the anesthesia services performed in your institution.

The failure to achieve accreditation is equally hazardous if the facility or the director admits that an accreditation survey was conducted and the anesthesia service was cited for numerous inadequacies when accreditation was denied. You can be certain that if a patient injury can be linked to any one of the inadequacies found by the accreditation survey team, the case is lost. There are facilities, however, that have never requested an accreditation survey be performed (accreditation is not presently a requirement for providing services). Although this in no way is a reflection on competency, not having to comply with standards of acceptable accrediting organizations may be viewed during a trial as providing a lesser quality of care.

Freestanding Center

What was stated in the preceding section is equally applicable to freestanding centers. An examination of the text of the accreditation standards published by the AAAHC reveals similarities with standards found in the JCAHO manuals (Accreditation Manual for Hospitals and Accreditation Manual for Ambulatory Health Care). There is no dispute as to the fact that one of the primary purposes of all such standards is the delivery of anesthesia to patients under conditions that are as safe as possible. However, these standards can become the proverbial sword of Damocles. One must comply to become accredited, but once one is accredited, full compliance is mandated not only to keep the accreditation, but also to ensure that patient safety is preserved. In the event of a mishap, these same standards then take on the role of the yardstick by which one's conduct will be measured.

One additional point needs to be stressed: From a legal standpoint, there is no justification for a difference in standards of anesthesia management in an ambulatory surgery center from those in a hospital. In the context of patient safety, the criteria for anesthesia management must be the same.

TRIAL EXCERPT INVOLVING INFORMED CONSENT: CAN ANESTHESIA STANDARDS DIFFER?

Q: Doctor, you have argued here that because of the nature of the ambulatory center and in an effort to provide a lower cost for your procedures, you are not able to provide the same level of patient safety in your anesthesia services as that provided by hospitals. Is that correct?

A: Yes.

Q: Now Doctor, before you gave this patient anesthesia, did you tell the patient that there was a risk of death, anoxia, hypoxia, brain damage, and other potential morbidities associated with general anesthesia even if you do everything as best you know how?

A: Yes.

Q: But Doctor, did you tell the patient that his risks were greater if he had the procedure done in your ambulatory surgery center because you, in an effort to lower costs, were not maintaining the same levels of patient safety in your center as would be available in a hospital?

A: No.

Q: Would you then agree, Doctor, that this man did not know of that risk (because you didn't tell him) when he agreed to be anesthetized in your center?

A: Yes.

If the criteria for anesthesia management are not the same, is it possible to overcome the informed consent problem? It is if you want to announce publicly that it is less safe to have anesthesia in your ambulatory surgery center than it is in a hospital. Why don't you just close the front door and sell the building now before the word gets out! The conclusion is obvious: There should never be and cannot defensibly be two disparate levels of patient care, management, and safety between the ambulatory center and the hospital inpatient administration of anesthesia services.

Office-Based Surgery

Recently, some third-party payors have been giving financial encouragement to surgeons to perform certain procedures in their offices by agreeing to a higher level of reimbursement. To the extent that a particular surgeon is highly judicious in the selection of patients and of the procedures he or she will perform in the office setting, this monetary incentive may be appropriate. To the extent that it affords some semblance of propriety to such locations of surgery, it may ultimately be a disaster in terms of patient safety, for standards of care provided in an office surgery suite are not addressed.

Peer review is one way a patient is protected from doctors who may be marginally competent. However, who reviews a physician's competency in his or her own office? Who says what procedures he or she can or cannot do? Who determines whether a given patient has been properly evaluated in accordance with some predetermined preoperative criteria? Are these problems peculiar to surgeons? What about the anesthesiologist who goes into such an office to participate in a procedure? What responsibility does such an anesthesiologist bear?

What about the JCAHO or AAAHC safety standards in such a setting? Are they no longer applicable? Are the guidelines for equipment (see Chapter 1, Table 1–7) recommended by the American Society of Outpatient Surgeons (ASOS)* comprehensive and thorough enough to ensure optimal patient care? These are just a sampling of the many, diverse issues that confront anesthesia practitioners involved in the performance of office-based procedures.

The obligations imposed on an anesthesiologist in an office setting may, in fact, be greater and involve a greater risk of being sued. In an office setting, an anesthesiologist may not have all the support personnel to assist in an emergency, and consequently, the risk of harm to the patient in the event of an anesthesia emergency may be greater. What about resuscitation equipment, medications, monitoring equipment, and the like? Is it not the responsibility of the anesthesiologist to adequately monitor a patient during a procedure and to treat that patient if respiratory function ceases or another emergency arises? What about transport arrangements and access to hospital facilities? Suppose the surgeon is not on the staff of any hospital in town.

The anesthesiologist has to protect the patients as well as himself or herself. Patients must be carefully evaluated, and all pertinent medical factors must be weighed and considered. The anesthesiologist should not accept any patient who is at greater risk in an office setting than he or she would be in an inpatient facility. If all the procedures are minor and the patients are all in excellent health, there may be less risk of having to use resuscitation equipment, but is that an acceptable basis for having less emergency equipment? If the patients are not all young and healthy and the procedures are not all quick and innocuous, the need increases to have all the requisite equipment and personnel to promote the interests of patient safety. If a patient gets into anesthesia-related trouble, remember that it will be the surgeon who will testify that he or she relied on the anesthesiologist to clear the patient for the procedure and to determine what, if any, equipment was necessary. Frequently, a surgeon will tell a jury that if the anesthesiologist had mentioned that he or she did not think the procedure was safe, the surgeon would never have operated in the first place.

An anesthesiologist cannot stop a surgeon from doing any procedure in his or her own office, but he or she does not have to participate. The anesthesiologist should carefully assess all the personnel, equipment, supplies, medications, and so forth, and if he or she finds them inadequate, he or she should refuse to participate in any procedure until the deficiencies have been corrected. This is probably the biggest favor an anesthesiologist will ever do for a patient and for himself or herself. Since the risks associated with anesthesia are the same regardless of whether the patient is admitted to a hospital or operated on in an office, the standards must be the same.

Ways to Avoid Legal Hazards
The preceding sections have addressed this issue in part. Basically, a starting point has to be to sit down and read the accreditation standards (see footnotes

*The American Society of Outpatient Surgeons, P.O. Box 33185, San Diego, CA 92103, (619) 692-9918.

on pp. 31, 34, and 38). The American Society of Anesthesiologists also has policies, guidelines, and standards for anesthesia care.* Then careful consideration of your practices and procedures in the context of these standards should be undertaken. Do you, in fact, have the written policies and regulations the standards require? Weigh all such procedures and regulations in the context of patient safety. Are they as current and appropriate as they should be? Can they be improved? When was the last time they were reviewed with the anesthesiologists and nurse-anesthetists who work in the ambulatory center? Is your equipment given regular inspections and maintenance checks? To whom do you report suspected problems? If you suspect an equipment problem, do you take the device out of service until the suspected problem can be checked?

There is no magic formula to avoid legal risks—certainly not a mechanical adherence to a lawyer's checklist. Patient care and the safe management of anesthesia service for ambulatory surgery, wherever it is performed, must become an overwhelming consideration in everything you do. It must be the cornerstone of your mental examination and inspection of your staff, facilities, and daily operations. It must be the touchstone by which you evaluate the procedures that should or should not be attempted in your facility. And finally, and perhaps most important, it must be the litmus paper by which you decide whether each patient has been appropriately selected, tested, and informed before any procedure is undertaken. If any of these factors, when weighed against the overriding factor of patient safety, tips the scale in such a way that the patient being given anesthesia is placed at greater risk in an ambulatory center than in an inpatient facility, then do not administer the anesthesia. Resolve all such doubts in favor of the patient's safety or transfer to an inpatient facility.

Finally, all conduct by health care providers is evaluated in court in terms of its degree of consistency with applicable prevailing standards of conduct at the time the treatment was rendered. There may be many physicians who are willing to testify as expert witnesses that ambulatory centers or physicians' offices are not as safe as inpatient facilities. It does not matter whether such testimony is biased, based on ignorance of ambulatory surgery, or even inaccurate. It will still be heard by the jury because the judge is not medically qualified to the point where he or she can substitute his or her opinion for that of the physician-witness. It is therefore urgent that in the ambulatory center there be as little difference as possible in the level of patient care and that, in all respects, the anesthesia management of the patient be as good as or better than its inpatient counterpart.

PREANESTHESIA VISIT
Definition and Purpose
The *preanesthesia visit*, or *patient interview* as it is commonly called, serves as a vehicle to facilitate the exchange of information between the anesthesiologist and

---

*Peer Review in Anesthesiology (monograph). The American Society of Anesthesiologists. 515 Busse Highway, Park Ridge, IL 60068, (708) 825-5586.

the patient (see *JCAHO Accreditation Manual for Hospitals*, 1990, standard SA.1.5, Surgical and Anesthesia Services). In essence, there are two objectives the anesthesiologist should seek to accomplish during this meeting with the patient. First, this initial interview is the appropriate forum to elicit relevant information from the patient about his or her present state of health, past medical history, prior reactions to any medication or anesthetic agent, and any other information that may be pertinent to the form of anesthesia contemplated. Second, the anesthesiologist should educate the patient during the patient interview about all the relevant information necessary in order for the patient to give a truly informed consent (the specifics of this issue are addressed later in the section "Informed Consent").

As illustrated earlier, the anesthesiologist should strive to impart as well as to extract information during the patient interview. In this fashion, the anesthesiologist will learn of the likely difficulties and problems that may be encountered with this individual and the patient will have a genuine awareness and understanding of the anesthesia aspect of the procedure he or she is about to undergo. Proper use of the patient interview will, in many instances, forestall litigation not only by averting anticipated complications through advance preparation, but also by removing liability for medical risks by making the patient aware of what might occur.

When and Where

Unquestionably, every patient deserves an ample amount of time to consider and reflect on the risks, benefits, and alternatives associated with the planned anesthetic agent as well as with the method by which it is to be administered. Similarly, the anesthesiologist needs time to analyze, evaluate, and deliberate about the information received from the patient. Depending on the data that have been elicited, ordering past medical records or contacting prior treating physicians may be indicated.

The benefits to be gained from the preanesthesia visit can be achieved only if sufficient time for contemplation and deliberation is afforded both the patient and the anesthesiologist. For inpatients, who are generally the higher-risk patients, the preanesthesia conference frequently occurs on the evening before surgery. It is not surprising, therefore, that in ambulatory surgery centers, the preanesthesia visit normally occurs on the day of the procedure. However, this visit should be conducted as soon as the patient arrives so that as much time as possible is gained for thought and reflection. A good surgeon who really knows the patient and who is concerned about that patient's welfare should notify the anesthesiologist far in advance of the upcoming procedure. This will allow the anesthesiologist to call the patient several days before the procedure to review the relevant information or to retrieve the patient's records. Prior notice of suspected problems may avert last-minute postponements and consequent patient displeasure.

Quite clearly, a meeting with the patient in the operating room itself just before the surgical procedure is unacceptable. These are a few of the many problems with this practice:

> A meaningful exchange of information is rendered more difficult owing to the patient's anxiety about the imminent surgical procedure.
>
> The anesthesiologist has foreclosed the opportunity for investigation of significant risk factors that might have been elicited during the interview.
>
> A truly informed consent may not be obtainable because the anesthesiologist has not had sufficient time to adequately analyze the risks, benefits, and alternatives associated with the planned anesthesia management, and perhaps more important, the patient has not had an opportunity to make a meaningful choice as to whether the contemplated anesthesia plan is acceptable.

All these problems can be obviated if the patient interview is conducted in advance of the surgical procedure. There is no question that this will involve additional time, effort, and planning. However, in the long run, it may save the time, energy, and expense associated with litigation of a malpractice suit.

There is no one right answer to the question of where and how the preanesthesia interview should be held. The optimal encounter would involve a face-to-face meeting between the anesthesiologist and the patient in a separate anesthesia screening office or in some other private space at the surgery center. This has the advantage of allowing the two to meet in a relaxed atmosphere and develop some sort of rapport before the anesthesia is administered. In addition, there is a greater opportunity for follow-up questions by both parties about the information exchanged.

In situations where a face-to-face meeting is not possible, either because of space restrictions or scheduling problems, a telephone conference may be substituted. Again, the telephone interview should take place as long before the scheduled surgical procedure as possible.

Some type of direct contact between the patient and the anesthesiologist should take place before surgery. Some institutions, as a time-saving measure, have resorted to preprinted forms and questionnaires to obtain informed consent and pertinent medical history from patients. These are appropriate measures, but they should always be reviewed personally with the patient on the day of the procedure. Such an approach promotes a meaningful exchange of information between a physician and the patient. Forms alone should never be used in lieu of a complete preanesthesia interview by the anesthesiologist.

Finally, the patient's medical record should contain the significant aspects of the medical history and physical examination. It is extremely important to record what the patient admits as well as what he or she denies. A simple note, such as "Denies S.O.B., allergies, asthma, or other respiratory problems," may save the day if the patient subsequently claims to have advised the anesthesiologist of such a problem and the procedure went forward with untoward consequences. The note should clearly reflect that there also was a detailed discussion of the risks of anesthesia and that the patient understood the discussion and consented. A listing of the most critical risks is particularly helpful: "Death, respiratory arrest, infection, hemorrhage," and so on. The point is simple. Let's assume

Mrs. Lange sustains a pulmonary problem that requires medication, postprocedure radiography and follow-up, and perhaps even a prolonged admission. The
patient claims that she was never told of this remote and unusual risk and that
she would not have undergone the procedure had she been so advised. If the
anesthesiologist can then present a note in the medical record stating that the
patient was willing to run the serious risk of hemorrhage and even death, it is
much easier to convince the jury that a person who is willing to risk death would
have accepted the risk of a relatively benign complication that might have occurred. Getting the patient to sign the note in the medical record as well as a
written consent form is highly recommended.

APPROPRIATE PREANESTHESIA LABORATORY TESTS

The use of mandatory preoperative or preanesthesia laboratory tests is meeting
with increasing disfavor. The cost of these tests outweighs their limited usefulness and the information they provide. The American Society of Anesthesiologists
addresses appropriate indications for ordering tests in its *Statement on Routine
Preoperative Laboratory and Diagnostic Screening* (see Chapter 3, Appendix 3A).
The ambulatory center has the responsibility to state what tests it will require
before the patient undergoes a given procedure. It must be emphasized, however,
that these are minimum requirements. At no time should the ambulatory center
appear to be inhibiting a physician from doing any further testing he or she
believes is medically indicated. This caveat is based on the simple fact that in
certain cases in which physicians did not perform indicated tests, they have
sometimes sought to extricate themselves by arguing that the hospital or other
facility had dissuaded them from doing the tests because of the institution's financial concerns. They have even gone so far as to suggest that they were in fear
of losing staff privileges if they performed more than the specified minimum
tests. Defendants in lawsuits take strange positions when trying to defend their
professional reputations and their assets. They are not above distorting sound
restrictions into total bans. It is therefore important to state unequivocally in the
written regulations of the center that the required preoperative and preanesthesia tests are minimums and that the ultimate responsibility for the medical
judgment as to what additional tests are required for a particular patient remains
with the attending surgeon and anesthesiologist.

Hospital Units

There are potential legal pitfalls if there are variations in treatment between hospital inpatients and patients undergoing the same procedures in hospital ambulatory centers. However, there are good reasons why a hospital, for its anticipated inpatient population, may specify a much more intensive program of
preoperative testing. Major teaching institutions may permit or encourage the
performance of numerous preoperative procedures or tests on their inpatients
as part of the teaching process. In fact any patient, regardless of age, who is at a
high risk for complications should be admitted to a hospital's inpatient surgery
service rather than to its ambulatory center for the procedure. There are many

operative procedures that cannot and should not be performed in an ambulatory center.

It is the responsibility of the surgical and anesthesia staffs in the hospital ambulatory facility to specify which procedures and which patients are appropriate. It is very important in a hospital setting that the staffs of both the inpatient unit and the ambulatory unit carefully review, procedure by procedure, their recommendations as to preoperative testing. In so doing, however, the temptation to become dogmatic must be avoided. "This is how we do it in the inpatient service and therefore this is the way it must be done in the hospital ambulatory unit."

If a real difference between patients receiving the same procedure does not generally exist, there should not be a lesser standard of preprocedure testing in the hospital ambulatory unit. On the other hand, if patients who have their procedure in the ambulatory unit are materially different from their inpatient counterparts in terms of age, health, or other relevant criteria, then there may be a rational, medically justified basis for a less intense testing protocol. Protocols should never be followed blindly. Again, they are minimum recommendations and not a prohibition for aggressively testing a patient whose signs, symptoms, medical history, and so forth suggest that greater caution is indicated.

Freestanding Ambulatory Centers

The ability of a freestanding center to screen its patients and surgeons may justify its adopting a less intensive program of mandatory preprocedure testing. In so doing, however, the center exposes itself to the argument that it practices "inferior medicine" because it did not work up the patient with the same level of care as the patient would have received at a hospital. The plaintiff will moan that if he or she had been told the tests were not going to be performed in the same careful manner as inpatients can expect at the hospital, he or she would never have agreed to go to the center. Then comes the critical testimony of the professional witness or, worse yet, the surgeon or anesthesiologist from a competing hospital, and the stage is set for a potentially costly loss. The loss is not just a monetary one; it is also a setback for a center's attempts to reduce costs and unnecessary procedures and will undoubtedly have an adverse impact on the center's reputation.

It is with reluctance, therefore, but with legal survival paramount in mind, that the directors of freestanding centers will have to measure the legal climates in their communities to determine whether their preoperative and preanesthesia testing can vary from that of the inpatient surgery services at nearby hospitals or even hospital-affiliated ambulatory surgery centers with which they are comparable in terms of procedures and patient selection. If the inpatient hospital surgery services and physicians are supportive of the center and its approach to the delivery of quality medical services, then a variance is possible without a severe increase in the legal risks. It may be advisable, to the extent possible, to have some of the hospital-based physicians review, in an advisory role, the proposed testing protocols for the freestanding center if for no other reason than such an approach might neutralize any criticism from them in the event of a maloccurrence. It is also important to note that in some states, freestanding centers may be required by law to perform certain minimum preprocedure testing. Illinois, for example, requires a hemoglobin, hematocrit, and urinalysis for any patient having an anesthetic at a freestanding ambulatory surgery center. The director or administrator of any freestanding center should be certain that the center's protocols for preprocedure testing are in strict compliance with all applicable state laws and department of health rules and regulations.

The specific enumeration of tests that should be done by an ambulatory center or those which can or should be dispensed with is not a legal question but rather a medical one and thus is not pertinent or appropriate for this discussion. Other chapters in this text deal with the medical aspects of this issue. Medical practitioners will continue to develop guidelines as to specific test procedures, and these guidelines will be further modified in accordance with future clinical experience.

Office-Based Surgery
Because the risk of harm in the event of a severe complication during a surgical procedure is potentially greater in a physician's office than in other facilities, greater caution in patient evaluation and selection is mandatory. This, by definition, may require additional testing. However, unlike the ambulatory center, which can mandate certain tests as a prerequisite for doing a certain procedure, a physician is free to decide in his or her own office what will or will not be done. The physician makes the selection at his or her own risk. However, what about the anesthesiologist who, sight unseen, is asked to anesthetize the patient?

In view of the foregoing, the anesthesiologist is strongly urged to develop his or her own preanesthesia minimal testing protocol. This protocol should be no less intensive than that of the ambulatory surgery center for the same operative procedure, and there may be justification for making it even more intensive, depending on the anesthesiologist's experience with each particular surgeon. The more cautious and careful the surgeon is in the preprocedure workup, the easier is the burden on the anesthesiologist. Clearly, however, this situation demands a close working dialogue between the two physicians. A continuous reassessment of working protocols is required, and each patient must be strictly followed in accordance with those protocols. If the surgeon is unwilling to adhere to the suggested protocols, the anesthesiologist is advised to terminate the relationship with the surgeon's office.

Conclusion
The one element of legal risk that is common to the hospital-affiliated ambulatory center, the freestanding center, and the physician who operates in his or her own office is the failure to adhere religiously to whatever protocols of testing and evaluation have been adopted. If you yourself have said that a particular combination of tests, at a minimum, is necessary for a safe and adequate evaluation of a patient, then how do you justify going forward with a procedure without performing those tests?

Make up your mind to follow a "no exceptions" policy. Specify how soon before the procedure the tests must be done and the results must be available. Doing the tests but then going forward with surgery without the results being on the chart is the equivalent, from both a legal and a common-sense point of view, of not doing the tests at all. If the results are not there, postpone the procedure. Remember, the accreditation standards mandate that a facility is responsible for its regulations and procedures and must enforce what it has adopted. If the parent of a minor scheduled for surgery did not sign the operative consent, you would not operate. Likewise, if other preanesthesia requirements are not met, cancel the procedure. Preoperative and preanesthesia testing is no less legally significant than consent.

INFORMED CONSENT
Background and Philosophy
A patient's consent to medical treatment has been a legal requirement for centuries. However, the consent required in the 1800s differed substantially from that required today. Formerly, a physician was required only to obtain the patient's "authorization" to treat. The only explanation that was required involved providing information about the nature of the treatment (i.e., the type of procedure to be performed). Today, however, it is incumbent upon a physician to explain to a patient not only the nature of the proposed treatment, but also the risks, benefits, and alternatives associated with it. Standards developed by the AAAHC specifically provide that "the informed consent of the patient or, if applicable, of the patient's representative [be] obtained before an operation is performed." Many physicians are unaware of this modern standard of care, and it is for this reason that informed consent is rapidly becoming the most popular theory of liability used against physicians in malpractice actions.

In today's society, the patient is given an important role in the medical decision-making process. Many recent court opinions have stressed that the patient's individual right to self-determination of treatment includes his or her right to refuse treatment, even if such refusal will have deleterious effects on his or her physical well-being. The law has created an innate conflict between the patient's right to decide on a course of treatment and the physician's right to treat the patient in the manner he or she feels is most appropriate. Such a conflict is difficult, if not impossible, to resolve without a cooperative working relationship between the physician and the patient.

How to Obtain an Informed Consent
Inherent in the concept of patient determination of treatment is the assumption that physicians will give patients the requisite information necessary to make an informed decision. This is the touchstone by which all informed consent cases are judged.

Generally, a physician risks civil action by withholding any facts that are necessary for the patient to form an intelligent decision as to whether or not to undergo the proposed treatment. Such a disclosure involves a discussion of the risks, benefits, and alternatives associated with the contemplated treatment. In the context of anesthesia, the following checklist details the proper procedure for obtaining a patient's informed consent:

1. Provide a simple and concise explanation of the type of anesthesia to be administered, as well as the method of its administration.
2. Explain why you think the anesthetic agent and its method of administration are the most appropriate in this instance.
3. Provide a thorough explanation of alternative types of anesthesia and methods of administration that might be appropriate.
4. Disclose any material risks associated with the anesthetic agent or its method of administration.
5. Disclose and discuss any material risks relevant to the particular patient's past or present medical history, signs, symptoms, clinical findings, radiograms, or other diagnostic tests.
6. Answer any questions the patient has about the proposed anesthesia management.

In the vast majority of cases, litigation arises out of a failure to discuss the risks associated with the anesthetic agent or its method of administration. Obviously, a patient does not ordinarily sue his or her anesthesiologist unless there has been a maloccurrence. In many instances, this maloccurrence falls within a risk category associated with the use of a particular anesthetic agent or its method of administration. If the anesthesiologist has failed to inform the patient of this risk before administration of the anesthesia, it is going to be very difficult to convince the members of a jury that they should not find the physician liable for proceeding without the patient's informed consent.

The law does not require an anesthesiologist to disclose all risks no matter how minute or remote. The only risks that must be disclosed are those which a reasonable anesthesiologist would have disclosed (*i.e.*, material and probable risks). In addition to warning about the general category of risks to which all patients are susceptible, the anesthesiologist has a duty to warn a patient of any additional risks to which the patient might be particularly susceptible. Examples include risks associated with the administration of anesthesia to an anemic patient, an obese patient, a patient with respiratory or coronary impairments, a pregnant patient, and a patient with abnormal blood study results. An anesthesiologist can be apprised of such patient peculiarities only if the proper studies and laboratory work are performed before surgery. For this reason, it is absolutely essential that a *clinically indicated* preoperative workup be undertaken for every patient. Only then can the anesthesiologist explain the probable and material risks to the patient and be assured that a truly informed consent has been obtained.

The phraseology and semantics of an informed consent conference with the patient are extremely important. Simple, plain, layperson's language must be used. Even a signed consent form is not going to provide a defense if a patient with a third-grade education tells a jury that every word you spoke had ten syllables and that he or she had no understanding of the medical terminology you used. If indicated, use an illustrative diagram to demonstrate where problems might be encountered with intubation or where other complications might arise. Above all, use *plain English* (*e.g.*, say "swelling" rather than "edema"; say "numbness" rather than "paresthesia").

Documentation of Informed Consent

Even the most thorough and comprehensive informed consent discussion with a patient will not be of any benefit to you years down the road when litigation has been instituted unless you can demonstrate that it actually occurred. Many patients and physicians conveniently "forget" that the discussion ever took place, and others genuinely do not have a clear recollection of the event years after the fact. In any case, the more facts you have to substantiate that an informed consent conference did take place, the better your chances are of achieving a favorable verdict in a litigation forum.

It is advisable to have a member of your staff (RN, CRNA, and so on) be present during the preanesthesia interview. Also, if the patient has brought a family member or friend along, encourage that person to attend the meeting. In this way, you have a number of witnesses to attest to the fact that the patient was given information about the risks and alternatives associated with the contemplated anesthesia treatment. Document in the patient's chart that an informed consent conference was held, that there were witnesses (note their names), and that the patient gave his or her written consent to proceed with the proposed anesthesia plan. In addition, if a patient was advised of a susceptibility to certain peculiar risks, note these risks on the chart. After conferring, have the patient sign an informed consent form on which you have listed all significant risks and alternatives about which the patient was informed. Also, make sure the form is dated.

These measures often deter a plaintiff's attorney from proceeding against an anesthesiologist on an informed consent theory, since any hope for recovery is slim in view of the documented preanesthesia interview with the patient.

Time Considerations

As discussed earlier under "Preanesthesia Interview," the timing of the informed consent discussion between the physician and the patient is crucial. Bear in mind that an ambulatory surgery center is an unfamiliar setting for most patients and frequently evokes feelings of fear, uncertainty, and anxiety. All these emotions are intensified on the day of the procedure when surgery is imminent. For this reason, an informed consent discussion should be held in the most relaxed setting the facilities at the unit permit. Obviously, the discussion should be held outside the operating suite itself. It must be held before the patient is premedicated with any sedative. If the patient is elderly, retarded, or a minor, or if he or she appears confused, the discussion must be held with a spouse, parent, or guardian present. The atmosphere should be relaxed, but there should be no attempt to downplay the seriousness of the discussion by jokes or excessive informality, and there should be no attempt to minimize the importance of the discussion by saying, "The lawyers make me do this, so don't worry about it." Such a comment has been held by one court to destroy the consent. Always record who was present during the discussion. Document their presence and consent by asking them to sign the consent form along with the patient.

Inherent in the concept of informed consent is the assumption that the patient will have an informative, noncoercive discussion with the physician about the proposed treatment and, thereafter, will have the opportunity to make a decision, without pressure, as to whether he or she wishes to proceed in view of the explanation of risks and alternatives.

The case law in this country is replete with examples of patients who have been awarded damages under a theory of lack of informed consent in which the alleged "informed" consent was obtained by the physician in the operating room immediately before the operation. A patient already in a gown, lying on a stretcher, who has been premedicated, and who is scheduled to undergo surgery in the next few minutes is not in any condition to make decisions that involve potential loss of life or limb. Because of the tension and anxiety associated with the impending surgical procedure, the patient's reasoning process may be temporarily impaired, and he or she may be unable to assimilate much of the medical information that has been communicated to him or her. Such a state of mind is not conducive to making calm and reasoned decisions. Unless a patient is given adequate time for contemplation and deliberation, a physician can, at best, hope to obtain a mere "authorization" to treat and not the informed consent required by law.

All the aforementioned problems can be eradicated by adoption of a simple technique: Conduct informed consent conferences as far in advance of surgery as time and circumstances permit. The extra time and effort required to implement this scheduling procedure are a small price to pay for the confidence that you have obtained a truly informed consent.

Some patients or even their surgeons may request a conference before the day of the procedure. This request should be accommodated. If the patient is this concerned, there may be some problem he or she wants to specifically discuss. This may lead to disclosure of a problem that may cause the procedure to be canceled. If this is going to happen, it is better to know it in advance and thus not lose valuable operating room time on the schedule. For example, suppose the conference discloses an extremely frightened patient who has a past medical history that requires a very prolonged discussion to allay his or her fears and to explain all the risks. If the anesthesiologist were confronted with such a patient on the morning of the procedure, the entire schedule for that day could be delayed. On the other hand, the anesthesiologist, as a result of seeing the patient a few days before the surgery, could decide that this patient belongs on an inpatient service. Clearly, everyone has benefited in such a situation. A good informed consent discussion can disclose all the reasonably foreseeable risks and yet be done in such a manner as not to frighten the patient, and it also can help to allay unreasonable fears. However, if a patient's fears are not allayed and he or she decides the next day not to undergo the procedure or opts to be admitted to an inpatient facility, then the extra time for this preprocedure visit was well spent indeed.

DISCHARGE FROM AN AMBULATORY SURGERY CENTER

While in the center, a patient is subject to your direction and control, but after the patient leaves, you no longer have any control. This is true because once the patient is discharged, usually within a few hours after the procedure, he or she must be relied on to monitor signs, symptoms, or complications. To be able to do this, a patient needs very careful instructions and predetermined lines of communication as well as immediate access, if necessary, to alternative medical centers. Perhaps discharge is not even feasible, and an immediate admission or transfer is in order. These are critical decisions, and various people must play important roles in making them. The wrong people should not be asked to serve inappropriate roles.

Standards for Discharge

The ultimate standard is whether it is medically appropriate to discharge a patient. The JCAHO anesthesia standards suggest that it may be appropriate to develop discharge criteria approved by the medical staff to ensure the same standard of care for all patients. If it is deemed appropriate to develop such criteria for inpatient hospital-affiliated anesthesia services, it is certainly appropriate to do so in the ambulatory center. The bottom line, however, is that if such criteria are developed, they *must* be rigidly enforced.

Status of the Patient

Discharge decisions must be based on the status of the patient at the time the decision to discharge is made. The decision should not be made hours in advance because the patient's status may have deteriorated during the interim. It is therefore important to evaluate the patient just before the patient leaves the facility. The patient's status must meet all the discharge criteria. Unexplained symptoms, fluctuations in blood pressure, temperature elevations, sensations of dizziness, or other significant findings should not be ignored or downplayed. Sometimes there is nothing more suspicious than the fact that the patient "looks funny." Keeping the patient a little longer for observation may be the best medicine you have practiced all day. If the patient does not improve, you have time to start alternative planning, including transfer to an inpatient facility. Admission to such a facility is a lot safer, legally, than gambling on a discharge under questionable clinical conditions.

Patient's Educational Level

The patient's level of education may be an important variable in the discharge equation. It may affect the patient's ability to comprehend what is happening. It will determine the kinds of instructions to be given to the patient. If the patient is unable to understand detailed and vital instructions, the risk is too great that he or she will not follow them. In order to protect the patient, such a risk should not be undertaken, and admission should be considered. If a responsible adult is present and indicates that he or she understands and is capable of carrying out the instructions for the patient, then the decision may be resolved in favor of discharge. Discharge evaluation and instructions as to outpatient care and monitoring of symptoms play an important role in patient discharge. It is the physician's responsibility both to evaluate and to instruct the patient in a timely and appropriate fashion. The instructions must be tailored to the patient's education level. It may be necessary to give a simple set of general written instructions. The telephone numbers of the physician and of the center should be included if the patient seems in any way confused or uncertain. In the case of a freestanding center, the telephone number of a transfer hospital should be supplied. It is also important to note that centers that treat patients who are not proficient in the English language have a duty to ensure that these patients are given discharge instructions in their own language so that they understand how to proceed after surgery. Centers that cater to a large foreign-speaking population also should have an interpreter as a member of their staff and should have written discharge instructions printed in the language or languages of their patients.

Accessibility to Emergency Facilities
Another factor to be weighed is the patient's ability to gain access to emergency facilities. Measuring this factor correctly requires knowledge of the transportation facilities available, including public emergency transportation, as well as the time and distance necessary to reach them. These factors are too varied and too important to leave to the last five minutes before the patient goes home. These and all discharge-related procedures should be discussed and explained before the patient arrives at the center for the procedure. Preadmission discharge planning may eliminate most problems. Clearly, the presence of a responsible adult to assist the patient home, to review the discharge instructions, and to be ready to summon aid if an emergency develops is indispensable. If it appears that, in the event of a foreseeable emergency, there is significant risk that the patient could not reach the emergency facility, then discharge is not indicated. This, of course, involves weighing the patient's status against the risk that the patient could not reach an emergency facility if a complication developed. The ultimate decision to discharge must involve considerations of the procedure the patient underwent, the patient's general health, risk factors disclosed by the patient's preprocedure testing, the patient's present status, and the accessibility of emergency facilities in the event of a complication.

Inpatient Admission
A great part of the discussion of legal risks has been devoted to the prevention of harm by opting for the course of conduct that is safest for the patient. Specific rules have been avoided in an attempt to reinforce and teach a methodology of thinking. If one gets in the habit of resolving troubling conflicts, doubts, or risks by doing that which has the highest probability of patient safety, a significant amount of patient harm and legal culpability can be avoided. In this context, the difficult issue of discharge versus inpatient admission must be resolved. In most cases, there is no contraindication to discharge, and the decision is easy and appropriate. There will be cases, however, in which a minor concern about the patient's status is resolved in favor of discharge because of ready access to the

center or to other emergency care facilities and because the patient is sufficiently intelligent to know how to respond. If, however, the patient's status suggests a significant possibility of a postoperative complication that no degree of ready access to emergency facilities is going to prevent, the patient must not be discharged. An overnight admission may turn out to be an unnecessary precaution or it may save the patient's life. Patients do not sue you for taking great precautions to protect them—they sue you for not taking those precautions when they are reasonably indicated. When in doubt, admit! You and the patient may both sleep more peacefully that night.

JCAHO and AAAHC Standards

The role of the physician or other licensed independent practitioner in making the postanesthesia discharge decision is clearly defined in both the JCAHO and AAAHC standards. The standards speak of delaying the discharge decision until the patient is fully recovered from the anesthetic agent. The patient's anticipated recovery is not the criterion; rather, it is the status of the patient after he or she has recovered from the anesthesia that determines whether discharge is appropriate. Documentation of the patient's condition is mandated, and the identity of the person responsible for the discharge decision also should be clearly noted. Familiarity with the patient is desirable on the part of the individual who is asked to make the discharge decision.

When this book was originally published in 1985, the JCAHO (then the JCAH) standards for discharge provided that "the basis for a decision to discharge a patient from any postanesthesia care unit shall be made only by a physician ... and not by nursing service personnel...." In January of 1990, the JCAHO standards provide for discharge by a "licensed independent practitioner" (hereinafter LIP)* or, in the absence of an LIP, by nursing staff or house staff as long as they followed discharge criteria approved by the LIP staff. The relevant JCAHO standards are excerpted below:

> SA.1.5.6 A licensed independent practitioner who has appropriate clinical privileges and who is familiar with the patient is responsible for the decision to discharge the patient.
> SA.1.5.6.1 When the responsible licensed independent practitioner is not personally present to make the decision to discharge or does not sign the discharge order,
> SA.1.5.6.1.1 The name of the licensed independent practitioner responsible for the discharge is recorded in the patient's medical record; and
> SA.1.5.6.1.2 Relevant discharge criteria are rigorously applied to determine the readiness of the patient for discharge.
> SA.1.5.6.1.2.1 The discharge criteria are approved by the medical staff.
> SA.1.7 When surgery or anesthesia is performed, a physician is immediately available in the facility in sufficient time to provide care in the event of a medical emergency.

---

*An LIP is defined by the JCAHO as "any individual who is permitted by law and who is also permitted by the hospital to provide patient care services without direction or supervision, within the scope of his license and in accordance with individually granted privileges." Under some state laws, podiatrists, chiropractors, and optometrists fit the JCAHO's definition of an LIP.

SA.2.2 When surgical or anesthesia services are performed on an ambulatory basis, the patient is provided with written instructions for follow-up care.
SA.2.2.1 The instructions include information about how to obtain assistance in the event of postoperative problems.
SA.2.2.2 The instructions are reviewed with the patient or a person responsible for the patient.
SA.2.3 Patients who receive other than local anesthesia on an ambulatory basis are accompanied at discharge by a designated adult who is responsible for the patient.

The AAAHC standards are more rigid than those of the JCAHO. Standard 9(G) states:

Patients who have received anesthesia are evaluated by the operating surgeon, anesthesiologist, or dentist after recovery from anesthesia, prior to discharge.

Also see Standard 10(I), which provides:

An anesthesiologist, another physician, or dentist qualified in resuscitative techniques is present or immediately available until all patients operated on that day have been discharged.

To the extent that the AAAHC standards may be read as advocating a higher standard of care on the part of the center and its physicians, they should be followed more closely than the standards of the JCAHO. Under various state laws, chiropractors, optometrists, and other independent professionals may qualify as LIPs under the JCAHO standards, but it would be the unusual case indeed that these practitioners would be qualified to make discharge decisions. We advocate the approach of the AAAHC, which suggests that discharge decisions should be made by the operating surgeon, dentist, or anesthesiologist.

Responsibility for Patient Discharge
Who Should Examine and Discharge?

Many physicians write such orders as, "OK to discharge when stable." *Stable* in an ambulatory center should be clearly stated to be a medical decision to be made only by a physician. There are both sound legal and medical reasons for this. If a nurse were to discharge a patient before the patient was medically ready, the nurse might be culpable, but the center that employs the nurse and the physician who wrote the order would be liable as well. Why? Because when the nurse was so instructed by the physician, he or she became the physician's agent for that purpose. Similarly, the nurse is the agent of the center by virtue of being employed there. If the nurse acted negligently as an agent, then the principal of the agent is also liable under the theory of *respondeat superior.*

Since the physician is going to be legally culpable for a negligent decision, he or she should at least assume the medical responsibilities of discharging a patient. Consider that only the physician discussed the patient's history, symptoms, preprocedure consent, risks, benefits, discharge planning, and medical follow-up. Consider that discharging a patient involves weighing all of these factors. And consider that only a physician is medically qualified to assess all aspects of a patient's status. Under this criteria, it is not appropriate to impose this final discharge decision on nursing personnel.

We feel very strongly that the discharge decision must be made by a physician. No patient should be allowed to leave until a physician makes the final examination and gives clearance for the patient to be discharged. An ambulatory center's standards and guidelines should explicitly disallow its nurses to discharge patients. This position is in accordance with the present standards of the AAAHC but is more rigid than the standards of the JCAHO.

The more interesting question is, "Which physician should discharge?" More often than not the surgical criteria for discharge may be met upon completion of the procedure. The surgeon may thereafter leave the center or may be involved in another procedure when the discharge decision has to be made. It is therefore much more likely that the discharge evaluation will be made by the anesthesiologist. The discharge decision generally does not involve whether or not the patient is surgically recuperated. That process may take days or even weeks in some instances. Therefore, what is really being assessed in an ambulatory center is whether the patient has recovered from the anesthesia sufficiently to be able to return home to continue with his or her surgical recovery and to respond intelligently if a delayed complication of the surgery or anesthesia should develop.

Anesthesiologists are therefore definitely qualified to make the discharge decision. This also may involve discharge instructions to the patient about return visits to the surgeon, medication, home care, and so forth. The discharge conference is extremely crucial and can be legally very important for the center. Apart from performing an integral part of patient care for the center's legal protection, the anesthesiologist's discharge decision also involves the important function of ensuring patient safety. From a proprietary standpoint, it also should be noted that anesthesiologists often own the freestanding centers and certainly in terms of job security and preservation of their investment have a much greater interest in the survival of the center than does a single surgeon. In no way are we implying that surgeons are not qualified to perform a discharge examination and make a discharge decision; they certainly are qualified in this area. Being involved in the discharge decision serves to reinforce the role of the anesthesiologist as a physician in the broader sense. The anesthesiologist's role is too often limited in the minds of both laypeople and other physicians. Anesthesiologists are not "time passers" or the "gas guys," as many think. The more responsibility for patient care and safety they assume, the more they enhance their own medical image.

Manner of Discharge

The written policy of the ambulatory center about discharge should be adhered to in all respects. The requirements specified in that policy should be reviewed before the procedure so that there is no doubt that full compliance can be ensured. The policy should specify the decisions to be made by the surgeon and those which are to be made by the anesthesiologist. The center's director has the overall responsibility to make certain that these written requirements are, in fact, being complied with. Physicians who do not properly brief their patients in advance of admission about the discharge procedures and requirements should be identified and counseled about the importance of these procedures. Noncompliance should not be condoned.

Discharge by Written Policy
The policy should state what discharge orders must be written and should particularly insist on clear identification of who will follow the patient on what date and where. The policy may insist that the information be given to the patient in written form. The individual discharging the patient should verify that the patient and responsible person have been instructed about the medication and understand those instructions. Particular procedures may lend themselves to a checklist of signs and symptoms to watch for, and if reduced to written instructions, the center may direct, in its discharge regulations, that such materials be given to the patient. The patient, as a matter of policy, should be encouraged to report to the surgeon, the anesthesiologist, or the center any changes in his or her status after discharge.

Nurses in hospital-affiliated ambulatory centers should not be given any greater role in the discharge instruction process than would be given to their inpatient counterparts. Many inpatient facilities do not permit nurses to give medications, decide dosages, or give instructions about side-effects and contraindications. Nurses may remind the patient to follow the physician's instructions or remind the patient that the particular medication should be taken with or without food, without dairy products, and so forth. However, the nursing role should not be expanded in the ambulatory center for the sake of expediency or to cut costs.

Discharge by Phone Order
In our opinion, discharging by phone should not be encouraged. It should be a rare exception if it is permitted at all. If the surgeon or anesthesiologist is unable, because of an emergency, to examine the patient, another physician should be contacted to come and actually see the patient. Nurses should not be asked to report the patient's signs and symptoms to a physician over the phone and then receive a verbal order to discharge. This makes the center, as well as the physician, potentially liable if the nurse has incorrectly ascertained the patient's status. The decision to discharge should be an on-the-spot medical decision made by a physician after appropriate examination and observation. The foregoing discussion is completely in accordance with the standards set forth in the AAAHC guidelines. These mandates may sound drastic, but the single most frequently cited reason for patients suing their physicians and ambulatory centers is the patient's perception that once the operation was over, a physician was not around. In short, the patient felt abandoned, and when something adverse occurred, he or she blamed it on the lack of attention.

The JCAHO discharge standards, however, do not even require a phone order for discharge. The JCAHO guidelines permit nursing personnel and house staff to discharge as long as they are following discharge criteria approved by the medical staff. However, even in instances where the LIP has delegated the authority to make the discharge decision to nursing personnel or house staff, the ultimate responsibility for that discharge decision remains with the LIP. Even under these guidelines, however, the presence or immediate availability of a physician in the facility is required to provide care in the event of a medical emergency. Some commentators view the JCAHO standards as a breath of fresh air and believe that the new regulations provide a reasonable mechanism for providing safe care to the ambulatory patient by shifting the emphasis more to assessing the condition of the patient than to mandating the presence of a physician at the time of discharge. We take a contrary view and believe that the superior education, knowledge, training, and experience possessed by the anesthesiologist or operating surgeon make these physicians a necessary and desirable part of the discharge process.

If the anesthesiologist accepts the important role of discharge physician, which we advocate, patient fears are allayed in most instances. Patients are grateful for the fine professional attention and remember the physician who came to "see them off." If a patient later develops a surgical complication and decides to sue, it may be the final impression the patient formed of the anesthesiologist and the center that keeps these parties from also being named as defendants in the suit against the surgeon.

No Physician Available

The following question is frequently asked by administrators of ambulatory centers: "What policies can be established to protect the nursing personnel and the facility in the event of a discharge when no physician is available?" The response is to adopt regulations that guarantee, to the extent humanly possible, that this situation will never arise. This discharge decision responsibility rests with the admitting physician and the anesthesiologist and ultimately with the center's administration itself. The center should adopt regulations that until the last patient of the day has been discharged a physician skilled in resuscitative techniques must be on the premises in the event of a medical emergency. The regulations should further state that before any discharge is made in the absence of the admitting physician or the anesthesiologist, contact should be established with a physician and the appropriateness of the discharge, as well as that of the discharge instructions, should be reviewed. Finally, after-hours emergency care facilities should always be identified to the patient and the responsible adult.

At a recent seminar, one of the participants cited an instance in which the admitting surgeon scheduled a number of procedures and, with at least four patients still on the premises, signed out to a physician in another community some miles distant and left for the weekend. The surgeon on call was busy operating on his own patients and could not even come to the phone when one of his colleague's patients began to experience problems. There was no way he could assist the patient. The center's director, who was not a physician, refused to allow the discharge of any of the recalcitrant physician's patients under these circumstances and ordered that they all be admitted to the transfer hospital. As the reader can imagine, this stirred up quite a row with the patients and their surgeon. The patients refused to pay for their hospital admissions because they were caused by the surgeon going sailing, and ultimately, this situation cost the surgeon over $1000 in patient hospital bills and a lot of bad publicity in the community. This surgeon now discharges all his patients in person.

An important point to note is that the surgeon was not the only one who received adverse publicity. The patients also were critical of the center for allowing this situation to occur. There were several qualified anesthesiologists on staff and present in the center who were just as able as the surgeon to make the discharge decision—had they been asked. Likewise, in units that are directed by a physician, the director should be prepared, when necessary, to perform the discharge evaluation. It is one thing for the surgeon to drop the ball, but the idea is not to compound the error. The center has an equal responsibility with the surgeon for the quality of all aspects of the medical care of its patients. It also has an interest in creating a favorable impression among patients and should encourage its staff to become deeply involved in patient care. The anesthesiologist is the most likely candidate for this role and should welcome the additional patient contact.

Physician Attendance

There should always be at least one physician in attendance until the last patient has left the facility. AAAHC Standard 10(I) requires that an anesthesiologist or other physician qualified in resuscitative techniques be present until the last patient leaves. JCAHO Standard SA.1.17 has a similar requirement. In a hospital unit, the patients are generally given the telephone number of the physician on call as well as that of the hospital emergency room. Patients are told that if for any reason they need to be seen, then they should go to the emergency room. It is a good idea for the hospital unit to give the emergency room staff a list of that day's patients and their procedures so that the emergency room has access to their charts in the event they are needed.

In the freestanding unit, the discharge instructions should advise the patient of his or her surgeon's telephone number. It is important also to advise the patient that in the event of an acute problem, he or she should go to the nearest hospital emergency room. Since all freestanding units should have arrangements with a transfer hospital, that facility also should be identified by name, address, and telephone number. The transfer hospital should always have a list of the physicians who are on call for each date. If a patient should sustain a delayed reaction and no physician were available to attend to that patient, it would be very difficult to convince a jury that the center was providing an acceptable level of medical care.

Written Discharge Instructions

The three most recurrent excuses for patient delay in responding to a significant postdischarge change of symptoms are that the patient (1) did not know what to look for, (2) did not know the significance of what he or she subsequently found, and (3) did not know what he or she was supposed to do or whom to contact.

With medications, the claim is that the patient did not know when to take it, when not to take it, and when to stop taking it. To the physician, the patient is one of many, and the physician may not be able specifically to recall the discussion several years later. The physician is then forced to rely on what he or she "usually" tells patients. The plaintiff invariably contends that although the physician may "usually" give patients those instructions, he or she did not receive them and, furthermore, had he or she received the "usual" instructions, he or she would have followed them and would not have been harmed. Many plaintiffs' lawyers believe that any time they can reduce a case to a credibility question and get the jury to weigh the absolute denial by the plaintiff against the defendant's qualified "I usually tell my patients," the odds are overwhelmingly in favor of the plaintiff. In this context, the use of written discharge instructions is strongly recommended. The center should retain a copy of what was given to the patient, and the patient should sign the center's copy acknowledging receipt of the instructions.

Some centers are now using a two-part form with carbon inserts. The top part contains general information such as emergency numbers or who to call. The bottom part contains general cautions about possible side-effects, symptoms to watch for and to report, and so forth. There is a space to write in specific warnings and to detail discharge instructions about follow-up care and the use of prescribed medications. (See section on "Forms and Policies" at the conclusion of this book.) Some centers have developed separate instruction sheets tailored to each procedure performed in the center, which are then attached to these general forms.

It is important that these discharge instructions, in whatever form they may be used, are written in a concise, clear manner. Obviously they should be dated, and the time of discharge should be noted. Even if this type of form is not used, the same information should be imparted to the patient, and this process should be memorialized by an appropriate entry in the patient's chart, and the patient should be required to sign the chart acknowledging that these instructions were actually received and understood.

Follow-Up Phone Call

There is no case that states that a follow-up phone call is legally required. However, the patient response to such a call is so great and its cost in time and dollars is so small that the justification for the call is self-evident. The mere fact that somebody calls the patient just to see how he or she is recovering is a very positive statement about the center and its approach to medicine. It is not, however, just a great marketing and public relations scheme. The call should be documented on the chart. The recorder should note the patient's statement that "everything is fine" or "I'm doing great." On the other hand, if the patient is having some problem and has been reluctant or embarrassed to call, this affirmative reaching out to the patient may elicit the problem and prompt potentially life-saving activity. Even if the nurse who may make the call simply reports the problem to the physician or puts the physician on the line to discuss the problem with the patient directly, serious harm can be avoided and you have a great record of concern to submit to a jury if you are ever sued thereafter. Such a call may keep you out of the suit altogether simply because the patient feels, as a result of that call, that the center, if not its surgeon, really cared about him or her.

The postdischarge call is a very humane, considerate step that will pay dividends in a lot of ways. However, it must be done correctly. In other words, if the patient does relate a sign or symptom, it must be accurately recorded, reported to the surgeon, anesthesiologist, or other LIP, and acted on. Once you receive potentially adverse information, there is a corresponding duty to act on it in a timely fashion. It may be advisable to have one physician, with no other duty assignment, available for a half-hour or so each day to discuss any feedback as it is elicited from the patients by the center personnel who are placing the calls. It would not take much time to call the patients from the previous day and check out their condition. The overwhelming majority will be doing great. They require little of the caller's time and none of the physician's. The few who may be having a problem warrant the additional time of the caller, and their complaints should be brought to the attention of a physician. Sometimes it is the little personal touches that bring patients back, encourage them to recommend the center to their friends, and help prevent a lawsuit. If your center does not now have a routine postdischarge call policy, think seriously about implementing one. By the way, get your friendliest, cheeriest people to make the calls, and tell them the importance of what they are doing.

Some centers use a postcard system of follow-up. This is not as legally helpful as the phone call. The phone call is instant and can be verified and noted in the chart. When you mail a postcard, there is no proof that it was ever received. Most mail surveys indicate that the response rate, whether it be for a sale, a donation, a cocktail party, or whatever, is very low. Assuming the patient got the postcard, an effective follow-up requires the patient either too initiate a call or to mail the card back. Many patients will be inclined to do neither. Follow-up by the patient in response to the postcard may require further time and expense.

Some institutions give the patient a postcard at the time of discharge. It is self-addressed, and of course, postage is prepaid. It lists several questions about the patient's health and recovery as well as about the overall performance of the center. This has increased the response rate and overcomes the argument that the patient never received the follow-up inquiry. It is critical, however, that all such returned cards be carefully reviewed and follow-up initiated where indicated.

Many anesthesiologists are secure about their expertise in providing anesthesia services to patients during inpatient surgical procedures. Ambulatory surgery centers, on the other hand, are a fairly recent innovation and present an entirely new environment and experience to most anesthesiologists. For this reason, it is extremely important to stress that all anesthesiologists who intend to practice in an ambulatory setting are responsible for acquiring an awareness of the medical and legal considerations involved in providing anesthesia services outside an accredited hospital facility. An insightful comment by the editor of this book, Bernard V. Wetchler, aptly describes this responsibility: "As we [practicing anesthesiologists] spread our wings, we don't want them clipped."

The legal commentary that follows is comprised of 20 questions that were submitted by practicing anesthesiologists throughout the country. In this question-and-answer section, we have attempted to put the principles discussed earlier in this chapter into perspective and to demonstrate how these principles may be practically applied to everyday situations that commonly confront the practicing anesthesiologist.

LEGAL COMMENTARY: 20 QUESTIONS

1. *We do not premedicate our patients. Some of our anesthesiologists insist on performing their preanesthesia interview after the patient is in the operating room on the table. Is this appropriate?*

This procedure is not advisable for two reasons. The purpose of the preanesthesia interview is to obtain the information necessary to determine whether a patient is able to tolerate the anesthesia, to get a relevant past medical history of potential risks or complication factors, and to obtain an anesthesia-related informed consent. The dangers of the approach set forth in this question are (1) that there are too many diagnoses involved for the proper exercise of care and (2) that the patient's consent may not be truly informed.

In considering the first danger, the patient is at the center and is psychologically geared for the procedure, the surgeon is standing near and is ready to go, and all the pressures of the situation on both you and the patient are to go ahead no matter what is elicited in the interview. The overwhelming tendency is to downplay any risk factor that might otherwise cause you, in a less committed moment, to postpone the procedure. It may be infinitely easier to tell a patient in the waiting room while he or she is fully dressed that you are concerned about his or her history and want to get prior medical records and review them than to try to explain that to someone who has gone through the mental stress of getting undressed and being wheeled into the operating room. At this point, the patient just wants to get the procedure over with and go home. Just knowing this may induce you to forget about getting the prior chart or trying to track down the treating physician in another community. It is at this point that you start rolling the dice that the potential problem will not occur, but you are gambling with the patient's life, your reputation, and the center's financial survival. Give yourself and the patient a real opportunity—do not put either of you so far down the road that it becomes almost impossible to turn back. Get the interviews done outside the operating room as far in advance of surgery as is practically possible.

The second danger concerns the issue of consent. If you do not have the opportunity to even investigate the significant risk factors elicited during the interview, how can you give the patient a meaningful assessment of his or her particular risks in proceeding or not proceeding, benefits, alternatives, and so forth? Or suppose you tell the patient that you are concerned about some risk-related aspect of his or her history. This inappropriately drops the decision to proceed or not in the patient's lap. Many plaintiffs have told juries that when they went into the operating room they were so scared they did not know who they talked to, who talked to them, what was said, or what it all meant. They were confused and disoriented and could not remember their own names. Now you try to tell a jury that you had a meaningful discussion, without pressure or coercion, with such a patient and that that patient made a calm, rational decision about the potential risks of the procedure. Do you still want to do the interviews with the patient in the operating room lying on the table? No, you don't.

2a. What are our alternatives when Mr. Bradley insists on being admitted after an ambulatory surgical procedure?

If you have tried by persuasion and reassurance to get the patient to go home and he refuses, you have, practically speaking, no alternatives. You cannot abandon the patient or ask the police to evict him as a trespasser. If anything should happen to that patient in the immediate postoperative period, you can imagine the patient's anger as he tells his lawyer that he insisted there was something wrong and that he needed to be admitted while you ignored him. The problem is that if you do admit the patient, how do you get him out of the hospital? This question highlights the necessity of educating patients in advance about ambulatory surgery. If the patient balks at the idea of coming in and going home the same afternoon, that patient should not be treated in the ambulatory center. You are just asking for trouble by forcing such a patient to have the surgery in a setting that he already views with hostility. That patient is a lawsuit waiting to happen—to you.

2b. Who is responsible for payment of an overnight stay if we do admit a patient even though the admission is not medically indicated?

Absent some medical indication for the inpatient admission, no insurance company is going to reimburse the hospital stay. This fact must be stressed to the patient, and the patient must be informed that he or she will be responsible for all charges attributable to the hospital stay. Nine out of ten patients will suddenly feel much better and will decide that admission probably is not necessary after all. In conclusion, if there is a medical concern, admit the patient. If there is no medical indication, persuade the patient to continue in the plan for ambulatory surgery and discharge to home care. If this fails and the patient is becoming emotionally overwrought, permit the admission, but only after you document in writing that you informed the patient that he or she was financially responsible for all costs.

3a. We require a responsible adult to accompany a patient home after general or regional anesthesia. One adult came to get a patient after surgery and our recovery room nurse was sure he was intoxicated. What do we do?

To highlight this basic problem, let us assume that the adult was intoxicated and causes an accident en route to the patient's home, thereby injuring the patient, or perhaps gets the patient home, passes out, and is unresponsive when the patient is seriously harmed as a result of a significant delay in getting needed medical attention. The first question a lawyer is going to put to you will be, "What was the reason for insisting that a responsible adult come for the patient in the first place?" Your response has to be that, after surgery, because of pain or the effects of the anesthesia or medication, patients are often unable to properly drive or otherwise care for themselves en route home. Also, you will state that it is advisable to have someone observe a patient to make certain there is no delayed complication, such as a hemorrhage. A third reason is that if such a complication should arise, this adult could expedite the patient's return to the hospital or center or call emergency services to the patient's assistance. If you analyze these responses (and others equally valid that you might add), how can you entrust an impaired patient to an intoxicated person? Would you let such a person drive your children home in a school bus? You have a duty of due care for a patient's safety until he or she reaches home and is fully recovered (intellectually and functionally) from the procedure.

Placate the "drunk" and find some other adult to come for the patient. If there is an adult at home who is rational, coherent, and cooperative but does not drive or cannot come for the patient, then send the patient home in a cab or get some other family member who lives nearby to drop the patient off at home. In some communities, the local police force is willing to assist patients in getting to and from a hospital, and their assistance can be particularly helpful not only in getting the patient home, but also in getting the intoxicated person out of your center and to his or her own home.

We have been addressing the problem of an intoxicated person, but clearly the situation would be the same regardless of the cause of the mental or physical impairment.

3b. The "responsible adult" turned out to be a 17-year-old. In our state, she would be considered a minor. Could she qualify as a responsible adult?

The term *responsible adult* has been used not so much to specify an age, but to indicate the requisite level of maturity and ability to care for the patient. A *responsible adult* is a person who is physically and intellectually capable of taking care of the patient once he or she leaves the center. There are many 17-year-olds of both sexes who are more calm, caring, and intelligent than persons twice their chronological age. Statistically, however, judgment and maturity are correlated with advancing years, and so, obviously, in doing one's preadmission planning, emphasis should be placed on finding a person over the age of 18. However, if no such person is available and the only one available to help the patient is a 17-year-old who is capable, then there is no legal impairment to releasing the patient to the care of such a person. In many states, young people are granted drivers' licenses at 16 or 17 years of age. Many people at that age hold responsible positions in their schools or jobs. Many young women are married at that age and may have children of their own. It is therefore an individual judgment that should be made by the physician who knows the family or is persuaded by the parent that the teenager is capable of driving him or her home and is able to comprehend and carry out the discharge instructions. In this regard, the discharge instructions should be tailored to the degree of comprehension demonstrated by the young adult.

Obviously, the next question is, "If you accept an occasional 17-year-old, then how about someone who is 16 or 15 or 14?" The line has to be drawn somewhere, and arbitrarily, we have drawn it at the age a particular state grants an unlimited driver's license. In this way, there is a driver who can get the patient home and has met certain tests of maturity and judgment. However, the mere fact that a person has a driver's license is not enough. There must be some additional evidence that the young person is capable of understanding the medical realities and is going to be present to assist the patient for the initial period following surgery.

4. What are the legal implications of obtaining a pregnancy test on women of childbearing age scheduled for general anesthesia?

The implications cut both ways, that is, doing or not doing the test. If you do the test, there is the legal requisite that it be done early and accurately and that the patient be told of the significance of the test, particularly if it is positive for pregnancy. Obviously, greater care must be exercised for the safety of the fetus, particularly in the choice of anesthesia methods and the selection of preoperative or postoperative medications. This is especially true with respect to certain anesthetic agents administered during the first three months of pregnancy that can pass through the placental barrier and may have an effect on fetal development.

In elective cases, the choices may include not doing the procedure at all. The problem is, of course, easier when the patient is an adult and can make the choice for herself. However, when the patient is a 14-year-old girl, the parent is still the legal guardian, and the parent cannot give an informed consent if there is any attempt to conceal a pregnancy from the parent. There are many physicians who believe that there is no legal obligation to inform a parent in this situation, but this is simply not true in most states, and the physician is taking a significant legal risk by participating in an operation on a pregnant teenager without notifying the parents of all the relevant facts. If a complication associated with the pregnancy occurs, there is no legal defense. The child is a minor incapable of consent, and the physician has committed a concealment from the parents.

What do you think the attitude of the other parents who may be on the jury will be? Do you really believe that parents think it is acceptable for a physician to substitute his or her judgment for theirs as to what is best for their child?

What about not doing the pregnancy test? Is ignorance bliss? It never really is. Does this mean that every female patient between the ages of 13 and 55 has to have a pregnancy test? Clearly not.

What is needed is to develop a protocol based on the nature of the proposed procedure and the type of anesthesia that is contemplated. For example, if an 18-year-old girl comes in to have a mole removed from her back under local anesthesia and is otherwise asymptomatic, it seems unnecessary to do a routine pregnancy test. On the other hand, if a woman in her thirties wants a tubal ligation and has been having some vague pelvic problems and has a slightly enlarged uterus, no one should operate or anesthetize such a patient without first checking to see if she is pregnant. It comes down to the patient's medical history and symptoms, the proposed procedure, and whether it involves local, spinal, caudal, or general anesthesia.

The worst possible case would be a procedure done under general anesthesia on a woman with an undiscovered pregnancy and as a result of a complication associated with the pregnancy, the mother and child are both lost. How many expert witnesses could the plaintiff find to testify that you never submit a woman of childbearing age to such a procedure under general anesthesia without first determining whether she is or is not pregnant? Can you think of one responsible physician who would testify on your behalf that there is no deviation from accepted standards in operating or administering anesthesia to a pregnant woman when you did not even endeavor to determine that factor in assessing the patient preoperatively?

We further note that the American College of Obstetrics and Gynecology (ACOG) does not require mandatory pregnancy testing of all females of childbearing age but does recommend testing if there is *any* question after a thorough history or in the event of suggestive signs or symptoms.

5. We require a pregnancy test on women of childbearing age (12–50 years) scheduled for general anesthesia. A 16-year-old girl is having a breast biopsy. Her mother is furious that we are going to do the test and refuses to have the test done. What do we do?

Obviously, if the center decides, upon due reflection, that the risk of pregnancy is sufficiently serious that all women should be tested before receiving anesthesia, then there is a valid reason for the rule. Once you admit that the risk justified the adoption of the rule, then how do you explain not following your own rules?

Patients are notorious for urging their physicians to accommodate them. They do not want to come back as frequently as they should be seen. They want renewable prescriptions so they do not have to make return visits. They do not want certain tests, but they want the surgery. Whose neck are they asking to be put in the noose? Not theirs! It is always the physician or the ambulatory center's staff that will ultimately be put in the position of trying to explain why they deviated from a rule they insisted upon enacting for the safety of their own patients.

Since there is no reason to have a rule and then ignore it or bend it to suit every patient, the solution is simple. Explain to the parent that the reason for the test is patient safety and that you are not going to practice in what you consider to be an inappropriate manner. In short, if local anesthesia cannot be agreed on as a satisfactory substitute for general anesthesia, then the patient either agrees to the test or goes somewhere else.

6a. A 6-year-old scheduled for a scar revision was accompanied by his mother and grandmother. The mother signed the consent form and left for work. Is a preanesthesia interview with the grandmother and patient appropriate?

The key to this question is the second sentence. The mother apparently came into the facility and was given a preprinted form with no discussion and no informed consent as that term is intended. An informed consent is not synonymous with signing a piece of paper. The written piece of paper is important only to the extent that it memorializes a discussion with the responsible person, in this case, a parent, as to the relevant risks, alternatives, and benefits of the procedure and, indeed, with regard to the administration of anesthesia itself. Since there was no discussion with the mother, what good is the written paper?

If the subsequent discussion, which is entitled a "preanesthesia interview," is intended to imply a meaningful discussion about the risks, alternatives, and benefits, then the question arises as to whether the grandmother is able to fully supply an accurate medical history and current health status concerning the child sufficient to enable the physician who is going to obtain the anesthesia consent to assess properly what the risks, benefits, and alternatives may be. If the grandmother indicates that she is not really certain about the child's health, medications the child is taking, past surgical history, the response of the child to prior anesthetic agents, and so forth, there is no way that a realistic evaluation of these factors can be undertaken.

Let's assume, however, that the grandmother is a terrific historian and gives very accurate information but then says, "I don't think that I should be the one to make the decision whether to go forward or not because of the risks that you have just outlined to me." In this situation, the parent is the one who must be notified and thereafter give consent. If the grandmother gives consent and an unfortunate event should occur, the facility may not be protected because the mother is going to state that she was the one who signed the consent form and that signifies that the facility understood that she was the one who had the right to consent or not to consent. Since the facility chose to obtain her signature without really giving her the explanation, it is at risk of the mother indicating after the tragic event that had she been told of these risks, she would never have given consent. She will, no doubt, testify under these circumstances that the grandmother was left simply so someone could accompany the child home after the procedure and be with the child while awaiting the start of the procedure. She may indicate that she never gave permission for the grandmother to consent, nor did she indicate that the grandmother was an appropriate person for such an important discussion.

All this points out the need to have meaningful discussions with the parent or parents of a minor in advance of the scheduled procedure so that you do not have situations like the one described here.

6b. *A 10-year-old boy is scheduled for bilateral myringotomy with tubes. After the interview with the anesthesiologist, and after signing the operative consent, the mother announces that she is leaving. She will come back after surgery to be with her son and take him home. Should we proceed on a minor without the responsible adult being present?*

Technically, the legal answer is no. Practically speaking, there may be acceptable compromises. If the mother agrees that she will be constantly available by phone and is only a short distance away, then the procedure could be done. However, a special consent form should be used in addition to the regular procedure consent form. A sample special consent form is given in Appendix 2A. If the parent refuses to sign this consent, do not do the procedure unless the parent agrees to stay. This points out the necessity of questioning the responsible adult *before* the procedure is undertaken.

6c. ***A 4-year-old child scheduled for a T&A is brought in by her grandmother. The grandmother has taken care of the child since birth but is not her legal guardian. The mother lives in town but at a different address and, according to the grandmother, is "not interested in coming to the surgical facility to be with her daughter." Can we accept the grandmother's information regarding the health status of the child? Can we proceed without the written or verbal consent of the mother?***

No. The information given by the grandmother must be verified. The natural mother should be contacted and her consent obtained. If she refuses to give the consent or to discuss the surgery, a court order can be quickly obtained. This case is a classic example of the need for surgeons to address these issues with their patients before a procedure is scheduled or before the patients arrive in the unit. The only exception to this answer would be in the event that the procedure was truly emergent, that is, there was an *immediate* risk of death or serious harm to the child if the procedure were to be delayed. Then the surgeon should proceed immediately. In an emergency an informed consent is unnecessary.

7. *What are the legal precedents regarding preoperative workup for an outpatient who is about to undergo general anesthesia?*

There are no general legal precedents that would serve as an adequate response to this question. It must be remembered that each case decides only the issues that pertain to the particular patient at hand. In short, each malpractice case stands for the proposition that under the particular circumstances existing at that time, applicable to that patient, and to that proposed procedure and anesthetic administration, certain acts or omissions were or were not negligent. However, as a result of an analysis of these cases, certain general guidelines have been developed.

These general guidelines state that for each individual patient it is incumbent upon the surgeon who is going to operate on the patient and the anesthesiologist who is going to administer the anesthesia to conduct a thorough and appropriate physical examination germane to their specialty and to elicit a comprehensive medical history. They are also charged with the responsibility of conducting such inquiries, tests, studies, and so forth that are necessary to provide them with the information needed to fully assess the propriety of the proposed procedure and the propriety of administering a particular form of anesthesia or particular anesthetic agents to that patient. Obviously, such tests may differ from patient to patient. For example, a patient scheduled for a gynecologic procedure who has given a history of heavy menstrual bleeding may require hemoglobin and hematocrit tests. Another patient may disclose, under occupational history, that he or she works in an asbestos plant. Such a patient would be a candidate for a chest film. A patient who has a history of tuberculosis may require not only a chest film, but also a skin patch test in order to determine whether he or she is still suffering from active tuberculosis before exposing other patients and the operating room staff to the risk of contracting the disease. A pregnancy test may be appropriate for women of a certain age, but not for those beyond the child-bearing years. A history of an earache may require an ENT consultation. Complaints of burning urine would require a urinalysis and perhaps a culture. A history that disclosed the use of certain medications might indicate that it is not wise to use general anesthesia and that the procedure should be done under either local or spinal anesthesia, or perhaps that the procedure should be postponed for some additional period of time. An asthma history may be relevant for the purpose of determining whether certain additional tests should be carried out or whether the patient should simply be given anesthesia by mask rather than being intubated.

The usual reaction of most physicians to this approach is the suggestion that lawyers and judges are dictating the practice of medicine and mandating defensive medicine by imposing a burden to test, test, test, and test some more. The fallacy of this rebuttal is that it is not the lawyers or the judges who are getting sued when something happens to patients. If a particular test is suggested and the physician chooses to gamble on what the test might have disclosed by not ordering it, then that physician runs the risk of losing the gamble. The physician loses if he or she does not do the test and some injury occurs to the patient that could have been avoided if the test had been done and the condition found. The physician elected to gamble not only with the patient's safety, but also with his or her own legal safety by exposing himself or herself to a risk. It is recognized and admitted that this adds to the cost of medical care in this country. However, if a patient sustains harm because, without consulting the patient, you elected not to undertake a particular test and the patient sustains a severe injury as a result thereof, do you really think the patient, in retrospect, is going to concur with your decision because you saved him or her $7 on a blood test? More likely than not the patient will say, "If the doctor had told me that this risk could have been determined before the procedure by doing a simple $7 blood test, I would have paid for fifty such tests rather than have happen to me what did happen." Since the physicians do not pay for the tests, there is little likelihood that a jury observing a severely injured patient is going to have much regard for a physician who tried to save $7 by not doing a test when the patient is now stuck with a lifetime of medical expenses and pain and suffering. Applying a risk-benefit analysis to this situation yields the following result: The physician gambles by not doing the appropriate tests and gains nothing for himself or herself or the patient if he or she wins, but on the other hand, if the physician loses, he or she has not only hurt the patient, but also has put himself or herself and his or her own assets at risk.

The conclusion is, therefore, that if the patient's medical history, physical examination, or other data suggest that it may be appropriate to conduct a certain test in order to assess the risks, benefits, and alternatives for that patient fully and completely, then the test should be ordered regardless of the fact that it may result in a temporary postponement of the procedure or an increase in the patient's overall cost of medical care.

8. Dr. X, a surgeon, has a practice of not doing a procedure without first having the patient undergo a cardiogram as well as a CBC and a urinalysis in patients over 40 years of age. Mrs. Smith, a 45-year-old woman, arrives at the center with the report from her cardiogram, but did not have a chance to get to the laboratory to have the CBC and urinalysis performed. Dr. Y, the anesthesiologist for the procedure (which will require general anesthesia), reviews the chart, notes the preoperative orders by Dr. X, and realizes that the requested laboratory tests have not been carried out. Dr. Y speaks to the patient, who assures him that she is in excellent health and indicates that there has been no change in her physical status since the last time she had the tests carried out, which was 2 or 3 years ago. The surgeon, Dr. X, wants to go ahead with the procedure and assures the anesthesiologist, Dr. Y, that it is his (Dr. X's) decision to make and that he (Dr. X) "will take full responsibility" for the decision to proceed. Should Dr. Y go forward with induction of anesthesia?

No. This question raises several important issues. The first issue has been addressed throughout this chapter. If preoperative laboratory testing is ordered, it is fair to assume that the testing was ordered to enhance patient safety and to ensure that the patient has no contraindications for surgery or anesthesia. If the preoperative orders mandate certain minimal testing and that testing has not been completed, how can one justify going forward? This question becomes especially pertinent if there is a maloccurrence during the procedure that is later shown to have been due to risk factors that could have been identified by the preoperative laboratory testing that was ordered. Suppose the CBC testing would have revealed a white blood count of 25,000, which demonstrates that a systemic infection is underway, or suppose the CBC testing would have revealed a white blood count of 1,000. How do you think a jury is going to react when your only justification for going forward with the procedure is that the patient said she was in excellent health? Even a mediocre plaintiff's attorney is going to cut you to shreds by simply pointing out that patients often feel fine even in the presence of risk factors that contraindicate surgery, and it is for this very reason that preoperative laboratory testing is ordered.

How about Dr. X's assurance that the decision to proceed is his and that he will take full responsibility for the decision? Is this going to be a defense for a malpractice action instituted against Dr. Y by the patient, Mrs. Smith? Not a chance. The surgeon and the anesthesiologist are *jointly* responsible for the patient's safety. In effect, each is a check on the other because the procedure cannot go forward unless both participate. The anesthesiologist has a duty to the patient, independent of that of the surgeon, to ensure that all preoperative testing that has been ordered is completed prior to the start of the procedure. Risk factors that may be identified by such testing are as germane to the anesthesia management of the patient as they are to the surgical management of the patient.

9a. *A patient has no one to escort her home and stay with her after surgery and general anesthesia. She insists on taking public transportation. Our policy requires that a responsible adult escort a patient home. What do we do? What are our options and our liabilities?*

Before administering any anesthetic agent or performing any surgical procedure, the surgery center must ensure that the patient intends to meet all the facility's preoperative and postoperative requirements. If a patient cannot assure the discharging practitioner that she or he is prepared to comply with the unit's discharge criteria, as in this question, no treatment should be rendered.

The intention behind the requirement that a responsible adult accompany a patient home involves considerations of safety. A person's physical and mental capabilities are markedly reduced immediately after surgery under general anesthesia. The center's policy is obviously designed to ensure that a patient has available assistance, if needed, in traveling from the clinic to home and to ensure that there is a responsible person on hand to alert medical authorities in the event that a complication should occur.

If a patient lies and says that a responsible adult will be present after the surgery to provide the required supervision and no one shows up, the center is in a quandary. Every attempt should be made to induce the patient to call some responsible adult to accompany her or him home (e.g., relative, neighbor, or friend). Failing this, the question arises as to whether the patient should be discharged on her or his own recognizance, and if so, whether the patient should be permitted to take public transportation home.

As a practical matter, when the patient is young and healthy, the surgery minor, and the postoperative course (vital signs and so on) exemplary, such a discharge might be acceptable. However, this would be the exception rather than the rule. If a patient shows any questionable signs or symptoms, or if the patient is at risk of developing complications, admission to an inpatient facility is indicated. If the patient refuses admission and insists on leaving the center without accompaniment, the person should be discharged only after signing out "against medical advice."

It is certainly unwise to allow an unescorted patient to take public transportation home after a surgical procedure under general anesthesia. If a complication should arise while the patient is on a public bus or subway, there would be no one available who would know that the person had just undergone surgery and who could communicate this information to medical personnel once they arrived on the scene. Consequently, much valuable time might be lost as the medical team attempted to ascertain what was wrong with the patient. Another major concern is the utter indifference of many individuals, especially in large cities, to the plight of others. Many people simply do not want to get involved and are unwilling even to summon medical aid for one obviously in need. Such conduct could easily result in the loss of valuable time in treating the patient's complication. These problems can be averted if the patient is escorted home by a responsible adult. Obviously, it is not the type of transportation the patient takes home that creates potential legal hazards; rather, it is the patient's returning home unescorted, regardless of what mode of transportation is used.

Surgical centers that routinely allow patients to leave unaccompanied contrary to their own express regulations are inviting trouble. In a malpractice action against such a surgery center, there is very little that can be raised to rebut the contention that the center's conduct was negligent, since the patient was discharged without accompaniment, in direct contravention of the unit's own rules and regulations. Consequently, it is imperative that the facility abide by the guidelines it has established.

9b. *The patient's husband is the responsible person who will be accompanying her home. Our policy requires the responsible person to remain with the patient overnight. The husband works the second shift (3 to 11 P.M.). He states, "our kids are at home." The oldest is an 8-year-old. Can we discharge under these circumstances? What are our obligations to our patient's safety?*

No. This is again a situation that should not arise if the ground rules are clearly given to the patient before the procedure is scheduled. If this information is elicited before the procedure, do not do the procedure. An 8-year-old does not legally meet any definition of a responsible adult. If the patient conceals this information until after the procedure has been completed, insist that the husband get an adult to be with his wife when he leaves for work. Verify that such an adult will be present and give that adult the discharge instructions (a phone discussion would be appropriate). If no such adult is able to be in attendance, admit the patient and tell the husband that he will be financially responsible for the cost of admission. Serious consideration should be given to inserting the following statement in the preadmission literature: "The requirement that a responsible adult remain with the patient for 24 hours after the procedure will be strictly enforced. The failure to comply with this requirement will result in either a cancellation of the procedure or the overnight admission of the patient at the patient's sole expense. *Warning:* Your insurance will not cover the cost of such an admission, so your compliance is absolutely essential."

10. *A family practitioner who has no surgical privileges at our local hospital wants privileges in our freestanding unit to perform D&C procedures and lump and bump removals. What are the legal hazards of the situation? Is there a difference if this is a hospital satellite unit or a proprietary freestanding unit?*

Although there will be some dispute about this answer, the response is that a physician should not be permitted to do in a hospital satellite or a proprietary freestanding unit any procedure that he or she does not have privileges to do in a hospital. If the reputation, utility, and quality of ambulatory surgery are to be preserved, one of the first lines of defense has to be physician selection. If a physician does not have privileges to do a particular procedure at a hospital, then he or she should not be afforded such privileges in an ambulatory center. Ambulatory units require physicians of great skill, not second-class physicians.

If privileges were given to the family practitioner and during the course of a

D&C procedure the physician's technique produced a massive hemorrhage that he or she was not qualified to treat, or the hemorrhage required the performance of an emergency hysterectomy in order to save the patient's life and the physician was not trained in that procedure, a great tragedy could occur to the patient, and a lawsuit would undoubtedly be brought against the physician and the center. If the plaintiff were able to prove that the physician had been refused privileges at a number of hospitals because of inadequate skills, training, or education, but that the ambulatory center had granted privileges, there would then be a strong likelihood that the center would be held liable for placing that physician in a position in which he or she could undertake such procedures on patients. From a legal standpoint, the safest course always has to be that only those physicians who have been found qualified to do procedures in a hospital setting should ever be given privileges to do them in an ambulatory center. Taking this equation one step further, we do not recommend giving a physician any greater privileges in terms of the complexity of procedures in an ambulatory center than that physician is authorized to do in an inpatient setting.

There may be instances where a physician limits all procedures to his or her office or to a freestanding facility and therefore has no hospital privileges. How are privileges granted to this individual? Close scrutiny must be exercised over this individual's credentials before privileges are granted. The administration of the center must consider such factors as whether the physician is board certified, the nature and extent of the physician's prior experience, maloccurrences the physician has been involved with in the past, and the comments of other well-respected physicians in the area who have had contact with the practitioner seeking privileges. Keep in mind that the center may be held directly liable for the actions of an unqualified or underqualified practitioner under a theory of corporate negligence if it can be shown that the center did not carefully review the practitioner's credentials before granting privileges. This consideration, coupled with the consideration of patient safety, mandates a careful, comprehensive credentialing process, especially for those who do not have any hospital privileges.

11a. ***An independent, freestanding ambulatory center advertises to fill the position of an individual responsible for all discharge examinations and evaluations. Dr. Y., a chiropractor, applies for this position, citing the new JCAHO standard permitting a licensed independent practitioner to discharge patients. Under the law of the state in question, Dr. Y is licensed and is permitted to provide patient care services without direction or supervision. Should the center give serious consideration to Dr. Y's application?***

No. The new JCAHO standards define "licensed independent practitioner" (LIP) as "[a]ny individual who is permitted by law and who is also permitted by the health care organization to provide patient care services without direction or supervision, within the scope of his/her license and in accordance with individually granted clinical privileges" (see *JCAHO Ambulatory Health Care Standards Manual*, 1990). The JCAHO standards relating to discharge (SA.1.17–1.18) also make it clear that an LIP qualified in resuscitative techniques must be present or immediately available until all patients operated on each day have been evaluated and discharged.

Initially, one must assess what it is that Dr. Y is going to be called on to do each day as the person in charge of discharge decisions. Dr. Y will be required to evaluate, monitor, and make medical decisions regarding the patients who are entrusted to him. More important, Dr. Y may be called on to resuscitate a patient who has a cardiac or pulmonary arrest. Is Dr. Y qualified to perform these functions? We think not. A chiropractor is skilled in manipulation therapy but has little or no training or experience with medical treatment and evaluation of patients. Dr. Y's state license permits him to perform chiropractic services to patients, not to treat or evaluate them medically. His request for employment by the center exceeds the bounds of his qualifications. Even assuming that Dr. Y has had CPR training and other resuscitation training courses, no sound-thinking administrator should entrust the lives of patients to an individual whose training and experience are in an area that rarely, if ever, involves the types of decisions that Dr. Y will have to make on a routine basis as the person responsible for discharge decisions.

11b. Our center permits podiatrists to perform certain procedures. The OR schedule is arranged so that the podiatry procedures are always the last of the day. There is always at least one podiatrist on the premises until the center closes for the day. By the time the podiatric procedures are completed, there are usually many patients who have undergone nonpodiatric procedures still at the center awaiting discharge. Our surgeons and anesthesiologists all leave by 6:00 P.M., even if they have patients who have not yet been discharged. Their rationale is that under the new JCAHO standards, a podiatrist qualifies as an LIP and, therefore, is competent to discharge their patients. Last week, at 6:30 P.M., a nonpodiatric patient who was awaiting discharge arrested. All the surgeons and anesthesiologists had left for the day. Dr. Y., a podiatrist, was on the premises, but he refused to attempt to resuscitate the patient because such techniques are beyond his licensure and he has no training in them. Is the center in trouble?

Yes. The center is responsible to be certain that appropriate standards are in place and being complied with to ensure patient safety. At a minimum, the center must require the presence of an LIP who has knowledge, experience, and training in all aspects of the decision of discharge and in all aspects of resuscitation techniques. While Dr. Y may have had the ability to make discharge decisions on his podiatric patients, he clearly was not qualified to and, in fact, was unable and unwilling to even attempt resuscitation of a patient in extremis.

The center's conduct in this case is simply indefensible. The center should have been certain that it had rules and regulations in place to ensure that at least one individual trained and qualified to make discharge decisions and to perform resuscitation techniques was on premises at all times.

We stress our approval of the AAAHC standards that require discharge decisions to be made by the operating surgeon or the participating anesthesiologist.

12. In a freestanding unit (without a transfer agreement with a hospital), the responsible party leaves while the patient is in the recovery area. At discharge time, no one can be found to take the patient home. The patient now wants to leave unescorted. What are our alternatives?

The unit's policy of requiring all its patients to be accompanied home by a responsible adult is a sound one. In fact, standards promulgated by the AAAHC provide that "patients [should be] discharged in the company of a responsible adult, except when they have not received anesthesia or when they have received unsupplemented local anesthesia." You can never be certain which patients will develop complications or how serious those complications might be. Although the responsible adult may not be able to render appropriate medical treatment to palliate the patient's complication, appropriate medical aid can be summoned immediately. If the patient were alone, no one would be available to summon such aid.

This discussion demonstrates that safety considerations underlie the patient accompaniment rule. It is clear that in many cases it is unsafe to release a patient without someone to escort him or her home. If a patient's escort has disappeared, an attempt should be made to obtain a substitute (e.g., friend, neighbor, relative, or family member). If no substitute can be found, the patient should be examined very carefully, preferably by the operating surgeon. If the examining physician finds even the slightest untoward sign or symptom, the patient should be admitted to an inpatient facility.

If the patient objects to inpatient admission, there is no way that he or she can legally be forced to stay. However, if a patient insists on leaving, the patient should be made to sign out "against medical advice." Before discharge, the risks involved in leaving under such circumstances should be fully explained to the patient, and the patient's chart should reflect this discussion. In instances such as this where the patient discharges himself or herself, the patient has assumed responsibility if complications later develop, and the physician and surgical center have insulated themselves from liability.

Even if the patient does agree to an inpatient facility, there may be a problem, since the facts of this question indicate that the ambulatory center does not have a transfer agreement with a hospital. Since this is not an emergency case, there exists the possibility that the patient might have difficulty in gaining admission to a local hospital if it were nearing its patient capacity limit. Situations such as this should not be left to chance. It is recommended that all freestanding ambulatory facilities provide for implementation of a transfer agreement with a local hospital to ensure that their patients will have ready access to an inpatient facility if the need arises.

13. During the preanesthesia interview, the anesthesiologist discovers that the patient has no idea of the nature of the anticipated surgical procedure or

its risks, benefits, or alternatives. Is there any legal risk to the unit or the anesthesiologist in going forward with the procedure?

Yes. A physician has no right to touch a patient unless that patient has given an informed consent to being touched. Informed consent means that the patient has been fully briefed and understands the nature of the anticipated surgical procedure and its risks, benefits, and alternatives. As a necessary adjunct of surgery, the patient must be given anesthesia. In order to understand the anesthesia risks, the patient has to relate them to the surgical risks, and vice versa. Once the anesthesiologist becomes aware that the patient has not given an informed consent, then he or she should refuse to go forward with the procedure until the patient has been so informed.

In a nonemergency situation, the procedure should be postponed in order to give the surgeon an opportunity to hold an informed consent conference with the patient. If there is an emergency, the informed consent discussion may have to be held with the patient as soon as possible. If the emergency is such that no delay is possible, then the consent is deemed to be waived by virtue of the emergency, and obviously, in order to protect the patient, the procedure should be performed as soon as possible. However, in the case of nonemergency, elective surgery, the anesthesiologist is best advised to report the situation to the surgeon and to decline to administer anesthesia to the patient until a truly informed consent has been obtained.

14. While assisting a patient in getting ready for surgery, a nurse observed the patient taking some medication and returning the container to her purse. When the nurse questioned the patient, the patient assured her that it was just a "nerve pill" and refused to disclose what it was or who had prescribed it. The nurse reported this information to the anesthesiologist. The anesthesiologist said the center was legally protected in accepting the patient's description of the medication and ordered the procedure to go forward. Was the center legally protected under these circumstances?

No. This patient is about to undergo a surgical procedure under anesthesia. The purpose of obtaining informed consent from both the surgical standpoint and the anesthesiology standpoint is to fully assess all the risks, benefits, and alternatives associated with the surgical and anesthetic procedures to be undertaken. These risks may be directly affected by whatever medication the patient just put into her mouth. If the medication is contraindicated with one of the anesthetic agents, there might be a severe allergic response or the effect of either one of the drugs might be potentiated by the other. If the drug the patient just took has an effect on cardiac output or might otherwise depress respiratory functions, then that drug might pose a significant risk attendant to the procedure. Therefore, without knowing the nature of the drug, its dosage, and how many more such "nerve pills" the patient has taken in the last two or three hours, how can one say that there has been an accurate assessment of the risks?

Suppose the pill was, in fact, nitroglycerin and the patient was suffering from angina that had not heretofore been disclosed. This might be a very relevant piece of information that the physician should know before undertaking either to operate on or to anesthetize that patient. Indeed, one of the first questions that should be asked of all patients who come to the ambulatory center is, "What medications, if any, have you taken in the last two weeks?" If the patient is unsure, then the name of the physician who prescribed the medication should be obtained, and contact should be established with that physician. If the physician indicates that he or she has not seen the patient in a substantial period of time and was unaware that the patient was even taking the medication, then further caution has to be exercised, and it may necessitate putting the procedure off until such time as the patient makes a complete disclosure and the actual medications are reviewed and assessed.

If you need horror stories, the following actual case may be appropriate. A dentist who had substantial experience in extracting impacted wisdom teeth under sedation and nitrous oxide was performing such a procedure. Shortly after the extraction was begun, all the patient's respiratory functions ceased. Attempts to revive the patient were unsuccessful, and the patient was pronounced dead on arrival at the hospital. At autopsy, the toxicology report indicated that the patient had taken enough sedatives to put eight insomniacs to sleep for at least 48 hours. When that medication was superimposed on the effects of the other anesthetic agents administered in the dentist's office, the result was predictable and fatal. The award that was entered against the dentist was in seven figures simply because, before anesthetizing the patient, neither the dentist nor the nurse-anesthetist had ever questioned the patient about any other medications that might have been taken.

15. *Our freestanding surgery center does not presently have a transfer agreement with a hospital. However, all our surgeons have admitting privileges at local hospitals, and we have never encountered any problems with the admission of our patients to the emergency room of a local hospital when an emergency has developed. Do you think we need a transfer agreement in this situation?*

Yes. Even in this situation, a transfer agreement is necessary. The emergency cases are not usually going to present a problem. In an emergency, such as cardiac arrest or respiratory failure, the emergency room of any hospital will always take the patient in. However, suppose a patient wakes up after an operation and has a flaccid paralysis of an extremity. Clearly, this person is going to require observation, monitoring, intensive care, and possibly rehabilitation therapy. An ambulatory surgery center is not equipped to provide these services. The patient requires admission to a hospital to be properly treated and cared for. A surgical center must have some type of agreement with an inpatient facility so that patients who do not require immediate emergency care but still need observation, monitoring, and treatment can be admitted. Although the surgeons at the ambulatory center may have admitting privileges at a nearby hospital, in a nonemergency situation, the hospital can elect to reject admission of the patient.

This situation will never develop if the center and the hospital have a preexisting transfer agreement.

A brief example should serve to clarify this discussion. Suppose a patient undergoes afternoon surgery and is admitted to the recovery room. Upon observation, it is noted that his or her blood pressure remains low. Very possibly, this patient is going to be fine. However, the patient's situation requires cardiac monitoring for several hours. The surgical center closes at 5 P.M., so the patient cannot remain there. The center, in this situation, requires the use of a facility where the patient can be monitored and observed until recuperation. A transfer agreement with a local hospital is the perfect solution. Since it is worked out in advance, no time is spent worrying about which hospital the patient should be taken to, who is going to take care of the patient, and whether or not he or she will even be admitted. The transfer agreement provides an extra margin of safety for both the patient and the center and is indicated from both a medical and a legal standpoint.

16. One of our surgeons insists on using her own instruments and her own scrub nurse. We do not know the nurse's qualifications or the method of sterilization used by the surgeon for her instruments. If it can be documented that these are not the center's equipment or personnel, are we legally protected?

You may or may not be. However, before worrying about whether or not you are legally protected, note that as we have repeatedly emphasized, all accrediting organizations insist that ambulatory surgery centers develop their own criteria, regulations, personnel qualifications, and so forth. It is the center's right, duty, and obligation to make certain that no one comes onto its premises to do anything that has not been previously reviewed and approved of by the center. Under the circumstances suggested by this question, it is the center's prerogative and obligation to advise the surgeon that she will either provide proof of her scrub nurse's qualifications or perform procedures without her. If the center is satisfied by virtue of the nurse's background, qualifications, and experience that she is qualified, it is still entitled to a probationary period during which the nurse can be observed by one of the center's scrub nurses in order to make certain that she is currently qualified. Once this has been accomplished, then it may be appropriate to permit this physician to use her own scrub nurse.

The same is true of the instruments. If the physician can document to the center's satisfaction that the method of sterilizing the instruments meets the center's standards, then it may be appropriate for the physician to sterilize and use her own instruments during procedures. However, this matter should be documented. In other words, a letter should be sent to the surgeon indicating that she has represented and warranted to the center that she will sterilize instruments in a certain manner and that she assumes full responsibility for those instruments and their sterilization. The letter also should indicate that if the center is sued because it is determined that the surgeon's instruments were not appropriately sterilized, the center will seek indemnification for any sums it is compelled to pay.

17. Mr. Anderson was scheduled for an early morning procedure in our ambulatory surgery unit and was told to stay NPO from midnight on. On the morning of the procedure, the patient disclosed that he had not done so. What are our options? Would the answer be any different if the patient had traveled 40 or 50 miles to the center for the procedure?

Initially, it should be stressed that all patients who have been instructed to stay NPO must be carefully questioned in order to determine whether they have followed these instructions. Many patients do not realize the importance of remaining NPO (often because it has not been stressed by the surgeon or the anesthesiologist) and will have a bite to eat or something to drink on the morning of the procedure. These same patients are often reticent to volunteer to the anesthesiologist that they have had something to eat or drink because they do not want to be chastised for failing to follow instructions. In many cases, it is only through careful questioning that individuals who have failed to follow NPO instructions are identified. Keep in mind that unless these individuals are identified, this significant risk factor cannot even be taken into account in deciding whether or not to go forward with the procedure.

Throughout this chapter, we have stressed the necessity of closely following the procedures and regulations that have been adopted by a center to ensure patient safety. It is these procedures and regulations that will be the standard by which an anesthesiologist is judged. The policy of NPO from midnight on has obviously been implemented to prevent regurgitation and subsequent aspiration during a procedure. If Mr. Anderson discloses that he has failed to remain NPO from midnight and the anesthesiologist proceeds in spite of this, what justification does he or she have if, during the procedure, Mr. Anderson suffers a sudden airway obstruction and subsequent injury as a result of regurgitation of the stomach contents?

There is no hard and fast rule that can be applied to every situation. In each instance, various factors must be weighed and balanced before deciding whether to go through with a procedure as scheduled. What is the patient's present state of health? Is the contemplated procedure major or relatively minor? Is regional or general anesthesia to be administered? How do patients normally react to the anesthetic agent that is to be administered? Will the patient be intubated? Is the procedure elective? What did the patient ingest? Was it a trickle of water after brushing his or her teeth, a sip of coffee, a glass of orange juice, a donut, or an entire breakfast of bacon and eggs with toast? When was the food or liquid ingested?

Once an assessment of all these factors (as well as other equally valid factors you might add) is undertaken, an intelligent and reasoned medical determination can be made of the propriety of proceeding with the surgery. If there is any lingering doubt about whether complications might develop (e.g., the patient is elderly and in poor health, the patient consumed a large breakfast one hour before the scheduled surgery), cancel the procedure. It is far better to cause the patient the minor inconvenience of returning for surgery another day than to subject him or her to the possibility of permanent injury and yourself to the possibility of entanglement in a web of legal woes.

The answer to this question would not be any different even if Mr. Anderson traveled 50 miles to get to the ambulatory surgery center. This factor should have no bearing whatsoever on the decision of whether or not to go through with the procedure. A patient who has traveled two hours to the center should be evaluated in the same fashion as the one who has had to travel only two minutes. Inconvenience to the patient in canceling a scheduled procedure is simply not a relevant consideration in the medical decision-making process of whether or not a surgical procedure can be safely performed.

18. *A 17-year-old girl refuses to proceed with laboratory testing or anesthesia and surgery on the morning of surgery. She states that she has had a bad dream, that she believes that she is going to die from the anesthetic, and that she does not wish to proceed. Her mother insists that we proceed, stating that the daughter is not yet an adult and since she (the mother) is responsible for signing the consent form, she wants the surgery performed. Scheduled surgery is removal of four third molars. What should we do?*

This question raises the issue of the difference between informed consent and consent to undergo surgery. There is no question that the informed consent of a minor's parent(s) must be obtained before proceeding with surgery and anesthesia. The risks, benefits, and alternatives regarding anesthesia and surgery must be discussed. Consent to proceed with surgery also must be obtained from the parent(s) of a minor, but there is a very real question as to whether a parent's decision to proceed with surgery can override a contrary decision by a 17-year-old patient. Remember that in this example we are not dealing with a 4- or 5-year-old child who has limited reasoning abilities. We are dealing with a 17-year-old who, most probably, is a junior or senior in high school and is in a position to make an informed choice regarding whether or not to proceed with surgery. Many 17-year-olds hold drivers' licenses, are employed in part-time jobs, and maintain leadership positions in their high schools. Is it wise to deny such individuals a say in a decision that may have an impact on their physical well-being?

One might question the validity of the reasoning for this particular 17-year-old in refusing to permit laboratory testing and surgery (*i.e.,* a bad dream envisioning death by anesthesia), but on the other hand, the procedure in question is a relatively minor one that certainly is not emergent and could be rescheduled for another date when the patient is in a better frame of mind.

As a practical matter, what do you propose to do if you accede to the mother's wishes—physically restrain the child for the laboratory testing, get stat results, and then restrain the child again while general anesthesia is induced and the child is rendered unconscious? Aside from increasing the risk of harm to the struggling patient, how are you possibly going to explain your actions to a jury if the child's premonition comes to pass and she dies while under anesthesia? No jury is going to buy your legal defense that the mother alone was able to consent to proceed with surgery and anesthesia and that the minor patient was entitled to no say whatsoever, especially if, at trial, the mother relates the sequence of events in a light that is much more favorable to the patient than the events that actually transpired. The mother is going to be feeling an awful lot of guilt, much of which she will attempt to deal with by blaming the anesthesiologist and surgeon for proceeding against her daughter's wishes.

We advocate an approach of persuasion and reasoning with the child to assure her that her fears are not well founded. If this approach fails, cancel the surgery.

19. During the preanesthesia interview, the anesthesiologist discovers that the patient scheduled for laparoscopic tubal sterilization is a heroin abuser. After discussion with the patient, it is determined that a more extensive evaluation (i.e., liver profile, chest roentgenogram, and so on) is needed and that the patient should be admitted following her procedure. The patient voices concern about insurance coverage. A call to the insurance company brings the response, "For laparoscopic tubal surgery, coverage is provided for minimal basic laboratory testing, and only if the procedure is performed on an outpatient basis." What is the responsibility of the anesthesiologist in this situation?

This question raises financial, professional liability, and patient confidentiality issues. Obviously, the anesthesiologist cannot provide a lower standard of care simply because the insurance carrier wants to save money. The carrier is unlikely to authorize the additional testing and inpatient surgery without knowledge as to the reasons that require it. Disclosure of heroin abuse cannot be made to the carrier without the patient's written consent. A conference with the patient and all interested health care providers is necessary. If the patient authorizes the disclosure (get it in writing), then the carrier can be contacted, and hopefully reimbursement for the additional testing and the admission will be authorized. The patient should be told that disclosure will not guarantee a change in the carrier's position and may import on the patient's future insurability. If the patient refuses to authorize disclosure or the carrier refuses to accept the case as an exception to its reimbursement schedule, then the physician must work out with the patient an acceptable payment arrangement. Under no circumstances should there be a change in the medical management of the patient based on insurance considerations.

20. One of our surgeons refuses to have his patients sign a written consent form. He claims that he heard a "lawyer/commentator" state that they are not worth the paper they are written on in a court of law. Do you agree? What makes a written consent form enforceable?

If the only consent in a case consists of handing a patient a written consent form with the instructions that he or she sign it and date it, then the legal commentator made a valid point. The purpose of the written consent form is to document that there has, in fact, been a discussion with the patient and that certain specific areas were discussed with the patient as evidenced in the written consent form. The patient's signature is intended to document not only that he or she participated in a discussion, but also that there was an opportunity to read and review the contents of the written consent form, which may very well supplement and further highlight what took place in the discussion with the patient. The written consent form is, therefore, not the informed consent, but rather the evidence of informed consent.

The written consent form should identify the physician who had the discussion and provide an opportunity for that physician to record some of the principal risks, alternatives, and benefits that were discussed. Many institutions require a nurse to witness the signature. If the point of this policy is to verify that it was this particular patient who signed the consent form, there is no objection to this procedure. On the other hand, giving a pad of written consent forms to a nurse and instructing him or her to have every patient sign a form is utterly meaningless. The nurse, no matter how competent, is not deemed under the law to be an appropriate person to obtain an informed consent. It is the surgeon or other physician who is going to do the procedure or to administer the anesthesia who has the obligation, by virtue of superior knowledge and training in that particular specialty, to inform the patient of the risks, benefits, and alternatives and to respond to the patient's inquiries about those areas and to then make certain that, when the patient agrees to proceed with surgery, the consent is voluntarily and knowingly made.

The direct response to this question is that the discussion of the physician with the patient as capsulized or memorialized in the written consent form is what makes the consent form meaningful and therefore enforceable in an action that may thereafter be brought by the patient. Absence of some written documentation of the informed consent discussion is often argued by plaintiff's attorneys to be strong evidence that the discussion never took place. Therefore, it is highly recommended that a written consent form be signed by patients.

Appendix 2A

■ ■

CONSENT BY A PARENT LEAVING A CHILD IN THE UNIT

I, _____ , being the natural parent and legal guardian of _____
_____ , a minor, acknowledge that I have been informed that I should remain in the
ambulatory surgery unit throughout the operative procedure on my child and during the recovery
period. I have elected to leave the unit despite such advice and, therefore, agree as follows:

     1. I will be constantly available by phone at
       (   ) _____ .
       (area code)   number
     2. I will not be more than _____ minutes away from the unit (20 minutes max-
       imum)

  I hereby authorize the surgeon, anesthesiologist, the unit, and their agents, servants, and employees to carry out any emergency or nonemergency procedures that they deem necessary and appropriate for the proper medical care and safety of my child in my absence. This consent and authorization is unlimited in scope and is applicable whether I am reachable by phone or not.

                                        _____
                                         Parent Signature

Selection

3

■ ■

FREDRICK K. ORKIN, BARBARA GOLD

Everything has been thought of before, Goethe suggested, but the problem is to think of it again. And so it is with anesthesia for ambulatory surgery. However, only recently have we come to recognize the importance of the selection of appropriate surgical procedures, patients, patient preparation, and equipment, among other considerations, in the ambulatory setting. This chapter surveys this important but illusive and evolving aspect of ambulatory anesthesia care, in what is now one of the most rapidly developing subspecialties in clinical anesthesiology. Rather than present a series of static lists relating to the various selection decisions, this chapter emphasizes principles and approaches that will enable the reader to respond to the challenges of adpating his or her own practice to the ambulatory setting as it evolves. Selection decisions in the choice of anesthetic techniques and drugs, personnel, and facility design are discussed in greater detail throughout the rest of this book.

SELECTION AND THE EVOLUTION OF AMBULATORY ANESTHESIA
From Antiquity to 1900
Well before the first surgical procedures were undertaken, rudimentary ambulatory anesthesia was practiced. The ancients knew that alcohol and opium derivatives could produce unconsciousness as well as pain relief. Physical methods of producing anesthesia, such as strangulation and a blow to the head, were used routinely in biblical Egypt prior to circumcision, one of the earliest surgical procedures. The Edwin Smith Surgical Papyrus (3000 B.C.) depicts several dozen other surgical procedures, including treatment of flesh wounds, facial fractures, and long bone trauma. Primitive anesthesia for these procedures and the first

81

applications of ether anesthesia by Crawford Long in 1842 and William Morton in 1846 all involved *ambulatory* patients.[1] Necessarily, the emergent nature of most of the surgery and ignorance about pathophysiology and the pharmacology of anesthetics precluded consideration of selection in any aspect of the ambulatory surgical experience. With the introduction of aseptic surgical techniques in the last quarter of the 19th century, modern surgery began to develop and, simultaneously, to become an activity for which patients would be hospitalized for recuperation as well as for the surgery itself.

Twentieth-Century Pioneers

Yet even as modern surgery developed during the past hundred years, several courageous physicians laid the foundations for ambulatory surgery and, quite remarkably, offered some insight into the importance of selection of appropriate patients and facilities.

Against a tide of peer criticism, James Nicoll, a pediatric surgeon in Glasgow, noted in 1909 that the successful completion of 8988 ambulatory procedures during the preceding decade had convinced him that "the treatment of a large number of the cases at present treated indoors constitutes a waste of the resources" and "we keep similar cases in adults too long in bed." He advised that infants and young children be operated on preferentially in the ambulatory setting because, "with their wounds closed by collodion or rubber plaster, [they] are easily carried home in their mothers' arms, and rest there more quietly." Decades ahead of his time, he stressed that "sucklings and young infants should remain with their mothers after operation." As a corollary, he continued, "no children's hospital can be considered complete which has not, in the hospital itself or hard by, accommodation for a certain number of nursing mothers whose infants require operation"; he provided "a small house" nearby for postoperative nursing.[2]

Only seven years later, Ralph Waters, then an itinerant anesthesiologist, opened the Down-Town Anesthesia Clinic in Sioux City, Iowa, the prototype of the modern independent freestanding surgical facility. Following a morning of "hospital work," he provided anesthesia services and surgical facilities to suit local dentists and patients who "objected to going to the hospital because of the time and expense involved," as well as to surgeons who were "also anxious to establish extra hospital clinical facilities." He made "careful physical examination on all suspicious risks," noting that a "sphygmomanometer and stethoscope are constantly present and frequently used." In particular, he noted that "the well trained and alert assistant is useful [for he or she] often warns me that the next patient is short of breath or shows some other evidence of needing careful examination."[3]

Ambulatory Surgical Care Is Rediscovered

Despite these favorable early experiences, ambulatory surgery remained largely dormant until the mid-1960s, when specialized units were established at the University of California Medical Center in Los Angeles[4] and George Washington University Medical Center in Washington, D.C.[5] In the late 1960s, the concept of the independent freestanding surgery center was reborn with the establishment of the Dudley Street Ambulatory Surgical Center in Providence, Rhode Island, and the Surgicenter in Phoenix, Arizona. The latter facility has distinguished itself by having treated more than 120,000 patients without a death. The success of such hospital-independent, freestanding surgery centers, augmented by changes in health care reimbursement policies,[6] stimulated the establishment of 851 similar facilities by the end of 1987, where 1,476,236 procedures were completed (SMG Marketing Group, Inc., Chicago, Ill.); this volume constituted 6.3% of U.S. surgery. During this same year, about 95% of acute-care hospitals had ambulatory surgery programs, which accounted for 43.8% of U.S. surgery.[7,8] Only those hospitals with more than 500 beds reported completing less than 40% of their surgery on an ambulatory basis.[8] Although some regions currently report a 60% level of ambulatory surgery, the American Hospital Association's Division of Ambulatory Care and Health Promotion predicts that this will be the industry average by 1995. Even if recent changes in health care reimbursement policy[6,8] temper this prediction somewhat, a 50% level should be attained by the early 1990s.

Equally dramatic developments account for the recent rediscovery and growth of ambulatory surgery. These include improved anesthetic drugs, growing public interest in participating in personal health care, growing acceptance by surgeons, endorsement and encouragement by industry and health insurers, and the demonstrated safety of surgery in the ambulatory environment.[6] In turn, a most important ingredient in ensuring patient safety and overall quality of care in ambulatory surgery is careful selection of the patient and surgical procedure.

GENERAL CONSIDERATIONS
Selection Decisions as a Problem in Medical Decision Making
The often elegant basic medical sciences are frequently found wanting in the more complex, less structured clinical setting. Moreover, medical knowledge pertaining to a particular patient-management problem is usually incomplete. Yet decisions must be made. The physician necessarily makes medical decisions by blending the available information with clinical judgment and even some degree of intuition. Once decisions are made, however, the clinical outcomes of those decisions are rarely evaluated formally, and the opportunity to improve similar decision making in the future is lost. As a result, much dogma is carried along in medical practice, codified in authoritative statements that are based on clinical suspicion, anecdotes, or poorly designed studies. One need only recall some of the reversals that have occurred during the past ten years with regard to clinical practices widely accepted, in part, because they seemed obvious: chest radiogram, routine laboratory studies, and hemoglobin level of at least 10 g/dl before surgery. Clearly, decisions relating to medical care and related technology deserve the most objective decision-making process that we can muster.[9]

As in other aspects of health care, dogma exists in ambulatory anesthesia care but, through careful analysis of clinical experience, can be replaced by more rational methods of making decisions. For example, consider postoperative nausea and vomiting, certainly one of the more common minor problems associated with surgery and anesthesia, but one that can delay the patient's discharge home and sometimes prompt inpatient admission.[10-12] Dogma had suggested that even small doses of droperidol, a long-acting major tranquilizer that also happens to be an antiemetic, is contraindicated in the ambulatory setting because its long-lasting sedation would synergize with that from general anesthesia and delay the patient's return home. Yet careful clinical trials have documented that droperidol in low dosage not only treats nausea and vomiting effectively but also either does not materially delay discharge[13] or actually enables earlier discharge of the patient.[14] Similarly, ketamine, another long-acting drug that dogma suggests is contraindicated, has been shown to be satisfactory (although hardly ideal) for ambulatory anesthesia care when given by well-monitored infusion.[15] These studies suggest generally that *how* we do things, rather than *what* we do, is critically important in ambulatory anesthesia. Until more careful analysis of actual clinical practice is undertaken, most of what we do will continue to be dogma.

Selection and Cost-Effective Practice

Achieving more cost-effective practice has been one of the potent stimuli in the development of ambulatory surgery.[6,16] Apart from the obvious and considerable savings in the hotel component of hospital care, (a night or two in the hospital), little attention has been paid to the cost-effectiveness of this mode of care to society at large. Surely, on an individual case basis, it is less expensive to perform a given procedure in the ambulatory setting. However, unless the hospital bed that the given patient would have used is left empty, the health care system as a whole experiences *greater* costs because the system has effectively been enlarged. That is, in tandem with the remarkable growth in ambulatory surgery, even with a slight decrease in inpatient surgery, the per capita rate of surgery in the United States has increased, resulting in a greater overall number of surgical procedures (and medical care cost to the society). Thus true savings from ambulatory surgery can come only from a global effort to contain, if not shrink, the health care system. Some appropriate initiatives include a greater reduction in inpatient surgical caseloads through bed closures, conversion of some acute-care beds for chronic care, control of possibly excessive ambulatory surgery utilization, and a moratorium on, or at least a reduction in, future facility expansion.[17] Nonetheless, instead of waiting for what may be slow to occur, it is incumbent upon each of us to make selection decisions that put as much surgery as possible in the ambulatory setting without compromising quality of care.

Selection Decisions and Accreditation Standards

The delivery of quality care in the ambulatory surgery setting imposes the need for various selection decisions that are embodied in the unit's policies and procedures, which are discussed in this and succeeding chapters. The policies and procedures, like those relating to other institutional services, must meet the requirements of external agencies that accredit the institution. Standards of the accreditation program for hospital-sponsored ambulatory care services set forth by the Joint Commission on Accreditation of Healthcare Organizations (JCAHO) specifically address selection decisions relating to surgical procedures, anesthesia care, and postoperative recovery care, as follows[18]:

Surgical procedures:
    Types that may be performed
    Locations where they may be performed
Anesthesia care:
    Types of anesthesia services provided
    Locations where they may be provided
Transportation:
    Preoperative and postoperative transportation
Preoperative patient evaluation and preparation:
    Definition of appropriate history, physical examination, and laboratory and x-ray evaluation
    Method of intervention when designated evaluation and preparation are incomplete
Postoperative care:
    Guidelines for postanesthesia recovery care
    Role of family members in care
    Discharge criteria
    Responsible person to accompany patient home
    Written instructions for follow-up care and emergency physician contact

Similar JCAHO accreditation requirements have been promulgated for independent freestanding ambulatory surgery centers.[19] Voluntary accreditation standards for both freestanding and hospital-affiliated ambulatory surgery programs also have been prepared by the Accreditation Association for Ambulatory Health Care (AAAHC).

Equivalence of Ambulatory and Inpatient Policies
The JCAHO leaves to the discretion of the institution's medical staff and administration how each requirement will be met. However, the policies and procedures set forth for a hospital-affiliated ambulatory surgery program must be consistent with those applicable to inpatients undergoing the same procedures in the given facility.

Local Definition of Appropriateness
Regardless of the type of ambulatory unit and accreditation sought, the underlying goal of the policies and procedures is the maintenance of patient safety and quality of care. Apart from the general principle that ambulatory surgical care be equivalent to its inpatient counterpart (if any exists), the accreditation process generally leaves the explicit requirements to the facility's professional staff. Thus each facility is given the freedom to define the laboratory evaluation, among other aspects of the ambulatory surgical care, that is "appropriate" to the planned surgical procedure and anesthetic for a patient in a given state of health.

Other, more specific aspects of accreditation standards are discussed in this chapter (e.g., evaluating medical staff credentials, utilization review, quality assurance) and in subsequent chapters that discuss anesthesia care of adults and children and postanesthesia care unit management (e.g., postoperative care, role of the family, discharge criteria).

SURGICAL PROCEDURES

Lists of surgical procedures appropriate to the ambulatory unit abound. Typically, each year the lists grow as we continue to discover that we have not yet reached the boundaries of acceptability. Thus, as noted earlier, as we begin the 1990s, half of U.S. surgery is now performed in the ambulatory setting, that fraction having tripled since 1981. However, for specified procedures and groups of procedures (e.g., dilatation and curettage, breast biopsy), a far greater fraction is undertaken without the traditional overnight hospital stay.

General Characteristics of Acceptable Procedures

Given the rapid evolution of ambulatory surgical care, setting forth even the characteristics of acceptable procedures is hazardous. Any set of specific characteristics is likely to seem as "conservative" in a few years as those established by the then-pioneers only 15 to 20 years ago. Nonetheless, recognizing that today's characterization of acceptability is likely to be short-lived, we may note that the most appropriate procedures are *generally* those which are accompanied by minimal blood loss and physiologic derangements and are associated with minimal, or at least readily controlled, postoperative pain, nausea and vomiting, and other postoperative complications. Prohibitions relating to durations of surgery (e.g., performing only procedures lasting less than 60 to 90 minutes) no longer appear warranted, particularly because the relationship between anesthesia time and recovery time is weak.[20] Yet recent case-control studies indicate that longer procedures[21] and procedures ending late in the work day[22] are associated with an increased risk of unplanned hospital admission, an important end point in evaluating decision-making criteria. Thus, although the ambulatory setting is an increasingly important site for medical education, great care must be exercised so that procedures do not become unduly prolonged.

It must be recognized, however, that the actual list of "acceptable" procedures in a given ambulatory unit is established in an evolutionary process, with accretion of procedures often in a "trial and error" fashion. On a periodic basis, the medical director of the unit must decide which procedures (and which patients) are "appropriate" for the unit, given its equipment, staff and their capabilities, ability and reliability of the given surgeon, and medical condition of the particular patient. Over the long term, the medical director, in consultation with the administrative body to which he or she reports (e.g., ambulatory unit advisory committee, operating room committee), can modify the spectrum of permissible surgery on the basis of periodic quality assurance studies and other mechanisms (see the section at the end of this chapter).

Classification of Surgical Procedures

In the past, surgical procedures have been categorized simply as major or minor. Although subjective, this classification is no longer useful in classifying the diversity of surgery that is currently undertaken in a variety of settings. A *functional* classification and terminology of ambulatory surgery settings is presented in Chapters 1 and 10. A similar functional classification of surgical procedures is needed. At the outset, procedures should not be categorized according to the anesthetic technique used or whether the patient is ambulatory or an inpatient, because such categorizations are not useful inasmuch as they overlook critically important factors such as patient condition and other highly individual factors.

Recognizing these classification inadequacies, Davis and Detmer suggested in 1972 that *ambulatory surgery* be defined as "surgery of an uncomplicated nature that traditionally has been done on an inpatient basis but which can be done with equal efficiency and safety without hospital admission."[23] Their intention was to describe an intermediate level of surgical care that would fit between the more demanding surgery undertaken on inpatients and the less demanding, often "minor" procedures performed in a surgeon's private office or perhaps in an emergency room. Unfortunately, ambulatory surgery has been used synonymously with outpatient surgery (and similar terms) to describe procedures often of different complexities and requirements.

More recently, they have further defined the topology of surgical care[24–27] (Figure 3-1). Note that, in accordance with their earlier definition, ambulatory surgery ("intermediate surgery" in Figure 3-1) lies between minor surgery that is properly performed in the surgeon's office and major surgery that truly requires hospital supportive services and postoperative hospital care. The overlapping regions emphasize the need for judgment and flexibility; that is, depending on the patient and other factors, a given procedure may be appropriate for either of two settings. As an example, consider a dental extraction. If the patient is a healthy adult, this procedure is appropriately performed in the oral surgeon's or dentist's office; however, if the patient is moderately mentally retarded, the same procedure is more appropriately undertaken in the ambulatory surgery unit where more comprehensive anesthesia care is available. A diagnostic laparoscopy that might reasonably lead to immediate laparotomy (*e.g.,* ectopic pregnancy) is more appro-

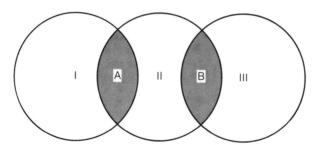

FIGURE 3-1. A proposed classification of levels of surgical care. Class I comprises *minor surgery,* or procedures appropriate for the surgeon's office, Class II is *intermediate surgery* that is appropriate for an ambulatory surgery unit, and Class III consists of *major surgery* that is undertaken on an inpatient basis. Subclasses A and B include procedures appropriate for either of their immediately adjacent classes, depending on the circumstances of the particular case. (SOURCE: Detmer DE, Buchanan-Davidson DJ: Ambulatory surgery. Surg Clin North Am 62: 685, 1982.)

priately performed in an inpatient environment than an ambulatory unit, regardless of the patient's general state of health. Similarly, another patient having an inguinal herniorrhaphy but whose social situation does not permit ambulatory care would have his or her surgery as an inpatient. Alternatively, given the incentives to decrease hospital stay, the patient might arrive at the hospital on the morning of the procedure ("A.M. admission"), have the procedure possibly in the hospital's ambulatory unit, and then be admitted to a hospital room. Finally, ambulatory units within the hospital can err on the liberal side in their selection decisions when uncertain whether a given procedure (or patient) is appropriate for the ambulatory setting, because of the ease with which they can admit the patient to a hospital room if it becomes advisable.

Current Spectrum of Ambulatory Surgery
The Procedure
Below is a list of procedures currently undertaken on an ambulatory basis. The list was generated from primary and secondary literature, as well as from anecdotal reports, and it captures the diversity of ambulatory procedures. A multitude of procedure lists have been promulgated by individual health care insurance entities, both private (e.g., Blue Cross/Blue Shield plans) and public (e.g., Medicare[28] and Medicaid programs), whose continual expansion has been an important stimulus to the recent growth of ambulatory surgery.[6]

The list is organized by medical subspecialties but in no way delineates what may be performed by a given discipline, for there are many procedures that overlap specialties. Moreover, the presence of a given procedure on this (or another) list does *not* indicate that it is appropriate for a given ambulatory surgery facility; such a judgment depends on characteristics of the given facility, as noted earlier in the discussion of general characteristics of acceptable procedures. For example, some very progressive facilities are performing cholecystectomy or vaginal hysterectomy in highly selected patients whose home situations afford the required nursing support. Finally, surgical complications may require additional, unlisted procedures (e.g., exploratory laparotomy to suture uterine perforation incurred during therapeutic abortion).

Oral and maxillofacial surgery:
  Closed reduction of jaw fracture (arch bar application)
  Dental restorations
  Intraoral biopsy
  Multiple dental extractions
  Odontectomy
  Open and closed reduction of zygomatic fracture
  TMJ arthroscopy
General surgery:
  Anal fissurectomy
  Anal fistulectomy

A-V fistula creation
Breast biopsy
Cholecystectomy
Debridement
Femoral herniorrhaphy
Ganglionectomy
Hemorrhoidectomy
Hydrocelectomy
Hypoglossal duct cystectomy
Incision and drainage, superficial abscess
Ingrown toenail excision
Inguinal herniorrhaphy

Lymph node biopsy
Partial mastectomy
Pilonidal cystectomy
Rectal biopsy
Small skin lesion excision
Thyroidectomy
Umbilical herniorrhaphy
Umbilical sinus excision
Varicose vein ligation/stripping
Varicocelectomy
Ventral herniorrhaphy
Gynecology:
Bartholin cystectomy
Breast biopsy
Cervical cone biopsy
Cervical polypectomy
Culdoscopy
Dilatation and curettage (D&C)
Dilatation and evacuation (therapeutic abortion)
Examination under anesthesia
Hymenotomy
Hysteroscopy
Pelvic laparoscopy (including lysis of adhesions, laser fulguration)
Tubal ligation (by laparoscopy, minilaparotomy, or transvaginally)
Vaginal hysterectomy
Vaginoplasty
Hematology-oncology:
Bone marrow aspiration (*e.g.,* iliac crest)
Bone marrow harvest
Lumbar puncture
Internal medicine/cardiology:
Angioplasty
Neurosurgery:
Intercostal neurectomy
Muscle biopsy (*e.g.,* biceps, quadriceps)
Nerve biopsy (*e.g.,* sural)
Nerve decompression (*e.g.,* median, ulnar)
Ulnar nerve transfer

Ophthalmology:
Cataract extraction, with or without lens implant
Conjunctival or corneal biopsy
Corneal transplant
Cryotherapy
Enucleation
Examination under anesthesia
Eyelid lesion excision (entropion, ectropion)
Fasanella procedure of lid
Incision and biopsy of chalazion
Keratotomy
Lacrimal duct probing
Mebelene sling to frontalis muscle
Peripheral iridectomy
Strabismus repair
Trabeculectomy
Orthopedics:
Arthroscopic debridement
Arthroscopic lateral release
Arthroscopic menisectomy
Arthroscopic shelf release
Bone biopsy
Bone-spur excision
Bunionectomy
Carpal tunnel release
Cast change, with or without manipulation
Closed reduction
Cyst removal (*e.g.,* Baker's cyst)
Debridement
Diagnostic arthroscopy
Epidural steroid injection
Excision and removal of foreign body
Excision of exostosis
Excision of ganglion
Excision of lesion
Fasciectomy (finger, palm)
Finger-joint replacement
Finger amputation and revision
Flexor tendon sheath release
Hammer-toe correction

Hardware removal
Joint manipulation
Median nerve decompression
Muscle biopsy
Olecranon bursectomy
Olecranon-spur excision
Open reduction/internal fixa-
    tion of fingers
Prepatellar bursectomy
Release of Dequervain's hand
Release of Dupuytren's con-
    tracture
Release of trigger thumb
Removal of foreign body
Removal of nails, pins, plates,
    screws, wires
Simple tendon repair
Syndactylization of toes
Synovectomy
Tendon exploration
Ulnar nerve transfer
Z-plasty
Otolaryngology:
    Adenoidectomy, with or with-
        out myringotomy
    Closed reduction of nasal frac-
        ture
    Ethmoidectomy
    Foreign-body removal (ear)
    Laryngoscopy, with or without
        polypectomy
    Mastoidectomy
    Myringotomy, with or without
        tubes
    Nasal polypectomy
    Pharyngoscopy
    Rhinoplasty
    Rhytidoplasty
    Rhytidectomy with blepharo-
        plasty
    Septorhinoplasty
    Stapedectomy
    Submucous resection
    Tonsillectomy, with or without
        adenoidectomy or myringot-
        omy
    Tympanoplasty

Pediatric surgery:
    Circumcision
    Excision of lesions
    Frenulectomy
    Inguinal herniorrhaphy
    Meatotomy
    Orchiopexy
    Suture of laceration
    Umbilical herniorrhaphy
    Urethral dilatation
Plastic surgery:
    Augmentation mammaplasty
    Basal cell carcinoma excision
    Blepharoplasty
    Cleft lip repair
    Contracture release
    Correction of prominent ears
    Fasciectomy
    Ganglionectomy
    Gynecomastia excision
    Laceration repair
    Otoplasty
    Pedicle-flap transfer
    Preauricular cyst excision
    Rhytidectomy
    Scar revision
    Skin-flap revision
    Skin graft
    Suction-assisted lipectomy
    Tendon repair
    Trigger-finger release
    Vermillionectomy
Thoracic surgery:
    Esophageal dilatation
    Pacemaker battery replacement
    Pacemaker insertion
Urology:
    Biopsy and/or fulguration of
        bladder tumor
    Circumcision
    Epididymovasostomy
    Fulguration of bladder neck
    Hypospadias repair
    Lithopexy
    Lithotripsy (renal)
    Orchiectomy
    Prostate biopsy

Meatotomy	Varicocelectomy
Testicular biopsy	Vasectomy
Testicular prosthesis insertion	Vasovasostomy

Surveying all U.S. hospitals, nine procedures appropriate to the ambulatory setting (in boldface) were among the 20 most commonly performed specific surgical procedures in 1986[29]:

Breast biopsy
Dilatation and curettage
Knee arthroscopy
Cystoscopy
Vaginal delivery
Myringotomy
Inguinal hernia repair
Tonsillectomy
Cataract procedures
**Fallopian tube ligation/
  destruction**
Appendectomy
Cesarean section
Hysterectomy
Transurethral resection of pros-
  tate
Bronchoscopy
Cholecystectomy
Laminectomy
Major joint procedures
Major artery/vein procedures
Coronary artery revascularization

The nine procedures listed in boldface comprised about 30% of total U.S. surgery. Among hospital-independent, freestanding ambulatory surgery centers, the mix of cases, by surgical subspecialty was already addressed in Chapter 1 (Table 1–6; SMG Marketing Group, Inc., Chicago, Ill., June 1989). Ambulatory surgery statistics have been similar in Canada.[30]

The More Common Procedures
Among the many procedures that are commonly undertaken in the ambulatory setting, a handful are mentioned here to highlight some of the underlying clinical considerations and possible problems. Some comments on anesthetic administration are unavoidable; more detailed coverage of anesthesia care is found throughout the rest of this text.

ORAL SURGERY. Historically, ambulatory anesthesia has been closely linked to oral surgery, and the association continues, the majority of procedures being performed in dental operatory units rather than ambulatory surgery units. The largest group of patients who require general anesthesia are those who have great fear of dental procedures; another group includes those requiring extensive or lengthy procedures that can be accomplished during one general anesthetic rather than several procedures under local anesthesia (children[31]); and the remaining patients include those who have allergies to local anesthetics, hyperactive gag reflexes, mental retardation precluding reasonable patient cooperation,[31,32] or spastic neuromuscular disorders. Although the patients may be reasonably healthy, the full spectrum of anesthetic-related morbidity and mortality occurs in ambulatory oral surgery, including malignant hyperthermia, muscle pains and prolonged apnea following succinylcholine, protracted nausea and vomiting, and sore throat.[33] Among the particularly common intraoperative problems are cardiac dysrhythmias, even in the young and healthy patient, regardless of whether a halogenated agent or narcotic technique is used.[34,35]

TONSILLECTOMY AND ADENOIDECTOMY. Tonsillectomy and adenoidectomy (T&A), with and without myringotomy, constitutes the majority of cases that an otolaryngologist might undertake in the ambulatory setting[36]; tonsillectomy, with or without other procedures, is the most common otolaryngologic operation. Yet T&As in the ambulatory surgery unit remain highly controversial, because of the potential for large, often unrecognized blood loss, which often occurs soon after surgery but may be delayed 12 to 24 hours, when the ambulatory patient is no longer closely observed in a health care setting. A national survey reviewing more than 1.3 million tonsillectomies found that 1.2% of patients experienced sufficient postoperative bleeding to warrant notation in the medical record, with 27 (0.002%) deaths.[37] Nonetheless, series of more than 40,000 T&As have been completed without mortality.[38] A recent review of 1,428 outpatient adenotonsillectomies documented a postoperative hemorrhage rate of 0.28% (and no deaths), which the investigators attributed to the use of bismuth subgallate for enhanced hemostasis; they concluded that the procedure is safe in the ambulatory setting.[39] Advocates of ambulatory surgery T&As place great emphasis on careful selection and, in particular, preoperative medical evlauation. Inappropriate patients for an ambulatory surgery T&A include those with a history of hemophilia, leukemia, other blood dyscrasias, and sickle-cell anemia, as well as those who take aspirin chronically. Since clinical experience indicates that inflamed tissue is associated with increased bleeding, patients acutely suffering from allergic disorders or those who have had an acute attack of tonsillitis within the past month or a "cold" within a week are also not candidates for the procedure on an ambulatory basis. Although coagulation studies (e.g., bleeding, clotting, prothrombin, and thrombin times and platelet count) have been recommended to screen for those likely to experience postoperative bleeding, careful analysis of clinical experience indicates that such testing is warranted only to *confirm* a suspected bleeding tendency that is identified when taking the history (e.g., "Do you bruise or bleed easily?") and performing the brief physical examination (e.g., ecchymoses). The clinical value of laboratory testing is discussed later in this chapter.

THERAPEUTIC ABORTION. Although the majority of voluntary interruptions of pregnancy in the first trimester are undertaken with sedation and local anesthesia, some of these therapeutic abortions are performed with general anesthesia, particularly when the uterus is larger and the risk of perforation is thereby greater. The common halogenated anesthetics (*i.e.,* halothane, enflurane, isoflurane) offer a more stable depth of anesthesia and a lower incidence of nausea and vomiting than fentanyl supplementation of nitrous oxide, but they risk a greater blood loss consequent to their dose-related uterine relaxation unless low inspired concentrations (less than 0.6 MAC value) are used.[40–42] The use of oxytocic agents is associated with diminished bleeding as well as with a higher incidence of nausea and vomiting. This is more true of ergonovine than of oxytocin.[43] Women undergoing a late midtrimester abortion, especially involving a technically difficult extraction, appear to be at increased risk for the development of disseminated intravascular coagulation and thus should be observed postoperatively for a minimum of two hours, with prompt evaluation of coagulation factors should increased bleeding occur.[44] Compared to a general anesthesia with a halogenated agent and nitrous oxide, following fentanyl and methohexital, a totally intravenous technique consisting of fentanyl (1.5 µg/kg) and methohexital (1.5 mg/kg) during oxygen supplementation seems to offer a prompter awakening, with fewer minor side effects, although acute memory for new facts is equally impaired transiently.[45] The new induction agent diisopropylphenol (propofol) promises an even shorter recovery time than methohexital.[46]

PELVIC LAPAROSCOPY. Laparoscopy is an increasingly common procedure that is performed principally to facilitate tubal sterilization but also to assist in the diagnosis and treatment of pelvic pain and infertility. Tubal ligation is now the most frequently performed procedure in women of reproductive age, and approximately 30% of these procedures are performed by means of laparoscopy.[47] The popularity and apparent simplicity of the procedure belie the numerous and diverse, potentially serious problems that may accompany it: pneumothorax,[48] bowel burns with electrocauterization (especially if nitrous oxide is the insufflating gas),[49] hypercarbia (especially during inadequate pulmonary ventilation), hypoxemia (especially in the obese and with an inadequately oxygen-enriched inspiratory mixture),[50] air embolism,[51] and gastric,[52] intestinal, and vascular perforation.[53] Controversy exists as to whether to undertake tracheal intubation in the majority of cases in which general anesthesia is used. Anesthesiologists in freestanding settings, where the procedure is often brief, have argued that patient comfort dictates that intubation be undertaken only when airway management is difficult, whereas representatives from hospital-affiliated units, where procedures tend to be longer, respond that a mild sore throat is a small price for an adequate airway, particularly in view of the impaired oxygenation associated with a steep Trendelenburg position, elevated diaphragms, and collapsed lower lobes. Undoubtedly, lean patients *may* be safely anesthetized without a tracheal tube during brief procedures; however, considerable expertise in airway management is required with the majority of patients. It is sobering to recognize that during the period 1977 through 1981, 29 deaths occurring during laparoscopic tubal ligations were reported to the Centers for Disease Control; 11 of these deaths were related to complications of general anesthesia, with 6 attributable to hypoventilation, which is generally preventable with tracheal intubation.[54]

BREAST BIOPSY. Breast biopsy under local anesthesia in the ambulatory setting has been advocated for almost 20 years.[55-57] Apart from the general benefits of ambulatory surgical care, its many advantages include a reduced need to confront the majority of patients (who have benign disease) with possible mastectomy and time for additional evaluation and planning should further surgery be necessary. There has never been documentation supporting a detrimental effect of several days' delay of definitive therapy.[58,59]

ARTHROSCOPY. Among the more recent, and now increasingly popular, additions to the ambulatory surgery caseload are arthroscopic procedures of the knee, as well as occasionally the wrist, temporomandibular, and shoulder joints. The majority of patients who undergo these procedures are young and healthy, if not athletic, with a localized problem, who are highly motivated to recover rapidly to normal functioning; in short, the ambulatory setting is ideal for these patients.[60] But the advantages of ambulatory care are also well suited to the carefully selected patient with rheumatoid arthritis who is having arthroscopy or finger-joint replacement (or a nonorthopedic procedure) and wishes to cope with his or her deformities in the privacy of his or her own home and family. Although local anesthesia has been used preferentially,[61] especially with a small needle-scope, general anesthesia and even regional anesthesia are now increasingly used.[60,62,63] A particular concern with regional anesthesia for knee arthroscopy is that with the use of the tourniquet, the block must be fairly high (at least at midthoracic level) to reasonably avoid tourniquet pain. The resulting extensive sympathetic block may delay the patient in tolerating ambulation, particularly with spinal anesthesia, in which the level of the sympathetic block is always several dermatomes higher than the sensory level,[64] as opposed to epidural anesthesia, which also offers greater flexibility in the duration of the anesthetic through the continuous (catheter) technique, but which requires more time before the patient is ready for the incision. Undergoing evaluation is continuous spinal anesthesia, which offers the reliability and shorter latency of spinal anesthesia, as well as the flexibility of the epidural technique.[65] Previously restricted to elderly patients, because the high incidence of postdural puncture headache is inversely related to patient age, this technique is likely to find wider acceptance because of the recent availability of catheters small enough to pass through 22-gauge (or smaller) needles, which are associated with a lower incidence of headache.

INGUINAL HERNIORRHAPHY. An accepted procedure in infants and small children for decades,[66,67] inguinal herniorrhaphy in ambulatory adults has achieved acceptance recently. Ambulatory herniorrhaphy in adults is not new, however, for Harvey Cushing described hernia repairs under cocaine infiltration half a century ago, and the Shouldice Clinic has performed more than 100,000 repairs under local anesthesia during the past 45 years. Rather, ambulatory herniorrhaphy in adults is receiving renewed interest as a result of its inherent potential for particularly large cost savings (several hospital days), the availability of a superior anesthetic technique, professional encouragement, and improved acceptance by both patient and surgeon.[68-73] In the current version of the Shouldice technique, the unmedicated patient walks to the operating room and has his or her hernia repair under a field block anesthetic with a large volume of bupivacaine, 0.25%, ensuring many hours' postoperative comfort, which, in turn, permits relatively pain-free immediate ambulation.[68–74] Depending on social supports, the patient departs for home or a convalescence unit near the hospital. Hernia recurrence rates are comparable to or better than those of inpatient procedures, although surgical experience is an important determinant of the actual rate.[70,75] The favorable experience with long-acting local anesthetics has prompted others to infiltrate wound margins in other surgical procedures and, where appropriate, subcostal nerves, with bupivacaine.[76] Still others have documented several days' analgesia from freezing the ilioinguinal nerve (cryoanalgesia) during inguinal herniorrhaphy, with improved appetite and mobility during recovery.[77] Alternatively, alone or as part of a field-block technique, one can administer iliohypogastric and ilioinguinal nerve blocks with bupivacaine.[78] However, bupivacaine should not be used for spinal and epidural anesthesia in the ambulatory setting because of the increased incidence of urinary retention.[79]

CATARACT EXTRACTION. Among the procedures particularly well suited to the ambulatory surgery setting and one of the most common performed in the elderly population, cataract extraction offers its own peculiar clinical challenges. Since the patients are generally elderly, one encounters a variety of important coexisting diseases, especially those affecting the cardiovascular and respiratory systems. Hence, regardless of the anesthetic technique chosen, one must be prepared to deal with acute episodes related to coronary artery disease, hypertension, and chronic obstructive lung disease, among other disorders. Of particular significance is that when matched according to age and gender with patients undergoing other procedures, cataract patients are found to experience a mortality rate (within 90 days of the procedure) that is about twice that of the reference patients; this suggests that the senile cataract represents a systemic phenomenon rather than merely a local disease.[80] Moreover, in addition to the various cardiovascular and other drugs these patients are taking, with which the anesthesiologist is often very familiar, these patients usually also take "eye drops." This seemingly localized therapy poses *systemic* problems as a result of interactions with drugs, particularly anesthetic drugs and adjuvants, patients may receive in association with their ambulatory surgery.[81] These ophthalmic drugs include timolol, a nonspecific β-adrenergic blocking agent that aggravates bronchospasm in susceptible patients, echothiophate, a long-acting anticholinesterase drug that has been associated with prolonged apnea following the use of succinylcholine, and atropine and scopolamine drops, which have been implicated in episodes of confusion, hallucination, restlessness, dysarthria, and, particularly in children, hyperthermia and coma. In addition, eye drops containing epinephrine and phenylephrine administered immediately before or during the procedure can enter the systemic circulation (by way of the conjunctival capillaries) and cause hypertension and coronary artery spasm.[81–83] Similarly, intraocular injection of acetylcholine in a patient receiving antihypertensive therapy that includes β-adrenergic blockade can precipitate bronchospasm.[84]

EXTRACORPOREAL SHOCK-WAVE LITHOTRIPSY (ESWL). Within a few years of the introduction of this remarkable technology for the noninvasive treatment of renal stones, ESWL not only has become the standard therapy, but also has moved largely out of the hospital into the ambulatory setting.[85-87] Despite the absence of a surgical incision, the procedure poses a variety of anesthetic concerns, including remote location from the anesthesiologist, and hemodynamic changes related to water immersion. There are two potential problems relating specifically to epidural anesthesia, a common technique: Contaminated lithotripter bath water can gain access to the epidural space by tracking along the indwelling epidural catheter; although the catheter can become colonized with flavobacteria or coagulase-negative staphylococci (16% in one small study[88]), there have been no apparent cases of epidural infection. The other potential problem is that air, injected when identifying the epidural space, can create an additional interface at which shock-wave energy is dissipated, causing damage to neural tissue; it is recommended that saline be used instead of air. Although a variety of general and regional anesthetic techniques can be used, they are equally satisfactory. Because perirenal hematoma, renal bleeding, ureteral and urinary obstruction, sepsis, and/or severe pain can occur postoperatively, the ambulatory patient must be reasonably close to medical care for 24 hours following discharge. Second-generation lithotripters, having no need for water immersion, are now available.

SUCTION-ASSISTED LIPECTOMY (SAL). An increasingly popular plastic surgical procedure for the removal of subcutaneous adipose tissue, SAL also may be undertaken with a variety of anesthetic techniques, depending on the site and area of the body.[90] Among the anesthetic concerns are the possible aggravation of preexisting hypertension and coronary artery disease by the epinephrine-containing hemostatic solution and the potentially large, largely unquantifiable blood loss during the procedure. The extent of blood loss is problematic because, with more extensive procedures and greater fluid loss, the hematocrit of the fluid removed is highly variable and, owing to the presence of fat globules, cannot be determined by routine clinical methods.[91] Postoperatively, there can be further bleeding and infection. Autologous blood transfusion ought to be considered when the proposed procedure is extensive.[92]

INVASIVE CARDIOLOGY PROCEDURES. Perhaps not unexpectedly, the ambulatory care movement is also having a great impact on invasive cardiology. Recently, there have been demonstrations of the safety of performing pacemaker[93,94] and peripheral angioplasty[95] procedures in selected ambulatory patients.

MAJOR SURGICAL PROCEDURES. As noted at the beginning of this section, when ambulatory surgery underwent its rebirth, the surgical procedures chosen included only the simpler ones, which had little impact on physiologic homeostasis. With the maturation of the field, physicians are attempting procedures in the ambulatory setting that only a few years ago seemed impossible. Examples include vitrectomy and retinal detachment repair, thyroidectomy,[96] and, with up to 24 hours' postoperative observation, cholecystectomy.[97] In each case, the patients are especially carefully chosen with regard to preexisting medical illnesses, anticipated difficulty of the surgery, and adequacy of social and nursing supports at home, among other considerations (see later sections of this chapter on patient selection and preparation; innovative postoperative care was discussed in Chapter 1). The surgical care also may be modified; for example, in the case of cholecystectomy, the surgeon may utilize a laparoscopic technique, or choose a less painful vertical incision, infiltrate the wound margins with bupivacaine, remove subcutaneous sutures and skin clips within 24 hours, eliminate drains when possible, use lower narcotic dosage, and arrange for visiting nurse care.

Nonsurgical Procedures

There are growing pressures to perform a variety of nonsurgical procedures, usually on an ambulatory basis, in ambulatory surgery units, solely because there is no other option in most hospitals. In addition, many of these "ancillary procedures" are viewed as important sources of additional revenue in all types of units. These diverse procedures include

Aspiration of breast mass
Bladder irrigation
Blood transfusion
Bone marrow aspiration[98,99] and harvesting[100]
Bronchoscopy (fiberoptic)[101]
Cardiac arteriography and catheterization[102,103]
Cardioversion
Chemotherapy, antineoplastic and antibacterial[104]
Colonoscopy
Cystoscopy
Dressing change
Electroconvulsive therapy[105]
Epidural blood patch
Esophageal variceal sclerotherapy
Esophagoscopy
Examination under anesthesia (gynecologic, ophthalmic, orthopedic)
Gastroscopy
Intercostal tube drainage for spontaneous pneumothorax[106]
Liver biopsy, percutaneous
Lumbar puncture, diagnostic
Nerve block, diagnostic or therapeutic
Ophthalmic examination
Paracentesis
Psychotherapy
Renal biopsy
Sigmoidoscopy
Thoracentesis

In general, the limiting factor in meeting this demand is the availability of appropriate staffing and equipment, as well as a clean, but not necessarily sterile, minor procedure room. However, vigilance must not be suspended, for many of these "minor" procedures entail substantial risk to the patient, either during surgery or for several hours afterward.

Nonsurgical Procedures That Involve Anesthesia Personnel

Anesthesia personnel may be requested to monitor and possibly administer sedation during many of these nonsurgical procedures and to be available for resuscitation. One example involving anesthesia personnel is presented here to highlight the clinical challenges posed by these seemingly minor cases.

ELECTROCONVULSIVE THERAPY. Increasingly used in the therapy of affective disorders and schizophrenia, electroconvulsive therapy (ECT) is accompanied by major disturbance in autonomic, cardiovascular, pulmonary, and neuromuscular function. Brief sinus bradycardia and hypotension are followed in succession by rapid sinus tachycardia and hypertension, apnea, hypoventilation, the desired cerebral stimulation with major motor seizure, and brief postictal coma. These disturbances are superimposed on what is necessarily a light general anesthetic—methohexital with succinylcholine—that is given principally to prevent dental injuries and compression fractures of the spine, as well as diminish the cardiovascular stress. In addition, since depression is more prevalent at advanced age, ECT is particularly likely to be performed in patients with clinically significant hypertension and cardiovascular disease. Thus this short and seemingly minor procedure poses a disproportionately great risk for a variety of acute medical problems, such as arrhythmias, severe hypertension, and myocardial ischemia and failure.[105] These patients require thorough medical evaluation before the procedure to ensure that they are in optimal condition.[108]

THE PATIENT

As was the case with acceptable surgical procedures, there have been numerous lists of essential characteristics of patients who are appropriate candidates for ambulatory surgery. When ambulatory surgery was reborn 25 years ago, when there was a need to gain credibility with both the medical community and the insurance industry, only the healthiest patients were deemed appropriate candidates. With the passage of time and the accrual of experience, however, the selection criteria have become increasingly liberal, so that we are no longer restricting this mode of care to only physical status 1 and 2 patients (Table 3-1). In fact, many patients in physical status 3—with insulin-dependent diabetes, coronary artery disease, asthma, moderate hypertension—are referred for ambulatory surgery because of the nature of their procedure (e.g., cataract extraction). Yet the price paid for relaxing selection criteria is an increased rate of unplanned hospital admissions (or transfers, in the case of the freestanding units), from 0.02% to 0.6%[108-110] for physical status 1 and 2 patients to 0.5% to 1.5%[21,22,104,110]

TABLE 3-1. The American Society of Anesthesiologists' Physical Status Classification

Classification	Description
Class 1	A healthy patient *Example:* Inguinal hernia in an otherwise healthy patient
Class 2	A patient with mild systemic disease *Examples:* Chronic bronchitis; moderate obesity; diet-controlled diabetes mellitus; old myocardial infarction; mild hypertension
Class 3	A patient with severe systemic disease that is not incapacitating *Examples:* Coronary artery disease with angina; insulin-dependent diabetes mellitus; morbid obesity; moderate to severe pulmonary insufficiency
Class 4	A patient with incapacitating systemic disease that is a constant threat to life *Examples:* Organic heart disease with marked cardiac insufficiency, unstable angina, intractable arrhythmia; advanced pulmonary, renal, hepatic, or endocrine insufficiency
Class 5	A moribund patient not expected to survive for 24 hours with or without operation *Example:* Ruptured abdominal aneurysm with profound shock
Emergency (E)	The suffix E is used to denote the presumed poorer physical status of any patient in one of these categories who is operated on as an emergency (*e.g.*, 2E).

when some of the physical status 3 patients are selected. Even with the inclusion of sicker patients, however, the hospital admission rate should be below 2%.[110]

General Characteristics of Acceptable Patients

Above all, the patient should be in reasonably good health. If the patient has systemic disease that places him or her in physical status 3 (see Table 3-1), the essential consideration is how stable his or her condition is. Would preoperative and/or postoperative hospitalization provide any benefit? Hospital units (integrated, separated) can often afford to accept a somewhat sicker patient than the freestanding facility because of the relative ease with which hospital admission can be arranged.

In addition to being in reasonably good health, the patient must truly accept, if not want, to have the procedure performed on an ambulatory basis; necessarily, the patient must understand the process fully. Since postoperative care will not be supervised and provided as it would be to an inpatient, the patient also must be able to understand and follow the instructions that are provided for postoperative care (see Chapter 7). Similarly, because even expertly administered sedation and general anesthesia impair mental acuity for much of the rest of the day, the patient must be accompanied by a responsible person who will transport the patient home and supervise his or her first day and night of home care. This person must be truly responsible enough to know when, how, and where to seek emergency postoperative treatment, if necessary, in accordance with the postoperative instructions. Thus it is essential that this person be intellectually as well as physically capable. Until very recently, the term *responsible person* was synonymous with *adult*; however, with emancipated minors and 16-year-old licensed drivers, one must take a broader, more functional perspective. Under no circumstances should a patient who has received sedation or general anesthesia be permitted to leave the ambulatory unit unaccompanied (see Chapter 2). Finally, the patient must live reasonably close to the ambulatory unit so that the trip home is not unduly long (individual facilities may wish to establish distance criteria based on local circumstances); traveling time to another medical facility for emergency care after hours should also be reasonably short.

The More Common "Problem" Patients

Only some of the more common patient-selection problems in the ambulatory setting are considered here. The specific issues posed in each situation are different, each within a given type of problem, and often must be evaluated on an individual basis. Nonetheless, with most of these problems, one should ask whether the patient's problem is in optimal control. If not, what can be reasonably done to improve his or her health status and thereby decrease the patient's risk of suffering a complication or decompensation?

THE PHYSICAL STATUS 3 PATIENT. Operative mortality increases geometrically with advanced physical status; not unexpectedly, although less studied, morbidity also increases dramatically with deterioration of health status.[111–116] A spate of recent books in the "medical care for the surgical patient" genre is testimony to the growing appreciation of the importance in identifying, monitoring, and improving the patient's other health problems perioperatively.[117–123] Generally, physical status 3 patients are appropriate candidates for ambulatory surgery only when their health problems are well controlled, plans have been made for the postoperative monitoring and treatment of those problems, and, of course, their home situation can accommodate their postoperative needs.

THE EMERGENCY PATIENT. Although almost all the procedures undertaken in the ambulatory surgery unit are both scheduled and elective, there are circumstances in which emergency procedures are entirely appropriate. These include dilatation and evacuation of the uterus following incomplete abortion, debridement and suturing of a hand laceration, and incision and drainage of a superficial abscess. Necessarily, the patient appears with little advance notice and must be evaluated without delay. Yet, unless the problem is truly urgent (*e.g.,* moderate ongoing blood loss with the incomplete abortion) and the planned schedule must be interrupted for the patient, there is sufficient time for the anesthesiologist to perform an adequate evaluation while waiting for a space in the schedule.

THE ELDERLY. As more procedures are mandated by third-party payors as outpatient procedures (*e.g.,* cataract extraction, D&C, hernia repair), a substantial number of geriatric patients are expected to undergo ambulatory surgery. The advantages the ambulatory surgery unit offers the elderly include a lower anxiety level, maintenance of their familiar family unit, and less disruption in their routines such as diet, medication, and sleep. Chronologic age should not be part of the selection criteria, for there are healthy old people and sick young people. Indeed, in studies that have evaluated the relationship between age and the rate of complications, the relationship was weak.[20-22] Instead, the emphasis must be placed on *physiologic* age, including *functional* state. That is, can the patient undertake all the activities appropriate to his or her age? If not, what is the nature of the limitation? Is there anything that can reasonably be done to improve the patient's health status prior to elective surgery? Would preoperative or postoperative hospitalization substantially help the patient? Particular attention must be directed toward learning all the many medications the elderly patient may be taking, because, with a greater number of drugs, there is an increased risk for drug interactions. A greater effort must be made also to make certain that the patient and his or her responsible person understand fully what to expect before and after the procedure. (Geriatric patients will be discussed in greater detail in Chapter 5.)

THE VERY YOUNG. Infants should not be denied required ambulatory surgery solely because of their age if the anesthesiologist and other personnel feel comfortable. However, infants with a history of respiratory distress syndrome, particularly those born prematurely and less than 60 postconceptual weeks old, are at greater risk of developing life-threatening perioperative apnea; their procedures should be postponed until they have reached a more appropriate age and level of maturity.[124] Patients considered at risk are those with anemia, a history of prematurity, or apnea or aspiration with feeding. (These patients are discussed further in Chapter 4.)

THE INSULIN-DEPENDENT DIABETIC. Insulin-dependent diabetes spans a broad spectrum of disease severity. At one extreme is the juvenile diabetic, whose control is often brittle, with premature vascular disease affecting major organ systems. At the other extreme is the elderly patient who may have developed relatively mild diabetes only late in life but who is likely to have clinically important coexisting diseases such as hypertension, coronary artery disease, and chronic obstructive pulmonary disease. Although the latter patient would be a suitable candidate for an ambulatory surgical experience if his or her diabetes and other disorders have been well controlled, the former is likely to drift out of control during the ambulatory surgical visit, if not just before arrival, because of the effect of the increased stress, unless unusual efforts are made. Efforts necessary to maintain these patients in good control include very close collaboration between the anesthesiologist, surgeon, and internist, scheduling the procedure as the first case of the day, and monitoring the blood glucose level on arrival and frequently (e.g., every two hours) thereafter. Rather than taking the morning insulin dose while fasting and then traveling to the surgery facility, patients should be instructed to bring their insulin with them so that it can be taken in the ambulatory unit after an intravenous infusion has been started. Through the close collaboration among the physicians must come a plan for the perioperative care, including the preoperative insulin dosage, infusion of a glucose-containing fluid with supplemental potassium until the patient can resume oral intake, and postoperative surveillance and therapy to maintain control. In addition, nausea and vomiting must be treated promptly and vigorously to prevent dehydration and to ensure an early return to a normal oral caloric intake. If a given ambulatory unit cannot meet the greater requirements of the insulin-dependent diabetic, it simply should not treat them. Hospital units (integrated, separated) are likely to feel more comfortable with these patients, again because of the relative ease with which inpatient admission can be arranged.

THE OBESE. Some degree of obesity is common in an economically advanced society, but when is a patient too obese for ambulatory surgery? Since *obese* refers subjectively to excessive weight relative to the individual's height, weight and height must be standardized. One such standardizing approach is the body mass index (BMI):

$$\text{Body mass index} = \frac{\text{weight in kilograms}}{(\text{height in meters})^2}$$

One also may estimate the patient's ideal body weight, as follows:

Men: Ideal body weight (kg) = height (cm) − 100

Women: Ideal body weight (kg) = height (cm) − 105

Patients who are modestly overweight (e.g., BMI 26–29, or weight 30% above "ideal") experience minimal increased excess mortality, whereas those more obese (e.g., BMI >30, or 35%–40% overweight) experience increased mortality following inpatient surgery.[125,126]

The implications of obesity are far-reaching, for it often exists as a predisposing disorder for the development of a variety of important chronic illnesses such as diabetes mellitus, cholelithiasis, cerebrovascular disease, hypertension, cirrhosis, and cardiac disease. Although its precise role is unclear, obesity appears to enable the chronic illness to begin prematurely, progress more rapidly, and become life-threatening more often.[125] Obesity stresses the cardiopulmonary systems because the increased carbon dioxide load (produced metabolically by the increased body mass) must be transported by an increased cardiac output and excreted by an increased pulmonary ventilation. When myocardial oxygen utilization exceeds supply, evidence of cardiac disease develops; similarly, those who are sufficiently overweight to be termed *morbidly obese* (i.e., body weight greater than twice ideal) are also close to the point of respiratory failure. These patients often become hypoxemic in the supine position because their abdominal corpulence pushes the diaphragm higher into the chest, collapsing lower lobes further and thereby producing a greater degree of shunt. Obese patients are also at greater risk for pulmonary aspiration because they tend to accumulate a larger gastric volume whose acidity is below the critical level for the development of aspiration pneumonitis.[127] In varying degrees, obese patients also present the anesthesiologist with a variety of acute problems that include difficulty in establishing intravenous access and in measuring blood pressure, propensity for airway obstruction and bronchospasm, and relative tolerance for anesthetics.

The pathophysiology of obesity nonwithstanding, remarkably little is known about the safety of treating these patients in an ambulatory surgery center. One study of women having pelvic laparoscopy concluded that obese patients are appropriate candidates as long as they can be classified as physical status 1 and 2. Although recovery time did not differ materially by body weight, the rate of unplanned hospital admission did. Only 0.7% of patients with a BMI below 27 required admission, whereas 2% of those with a BMI of 27 to 30 and 3% of those with greater values did. Although the incidence of emesis was related to body weight, the principal reason for admitting the more obese patients was surgical (need to resort to minilaparotomy).[109] Other studies have shown that obesity is a risk factor for developing intraoperative and postoperative hypoxemia as measured by pulse oximetry.[128,129] Additional studies are needed to define further what degree of obesity (and with what severity of which associated medical disorders) is appropriate for the ambulatory setting.

THE BRONCHOSPASTIC PATIENT. Despite their many differences, children and younger adults with asthma and the cigarette smoker with chronic obstructive pulmonary disease share a common feature—a very reactive airway. The spectrum in disease severity is sufficiently broad that some of these patients do not require chronic medication, whereas others are taking bronchodilators daily and still others are dependent on steroids as well as bronchodilators. Hence it is essential that each of these patients be considered individually. The history and physical examination are the most important parts of the evaluation of these patients: Does the patient have a reasonable exercise tolerance for his or her age? Has there been a recent productive cough? How frequent are the episodes of bronchospasm, what are the precipitating factors, and how have they been treated? When was the last attack, and does the patient feel fully recovered? Are there rhonchi, wheezes, or other auscultatory abnormalities? Is there any evidence of congestive heart failure? These patients should have a chest radiograph unless they appear asymptomatic and a film was normal within the past six months. In the end, the decision to treat these patients in an ambulatory surgery unit rests with how well controlled their bronchospasm is and how stable they have been on their therapeutic regimen. If one opts to treat them in the unit, one must collaborate closely with the patient's internist regarding optimal preoperative preparations and postoperative care; some patients may require a short preoperative course of steroids or antibiotics to treat residual bronchospasm. A halogenated agent (for bronchodilatation) should be used if general anesthesia is chosen. Airway manipulations (e.g., insertion of oropharyngeal airways, tracheal tubes) must be avoided under light anesthesia. And bronchospasm must be treated promptly by deepening anesthesia or using inhaled β-adrenergic receptor agonists. Where appropriate, regional anesthetic techniques such as spinal, epidural, or axillary block also should be considered to avoid airway manipulation.

THE COMMON COLD. Coryza occurs so frequently among school-age children that it is common to find that a seemingly well child has developed a "cold" in the short time since his or her ambulatory surgical care has been scheduled. Because of the more complicated social arrangements that must be made to treat children in the ambulatory surgery unit (because two adults are generally required for the trip home), the temptation is to proceed with "a little runny nose." Temptation must be resisted if symptoms are acute, for the seeming innocent "postnasal drip" often results in laryngospasm during light levels of anesthesia. Although eminently treatable, this problem tends to recur throughout the anesthetic, threatening hypoxemia each time. Prospective studies of children with and without symptoms of upper respiratory tract infection have shown that symptomatic patients are at greater risk for developing intraoperative airway complications (e.g., laryngospasm, apnea, cyanosis) and postoperative hypoxemia. Clearly, this risk is unwarranted for elective surgery that can be postponed until the child is well or at least has a dry nose. (This is covered more fully in Chapter 4). Other concerns raised in connection with administering general anesthesia during an upper respiratory viral illness include the anesthetic-induced impairment (for hours) of mucociliary clearance that predisposes to spread of the disease process throughout the lungs.[132]

THE SICKLE-CELL PATIENT. Sickle-cell disease is actually a family of disorders in which an abnormal, genetically determined hemoglobin undergoes a change in its molecular shape, resulting, in turn, in the sickling of the red cell and secondary vaso-occlusive signs and symptoms.[133] The most serious disorder is sickle-cell anemia (hemoglobin SS disease), with a frequency in the U.S. black population of 1:625, which over time can be associated with hepatic and renal insufficiency, hemiplegia, severe infections, and congestive heart failure. Several other related hemoglobinopathies are less common and, fortunately, less severe and debilitating. Sickle-cell trait (SA disease) is present in 8% to 9% of black Americans but is not associated with sickling, other symptomatology, or anemia.[133,134] Sickling episodes are prevented by strictly avoiding precipitating factors such as acidosis, hypoxia, hypotension, stasis, and hypothermia. Clinically, this means that the patient must be kept warm, tourniquets should be avoided, and anesthetic management must scrupulously avoid hypotension and airway obstruction.[133–135] Clearly, the decision to treat a sickle-cell anemia patient in an ambulatory surgery unit must be made on an individual basis.

THE ALCOHOL AND DRUG ABUSER. Substance abuse is so common that we probably administer anesthesia to an occasional self-medicated patient unknowingly. Two aspects of substance abuse deserve emphasis. First, abuse patterns generally involve a combination of substances, which complicates the care of these patients (as well as precise discussion here). Second, a critical distinction must be made between acute and chronic ingestion of an abuse substance. The potential for diverse acute autonomic and cardiovascular effects is sufficiently great that elective surgery is contraindicated if recent substance abuse is reasonably likely. This is, in large part, due to the likelihood of serious drug interactions between the anesthetics and the abused substances. However, chronic abusers *may* be appropriate candidates for ambulatory surgery, but only if they are reasonably healthy and the likelihood of a withdrawal episode seems remote.

Chronic alcoholism is often associated with serious systemic disorders that adversely affect perioperative mortality (and presumably morbidity): hepatitis, cardiomyopathy, organic brain syndrome, anemia, thrombocytopenia, abnormal platelet function, prolonged prothrombin time, hypoglycemia, and lactic acidosis. Chronic abuse of illicit drugs is associated with an even more diverse set of medical problems: endocarditis, osteomyelitis, superficial infection, tetanus, septic emboli, pulmonary edema, chronic aspiration pneumonia and lung abscess, renal insufficiency, hepatitis, peripheral nerve injury, and thrombophlebitis. Although the chronic alcoholic is generally relatively tolerant of anesthetics, the response of the patient abusing other substances is more variable depending on the given substance or substances, as well as their overall health status. Narcotic addicts often require larger narcotic dosage for analgesia but reasonably normal anesthetic levels, whereas chronic amphetamine abuse is associated with reduced anesthetic requirement. Barbiturate abusers tend to require greater amounts of anesthetics.

Withdrawal from chronic substance abuse is a potentially life-threatening event whose manifestations differ according to the substance. Alcoholics develop tremors and irritability within hours of their last ingestion, and seizures occur within 24 to 48 hours. The characteristic abstinence syndrome delirium tremens—which includes fever, global confusion, hallucinations, and tachycardia—occurs within 48 to 72 hours of last ingestion but may be delayed a week or more. As might be expected, the withdrawal syndromes associated with the abuse of other substances are different depending on the class of substance. The barbiturate withdrawal syndrome resembles that of alcohol and can be treated acutely with short-acting barbiturates. Amphetamine withdrawal includes sleep and toxic psychosis. Narcotic withdrawal includes diverse visceral signs and symptoms that begin with yawning, diaphoresis, lacrimation, and rhinorrhea and progress after several days to myalgias, muscle cramps, vomiting, diarrhea, tachycardia, and hypertension; the syndrome is treated acutely with narcotics.[136]

THE MENTALLY RETARDED AND DISABLED. Except for the most severely retarded and those with other clinically important health problems (e.g., symptomatic congenital heart disease), the mentally retarded are usually most appropriately treated in the ambulatory setting, surgical or medical. The ambulatory setting causes the least interruption in their otherwise psychologically fragile existence, particularly because it involves minimal separation from a familiar family or guardian. Similarly, with the exception of the most severely affected, the disabled also should be preferentially treated in the ambulatory setting, which affords them greater privacy and a more rapid return to familiar, supportive surroundings.[32,137]

THE PHYSICIANS

The ambulatory surgery unit is clearly a dynamic setting that represents much more than the transplantation of traditional approaches. Indeed, the success of the freestanding units is due, at least in part, to their innovation and to their ability to involve personnel of different types into the development of the facility and thereby provide high-quality care in a cost-effective manner. In this pioneering environment, personal attributes that are important for the success of both the facility and the individual personnel include initiative, flexibility, versatility, and responsibility. In particular, a "think ambulatory" orientation on the part of all personnel is essential because what clearly differentiates this care from inpatient care is the ability to discharge the patient to his or her home safely within hours of the procedure.

Because the importance of personnel policies among other fundamentals of the successful facility is discussed in Chapter 10, this section will focus on selection decisions that relate to the physicians who work in the ambulatory unit and which facilitate development of the unit. First, as a way of encouraging a minimal level of quality control, accreditation bodies require that specific procedures be established for evaluating the credentials and delineating the privileges of the surgeons and anesthesiologists (also nurse-anesthetists) who work in the unit. No longer can the hospital extend "full privileges" to each practitioner, assuming that peer pressure and professional integrity will ensure that an individual does not attempt a procedure for which he or she lacks substantial proficiency. Neither can a hospital-independent, freestanding ambulatory unit extend the same privileges for its facility as might be appropriate for an inpatient setting without requiring that its physicians possess equivalent privileges at a local hospital (granting of appropriate privileges was discussed in Chapter 2); otherwise, a freestanding unit would tend to attract surgeons whose practices had already been limited or prohibited.[138] Instead, as a safeguard to ambulatory patients, accreditation bodies require that the facility's medical staff formally delineate the scope of professional practice of each member of the medical staff in its ambulatory setting. Although peer judgment is likely to be an important determinant in the delineation of clinical privileges, utilization review and quality assurance programs (see section at the end of this chapter) are likely to be important sources of documentation upon which to modify those privileges.

The Anesthesiologist

With advances in clinical monitoring and development of improved anesthetics and adjuvants, the anesthesiologist has the ability to render safer care to progressively sicker patients, some not too long ago regarded as "too ill" for surgery. An unfortunate corollary of this medical progress is that many anesthesiologists no longer find it necessary to communicate with their patients; instead, they function more as technicians, knowledgeable and skillful, but nonetheless operating in a largely technical role. Yet anesthesia for ambulatory surgery offers an unusual opportunity for anesthesiologists to relate to conscious patients and their families, become more active in their preoperative assessment, and once again function more fully as physicians. In addition, there is the increasingly important challenge of providing the same high-quality care most cost-effectively in this rapidly developing subspecialty area in anesthesiology.

The Anesthesiologist as Manager

Anesthesiologists *selected* for the ambulatory setting, then, should be fully capable of becoming active participants; they must not be castaways from the traditional operating rooms. Because of the anesthesiologist's constant presence in the operating room (as compared with surgeons), he or she also has a natural opportunity to assume a managerial role, usually as medical director, if the unit has such a designation. For this new role beyond the care of an individual patient, the anesthesiologist must have or develop skills that enable him or her to set specific goals and objectives that must be clear to others, evolve organizational strategies rather than act alone, become a good listener, encourage constructive suggestions, and enrich the jobs of others by delegating as much as possible without losing control.

The Anesthesiologist's Preoperative Evaluation

The ultimate success of the ambulatory surgery unit depends on its ability to provide cost-effective care without jeopardizing quality and patient safety. To accomplish this, the unit must *mesh* appropriate patients with appropriate procedures performed by cooperative surgeons who understand fully the foregoing prerequisites for these patients and procedures. Although the surgeon sees potential ambulatory surgery patients first and selects appropriate candidates, he or she necessarily uses an evaluation procedure set forth by the anesthesiologists at the ambulatory surgery unit who will be looking after the overall well-being of his or her patients. Thus, by setting forth the selection policies, in particular those relating to the patient evaluation, and by being available continuously at the unit, the anesthesiologist is truly a gatekeeper and guardian in the ambulatory surgical setting.

OBTAINING THE PREOPERATIVE PATIENT INFORMATION. Once the surgeon has decided to undertake an ambulatory procedure in a given patient (see "The Surgeon," below), the anesthesiologist must gather the requisite information that will allow him or her to assess the patient, too. In perhaps half the ambulatory units, patients are required to make a preoperative visit several days in advance of surgery, at which time they tour the facilities, meet many of the personnel who will be caring for them, and meet the anesthesiologist. In effect, they meet the anesthesiologist in a consultative role in what has been termed an *anesthesia screening clinic.* Here, in a relatively unhurried session, without the anxiety of an immediately impending surgical procedure, the patient undergoes a relevant history and physical examination, learns about anesthesia care, and has an opportunity to have questions answered. In other units, the necessary information is obtained from the surgeon's office or by a telephone interview in the days before the procedure or during an interview with the anesthesiologist on the day of the procedure. The timing of the preoperative evaluation depends largely on the patient population and the resources of the facility. Regardless of when it occurs, a thorough and consistent preoperative evaluation is necessary for all ambulatory patients, especially as this population broadens to include a greater number of the elderly and medically compromised. The overall strategy is improvement of patient outcome through the treatment of whatever modifiable risk factors for adverse outcome may be present.[139]

Although the time-honored complete history and physical examination provide the necessary information, a more focused history is usually obtained. But what pieces of information are most relevant to the decision whether to proceed with anesthesia in a given patient? A British study sought to establish the minimum amount of information that permits an accurate assessment of one's fitness for anesthesia. The following are the simple questions whose answers the researchers found correlated with peer consensus of fitness for anesthesia[140]:

1. Do you feel sick?
2. Have you had any serious illnesses in the past?
3. Do you get more short of breath on exertion than others of your age?
4. Do you have a cough?
5. Do you have a wheeze?
6. Do you have any (anginal) chest pain on exertion?
7. Do you have ankle swelling?
8. Have you taken any medications in the past three months?
9. Have you any allergies?
10. Have you had an anesthetic in the past two months?
11. Have you or your relatives had any problems with anesthesia?

Note how relevant each is to the patient's functional status. Using this set of questions, the authors noted there was agreement among ten anesthesiologists in 96% of 200 patients that they evaluated prospectively. They concluded,

> Patients who are thought to be perfectly fit on the basis of simple questions usually prove to be so after the traditional preoperative history and investigations. This suggests that a questionnaire might be developed for use in surgical outpatients to select patients for day surgery.

This provides the rationale for the patient information questionnaires that many ambulatory surgery units are using (see section "Forms and Policies" for examples of these questionnaires). The questionnaire can be completed in the surgeon's office, in the unit, or even over the phone. Affirmative answers serve as "flags" to alert physicians to obtain additional information in areas of relevance to anesthesia care.

ROLE OF THE MEDICAL CONSULTANT. Often when faced with the sicker patient, the anesthesiologist and the surgeon will consult the patient's physician, who is most familiar with the patient's medical problems, or perhaps another internist whose expertise might benefit the patient. Unfortunately, in too many cases the request for a medical consultation is termed "clearing the patient for surgery," as if, in a return to the ancient days of sorcerers and rituals, the physician is being called on for a symbolic blessing that all will go well for the patient. However, when performed in this fashion, the patient, surgeon, and anesthesiologist lose an opportunity to gain potentially valuable help. Thus "medical clearance" is truly outdated and counterproductive.[141] Instead, the anesthesiologist must ask the medical consultant focused questions that will help guide anesthetic management. In turn, the medical consultant must address the specific questions raised and provide a list of the patient's medical problems and an assessment of how well each is controlled. The consultant also should be available postoperatively.

ROLE OF THE CLINICAL LABORATORY EVALUATION. Laboratory tests may be used for two different purposes. One may search for unsuspected disease in all preoperative patients by subjecting them to a battery of laboratory tests. This is termed *screening*, and its underlying rationale is that finding an abnormality will be beneficial to the patient. On the other hand, knowing or suspecting from the history and physical examination that a given patient has a particular abnormality, one may obtain a specific test to confirm that suspicion. Which approach is more rational?

Because clinical laboratory studies consume a large and growing portion of health care expenditures, excessive and inappropriate preoperative testing is being scrutinized. Such testing necessarily must reflect the incidence of disease in the population, sensitivity of the given tests, and factors related to the proposed surgery and anesthesia. Although recommendations for more rational use of laboratory testing are evolving in general medicine,[142] progress has been a little slower in the area of preoperative testing.[143–145] Nonetheless, the methods for evaluating the usefulness and cost-effectiveness of tests are at hand.[146,147] From the application of these methods to a variety of screening procedures has come a large number of studies with the same conclusion: Abnormal test results do occasionally occur, generally much less often than we would expect; the large majority of the abnormalities identified do not lead to new diagnoses; and even in those few in whom a new diagnosis is established, there is generally no reason to alter the agreed-upon surgical plan. Thus, using panels of tests for screening asymptomatic, preoperative patients is not cost-effective and should not be undertaken.

The corollary of these studies is that the history and physical examination are the principal sources of data in the evaluation of the patient.[143–146,148,149] Individual tests may be helpful in *selected* circumstances, when guided by abnormalities noted in the history and physical examination.[150,151]

HEMATOCRIT. The determination of hematocrit (or hemoglobin) is so inexpensive, the incidence of undiagnosed anemia so relatively high, and the ability of the physical examination to detect anemia so limited that this test should be performed in all preoperative patients.[143] However, it must be acknowledged that there is no objective basis to support the oft-quoted need for a hematocrit value of, say, 30% to enable normal postoperative wound healing. Also, with 98.7% accuracy and half the errors being conservative, it is possible to differentiate "safe" hematocrit levels from those which are "unsafe" (e.g., less than 28%) by examination of the conjunctiva.[152] Thus it is not clear that the hematocrit (or hemoglobin), the only test recommended for all patients, is really needed.

URINALYSIS. Relatively unstudied, the urinalysis is occasionally found among recommendations for screening because it is also a relatively inexpensive test and the incidence of abnormalities detected is so great. For example, half the 10% of the general population with diabetes mellitus are undiagnosed, and glycosuria is reliably detected by the urinalysis. Yet recent study suggests that the use of urinalysis for screening can be eliminated without adversely affecting patient care or outcome.[148,149,153]

CHEST RADIOGRAPHY. Chest radiography is among the most commonly performed preoperative testing, yet its clinical usefulness for screening is also questioned.[144,154–156] For example, a large number of studies suggest that in asymptomatic persons under 40 years of age, more than half the "routine" radiographs reported to be abnormal are falsely positive. Furthermore, a chest radiograph would detect an abnormality that would alter anesthetic management in only 1.5% of the population under age 40.[144] Whether patient outcome would be different is unknown. Even in patients between 40 and 60 years of age, the yield from preoperative screening is inadequate to justify the practice.[155] The argument that these films offer medicolegal protection is fallacious because the total number of false-negative and false-positive results may exceed the total of the true positives.[144,145] Thus an expert panel (which included anesthesiologists, internists, surgeons and radiologists) convened by the U.S. Food and Drug Administration's Center on Devices and Radiological Health recommends that the preoperative chest film not be routinely obtained in the absence of a specific abnormality noted in the history or physical examination or in a selected population already shown to have significant yields of previously undiagnosed disease.[157] The House of Delegates of the American Society of Anesthesiologists (ASA) approved the recommendation in October of 1984. As with other tests, the substitution of selective ordering for routine ordering does not result in adverse patient care.[158]

ELECTROCARDIOGRAM. Despite its widespread use in evaluating specific cardiac problems, the usefulness of the electrocardiogram (ECG) as a screening tool has yet to be established.[159] It has only limited value in detecting ischemic heart disease in asymptomatic persons. Similarly, the value in obtaining a "baseline" ECG for possible subsequent comparison has never been established.[159,160] Although the ECG becomes increasingly valuable with older populations,[161,162] formal recommendations cannot be made without knowing the underlying prevalence of ECG abnormalities in a given population.

LIVER FUNCTION TESTS. Tests of hepatic function (e.g., SGOT, LDH, total bilirubin) have such a low yield that such routine testing is also apt to be unwarranted; when abnormalities are noted, many can be attributed to information already obtained from taking the patient's history.[143–146] Some argue that there is a medicolegal basis for obtaining such tests prior to general anesthesia which is felt to be possibly hepatotoxic, but this point of view has yet to be evaluated objectively.

COAGULATION STUDIES. Prothrombin time (PT) and partial thromboplastin time (PTT) have been recommended as screening tests to detect unsuspected bleeding disorders and thereby avoid hemorrhagic surgical complications, yet this clinical recommendation has never been validated. In a recent study of 750 preoperative inpatients, 139 patients (19%) were suspected of having a bleeding abnormality based on information obtained in the history or physical examination, of whom 25 (18%) were found to have an abnormal PT or PTT result. Of the 611 patients (81%) lacking an indication of a bleeding disorder, 480 had determinations of PT or PTT and 13 (2.7%) were found to have abnormal values. Of this latter group, 4 were found to have normal values on repeat testing, 8 were operated on uneventfully without retesting, and only 1 patient experienced a hemorrhagic complication, which was found at reoperation to have been caused by an unligated artery. In addition, the low yield of these tests was obscured by a larger number of false-positive results. The investigators concluded that these tests are useful only in those patients previously identified as having an increased risk of bleeding, based on abnormalities noted in the history and physical examination.[163] Other studies have corroborated these results.[164–169]

OTHER TESTS. Although not useful for screening, a variety of other tests are valuable in specific circumstances to evaluate clinical situations that cannot be assessed by other means. For example, a blood sugar determination is often valuable in patients with insulin-dependent diabetes; similarly, serum electrolyte determinations are useful in patients who are receiving chronic diuretic or digitalis therapy. Yet routine determination of pseudocholinesterase level prior to general anesthesia has such a low yield that it is unwarranted; more rational is a careful history of the patient's past anesthetic experiences.

A CLINICAL LABORATORY RECOMMENDATION. Given that screening with laboratory tests is not cost-effective but individual tests may be helpful in confirming clinical suspicion, it is clear that we must be more selective when we order tests. No longer are there "routine tests"; instead, there are specific recommendations according to the patient population and particular test. Moreover, tests should be obtained only when their results will actually be part of the decision making. Or, as aptly stated by Cochrane[170]:

> When considering whether to order a test, ask yourself what you would do if the test result were positive, and what you would do if it were negative. If the answers are the same, don't order the test.

Table 3-2 presents clinical recommendations for the laboratory evaluation of preoperative patients, both ambulatory and inpatient, based on current knowledge about these tests. Note that specific tests are obtained only for specific indications, based on abnormalities noted in the history and physical examination.

TABLE 3-2. A Recommended Schema for Minimal Preoperative Testing

Test to be → Obtained	HGB M	HGB F	WBC	PT/PTT	PLT, BT	Elect	Creat/BUN	Blood Gluc	SGOT/ALK PTASE	X-ray	ECG	Preg	T/S
Preop. conditions													
Suspected													
Surgical procedure:													
With blood loss	X	X											X
Without blood loss													
Neonates	X	X											
Age <40	X	X											
Age 40–59	X	X									±		
Age ≥60	X	X								X	X		
Cardiovascular disease							X				X		
Pulmonary disease										X	X		
Malignancy	X	X	*	*						X			
Radiation therapy			X							X	X		
Hepatic disease				X					X				
Exposure to hepatitis									X				
Renal disease	X	X				X	X						
Bleeding disorder				X	X								
Diabetes						X	X	X			X		
Smoking ≥20 pk-yrs	X	X								X			
Possible pregnancy												X	
Diuretic use						X	X						
Digoxin use						X	X				X		
Steroid use						X		X					
Anticoagulant use	X	X		X									

NOTE: M = male; F = female; HGB = hemoglobin; WBC = white blood count; PT = prothrombin time; PTT = partial thromboplastin time; PLT = platelet count; BT = bleeding time; Elect = electrolytes; Creat/BUN = creatinine or blood urea nitrogen; SGOT/ALK PTASE = serum glutamic oxaloacetic transaminase phosphatase; Preg = pregnancy test; T/S = blood typing and screen for unexpected antibodies; ± = possibly; * = leukemias only; X = obtain.

The ASA House of Delegates also has promulgated a statement relating to the appropriate use of laboratory testing (see Appendix 3A). Test results are acceptable for 30 days, unless the patient's underlying disease would dictate that testing be repeated closer to the scheduled procedure; chest radiographs and electrocardiograms taken within the past six months are acceptable if they were normal and the patient has no cardiorespiratory abnormalities. These recommendations for clinical laboratory testing should be considered optional, at the discretion of the surgeon, in the case of those patients who are scheduled to have procedures performed under local anesthesia *without* sedation.

Educating the Surgeon and the Office Staff

Since the preoperative assessment relates largely to the more global concerns of the anesthesiologist and the surgeon necessarily has first contact with the patient, it is encumbent upon the anesthesiologist to take the initiative in educating the surgeon and staff. The anesthesiologist should summarize briefly his or her approach to preoperative assessment (see preceding section) and make this information available to all surgeons (and their staffs) who are potential users of the ambulatory unit. In addition, the anesthesiologist should be available to answer questions. Recognizing that the surgeon often delegates many administrative aspects of patient preparation, representatives from the ambulatory unit also should meet with the surgeon's staff to answer their questions and establish rapport that can facilitate the implementation of future policy changes as the unit develops.

The Surgeon

Given the diversity of procedures currently undertaken in the ambulatory setting, and particularly the presence of some that are clearly *non*surgical, *surgeon* must be viewed rather broadly as any physician who performs a procedure. Thus, among the "surgeons" in the ambulatory unit are the neurologist performing a lumbar puncture and the pulmonologist undertaking fiberoptic bronchoscopy. A *sine qua non* is that the surgeon have sufficient skill to perform procedures effectively and within a reasonable time. During the early development of the ambulatory unit, his or her patience (and patients!), understanding, and support will be important in launching the unit. Although in most cases the surgeon no longer decides whether surgery is undertaken on an ambulatory basis, his or her cooperation will be amply repaid by his or her enhanced productivity, because the time previously spent in preoperative and postoperative hospital rounds will be spared and his or her surgical schedule will move along faster and generally with greater predictability. In return, the smallness of the ambulatory unit will be conducive to the delivery of efficient and high-quality care, largely because the surgeon will be working with the same small number of people who will become familiar with his or her needs.

Preoperative Assessment in the Surgeon's Office

The surgeon and staff must develop an appreciation of the importance of the preoperative assessment in appropriate selection of patients in the ambulatory setting. Although very familiar, of course, with the planned procedure and his or her needs, the surgeon may not have given sufficient thought to the procedure in the given patient. Concerned about the patient's particular surgical problem, the surgical specialist is apt to overlook general aspects of the patient's health or social setting that may make him or her a poor candidate for ambulatory care. What is the patient's physical status category? What are the coexisting diseases, and are they well controlled? How far from a hospital or physician's office does the patient live? Is the patient's family capable of providing postoperative care? Does he or she live alone? What preoperative laboratory testing should be obtained? The surgeon and staff must consider each of these questions.

Educating the Patient in the Surgeon's Office

Once the decision has been made to undertake the procedure on an ambulatory basis, the surgeon and staff must explain, emphasize, and restate the importance of following the instructions that are provided in a brochure prepared by the ambulatory surgery unit for patient guidance (Figure 3-2). The patient must be specifically told not to eat or drink after a certain hour, (e.g., midnight), but the patient should brush his or her teeth and take any usual medications with a sip of water unless specifically advised otherwise. These instructions should be reinforced by telephone the day before surgery. Experience indicates that such patient education, and, in particular, the repetition of important instructions, is invaluable in preventing unnecessary cancellations due to misunderstanding and nonadherence. The patient also should be advised about postoperative care so that when the nurse in the postanesthesia care unit dispenses discharge instructions, the patient is more likely to understand and comply.

Scheduling the Procedure

Recognizing that the patient is an appropriate candidate for the proposed ambulatory procedure, the surgeon or, more likely, his or her staff then calls the ambulatory unit to schedule the surgery. Although there are many administrative variations that suit local situations, the following is true of most units. Whether the unit uses "block scheduling" or schedules "as time and space are available" is largely dependent on the maturity of the unit, with the former predominating as the unit develops. Because of the need for a minimal two to three hours' postoperative recovery period following general anesthesia, cases involving general anesthesia are scheduled preferentially early in the day, with the last case starting no later than about 2 P.M. Cases involving either local anesthesia administered by the surgeon or sedation or regional anesthesia administered by anesthesia personnel may start later in the day, although they should end by midafternoon.

The patient is requested to arrive about an hour prior to the scheduled procedure, having completed preregistration (e.g., insurance forms) and having had any indicated laboratory testing. If the anesthesiologist has not interviewed the patient and undertaken preoperative assessment (see preceding section), he or she does so at this time; regardless, however, he or she confirms that the patient has not experienced some intercurrent illness that might warrant postponement. Also, adherence to "nothing by mouth" and the presence of a responsible person

WEEK BEFORE SURGERY

After your surgery has been scheduled, please come directly to the UCSF Surgery Center to register. You do not need an appointment for this visit, and you can come anytime between 8 a.m. and 5 p.m., Monday through Friday. During this visit, you will be issued a special yellow UCSF patient card valid for the day of your scheduled surgery. You will also consult with an anesthesiologist and receive specific instructions regarding your surgery—including information about any required laboratory tests. This visit will give you an opportunity to ask questions and discuss any concerns you may have.

Through our experience, we have found that this visit is particularly important for children because it enables us to prepare your child psychologically for anesthesia and surgery.

Be sure to bring your insurance card when you come to register if you wish us to bill your insurance company directly. If you wish us to bill you, please be prepared to make a cash deposit before surgery.

Please allow approximately one hour for this registration and consultation visit.

Interpreters are available for our non-English-speaking patients. We ask that you give us advance notice if you need an interpreter or a special telecommunications unit for hearing- or speech-impaired persons.

You must arrange for a friend or relative to drive and escort you home after surgery. **Your surgery will be cancelled if you have not arranged for someone to drive and escort you home.** For the convenience of your escort, we will be happy to estimate when you will be ready to leave the Surgery Center. If desired, your escort may wait for you in the Surgery Center Family Lounge.

DAY BEFORE SURGERY

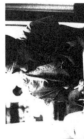

If you cannot keep your surgical appointment, or if your health or your child's health changes in any way (for example, if you develop a rash, cold or fever), please notify your surgeon and call the Surgery Center at 415/476-8384.

You will be contacted by telephone to verify your surgery time, review preoperative instructions, and answer any questions. If you have not been contacted by 4:00 p.m., please call the Surgery Center at 415/476-8384.

Plan to wear loose, comfortable, easy-to-remove clothing the day of surgery. Children may come in night clothing and bring a favorite toy or blanket. (If you are from outside of the Bay Area, remember that San Francisco weather is often much cooler than the surrounding area. Be sure to bring a coat or sweater.)

Adults and children 5 years and older must not eat or drink anything after midnight. Children under 5 may eat up to 6 hours before surgery and may have **clear** liquids (including breast milk) until 4 hours before surgery. Infants under six months may eat up to 4 hours before surgery and may have **clear** liquids (including breast milk) until 2 hours before surgery. If you are scheduled to have surgery after 2:00 p.m. or if you have diabetes, you may be given special instructions about eating and drinking. **Surgery will be cancelled if instructions about eating and drinking are not followed.** Unless you are told otherwise, you should take your regular medications by mouth with a very small sip of water.

Be sure to bring your UCSF patient card.

Plan to arrive at the UCSF Surgery Center one hour before the time your surgery is scheduled. Allow an extra 10 minutes to park in the Millberry Union Parking Garage.

Do not bring any jewelry (including wedding rings), money or credit cards. The UCSF Surgery Center cannot be responsible for storage of these items.

Do not wear makeup, hair pins, a wig or contact lenses.

DAY OF SURGERY

BEFORE SURGERY

- You will change into a hospital gown in your private room. Your clothing will be secured in a locker.

- You (or your parent or legal guardian) will sign the surgery consent form. Please feel free to ask any questions before signing this form.

- Your blood pressure, temperature and pulse will be taken, and any special preparations ordered by your doctor will be done.

- Your anesthesiologist will visit you.

- Your surgical nurse will accompany you to the Operating Room.

You will recover in the Postanesthesia Care Unit under the supervision of your nurse. You will spend about one to two hours there before being escorted to the Recovery Lounge where your friend or family member may join you. Parents will be reunited with their child as soon as possible.

Once you have recovered, we will help you dress. It is normal to feel somewhat sleepy for several hours after surgery.

Before leaving the Surgery Center, you and your escort will receive both written and verbal instructions regarding your postoperative care. We will be happy to answer your questions.

AFTER SURGERY

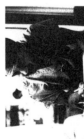

If you have any concerns about your medical condition after you arrive home, please contact your surgeon. His or her telephone number is on your instruction sheet. If you cannot reach your doctor, please call the Medical Center Emergency Department at 415/476-1037.

We will check on you the following day by telephone. You may expect our call between 9 a.m. and 5 p.m. Be sure to give us a telephone number where you can be reached.

FIGURE 3-2. Information given to patients before their ambulatory surgery. (SOURCE: UCSF Surgery Center, Medical Center at the University of California at San Francisco.)

are confirmed. Many ambulatory units require the patient arriving for surgery to sign a form on which he or she certifies that he or she understands the information provided, has provided correct information, has a responsible escort home, and has had nothing to eat or drink since midnight and acknowledges that he or she may not drive a car (or operate other dangerous machinery) or drink alcoholic beverages for 24 hours (see section "Forms and Policies"), must notify the physician immediately if unusual bleeding or other problems (the list often includes respiratory difficulties and acute pain) occur, and that he or she may have to be admitted to the hospital due to unforeseen circumstances.

EQUIPMENT
Operating Room Equipment
Although the risks to the patient associated with simpler, often minor surgery are generally smaller than those associated with inpatient procedures, the risks of anesthesia remain relatively constant and substantial. The same high quality of equipment is required in the ambulatory setting as in the inpatient facility; indeed, the JCAHO accreditation standards (see earlier section) require that the policies and procedures relating to the same surgical procedures be the same in both settings. This equipment includes a reasonably modern anesthesia machine capable of delivering the common anesthetic agents, a full complement of tracheal tubes and other artificial airways and laryngoscope blades, appropriate monitoring devices and resuscitative equipment, suction, conventional operating table, electrocautery machine, sterilizers, and surgical instruments and ancillary operating room equipment appropriate to the type of procedures performed (e.g., operating microscope or fluoroscopy). All this equipment must necessarily meet appropriate standards and guidelines, such as those relating to delivery and scavenging of anesthetic gases and to electrical safety.[171-173]

Monitoring Equipment
Physiologic monitoring entails the continual observation and assessment of the patient's condition and response to anesthesia and surgery. Advances in commercially available monitoring equipment during the past five years have been so dramatic that the sourcebooks on clinical monitoring published only a few years ago appear dated. As with operating room equipment, the choice of clinical monitoring devices in the ambulatory setting is no different from that in the hospital. The ASA House of Delegates has also promulgated standards for intraoperative patient monitoring (Appendix 3B).

EVALUATING AND MODIFYING SELECTION DECISIONS
Conscientious ambulatory anesthesia units will seek to maintain their ability to provide high-quality, cost-effective care by modifying their selection decision according to the outcome of their care. Ideally, this process should involve continuous data collection and periodic rigorous analysis, including double-blind clinical trials of alternative drugs or other modalities of care. Realistically, however, few units can muster such an intensive evaluation process. The majority of units

will find that criteria established through peer review of available literature, with adjustments to their local setting, can be modified by using the same process. Utilization review and quality assurance programs, mandated by accreditation standards, demonstrate how peer review can be used to modify selection decisions.

Utilization Review Programs

Utilization review (UR), another accreditation requirement, endeavors to ensure appropriate allocation of the hospital's resources so that high-quality care is delivered in the most cost-effective manner. Although external insurance and governmental entities have become increasingly involved, institutional UR programs specifically address overutilization, underutilization, and inefficient scheduling. In the context of ambulatory care, of course, UR programs have sought to shift the simpler, less complex elective surgery from expensive hospital operating rooms to less costly ambulatory surgery units. Among the most potent forces behind these efforts has been, not unexpectedly, the insurance industry, both private (e.g., Blue Cross/Blue Shield plans) and governmental (e.g., Medicare, Medicaid), which have successfully focused such UR programs on ambulatory surgery by using educational and financial incentive programs. Insurers have established lists of surgical procedures that are or could be performed on an ambulatory basis, distributed the lists to participating physicians and local hospitals, requested that the physicians perform them on an ambulatory basis unless there was a demonstrated need for hospitalization, and asked the hospitals to develop UR procedures relating to listed procedures that were being performed on an inpatient basis. The performance of listed procedures at a high rate among inpatients has prompted statewide programs to create preadmission screening criteria that assist in shifting appropriate cases to the ambulatory setting.

Preadmission screening criteria were not designed to be standards of care or to replace good clinical judgment. Rather, they served to assist UR personnel to evaluate whether hospitalization was warranted. In cases of dispute, a physician consultant within the facility reviewed the case. The implementation of such a program, augmented by changes in reimbursement for care,[6] resulted in a sharp decrease in the frequency of affected procedures being performed on an inpatient basis without compromising patient care. In this way, hospital admission criteria developed through peer review effectively augment the decision making regarding patient selection in the ambulatory setting. Recently, however, the utilization review process external to the health care facility has been strengthened by the insurers, with the development of preadmission certification programs. Under these programs, the surgeon must obtain preadmission approval from the insurer, regardless of the site of surgery. Thus decision making relating to whether—not just where—to do surgery is now influenced by external entities.

Quality Assurance Programs

Ambulatory surgery centers also can ensure that their selection decisions (among other aspects of their care) are maintaining patient safety and quality of care by conducting a quality assurance program. Given the growth and importance of

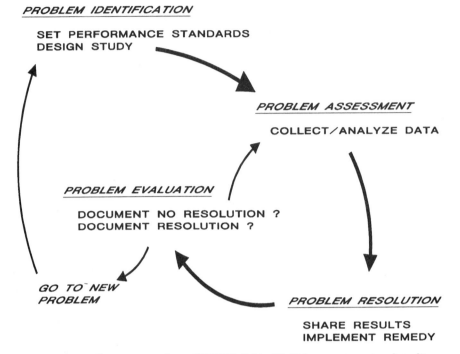

FIGURE 3-3. The quality assurance loop. (SOURCE: Orkin FK: Risk management and quality assurance in outpatient anesthesia care. Problems in Anesthesia 2: 152, 1988.)

ambulatory care, this activity is now a major focus of JCAHO accreditation.[18,174] The underlying rationale for a quality assurance program is simply the improvement in patient care. The components of such a program are the identification of patient-related problems, objective assessment of such problems, implementation of meaningful solutions, monitoring the effectiveness of the solutions, and finally, documentation of the effectiveness of the solutions in a cyclical fashion[175–177] (Figure 3-3).

Rudiments of a Quality Assurance Program
Individuality, creativity, and innovation are encouraged in the implementation of the program, which may include two approaches: The newer approach of monitoring and evaluation involves retrospective patient care evaluation that assesses the occurrence of clinically important postoperative problems (clinical indicators) such as the following over sequential time periods:

Respiratory symptoms
Excessive bleeding
Persisting nausea or vomiting
Circulatory or neurologic impairment
Excessive pain
Signs of infection

This patient-care evaluation can be facilitated with a form that the patient receives once home or by use of a phone call within a few days of the surgery. The older approach is the formal quality assurance audit that for many years JCAHO has encouraged hospitals to undertake periodically in relation to specific perceived problems. Operationally, however, the two approaches are often undertaken in series; the retrospective patient-care evaluation may suggest a problem that can be examined in detail through the quality assurance audit.[178]

Regardless of the approach, however, the program should stress objective outcome measures, such as

- Deaths
  Unplanned hospital admissions or hospital transfers
  Complications
  Cancellations and delays
  Blood transfusions
  Infection rates

Even patient and surgeon satisfaction can be assessed by using objective, criteria-based rating scales rather than diffuse, freeform, subjective comments. Tracking the incidence of objective adverse events will become the principal quality assurance activity in the early 1990s, when accreditation becomes outcome-based.[179]

Once a problem is identified, its causes are sought. Depending upon the nature of the problem, staff meetings, interviews, or perhaps some other approach is used. Often, however, with a little detective work, a cause seems obvious. For example, a disproportionate number of unplanned admissions occurring among patients with asthma might prompt a more stringent preoperative assessment of such patients (e.g., electing not to treat those requiring steroids and bronchodilators in the ambulatory setting). Following implementation of the revised preoperative assessment, an audit is performed to monitor the effectiveness of the new policy; if the new policy is found ineffective, other changes in the selection decisions might be tried and the audit repeated until effectiveness is documented. In this way, a cycle is completed (Figure 3-3) and care is improved. A quality assurance program thus becomes a mechanism by which selection decisions can be modified to improve patient care. (Quality assurance is discussed further in Chapters 8 and 10.)

REFERENCES

1. Keys TE: The History of Surgical Anesthesia, pp 3–31. Huntington, N.Y., Robert E Krieger, 1978
2. Nicoll JH: The surgery of infancy. Br Med J 2: 753, 1909
3. Waters RM: The Down-Town Anesthesia Clinic. Am J Surg (Anesth Suppl) 33: 71, 1919
4. Cohen DD, Dillon JB: Anesthesia for outpatient surgery. JAMA 196: 1114, 1966
5. Levy ML, Coakley CS: Survey of in and out-surgery—The first year. South Med J 61: 995, 1968
6. Orkin FK: Economic and regulatory issues. In White PF (ed): Outpatient Anesthesia. New York, Churchill-Livingstone 1990
7. Ambulatory care growth continues. Outreach 10(1); 1, 1989

8. Hospital Statistics, 1988, Text Table 12, Table 2A. Chicago, American Hospital Association, 1988
9. Orkin FK: Practice standards: The Midas touch or the emperor's new clothes? Anesthesiology 70: 567, 1989
10. Brindle GF, Soliman MG: Anaesthetic complications in surgical outpatients. Can Anaesth Soc J 22: 613, 1975
11. Natof HE: Complications associated with ambulatory surgery. JAMA 244: 1116, 1980
12. Levy M-L: Complications: Prevention and quality assurance. Anesthesiol Clin North Am 5: 137, 1987
13. Abramowitz MD, Oh TH, Epstein BS, et al: The antiemetic effect of droperidol following strabismus surgery in children. Anesthesiology 59: 579, 1983
14. Wetchler BV, Collins IS, Jacob L: Antiemetic effects of droperidol on the ambulatory surgery patient. Anesthesiol Rev 9(5): 23, 1982
15. White PF: Ketamine—Its use as an intravenous anesthetic. Clin Anesthesiol 2(1): 43, 1984
16. Gold B, Orkin FK: Cost-effectiveness of outpatient surgery. Curr Opinion Anaesthesiol 1: 76, 1988
17. Egdahl RH: Should we shrink the health care system? Harvard Business Review 61(1): 125, 1984
18. Joint Commission on Accreditation of Healthcare Organizations: Hospital-sponsored ambulatory care services. In Accreditation Manual for Hospitals, 1989, pp 55–65. Chicago, Joint Commission on Accreditation of Healthcare Organizations, 1988
19. Joint Commission on Accreditation of Healthcare Organizations: Accreditation Manual for Ambulatory Health Care. Chicago, Joint Commission on Accreditation of Healthcare Organizations, 1988
20. Meridy HW: Criteria for selection of ambulatory surgical patients and guidelines for anesthetic management: A retrospective study of 1553 cases. Anesth Analg 61: 921, 1982
21. Gold B, Kitz DS, Lecky JH, et al: Unanticipated admission to the hospital following ambulatory surgery. JAMA 262: 3008, 1989
22. Freeman LN, Schachat AP, Manolio TA, et al: Multivariate analysis of factors associated with unplanned admission in "outpatient" ophthalmic surgery. Ophthalmic Surg 19: 719, 1988
23. Davis JE, Detmer DE: The ambulatory surgical unit. Ann Surg 175: 856, 1972
24. Davis JE: The need to redefine levels of surgical care. JAMA 251: 2527, 1984
25. Detmer DE: Ambulatory surgery. N Engl J Med 305: 1406, 1981
26. Detmer DE, Buchanan-Davidson DJ: Ambulatory surgery. Surg Clin North Am 62: 685, 1982
27. Detmer DE, Buchanan-Davidson DJ: Ambulatory surgery. In Rutkow IM (ed): Socioeconomics of Surgery, pp 30–50. St. Louis, CV Mosby, 1989
28. Medicare Program: List of covered surgical procedures for ambulatory surgical centers (Final notice). Fed Reg 52(76): 13176, 1987
29. National Center for Health Statistics: Detailed diagnoses and procedures for patients discharged from short-stay hospitals, United States, 1986. Vital and Health Statistics, Series 13, no 95. Washington, U.S. Government Printing Office, 1989
30. Shah CP: Anaesthesia for day-case surgery: I. Day-case surgery in Canada. Can Anaesth Soc J 27: 399, 1980
31. Frassica JJ, Miller EC: Anesthesia management in pediatric and special needs patients undergoing dental and oral surgery. Int Anesthesiol Clin 27: 109, 1989
32. Indresano AT, Rooney TP: Outpatient management of mentally handicapped patients undergoing dental procedures. J Am Dent Assoc 102: 328, 1981
33. Kay M: General anaesthesia in the private dental office. Can Anaesth Soc J 30: 406, 1983
34. Heneghan C, McAuliffe R, Thomas D, et al: Morbidity after outpatient anaesthesia: A comparison of two techniques of endotracheal anaesthesia for dental surgery. Anaesthesia 36: 4, 1981
35. Willatts DG, Harrison AR, Groom JF, et al: Cardiac arrhythmias during outpatient dental anaesthesia: Comparison of halothane with enflurane. Br J Anaesth 55: 399, 1983
36. Bailey HAT Jr, Pappas JJ, Gay EC Jr: O.P.S.C.: Improving delivery of otolaryngological surgical care. Laryngoscope 88: 1612, 1978
37. Pratt LW, Gallagher RA: Tonsillectomy and adenoidectomy: Incidence and mortality. Arch Otolaryngol Head Neck Surg 87: 159, 1979

38. Chiang TM, Sukis AE, Ross DE: Tonsillectomy performed on an outpatient basis: Report of a series of 40,000 cases performed without a death. Arch Otolaryngol 88: 105, 1968

39. Maniglia AJ, Kushner H, Cozzi L: Adenotonsillectomy: A safe outpatient procedure. Arch Otolaryngol Head Neck Surg 115: 92, 1989

40. Cullen BF, Margolis AJ, Eger El II: The effects of anesthesia and pulmonary ventilation on blood loss during elective therapeutic abortion. Anesthesiology 32: 108, 1970

41. Hackett GH, Harris MNE, Planetvin OM, et al: Anaesthesia for outpatient termination of pregnancy: A comparison of two anaesthetic techniques. Br J Anaesth 54: 865, 1982

42. Sidhu MS, Cullen BF: Low-dose enflurane does not increase blood loss during therapeutic abortion. Anesthesiology 57: 127, 1982

43. Garrioch DB, Gilbert JR, Plantevin OM: Choice of ecbolic and the morbidity of day-case terminations of pregnancy. Br J Obstet Gynaecol 88: 1029, 1981

44. White PF, Coe V, Dworsky WA, et al: Disseminated intravascular coagulation following midtrimester abortions. Anesthesiology 58: 99, 1983

45. Ogg TW, Jennings RA, Morrison CG: Day-case anaesthesia for termination of pregnancy: Evaluation of a total intravenous anaesthetic technique. Anaesthesia 38: 1042, 1983

46. Fragen RJ (ed): Propofol: Clinical update and implications. Semin Anesth 7(1, Suppl 1): 1, 1988

47. Centers for Disease Control: Annual summary 1982: Reported morbidity and mortality in the United States. MMWR 31(54): 134, 1983

48. Denlinger JK: Pneumothorax. In Orkin FK (ed): Complications in Anesthesiology, 2d ed. Philadelphia, JB Lippincott (in press)

49. Knickerbocker GS, Neufeld GR: Burns and electrocution. In Orkin FK (ed): Complications in Anesthesiology, 2d ed. Philadelphia, JB Lippincott (in press)

50. Don H: Hypoxemia and hypercapnia during and after anesthesia. In Orkin FK (ed): Complications in Anesthesiology, 2d ed. Philadelphia, JB Lippincott (in press)

51. Bedford RF: Air embolism. In Orkin FK (ed): Complications in Anesthesiology, 2d ed. Philadelphia, JB Lippincott (in press)

52. Reynolds RC, Pauca AL: Gastric perforation, an anesthetic-induced hazard in laparoscopy. Anesthesiology 38: 84, 1973

53. Spielman FJ: Laparoscopic surgery. Prob Anesth (3(1): 151, 1989

54. Centers for Disease Control: Annual summary 1981: Reported morbidity and mortality in the United States. MMWR 30(54): 126, 1982

55. Abramson DJ: 857 breast biopsies as an outpatient procedure. Ann Surg 163: 478, 1966

56. Mitchell GW, Homer MJ: Outpatient breast biopsies on a gynecologic service. Am J Obstet Gynecol 144: 127, 1982

57. Stein HD: Ambulatory breast biopsies: The patient's choice. Am Surg 48: 221, 1982

58. Jackson DP, PItts HA: Biopsy with delayed radical mastectomy for carcinoma of the breast. Am J Surg 98: 184, 1959

59. Pierce EH, Clagett OT, McDonald JF, et al: Biopsy of the breast followed by delayed radical mastectomy. Surg Gynecol Obstet 103: 559, 1956

60. Miller LB: Orthopedic patients in an ambulatory surgery facility. Nurs Clin North Am 16: 749, 1981

61. Miller LB: Orthopedic patients in an ambulatory surgery facility. Nurs Clin North Am 16: 749, 1981

62. Falstie-Jensen S, Jensen UH, Sondergaard-Petersen PE, et al: Arthroscopy: Should it be done as an outpatient procedure or during hospitalization? Acta Orthop Scand 54: 131, 1983

63. Rosenberg TD, Wong HC: Arthroscopic knee surgery in a freestanding outpatient surgery center. Orthop Clin North Am 13: 277, 1982

64. Greene NM: Physiology of Spinal Anesthesia, 3d ed, p 27. Baltimore, Williams & Wilkins, 1981

65. Gold B, Bogetz MS, Orkin FK: Continuous spinal anesthesia for ambulatory surgery. Anesthesiology 71: A722, 1989

66. Herzfeld G: Hernia in infancy. Am J Surg 39: 422, 1938

67. Othersen HB, Claworthy HW Jr: Outpatient herniorrhaphy for infants. Am J. Dis Child 118: 78, 1968

68. Glassow F: Short stay surgery (Shouldice technique) for repair of inguinal hernia. Ann R Coll Surg Eng 58: 123, 1976

69. Flanagan L Jr, Bascom JU: Herniorrhaphies performed upon outpatients under local anesthesia. Surg Gynecol Obstet 153: 557, 1981

70. Abdu RA: Ambulatory herniorrhaphy under local anesthesia in a community hospital. Am J. Surg 145: 353, 1983

71. Flanagan L Jr, Bascom JU: Repair of the groin hernia: Outpatient approach with local anesthesia. Surg Clin North Am 64:257, 1984

72. Lee RH, Marzoni FA, Cannon WB, et al: Outpatient adult inguinal-hernia repair. West J Med 140: 905, 1984

73. Statement on cost containment. Bull Am Coll Surg 64(7): 3, 1979

74. Ponka JL, Sapala JA: Bupivacaine as a local anesthetic for hernia repair. Henry Ford Hosp Med J 24(1): 31, 1976

75. Kingsnorth AN, Britton BJ, Morris PJ: Recurrent inguinal hernia after local anaesthetic repair. Br J Surg 68: 273, 1981

76. Humphreys CF, Kay H: The control of postoperative wound pain with the use of bupivacaine injections. J Urol 116: 618, 1976

77. Wood GJ, Lloyd JW, Bullingham RES, et al: Postoperative analgesia for day-case herniorrhaphy patients: A comparison of cryoanalgesia, paravertebral blockade and oral analgesia. Anaesthesia 36: 603, 1981

78. Ericksson E (ed): Illustrated Handbook in Local Anaesthesia, 2d ed, pp 52–54. Philadelphia, WB Saunders, 1980

79. Ryan JA, Adye BA, Jolly PC, et al: Outpatient inguinal herniorrhaphy with both regional and local anesthesia. Am J Surg 148: 313, 1984

80. Hirsch RP, Schwartz B: Increased mortality among elderly patients undergoing cataract extraction. Arch Ophthalmol 101: 1034, 1983

81. Adler AG, McElwain GE, Merli GJ, et al: Systemic effects of eye drops. Arch Intern Med 142: 2293, 1982

82. Cass E, Kadar D, Stein HA: Hazards of phenylephrine topical medications in persons taking propranolol. Can Med Assoc J 120: 1261, 1979

83. Solosko D, Smith RB: Hypertension following 10% phenylephrine ophthalmic. Anesthesiology 36: 187, 1972

84. Rasch D, Holt J, Wilson M, et al: Bronchospasm following injection of acetylcholine in a patient taking metoprolol. Anesthesiology 59: 583, 1983

85. London RA, Kudlak T, Riehle RA: Immersion anesthesia for extracorporeal shock wave lithotripsy. Urology 28: 86, 1986

86. Burns JR, Breaux EF, Crowe AD: Practical aspects of outpatient extracorporeal shock-wave lithotripsy. Urol Clin North Am 14: 73, 1987

87. Zeitlin GL, Roth RA: Effect of three anesthetic techniques on the success of extracorporeal shock wave lithotripsy in nephrolithiasis. Anesthesiology 68: 272, 1988

88. Cooper GL, Roberts JT, O'Brien A, et al: Microbial examination of kidney lithotripter tub water and epidural anesthesia catheters. Infact Control 7: 216, 1986

90. Klein JA: Anesthesia for liposuction in dermatologic surgery. J Dermatol Surg Oncol 14: 1124, 1988

91. Goodpasture JC, Bunkis J: Quantitative analysis of blood and fat in suction lipectomy aspirates. Plast Reconstr Surg 78: 765, 1986

92. AMA Council on Scientific Affairs: Autologous blood transfusions. JAMA 256: 2378, 1986

93. Hayes DL, Vlietstra RE, Trusty JM, et al: A shorter hospital stay after cardiac pacemaker implantation. Mayo Clin Proc 63: 236, 1988

94. Belott PL: Ambulatory pacemaker procedures. Mayo Clin Proc 63: 301, 1988

95. Lemarbre L, Hudon G, Coche G, et al: Outpatient peripheral angioplasty: Survey of complications and patients' perceptions. AJR 148: 1239, 1987

96. Steckler RM: Outpatient thyroidectomy: A feasibility study. Am J Surg 152: 417, 1986

97. Moss G: Discharge within 24 hours of elective cholecystectomy: The first 100 patients. Arch Surg 121: 1159, 1986

98. Evans DIK, Morris Jones P, Morris P, Shaw EA: Outpatient anaesthesia for a children's leukaemia clinic. Lancet 1: 751, 1971

99. Fisher DM, Robinson S, Brett CM, et al: Comparison of enflurane, halothane, and isoflurane for diagnostic and therapeutic procedures in children with malignancies. Anesthesiology 63: 647, 1985

100. Brandwein JM, Callum J, Rubinger M, et al: An evaluation of outpatient bone marrow harvesting. J Clin Oncol 7: 648, 1989

101. Ackart RS, Foreman DR, Klayton RJ, et al: Fiberoptic bronchoscopy in outpatient facilities, 1982. Arch Intern Med 143: 30, 1983

102. Cardiac catheterization plan cuts hospitalization. Hosp Pract [Off] 17(3): 51, 1982

103. Gavin WA, Stewart DK, Murray JA: Outpatient coronary arteriography. Cathet Cardiovasc Diagn 7: 347, 1981

104. Poretz DM, Eron LJ, Goldberg RI, et al: Intravenous antibiotic therapy in an outpatient setting. JAMA 248: 336, 1982

105. Drop LF, Welch CA: Anesthesia for electroconvulsive therapy in patients with major cardiovascular risk factors. Convuls Ther 5: 88, 1989

106. Mercier C, Page A, Verdant A, et al: Outpatient management of intercostal tube drainage in spontaneous pneumothorax. Ann Thorac Surg 22: 163, 1976

107. Elliot DL, Linz DH, Kane JA: Electroconvulsive therapy: Pretreatment medical evaluation. Arch Intern Med 142: 979, 1982

108. Jensen S, Wetchler BV: The obese patient: An acceptable candidate for outpatient anesthesia. JAANA 50: 369, 1982

109. Porterfield HW, Franklin LT: The use of general anesthesia in the office surgery facility. Clin Plast Surg 10(2): 289, 1983

110. Wetchler BV: Anesthesia for outpatients. In Mauldin BC (ed): Ambulatory Surgery: A Guide to Perioperative Nursing Care, pp 111–158. New York, Grune & Stratton, 1983

111. Goldman L, Caldera DL, Nussbaum SR, et al: Multifactorial index of cardiac risk in noncardiac surgical procedures. N Engl J Med 297: 845, 1977

112. Lewin I, Lerner AG, Green SH, et al: Physical class and physiologic status in the prediction of operative mortality in the aged sick. Ann Surg 174: 2, 1971

113. Marx GF, Mateo CV, Orkin LR: Computer analysis of postanesthetic deaths. Anesthesiology 39: 54, 1973

114. Schneider AJL: Assessment of risk factors and surgical outcome. Surg Clin North Am 63: 1113, 1983

115. Vacanti CJ, Van Houten RJ, Hill RC: A statistical analysis of the relationship of physical status to postoperative mortality in 68,388 cases. Anesth Analg 49: 564, 1970

116. Cohen MM, Duncan PG: Physical status score and trends in anesthetic complications. J Clin Epidemiol 41: 83, 1988

117. Goldmann DR, Brown FH, Levy WK, et al (eds): Medical Care of the Surgical Patient: A Problem-Oriented Approach to Management. Philadelphia, JB Lippincott, 1982

118. Kammerer WS, Gross RJ (eds): Medical Consultation: Role of the Internist on Surgical, Obstetric, and Psychiatric Services. Baltimore, Williams & Wilkins, 1983

119. Lubin MF, Walker HK, Smith RB III (eds): Medical Management of the Surgical Patient, 2d ed. Boston, Butterworths, 1988

120. Molitch ME (ed): Management of Medical Problems in Surgical Patients. Philadelphia, FA Davis, 1982

121. Stoelting RK, Dierdorf SF, McCammon RL (eds): Anesthesia and Co-Existing Disease, 2d ed. New York, Churchill-Livingstone, 1988

122. Vandam LD (ed): To Make the Patient Ready for Anesthesia: Medical Care of the Surgical Patient, 2d ed. Menlo Park, Calif., Addison-Wesley, 1984

123. Vickers MD (ed): Medicine for Anaesthetists, 3d ed. Oxford, England, Blackwell Scientific Publications, 1989

124. Kurth CD, Spitzer AR, Broennle AM, et al: Postoperative apnea in preterm infants. Anesthesiology 66: 483, 1987

125. Vaughan RW: Definitions and risks of obesity. In Brown BR Jr (ed): Anesthesia and the Obese Patient, pp 1–7. Philadelphia, FA David, 1982

126. Pasulka PS, Bistrian BR, Benotti PN, et al: The risks of surgery in obese patients. Ann Intern Med 104: 540, 1986

127. Vaughan RW, Bauer S, Wise L: Volume and pH of gastric juice in obese patients. Anesthesiology 43: 686, 1975

128. Raemer DB, Warren DL, Morris R, et al: Hypoxemia during ambulatory gynecologic surgery as evaluated by the pulse oximeter. J Clin Monit 3: 244, 1987

129. Morris RW, Buschman A, Warren DL, et al: The prevalence of hypoxemia detected by pulse oximetry during recovery from anesthesia. J Clin Monit 4: 16, 1988

130. Liu LMP, Ryan JF, Cote CJ, et al: Influence of upper respiratory infection on critical incidents in children during anesthesia. In Abstracts of the Ninth World Congress of Anaesthesiologists, A0786, May 1988

131. DeSoto H, Patel RI, Soliman IE, et al: Changes in oxygen saturation following general anesthesia in children with upper respiratory infection signs and symptoms undergoing otolaryngological procedures. Anesthesiology 68: 276, 1988

132. Forbes AR, Gamsu G: Mucociliary clearance in the canine lung during and after general anesthesia. Anesthesiology 50: 26, 1979

133. Platt OS, Orkin FK: Difficulties in sickle cell states. In Orkin FK (ed): Complications in Anesthesiology, 2d ed. Philadelphia, JB Lippincott (in press)

134. Gibson JR: Anesthesia and hemoglobinopathies. Semin Anesth 6: 27, 1987

135. Esseltine DW, Baxter MRN, Bevan JC: Sickle cell states and the anesthetist. Can J Anaesth 35: 385, 1988

136. Levy WK: Alcohol and drug abuse in the surgical patient. In Goldmann DR, Brown FH, Levy WK, et al (eds): Medical Care of the Surgical Patient: A Problem-Oriented Approach to Management, pp 568–577. Philadelphia, JB Lippincott, 1982

137. Stiles CM: Anesthesia for the mentally retarded patient. Orthop Clin North Am 12: 45, 1981

138. Sieverts S: Ambulatory surgery and health insurance. In Burns LA (ed): Ambulatory Surgery: Developing and Managing Successful Programs, pp 177–194. Rockville, Md. Aspen Systems, 1984

139. Glaser R: Preoperative assessment: Impact on patient outcome. Semin Anesthesiol 7: 251, 1988

140. Wilson ME, Williams NB, Baskett PJF, et al: Assessment of fitness for surgical procedures and the variability of anaesthetists' judgments. Br Med J 280: 509, 1980

141. Choi JJ: An anesthesiologist's phiosophy on "medical clearance" for surgical patients. Arch Intern Med 147: 2090, 1987

142. Sox HC Jr (ed): Common Diagnostic Tests: Use and Interpretation. Philadelphia, American College of Physicians, 1987

143. Roizen MF: Optimizing preoperative evaluation. In Miller RD (ed): Anesthesia, 3d ed, New York, Churchill-Livingstone, 1990

144. Roizen MF, Kaplan EB, Schreider BD, et al: The relative roles of the history and physical examination, and laboratory testing in preoperative evaluation for outpatient surgery: The "Starling" curve of preoperative laboratory testing. Anesthesiol Clin North Am 5: 15, 1987

145. Roizen MF: The compelling rationale for less preoperative testing. Can J Anaesth 35: 214, 1988

146. Carson JL, Eisenberg JM: The preoperative screening examination. In Goldmann DR, Brown FH, Levy WK, et al (eds): Medical Care of the Surgical Patient: A Problem-Oriented Approach to Management, pp 16–30. Philadelphia, JB Lippincott, 1982

147. Galen RS, Gambino SR: Beyond Normality: The Predictive Value and Efficiency of Medical Diagnoses. New York, Wiley, 1975

148. Kaplan EB, Sheiner LB, Boeckmann AJ, et al: The usefulness of preoperative laboratory screening. JAMA 253: 3576, 1985

149. Johnson H, Knee-loli S, Butler TA: Are routine preoperative laboratory screening tests necessary to evaluate ambulatory surgical patients? Surgery 104: 639, 1988

150. Blery C, Charpak Y, Szatan M, et al: Evaluation of a protocol for selective ordering of preoperative tests. Lancet 1: 139, 1986

151. Charpak Y, Blery C, Chastang C, et al: Usefulness of selectively ordered preoperative tests. Med Care 26: 95, 1988

152. Ashcraft KE, Guinee WS, Golladay ES: Clinical assessment of hematocrit and hemoglobin. Anesthesiol Rev 9(2): 37, 1982

153. Akin BV, Hubbell FA, Frye EB, et al: Efficacy of the routine admission urinalysis. Am J Med 82: 719, 1987

154. Abrams HL: The "overutilization" of x-rays. N Engl J Med 300: 1213, 1979
155. Tape TG, Mushlin AI: The utility of routine chest radiographs. Ann Intern Med 104: 663, 1986
156. Robin ED, Burke CM: Routine chest x-ray examinations. Chest 90: 258, 1986
157. U.S. Department of Health and Human Services, Food and Drug Administration, Center for Devices and Radiological Health: The Selection of Patients for X-Ray Examinations: Presurgical Chest X-Ray Screening Examinations, HHS Pub. FDA 86-8261. Washington, U.S. Government Printing Office, 1986
158. Charpak Y, Blery C, Chastang C, et al: Prospective assessment of a protocol for selective ordering of preoperative chest x-rays. Can J Anaesth 35: 259, 1988
159. Goldberger AL, O'Konski M: Utility of the routine electrocardiogram before surgery and on general hospital admission. Ann Intern Med 105: 552, 1986
160. Rubenstein LZ, Greenfield S: The baseline ECG in the evaluation of acute cardiac complaints. JAMA 24: 2536, 1980
161. Ferrer MI: The value of obligatory preoperative electrocardiogram. J Am Med Wom Assoc 33: 459, 1978
162. Rabkin SW, Horne JM: Preoperative electrocardiography: Its cost-effectiveness in detecting abnormalities when a previous tracing exists. Can Med Assoc J 121: 301, 1979
163. Eisenberg JM, Clark JR, Sussman SA: Prothrombin and partial thromboplastin times as preoperative screening tests. Arch Surg 117: 48, 1982
164. Borzotta AP, Keeling MM: Value of the preoperative history as an indicator of hemostatic disorders. Ann Surg 200: 648, 1984
165. Redding SW, Olive JA: Relative value of screening tests of hemostasis prior to dental treatment. Oral Surg Oral Med Oral Pathol 59: 34, 1985
166. Suchman AL, Mushlin AI: How well does the activated partial thromboplastin time predict postoperative hemorrhage? JAMA 256: 750, 1986
167. Suchman AL, Griner PF: Diagnostic uses of the activated partial thromboplastin time and prothrombin time. Ann Intern Med 104: 810, 1986
168. Manning SC, Beste D, McBride T, et al: An assessment of preoperative coagulation screening for tonsillectomy and adenoidectomy. Int J Pediatr Otorhinolaryngol 13: 237, 1987
169. Rohrer MJ, Michelotti MC, Nahrwold DL: A prospective evaluation of the efficacy of preoperative coagulation testing. Ann Surg 208: 554, 1988
170. Cochrane AL: Effectiveness and Efficiency: Random Reflections on Health Services, Chap 5. London, Nuffield Provincial Hospital Trust, 1972
171. American National Standards for Anesthetic Equipment—Scavenging Systems for Excess Anesthetic Gases, ANSI Z79.11-1982. New York, American National Standards Institute, 1982
172. American Society of Anesthesiologists' Ad Hoc Committee on Effects of Trade Anesthetic Agents on Health of Operating Room Personnel: Waste Anesthetic Gases in Operating Room Air: A Suggested Program to Reduce Personnel Exposure. Park Ridge, Ill., American Society of Anesthesiologists (undated)
173. Knickerbocker GS, Neufeld GR: Electrotrauma in the operating room: Shock, electrocution, and burns. In Orkin FK (ed): Complications in Anesthesiology, 2d ed. Philadelphia, JB Lippincott (in press)
174. Joint Commission on Accreditation of Healthcare Organizations: Surgical and anesthesia services, Hospital-sponsored ambulatory care services. In Accreditation Manual for Hospitals, pp 269–279. Chicago, Joint Commission on Accreditation of Healthcare Organizations, 1988
175. Buske SM: A quality assurance program for ambulatory surgical services. In Burns LA (ed): Ambulatory Surgery: Developing and Managing Successful Programs, pp 63–81. Rockville, Md., Aspen Systems, 1984
176. Palmer RH: Ambulatory Health Care Evaluation: Principles and Practice. Chicago, American Hospital Association, 1983
177. Orkin FK: Risk management and quality assurance in outpatient anesthesia care. Probl Anesth 2: 152, 1988
178. Brown EM: Quality assurance in anesthesiology—The Problem-oriented audit. Anesth Analg 63: 611, 1984
179. O'Leary DS: The Joint Commission looks to the future. JAMA 258: 951, 1987

Appendix 3A

STATEMENT ON ROUTINE PREOPERATIVE LABORATORY AND DIAGNOSTIC SCREENING
(Approved by American Society of Anesthesiologists' House of Delegates on October 14, 1987)

Preanesthetic laboratory and diagnostic testing is often essential; however, no routine* laboratory or diagnostic screening** test is necessary for the preanesthetic evaluation of patients. Appropriate indications for ordering tests include the identification of specific clinical indicators or risk factors (e.g., age, pre-existing disease, magnitude of the surgical procedure). Anesthesiologists, anesthesiology departments, or health care facilities should develop appropriate guidelines for preanesthetic screening tests in selected populations after considering the probable contribution of each test to patient outcome. Individual anesthesiologists should order test(s) when, in their judgment, the results may influence decisions regarding risks and management of the anesthesia and surgery. Legal requirements for laboratory testing where they exist should be observed.

*Routine refers to a policy of performing a test or tests without regard to clinical indications in an individual patient.
**Screening means efforts to detect disease in unselected populations of asymptomatic patients.

Appendix 3B

STANDARDS FOR BASIC INTRA-OPERATIVE MONITORING
(Approved by American Society of Anesthesiologists' House of Delegates on October 18, 1989)

These standards apply to all anesthesia care although, in emergency circumstances, appropriate life support measures take precedence. These standards may be exceeded at any time based on the judgement of the responsible anesthesiologist. They are intended to encourage high-quality patient care, but observing them cannot guarantee any specific patient outcome. They are subject to revision from time to time, as warranted by the evolution of technology and practice. This set of standards addresses only the issue of basic intra-operative monitoring, which is one component of anesthesia care. In certain rare or unusual circumstances, 1) some of these methods of monitoring may be clinically impractical, and 2) appropriate use of the described monitoring methods may fail to detect untoward clinical developments. Brief interruptions of continual[1] monitoring may be unavoidable. *Under extenuating circumstances, the responsible anesthesiologist may waive the requirements marked with an asterisk (*); it is recommended that when this is done, it should be so stated (including the reasons) in a note in the patient's medical record.* These standards are not intended for application to the care of the obstetrical patient in labor or in the conduct of pain management.

STANDARD I
Qualified anesthesia personnel shall be present in the room throughout the conduct of all general anesthetics, regional anesthetics and monitored anesthesia care.

Objective
Because of the rapid changes in patient status during anesthesia, qualified anesthesia personnel shall be continuously present to monitor the patient and provide anesthesia care. In the event there is a direct known hazard, e.g., radiation, to the anesthesia personnel which might require intermittent remote observation of the patient, some provision for monitoring the patient must be made. In the event that an emergency requires the temporary absence of the person primarily responsible for the anesthetic, the best judgement of the anesthesiologist will be exercised in comparing the emergency with the anesthetized patient's condition and in the selection of the person left responsible for the anesthetic during the temporary absence.

STANDARD II
During all anesthetics, the patient's oxygenation, ventilation, circulation and temperature shall be continually evaluated.

Oxygenation
Objective
To ensure adequate oxygen concentration in the inspired gas and the blood during all anesthetics.

Methods

1. Inspired gas: During every administration of general anesthesia using an anesthesia machine, the concentration of oxygen in the patient breathing system shall be measured by an oxygen analyzer with a low oxygen concentration limit alarm in use.*

2. Blood oxygenation: During all anesthetics, a quantitative method of assessing oxygenation such as pulse oximetry shall be employed.* Adequate illumination and exposure of the patient are necessary to assess color.*

Ventilation
Objective

To ensure adequate ventilation of the patient during all anesthetics.

Methods

1. Every patient receiving general anesthesia shall have the adequacy of ventilation continually evaluated. While qualitative clinical signs such as chest excursion, observation of the reservoir breathing bag and auscultation of breath sounds may be adequate, quantitative monitoring of the CO_2 content and/or volume of expired gas is encouraged.

2. When an endotracheal tube is inserted, its correct positioning in the trachea must be verified. Clinical assessment is essential and end-tidal CO_2 analysis, in use from the time of endotracheal tube placement, is encouraged.

3. When ventilation is controlled by a mechanical ventilator, there shall be in continuous use a device that is capable of detecting disconnection of components of the breathing system. The device must give an audible signal when its alarm threshold is exceeded.

4. During regional anesthesia and monitored anesthesia care, the adequacy of ventilation shall be evaluated, at least, by continual observation of qualitative clinical signs.

Circulation
Objective

To ensure the adequacy of the patient's circulatory function during all anesthetics.

Methods

1. Every patient receiving anesthesia shall have the electrocardiogram continuously displayed from the beginning of anesthesia until preparing to leave the anesthetizing location.*

2. Every patient receiving anesthesia shall have arterial blood pressure and heart rate determined and evaluated at least every five minutes.*

3. Every patient receiving general anesthesia shall have, in addition to the above, circulatory function continually evaluated by at least one of the following: palpation of a pulse, auscultation of heart sounds, monitoring of a tracing of intra-arterial pressure, ultrasound peripheral pulse monitoring, or pulse plethysmography or oximetry.

Body Temperature
Objective

To aid in the maintenance of appropriate body temperature during all anesthetics.

Methods

There shall be readily available a means to continuously measure the patient's temperature. When changes in body temperature are intended, anticipated or suspected, the temperature shall be measured.

¹Note that "continual" is defined as "repeated regularly and frequently in steady and rapid succession" whereas "continuous" means "prolonged without any interruption at any time."

Addendum: The Board of Directors of the American Society of Anesthesiologists at its March 1990 meeting accepted a proposed modification of the following standard.

Ventilation

2. When an endotracheal tube is inserted, its correct positioning in the trachea must be verified by clinical assessment and by identification of carbon dioxide in the expired gas.* End-tidal CO_2 analysis, in use from the time of endotracheal tube placement, is encouraged.

The above modification will not become part of the Standards for "Basic Intra-Operative Monitoring" until final action by the House of Delegates in October 1990. If approved, date of implementation will be determined by the House of Delegates.

The Pediatric Patient

4

■ ■

RAAFAT S. HANNALLAH, BURTON S. EPSTEIN

The concept of ambulatory or same-day surgery in infants and children is not new. Outpatient pediatric anesthesia was reported as early as 1909 by Nicoll[1] and by Herzfeld in 1938.[2] The more recent "discovery" and growing popularity of ambulatory surgery, particularly for pediatric patients, have been dictated by our current social and fiscal needs and have created new challenges and rewarding opportunities for the pediatric anesthesiologist. This chapter reviews the fundamentals of the safe practice of pediatric anesthesia in the ambulatory surgery setting. It is based on a review of the literature, discussions with professionals who have had extensive experience with the subject, and our own personal experience.

Many authors believe that up to 50% of all surgical procedures in children can be performed safely on an outpatient basis. A survey by the American Academy of Pediatrics confirmed that a substantial amount of surgery is indeed being done this way.[3] Of the pediatric anesthesiologists responding to the survey, 97% reported that they perform outpatient anesthesia at their institutions. Forty percent of the respondents noted that outpatients represented 20% or less of their practice; 50% stated that such patients constituted 20% to 40% of their practice; and 6% said that outpatients accounted for some 40% of their cases.

ADVANTAGES
Some of the reasons for performing surgery on an outpatient basis are the same in both children and adults. These include:

131

Reducing the cost of medical care
Increasing the availability of hospital beds for those who truly need them
Offering a level of care comparable to that received by the inpatient with-
    out its inconveniences and potential hazards

At the same time, however, ambulatory surgery has several distinct advantages
that are unique to the pediatric patient:

Children rarely have systemic disease and are good anesthetic risks.
Many common surgical procedures such as herniotomy and myringot-
    omy are simpler to perform in children than in adults and are associ-
    ated with a shorter, less complicated convalescent period.
Separation from the parent is minimized.[4]
Hospital-acquired infections are reduced.[5]
The feeding schedule is less severely disrupted.

For children, the two greatest advantages of ambulatory surgery are the reductions in separation anxiety and nosocomial infections. Steward has noted that in
a well-organized program it should not be necessary to separate parent and child
for much longer than the duration of anesthesia.[6] Minimizing separation from
family, home, and friends is particularly beneficial for the preschooler who still
depends on his or her mother as the ultimate security object during times of
stress.[7] Most parents are usually enthusiastic about participating in the preparation and postoperative care of the child and prefer this to having the child
admitted to the hospital. The experience may be of benefit to the whole family
unit.[8]

The reduction in nosocomial infections is particularly important in infants.
Othersen cites two of the few available studies concerning this issue.[5] The first,
reported by Izant in 1957, involved a group of infants admitted for "clean" elective
operations, of whom 17% developed signs and symptoms of enteric or respiratory infection while hospitalized or within 3 days of discharge. Izant also noted
that during a two-day hospitalization for elective herniorrhaphy, an average of 25
different potentially contaminated hospital personnel touched each infant or his
or her bed. Twenty-three additional individuals were intimately involved with the
care of the infant during a single visit to the operating and recovery rooms. In
the second study cited by Othersen, Mintor compared 68 infants admitted for
inpatient herniorrhaphy with 26 similar infants undergoing the same procedure
as outpatients. He found that the incidence of postoperative cross-infection was
50% to 75% lower in the outpatient group. Although the evidence seems convincing, there are no recent studies on large groups of patients that verify a reduction in cross-infection among ambulatory surgical patients.

LIMITATIONS

Although the advantages are striking, pediatric ambulatory surgery also can have
its problems. Unfortunately, there is a tendency to associate outpatient surgery

with "minor procedures" and "healthy patients" and to assume that all children about to undergo minor operations as outpatients have no concurrent medical problems and are psychologically well adjusted. This assumption does a disservice to those who require special consideration. When the emphasis is on increasing speed, reducing turnaround time between procedures, and minimizing the length of hospitalization, children have less time to adjust to the hospital environment. As a matter of fact, there is evidence that from the psychological point of view, for some children hospitalization may actually be an experience that is not at all detrimental to mental health, particularly if the stay is less than two days.[9] This subject is further discussed under the heading "Psychological Preparation."

Assuming that all short-stay patients are a healthy and uniform group medically is a common misconception that leads to problems. Patients who have undiagnosed acute diseases such as upper respiratory infections (URI) or diarrhea or asymptomatic patients with a previously diagnosed or even undiagnosed chronic problem such as heart disease may be scheduled at ambulatory surgery facilities. Unfortunately, the record of a previous consultation report, if performed, including diagnosis and recommendations for therapy, may not always be available for these patients. This usually leads to delays and hard feelings between physicians and parents.

Another potential problem results from the stipulation by many ambulatory surgical facilities that one or both parents remain with the child throughout the stay in the center. This may require that one or both parents take leave from work and that siblings at home be cared for by others. In some cases, the inconvenience and out-of-pocket expense to the parents caused by this practice may be greater than the cost of hospitalization to them. In addition, some parents are apprehensive about caring for their child at home after discharge.[4] This is particularly true if the child is very young or if any problems have arisen during the recovery stay. The lack of privacy of outpatient accommodations and the potential necessity for extra visits to the facility to obtain preoperative screening and consultations are also annoying for pediatric ambulatory surgery patients. A long distance between the home and the facility causes many inconveniences, especially when surgery is scheduled early in the morning and the family is required to leave home several hours earlier.

The question of reducing the cost of medical care to a given patient versus the overall cost to an institution or community whose inpatient census declines because of the advent of ambulatory surgery is yet another complex issue that has generated great debate.[10]

FACTORS IN SELECTION OF PATIENTS

The criteria for selecting patients and procedures for pediatric ambulatory surgery vary greatly among institutions. They are usually influenced by the condition of the patient, the attitude of the parents, the type of surgical procedure, and any special considerations for anesthetic management and recovery.[11] Since the surgeon initiates the entire process, he or she must cooperate with and un-

derstand the overall process completely. Some of the most important considerations are as follows.

THE PATIENT

The child should be in good health or any systemic disease he or she has must
be under good control. Some anesthesiologists still restrict ambulatory surgery
to patients classified as ASA physical status 1 and 2, while others[8,12,13] may accept
ASA physical status 3 patients under special circumstances. This usually requires
prior consultation with a member of the anesthesia staff and a current written
statement from the attending physician about the nature of the illness and recommended therapy. Patients with a controlled convulsive disorder or well-reg-
ulated diabetes, for example, may be acceptable, while those with a bleeding
tendency, liver insufficiency, incipient heart failure, uncontrolled diabetes, or infectious diseases are not. Many children with chronic diseases benefit substantially from outpatient treatment.[8] Hospital-acquired infections are a specific risk
to these children, as is the emotional trauma of repeated hospitalization. A child
with leukemia or one who is receiving immunosuppressant medication is particularly suitable for outpatient care. Physically handicapped, psychologically disturbed, or mentally retarded children benefit tremendously from the lack of separation and continued support of a parent or guardian that is usually fostered in
outpatient facilities.

Special Problems
The Child with a Runny Nose
One of the most perplexing issues that commonly faces the anesthesiologist is
the child who presents with a runny nose. Since probably 20% to 30% of all
children have a runny nose a significant part of the year, the practice of *auto-
matically* canceling all children with a runny nose would result in inordinate
hardships on the parents, the child, and the medical system. Every child with a
runny nose must be evaluated on an individual basis. The subject has been recently reviewed by Berry[14] and is summarized here.

The points to consider before making a decision are that a child who presents
with a runny nose may have either a completely benign, noninfectious condition,
in which case elective surgery may safely be performed, or the runny nose may
be a prodrome to, or actually be, an infectious process, in which case elective
surgery should be canceled. Examples of these conditions are shown below.[14]

        Noninfectious runny nose:
          Allergic rhinitis:
            Seasonal
            Perennial
          Vasomotor rhinitis:
            Emotional (crying)
            Temperature

Infectious runny nose:
  Viral infections—*e.g.*, nasopharyngitis (common cold), contagious diseases (chicken pox/measles)
  Acute bacterial infections (*e.g.*, streptococcal tonsillitis, meningitis)

The preanesthetic assessment of these patients consists of obtaining a complete history, performing a physical examination, and examining certain laboratory data. Early in the clinical course, the history will be the most important single factor in the differential diagnosis. Specifically, allergic problems such as hay fever, sinusitis, asthma, and recurrent bronchitis should be actively sought. A history of an infectious illness in other members of the family or in the community is important. Parents are usually well aware and can tell whether their child's runny nose is "the usual runny nose" or something different. The following questions need to be answered by the parents: *Is this the usual runny nose, or is it something different? Does the child have his or her normal appetite? Is the child playing and sleeping normally?* If the parents say that this condition is not the usual runny nose and that it is something different, then this, by itself, is sufficient cause to cancel elective surgery. The physical examination is not always conclusive. Normal findings may be present during the early part of an infectious process. Chronic allergic rhinitis, on the other hand, may be associated with local infections within the nasopharynx resulting in purulent nasal discharge. Again, the parents can be helpful in establishing whether this is the usual discharge or not. If the remainder of the physical examination and history are normal, elective surgery may be performed. However, if there are obvious findings on physical examination such as a temperature of 38°C or higher, viral ulcers in the oropharynx, tonsillitis, or rales, the child is considered to have an infectious process and elective surgery is canceled.

Useful laboratory data include a complete blood cell count and, if indicated, a chest radiograph. A white blood cell count $\geq$ 12,000 to 15,000 with a shift to the left suggests an infectious process. If a child has a runny nose and a cough and there is still a question of an infectious process, a chest radiograph may be indicated before proceeding with elective surgery.

The risk associated with anesthetizing a child who has had a URI may be present for up to 4 to 6 weeks after an apparent recovery. Although well-controlled studies are still lacking, this appears particularly true after a flulike syndrome that involves both the upper and lower respiratory tract. In such a case, there are symptoms of the common cold plus the constitutional signs and symptoms of chills, fever, myalgias, and often a severe cough. In children who have these syndromes, perioperative respiratory complications such as laryngospasm and bronchospasm were reported during anesthesia by Tait and coworkers.[15] McGill and coworkers[16] noted atelectasis, which was probably related to inspissation of secretions because of residual reduction in ciliary activity caused by the previous URI.

Because of these studies it is recommended that a careful history of a URI (flulike syndrome) in the past 4 to 6 weeks be elicited. If doubt exists as to its resolution, the surgery should be postponed for at least a month following recovery. If symptoms persist, a preoperative chest radiograph should be obtained. If radiography is positive, surgery should be canceled; if it is negative, the anesthesiologist should still be alert for signs of an irritable airway or atelectasis during or following surgery.

A common situation that poses a difficult decision is that of a child with a runny nose presenting for relatively brief or low-risk procedures such as the insertion of ventilation tubes for chronic serous otitis media. Many such children make multiple trips to the hospital for ventilation tubes, but the procedures are canceled because of a runny nose. Many anesthesiologists are willing to proceed with this group of patients,[14,15,17] and some have reported no increase in perioperative complications associated with uncomplicated URIs.[15,17] Although one must be prepared to face the consequences of anesthetizing a child with an irritable airway such as cough, breath holding, and laryngeal spasm, one study recently suggested that the majority of complications were associated with endotracheal intubation.[15] In our experience, a gentle induction with an intravenous or inhalational agent is most appropriate. Procedures of brief duration or those in which the airway is not very reactive can usually be managed without intubation. If endotracheal intubation is otherwise indicated or is needed because of difficulty with airway management, then the endotracheal tube should be inserted early. Muscle relaxants are usually needed in this situation to facilitate early endotracheal intubation. At the termination of surgery, the airway should be cleared of secretions, and the endotracheal tube should be removed only after the child is fully awake. Because some of these children may be at increased risk of developing transient postoperative hypoxemia, they should be given supplemental oxygen and/or have their oxygen saturation monitored during transport and in the postanesthesia care unit (PACU).[18]

The Ex-premie

The age of the child is usually not a limiting factor in scheduling surgery on an ambulatory basis at most institutions.[4,6,8,19,20] At Children's National Medical Center (CNMC), 14 days is arbitrarily selected as the minimal age for considering an otherwise healthy full-term infant suitable for ambulatory surgery. Some major pediatric centers, however, are reluctant to discharge even a previously healthy full-term infant less than three to six months of age on the day of surgery. This may be due to the possible association of postoperative respiratory problems with sudden infant death syndrome (SIDS) in this group. The premature infant, however, is unsuitable for ambulatory surgery because of potential immaturity of temperature control, respiratory center, and gag reflexes. Hypothermia, irregular breathing, apnea, laryngeal spasm, and aspiration of liquid or food are common and may occur in the immediate postoperative period. Infants who are anemic or who have a history of apnea or aspiration with feeding, as well as survivors of respiratory distress syndrome, are considered to be especially at risk. Those who have required endotracheal intubation, with or without mechanical ventilation, for treatment of respiratory insufficiency following birth may have abnormal blood gases and pulmonary function tests for six months to a year following termination of therapy.[21] Recent studies have reported perioperative complications such as apnea even in the absence of a history of respiratory distress syndrome.

In a retrospective chart review of healthy infants undergoing herniorrhaphy, Steward[22] reported that preterm infants who require surgery during the first months of life are more likely to develop respiratory complications during and following anesthesia than are full-term infants. He found that 12% of preterm infants were observed to have prolonged apnea during and up to 12 hours after anesthesia. None required mechanical ventilation postoperatively. In the prospective study by Liu and coworkers,[23] six infants with a history of apnea and a conceptual age below 46 weeks (Fig. 4-1) were observed to have prolonged apnea after anesthesia and surgery. Seven infants who had a preoperative history of apnea but a conceptual age of 46 to 80 weeks were not observed to have apnea postoperatively. A large number of patients in this study required mechanical ventilation for other, preexisting conditions (e.g., brain damage), and therefore, the true incidence of apnea that is precipitated by anesthesia and surgery in this subgroup remains unknown.

In a study of 86 otherwise healthy infants of less than 12 months postnatal age undergoing general anesthesia for herniorrhaphy, Welborn and coworkers found no incidents of apnea or periodic breathing with bradycardia on postoperative pneumograms, even in patients who had a history of preanesthetic apnea and who were being monitored for apnea at home. Periodic breathing without bradycardia, however, was found in 14 of 38 preterm infants during the postoperative period. In 4 of the 14 there was no preoperative history of apnea. Periodic breathing occurred as late as five hours postoperatively and was more frequent the more immature the baby. Apnea and/or periodic breathing did not occur in former premature infants whose conceptual age was more than 44 weeks and who were without any major systemic disease at the time of surgery.

In a later study, however, Welborn reported a 73% incidence of postoperative prolonged apnea with bradycardia in a similar group of infants whose conceptual age ranged between 35 to 44 weeks.[25] In still another prospective study using pneumography, Kurth and coworkers[26] observed a 37% incidence of postanesthetic prolonged apnea limited to 47 former preterm infants whose conceptual

HOW OLD IS YOUR PATIENT?

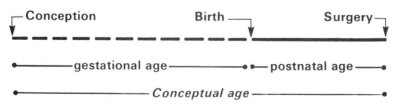

FIGURE 4-1. How the conceptual age of a prematurely-born infant is calculated.

ages varied from 32 weeks to as old as 55 weeks. These authors also demonstrated that the initial episode of apnea could occur as late as 12 hours after anesthesia.

Mestad and coworkers[27] reported an 18% incidence of apnea following discharge from the PACU in a group of former preterm infants who underwent general anesthesia for repair of inguinal hernia or lacrimal duct probing. Infants who developed apnea were less than 39 weeks post-conceptual age, and 89% had a history of apnea and/or lung disease. Patients with conceptual ages of more than 40 weeks without a prior history of apnea or lung disease did not develop apnea postoperatively. Recently, Tetzlaff and coworkers[28] reported a full-term infant who had prolonged and repetitive apneic episodes following anesthesia for eye surgery at a post-conceptual age of 42 weeks and a post-natal age of 21 and 27 days.

This brief summary emphasizes the difficulty of interpreting and objectively comparing much of the existing literature. Each of these studies has limitations. Although the sum total of cases reported in the literature is approximately 300, no one study has a large series of ASA physical status 1 or 2 patients undergoing the same operative procedure with the same anesthetic technique by the same anesthesiologist and the same surgeon and under the same operating room conditions.[29] Many of the data are derived from retrospective reviews of complications or from patients with preexisting disease who underwent complex surgical procedures. Therefore, it is difficult to make definitive statements that apply to all conditions. Moreover, the significance of apneic episodes that are long enough to result in bradycardia and arterial oxygen desaturation but eventually self-correct before cardiorespiratory arrest develops remains enigmatic.[30] While one may argue that the spontaneous return of respiration is the most likely outcome in these infants, potential deleterious hypoxic-ischemic effects on the brain or even a relationship to SIDS in many children has been suggested. Failure to detect and treat breathing irregularities in these high-risk infants may increase the likelihood of sudden death. The bottom line is that a history of prematurity is a red flag that means these infants must be observed very carefully for episodes of postoperative apnea.[29]

The age at which the premature infant attains physiologic maturity and no longer presents an increased risk must be considered individually, with attention given to growth and development, persistent problems during feeding, time to recover from upper respiratory infections, apneic history, and presence or absence of metabolic, endocrine, neurologic, or cardiac disorders.

It is generally considered that the infants at greatest risk are those younger than 46 weeks post-conceptual age with a preoperative history of apnea. Obviously, there must be a middle ground between the conservative 60 weeks recommended by Kurth and coworkers and the recommendations by Liu et al. and Welborn et al. of 44 to 46 weeks. It appears that as the child matures, the tendency toward apnea greatly diminishes, but no one knows the age when all babies may be safely anesthetized. Therefore, until more extensive, meticulous, prospective studies are carried out, it seems prudent to admit to the hospital all ex-premature infants less than 50 weeks post-conceptual age so that they may be monitored for possible apnea, bradycardia, and oxygen desaturation. It is also appropriate to individualize this decision and, when in doubt, to err on the side of conservatism. If the infant has bronchopulmonary dysplasia (BPD), this period should be extended for as long as the infant is symptomatic. Should any questions arise, inpatient care is recommended (see additional discussion, Chapter 9, case 7).

By far the most common elective surgical procedure performed on infants three to six months of age is repair of an inguinal hernia—a procedure perfectly suited for ambulatory surgery. Since preterm infants have a substantially higher incidence of inguinal hernias than term infants, the former represent a significant number of those who appear on the surgical schedule for operative repair. Because of the risk of incarceration, the patients usually require "urgent" surgery. Also, because of the many medical and economic benefits of day surgery, pressure exists to send these infants home on the same day of surgery.[31] The responsibility of the medical team is to screen these patients who are considered high risk. Ideally, this is done by the surgeon's office or the screening clinic before the day of surgery. Cases that are undetected during the initial screening must be identified on the day of surgery. Parents of any infant under six months of age must be specifically asked about history of prematurity. If the child was born prematurely, then the immediate postnatal history must be carefully reviewed: *Did the child have any respiratory difficulty? Did he or she need supplemental oxygen, endotracheal intubation, mechanical ventilation, and so forth? Is there a history of apnea? Was an apnea monitor needed in the hospital or at home? Is there a history of feeding difficulty, aspiration, repeated lung infections, or wheezing?* This information is vital before a decision can be made to proceed with ambulatory surgery in an infant who was premature, and therefore cannot be left to parents to volunteer such information spontaneously.

Two recent reports by Welborn and coworkers[25,30] suggest that the use of a single intravenous dose of caffeine at the beginning of surgery may be effective in the control of postanesthetic apnea in former premature infants. When a 5-mg/kg dose was used, no infant developed prolonged apnea with bradycardia.[25] Complete abolition of all types of apnea, however, was not seen. In a later study, the authors reported that a 10-mg/kg dose of caffeine was effective in the control of all types of apnea in these infants.[30] It is still recommended that until more extensive experience with this approach is available, all infants at risk should be monitored for apnea and/or bradycardia following anesthesia.

The Child with a Heart Murmur

A common problem in pediatric outpatient anesthesia is the child in whom a previously undiagnosed cardiac murmur is first heard during the preanesthetic examination. Even if the child is active and shows no signs of cardiac disease such as cyanosis, clubbing of the fingers, or congestive heart failure, it is imperative that the cause of the murmur be correctly diagnosed prior to anesthesia and surgery. A recent study has shown that a pediatric cardiologist may be the only person who can confirm that a murmur is innocent by physical examination alone.[32] At CNMC, the following grid serves as a guide as to when a cardiology consultation is needed before proceeding with surgery:

The Child with a Heart Murmur

By Whom?	Clinical Diagnosis	No heart disease	Possible heart disease		Definite heart disease
Anesthesiologist		Yes	Yes	No	Yes
Pediatrician		Yes	No	Yes	Yes
Cardiology consult		No	Yes		Yes

A child with a confirmed cardiac lesion may not require specific preoperative cardiac therapy or even a modification in the selection of anesthetic agents and technique, but he or she usually needs antibiotic prophylaxis to prevent subacute bacterial endocarditis. To prevent delays and cancellations, surgeons and pediatricians must be told to have a child with a murmur fully evaluated prior to the day of surgery. The specific diagnosis, and recommendations for therapy, if any, should be known by the anesthesiologist in advance. For quick reference, every department of anesthesiology should have available the most recent American Heart Association's guidelines[33] for prevention of bacterial endocarditis. The instruction card used at CNMC gives the following protocol:

Bacterial Endocarditis Prevention in Pediatric Patients

*For Dental Procedures and Surgery of the Upper Respiratory Tract**

1. Parenteral: Aqueous crystalline penicillin G, 50,000 units/kg IV during induction or IM, 30–60 min before procedure and then 25,000 units/kg IV or IM 6 hr later. Oral penicillin V (1 g for children > 27 kg or 500 mg for those < 27 kg) may be used for the second dose.
2. Oral: Penicillin V, 2 g orally 1 hr before procedure, then 1 g 6 hr later. For children < 27 kg, use 1 g orally 1 hr before procedure, then 500 mg 6 hr later.

For children allergic to penicillin: Erythromycin, 20 mg/kg orally, 1 hr prior to procedure, then 10 mg/kg 6 hr later.

For Gastrointestinal and Genitourinary Tract Surgery and Instrumentation

Ampicillin, 50 mg/kg, IV or IM

Plus

Gentamicin, 2 mg/kg IM or IV
Give initial dose 30 min prior to procedure, then 1 g oral penicillin V 6 hr later. The parenteral regimen may be repeated once 8 hr later.

For children allergic to penicillin: Vancomycin, 20 mg/kg, given IV slowly over 1 hr, starting 1 hr *before* procedure. No repeat dose is necessary.

*NOTE: Another regimen is used for children with prosthetic heart valves.

THE PARENT

In the past, the choice of outpatient care has been largely influenced by parents' wishes and the experiences of friends and family. Third-party payors are now increasingly reluctant to comply with parents' demands for hospitalization of a healthy child who is having a relatively minor superficial operation. Parents of pediatric outpatients, however, should be capable of understanding and willing to follow specific instructions related to ambulatory surgery. In most cases, it is up to the physician to educate them and make them feel secure and comfortable.

THE PROCEDURE

The planned surgical procedure should be brief and should be associated with only minimal bleeding and minor physiologic derangements. Reed and Ford stated that almost any operation that does not require a major intervention into the cranial vault, abdomen, or thorax can be considered.[34] Superficial procedures are selected most often. Septic cases are rarely considered because of the need for separate facilities in the recovery room.

A representative list of procedures that are commonly performed at CNMC is given below. Of these, the five most frequently performed operations during the past two years were herniorrhaphy, myringotomy, adenoidectomy with or without myringotomy, circumcision, and eye-muscle surgery.

General surgery:
  Hernia repair
  Excision of cyst, ganglion, skin
    lesion, breast mass
  Suture of lacerations; removal
    of sutures
  Dressing change
  Muscle biopsy
  Sigmoidoscopy, bronchoscopy,
    esophagoscopy and
    dilatation
  Incision and drainage of
    abscess
  Protologic and vaginal
    procedures
Otolaryngology:
  Adenoidectomy
  Myringotomy and insertion of
    tubes
  Removal of foreign body from
    ear
  Frenulectomy
  Laryngoscopy
  Closed reduction of nasal
    fracture

Ophthalmology:
  Examination under anesthesia
  Eye-muscle surgery
  Lacrimal duct probing
  Excision of chalazion
  Insertion of lens or prosthesis
Dental:
  Extraction
  Restoration
Orthopedic:
  Cast change
  Arthroscopy
  Closed reduction of fracture
  Manipulation
Urology:
  Cystoscopy
  Meatotomy
  Orchiopexy
  Circumcision
  Hydrocelectomy
  Testicular biopsy
Plastic surgery:
  Otoplasty
  Scar revision

At the Surgicenter in Phoenix, Arizona, a mixed pediatric-adult surgical setting where children less than 12 years of age comprise 30% of the population, two of the five most commonly performed operations are myringotomy with or without adenoidectomy and herniotomy. Since the customary dividing line between pediatric and adult patients is defined as 17 to 18 years of age, it is no wonder that many children's hospitals and mixed facilities report that over 40% of the pediatric surgery is being performed on an ambulatory basis.

Private insurance and Medicaid guidelines in some states mandate that certain surgical procedures be performed on an ambulatory basis unless factors exist that prohibit this form of care.[35] If these procedures are performed as inpatient surgery, reimbursement to the hospital for room and board is not provided. Special, individual consideration for reimbursable hospitalization is given, however, under the following conditions:

> Patients with coexisting medical conditions, such as severe diabetes or
>   heart disease, that make prolonged postoperative observation by a
>   nurse or skilled medical personnel a necessity
> Patients who will simultaneously undergo an unrelated procedure that
>   itself requires hospitalization
> Patients who lack proper home postoperative care
> Patients in whom there is a possibility that more major surgery could
>   follow the initial procedure
> Technical difficulties, as documented by admission or operative notes

Because of the increased risk of hemorrhage, there is a continuing debate as to the advisability of performing tonsillectomy with or without adenoidectomy as an outpatient procedure. This procedure is not currently performed on an ambulatory basis at CNMC. In 1968, however, Chiang and associates[36] reported 40,000 outpatient tonsillectomies and adenoidectomies (T&As) without death. In order to decrease the risk of hemorrhage, they emphasized careful selection of cases and preoperative evaluation to eliminate patients with bleeding tendencies and cardiopulmonary disease. Also, no "allergic" patient was operated on during the pollen season, and no operation was performed until 4 to 5 weeks after an acute attack of tonsillitis.

More recently, Maniglia and coworkers[37] reported a series of 1428 cases of adenotonsillectomies performed on outpatients. Two cases (0.14%) of immediate (within 24 hours) bleeding and two late (after 24 hours) episodes occurred. The two incidents of immediate bleeding occurred within the first hour following the surgical procedure. The authors concluded that outpatient adenotonsillectomy is safe and cost-effective and that there was little benefit in keeping patients in the hospital more than a few hours after surgery.

A particularly informative discussion of the T&A question was provided by Ahlgren and coworkers.[19] Of the 977 cases they reported in 1969, 184 were T&As. Average recovery-room time for these patients was more than twice that for patients undergoing other procedures (233 versus 102 minutes). The most common complication was vomiting, usually of old blood. Of the 33 patients who developed laryngeal stridor, 7 were in the T&A group. The authors noted, however, that 15% of the patients undergoing eye-muscle procedures had stridor, compared with 4% in the T&A group. Three of the ophthalmologic patients and one T&A patient who developed this complication required hospitalization. The authors concluded that since only 2% of the T&A group required admission for bleeding (4 of the 184 patients), the incidence was not high enough to eliminate the procedure from an outpatient setting. It must be noted, however, that of the 17 patients in their series requiring hospitalization, 5 were in the T&A group.

PREOPERATIVE PREPARATION AND SCREENING

From the anesthesiologist's point of view, the essential preoperative requirements for safe conduct of anesthesia in pediatric outpatients are the same as those for inpatients. A complete history and physical examination (H&P) performed by a member of the medical staff, appropriate laboratory tests, consultations when indicated, an appropriate fasting period, and a chance to personally evaluate and establish rapport with the child and the parents are the standard preanesthetic requirements. *The special challenge in ambulatory surgery, however, is to accomplish as many of these steps as possible before the child arrives at the facility for surgery and therefore to minimize delays and last-minute cancellations.* This requires proper planning and organization.

Since the surgeon is the first member of the team the parents will meet when ambulatory surgery is scheduled, the smoothness and success of the whole experience will depend on the conduct of the first visit. Because of the very brief encounter on the day of surgery, the parents (and the child, when appropriate) must have the procedure explained and have as many of their questions as possible answered in the surgeon's office. Assured, relaxed parents will be more supportive and reassuring to the child. Arrangements for preoperative laboratory testing can be made at this time, and detailed written instructions can be given about fasting, where and when to report on the day of surgery, and whom to call for further instructions if the child develops a cold, fever, or any unexpected illness while waiting for surgery.

Since the appropriate period of preoperative fasting varies with age, it is often useful to prepare a few sets of instructions for different age groups and hand (or mail) them to parents as appropriate. A child should not be made to fast for a prolonged period of time (beyond what is safe for his or her age). Besides the possible risk of dehydration, or hypoglycemia in young infants, children are usually more irritable and upset when hungry or thirsty. On the other hand, one should allow for some flexibility in scheduling the child for surgery earlier in the day should an unexpected cancellation occur. Jensen and coworkers recently measured blood glucose concentrations in a group of children six months to nine years of age undergoing inpatient and outpatient anesthesia. They reported only one case (1%) of hypoglycemia in an inpatient who fasted overnight. They concluded that in order to minimize the risk of hypoglycemia and inhalation of vomitus on the induction of anesthesia, children older than six months should fast overnight and be operated on in the morning.

It is interesting to note, however, that more recent studies suggest that a shorter period of fasting may be acceptable. The effect of 3 ml/kg of apple juice given 2.6 ± 0.4 hours preoperatively was investigated in 80 healthy children of ages five to ten years in a prospective, randomized, single-blind study.[39] The children who drank apple juice preoperatively had decreased gastric volume, thirst, and hunger ($p < 0.05$). The gastric volume in the control group was 0.43 ± 0.46 ml/kg, and in the patients who received apple juice, the gastric volume was 0.24 ± 0.31 ml/kg. The gastric pH was not significantly different, with the control group's pH being 1.7 ± 0.6 and the treated group's pH being 2.2 ± 1.2. Although it may be premature to change our anesthetic practice based on the results of studies on a small series of patients, this and similar findings are important starting points for future investigations.[40] Large, well-controlled studies may result in significant modification of current fasting guidelines and may make anesthesia safer and less difficult for children (and adults).[40] Current NPO requirements at CNMC are found in Table 4-1. Examples of the instruction sheets handed to parents can be found in the section "Forms and Policies" at the end of the book. At the Hospital for Sick Children (HSC) in Toronto, Canada, the preoperative fasting period is shorter, and most children undergoing minor surgery as outpatients do not receive infused fluids. For comparison the preoperative fasting orders for outpatients in the HSC (1984) are as follows:

> Infants under two years of age should be given clear fluids until four hours before surgery. Other feedings must be discontinued at least six hours before the induction of anesthesia.
> Children over two years of age must have no food on the day of operation but may be offered clear fluids up to 4 hours preoperatively.

Various medications have been reported to decrease the volume of gastric contents in pediatric patients. The oral administration of such drugs as cimetidine (2.5–7.5 mg/kg),[41] ranitidine (2.5 mg/kg),[42] or sodium citrate (0.4 ml/kg)[43] can reduce the volume and/or the acidity of gastric contents. However, since the actual risk of aspiration in the healthy fasting pediatric outpatient is believed to be very small, the routine use of these agents has not been widespread.

The actual laboratory data required in children, as well as the length of time specimens can be analyzed prior to surgery, vary between hospitals. Complete blood count (CBC) and urinalysis are the usual requirements; however, a few pediatric institutions either do not demand a urinalysis or request it only when

TABLE 4-1. NPO Orders at CNMC

Age	Interval between Solid Food*	Interval between Clear Liquids†
<1 yr	6 hr	4 hr
1–6 yrs	MN	6 hr
>6 yrs	MN	8 hr

*Includes milk or milk products.
†Includes breast milk.

TABLE 4-2. Normal Hematocrit Values

Age	Mean	Range
Birth	54	45–65
3 mos	36	30–41
5 mo–6 yrs	37	33–42
6–12 yrs	38	35–42

SOURCE: Berry.[46]

there is a history of genitourinary disease. A "routine" preoperative chest radiograph is rarely a requirement in pediatric anesthesia.[44,45]

The minimum acceptable hematocrit value for an otherwise healthy child varies with age. If the hematocrit is not in the normal range for a given age group (Table 4-2), an appropriate medical workup should be performed and elective surgery postponed. Children with underlying medical conditions such as renal disease or leukemia may consequently have long-standing anemia and are usually accepted if otherwise suitable for a brief ambulatory procedure.

Busy day-surgery units cannot rely on the surgeon alone to present them consistently with a fully evaluated and prepared child. This is especially true when a large number of surgeons with varying interests and attitudes have privileges to practice in the unit. In order to expedite the evaluation process and ensure some degree of uniformity in the preoperative preparation of the child, personnel other than surgeons in some facilities have found it useful to participate in the preoperative screening process. The degree of involvement varies from a simple phone call to the parents by the unit clerk a day or two prior to surgery to the establishment of a formal screening clinic to clear all patients before admission into the operating suite.

We feel that the process proceeds most expeditiously when there is a screening clinic primarily staffed by a pediatric nurse practitioner or a physician's assistant who is responsible to, and remains in close contact with, the department of anesthesiology. One of the functions of the clinic is to telephone the parents. The parents of each child are contacted initially by telephone shortly after the operation has been posted and a second time within 48 hours of the scheduled surgery. The initial telephone interivew is highly specific and is directed at identifying any past or present risk factors such as the following (see also the preoperative telephone screening questionnaire in the section on Forms and Policies at the end of the book):

> Breath-holding spells (apnea)
> Cardiac, respiratory, and other problems
> History of prematurity:
> > Was oxygen required?
> > Was child intubated?
> > Lasting effects?
> Muscular problems
> Developmental delays

Significant findings are reported to the anesthesiologist who can then determine whether additional preoperative evaluation is required in advance of surgery and/or question the suitability of performing the procedure on an ambulatory basis. During the subsequent phone call, NPO orders should be reinforced, a reassessment of the patient's present health made, and any social questions answered about parking, what to bring to the hospital, the rules of the short-stay recovery unit, and so forth.

The clinic also functions as an area in which families are seen and services are arranged:

On the day before surgery or earlier if needed: Clinic services are available for families whose children do not have their own pediatrician to perform the H&P or for those who prefer to have the child come to the hospital in advance of the day of surgery for any other reason. Personnel in the clinic obtain all necessary information to preregister the child, perform a definitive H&P, and arrange for any needed consultations and laboratory tests. This earlier visit, which is optional for a healthy child, is mandatory for any child who has a history of a chronic disease process that requires consultation or special management.

On the day of surgery: Children who have not been seen before the day of surgery are fully evaluated (H&P, laboratory, and so on). *All* patients are screened for acute illness (e.g., URI) and NPO status. Consultation reports are evaluated, and the need for any special preoperative psychological or pharmacologic treatment is considered before the child is routed to the operating room. The patient therefore always arrives in the operating room with a complete evaluation, including a valid permit for anesthesia and surgery. This avoids unnecessary delays and frustrations.

PREPARATION OF THE CHILD FOR AMBULATORY SURGERY
Psychological Preparation
From a psychological point of view, anesthesia and surgery on an outpatient basis can be a mixed blessing. The short stay in the hospital or surgery facility has the definite advantage of minimizing or even eliminating the trauma of separating child and parent; however, it may present other emotional problems.

Many of these problems result from the child's lack of familiarity with the hospital environment and the very brief exposure that precedes the induction of anesthesia. In many centers, the child may be taken to the operating room within 30 to 45 minutes of admission—hardly enough time for the child to become familiar with the new surroundings or to establish a rapport with the staff. In this respect, the inpatient who spends the night before surgery in the hospital has some advantage. This is especially true in institutions that offer "rooming in" accommodations for a parent who wishes to remain with the hospitalized child overnight. Once in the ward, the inpatient gets to know the hospital routine, meets the nurses and doctors, and sees children who are recovering from surgery and who are wearing hospital gowns, bandages, and the like. The child and parents have a good chance to ask questions and get reassuring answers. This experience, which takes away some of the fears of the unknown, may make the induction of anesthesia much smoother and also makes the postoperative period less frightening.

The outpatient deserves the same opportunity. This is why preparation should start a few days before surgery, with a visit to the hospital, a tour of the facility, and a movie or a puppet show that illustrates the entire procedure in language the child understands.

At CNMC, and in many other pediatric institutions, the children and parents are invited for a preoperative visit to the hospital. A puppet show or a movie is followed by a short tour of the hospital, conducted by a caring staff who are trained to answer all questions honestly, to familiarize the child and his or her parents with what will happen on the day of surgery. The tour is oriented to the child and is conducted in a friendly, playful fashion with special attention paid to the following areas:

1. *Preoperative encounters:* The tour guide must carefully ascertain that the child actually knows he or she will be coming to the hospital for surgery. This is a bad time to first inform an unsuspecting child that he or she is not really here to "have a picture taken." The admission procedure and the need for laboratory tests are explained, and the wearing and use of identification bands and hospital gowns are stressed. Finally, the actual waiting area, or playroom, where child (and parents if appropriate) will eventually go on the day of surgery is visited. The child is encouraged to bring along a favorite toy or comforter. Some children might want to try on a hospital gown at this time and get the other children to become familiar with its appearance. (For many young children, having to undress and wear that strange gown is one of the worst events they remember about the day of surgery.)

2. *The operating room:* The child is shown either a special operating or induction room or an anesthesia machine that has been set aside for this purpose. The child is allowed to handle the machine, breathing circuits, masks, syringes, and so forth. Although it is often difficult to spot an unusually fearful child at this time, any such patient should be brought to the attention of the department of anesthesiology for "extraspecial handling."

3. *The recovery area:* Both the recovery room and the location where the child will stay until fit for discharge should be shown. The fact that the child may be hurting after surgery should be mentioned, with the reassurance that measures will be taken to minimize the discomfort. Any special equipment such as an intravenous line, oxygen tubing, and thermometer should be demonstrated. The child should be told where and when he or she will meet the parents, and it should be emphasized that the stay will last only one day.

Included in the tour is either a live or videotaped puppet show depicting "Clipper" undergoing the hospital experience, including anesthesia, surgery, and recovery (Fig. 4-2). In group tours, the children seem to like the puppet shows

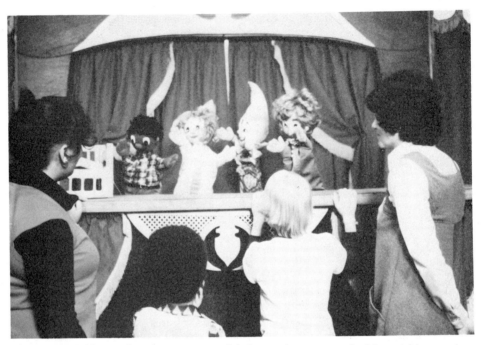

FIGURE 4-2. Children and parents get many of their questions answered while watching a puppet show during the preoperative tour at CNMC.

and can participate when the group is asked to sing along. This is followed by punch and cookies in the hospital cafeteria, where children and their parents have plenty of time to ask questions.

Although there is a general consensus that this kind of preparation program is useful, there are few studies that document its value. Rosen and coworkers[47] studied anesthesia induction in 500 unpremedicated children between the ages of 2 and 12. They found that children who attended a preadmission orientation program (including a puppet show) did significantly better during the induction of anesthesia than those who did not attend. We need to be careful, however, when interpreting these results. Parental motivation, traveling distance, socioeconomic conditions, and the child's age are some of the factors that motivate the parents to bring their children to the program. These factors may in themselves lead to better cooperation. Additionally, children who have undergone previous anesthetics rarely returned to attend the program, and these children were shown to have poorer cooperation rating.

It would be very desirable to have different preoperative programs for adolescents and handicapped children. At the Children's Hospital of Denver, for example, a separate program for adolescents was instituted in response to complaints that some of the teenagers were insulted by terms such as *magic gas*, which are often used to explain anesthesia induction to preschool children.

Although these recommendations represent an ideal comprehensive approach

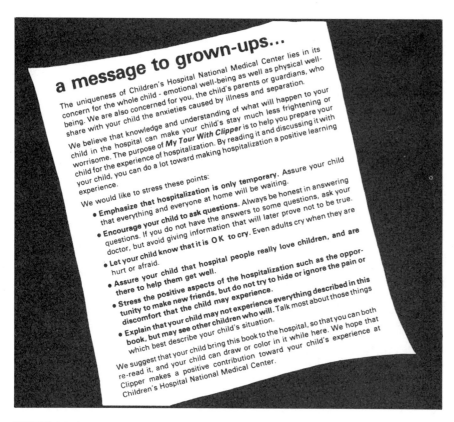

a message to grown-ups...

The uniqueness of Children's Hospital National Medical Center lies in its concern for the whole child - emotional well-being as well as physical well-being. We are also concerned for you, the child's parents or guardians, who share with your child the anxieties caused by illness and separation.

We believe that knowledge and understanding of what will happen to your child in the hospital can make your child's stay much less frightening or worrisome. The purpose of *My Tour With Clipper* is to help you prepare your child for the experience of hospitalization. By reading it and discussing it with your child, you can do a lot toward making hospitalization a positive learning experience.

We would like to stress these points:

- **Emphasize that hospitalization is only temporary.** Assure your child that everything and everyone at home will be waiting.
- **Encourage your child to ask questions.** Always be honest in answering questions. If you do not have the answers to some questions, ask your doctor, but avoid giving information that will later prove not to be true.
- **Let your child know that it is O K to cry.** Even adults cry when they are hurt or afraid.
- **Assure your child that hospital people really love children, and are** there to help them get well.
- **Stress the positive aspects of the hospitalization such as the opportunity to make new friends, but do not try to hide or ignore the pain or** discomfort that the child may experience.
- **Explain that your child may not experience everything described in this book, but may see other children who will.** Talk most about those things which best describe your child's situation.

We suggest that your child bring this book to the hospital, so that you can both re-read it, and your child can draw or color in it while here. We hope that Clipper makes a positive contribution toward your child's experience at Children's Hospital National Medical Center.

FIGURE 4-3. A message to grown-ups. The inside cover of the "coloring book" information booklet mailed to children before surgery.

to the psychological preparation of the child for ambulatory surgery, some institutions are unable or unwilling to provide this service. In these cases, the surgeon's office usually undertakes this function. Books, pamphlets, and handouts are available that can help the parents understand their child's forthcoming surgery. The surgeon and other members of the health care team should be aware of these publications and their availability.[48] Ideally, a description of the process at the particular hospital in which the operation is scheduled should be distributed to the parent by the surgeon in the office at the time the surgery is scheduled. At that time, some of the important features of the forthcoming procedure can be discussed, and the pamphlet can be reviewed later at home by the parents and child. An example of the introductory remarks from the coloring book used at CNMC outlines its purpose (Fig. 4-3).

PHARMACOLOGIC PREMEDICATION

The value of and need for pharmacologic premedication in pediatric day-surgery patients is a difficult question to answer in a general way. With modern agents and techniques, it is now possible to anesthetize an unmedicated, struggling, screaming child in a few minutes with no apparent physical or physiologic harm.[49,50] As a result, premedication has now assumed more value for the emotional protection of the child rather than as an adjunct to anesthesia. Although most authors usually state that if the child has been properly prepared, premedication is not necessary,[6,51] or is even undesirable if it prolongs recovery and delays discharge home, others feel that some form of sedation is advantageous[52-55] to facilitate anesthesia induction.

A close look at some representative studies illustrates the nature of this controversy. In a recent study of oral premedication in 143 children, preoperative and postoperative sedation was compared following oral trimeprazine (4 mg/kg) versus diazepam (0.25 mg/kg) with and without added droperidol (0.2 mg/kg).[56] Trimeprazine produced significantly more preoperative sedation and postoperative analgesia with less vomiting than did diazepam. The addition of droperidol only marginally improved the performance of these drugs but further delayed discharge times. It is worth noting, however, that the dose of trimeprazine used in this study frequently produced sedation lasting several hours into the postoperative period. While this is an obvious disadvantage in ambulatory patients, smaller doses of trimeprazine produce a less predictable result and may even have a hyperexcitable effect.

Although narcotics alone usually do not effectively reduce preoperative anxiety, satisfactory results have been obtained by using combinations of narcotics and sedatives or tranquilizers. In one study,[52] children who were given an oral preparation of meperidine, diazepam, and atropine in doses of 1.5, 0.2, and 0.02 mg/kg, respectively, exhibited a significantly lower incidence of crying and secretions upon arrival in the operating room—conditions that are favorable for smooth mask induction—than those who did not receive premedication (19% vs. 34%). There was no difference in the total recovery time from anesthesia to discharge home between the medicated and the control groups (147 ± 80 min vs. 156 ± 78 min, respectively). Another study,[51] however, found that the oral administration of hydroxyzine, promethazine, or diazepam was no better than placebo in easing the induction of anesthesia or protecting against psychological reactions in the early postoperative period. Of the inductions in these cases, however, 73% were with intravenous thiopental sodium. In no case did any of the oral preparations used for premedication cause a significant delay in recovery from anesthesia or discharge home.

In another study where intravenous thiopental was used for induction, Booker and Chapman[57] found no difference in the incidence of unacceptable behavior during induction between one group of children medicated with intramuscular morphine/atropine and another who received an oral preparation of dichloral-phenazone and paracetamol. Morphine, however, had a pronounced emetic effect that lasted into the period following surgery, and many children remarked that the intramuscular injection before the operation was the worst thing that happened to them in the hospital. Children premedicated with morphine were significantly more drowsy at home, especially following pain-free procedures, than those who received no narcotics or even those who received intravenous fentanyl (3 µg/kg) intraoperatively for more painful operations. Of particular interest in this study was the observation that 25% to 38% of the children who had exhibited an unacceptable demeanor during induction had received their premedicant drug too late to allow for full sedating effect—a common problem, especially in outpatient practice. Still another study[58] found intramuscular ketamine (3 mg/kg) to be an effective premedicant in children under two years of age who were given thiopental, nitrous oxide, oxygen, succinylcholine anesthesia for elective outpatient adenoidectomy. It was more than three times as effective as narcotic (meperidine, 1 mg/kg) in calming or sedating a child, with no prolongation in recovery time, and no difference in the emotional state following recovery.

The use of midazolam, a water-soluble benzodiazepine, has been advocated for preoperative sedation in children. In a study of 90 children 1 to 15 years of age scheduled for ambulatory surgery, Rita et al.[59] found that patients 1 to 5 years old who received midazolam (0.08 mg/kg IM) were significantly more sedated preoperatively than patients who received morphine (0.15 mg/kg IM) or placebo. They also found that smooth induction of anesthesia occurred more frequently in children who were given midazolam than in patients sedated with morphine or control. The midazolam group had shorter lengths of stay in the PACU and a lower incidence of vomiting and sleepiness postoperatively.

In a different study,[60] midazolam (0.2 mg/kg) was compared with papaveretum (0.4 mg/kg) and scopolamine (0.008 mg/kg) as an intramuscular premedication in small children (2 to 10 years of age). Midazolam produced satisfactory sedation and anxiolysis, and during the early postoperative period, patients were significantly more awake.

The major problem, however, in applying the results of such studies to clinical practice is that they merely compare the effects of different premedication regimens or a placebo on a mixed group of children. The results cannot be used to predict a similar effect when dealing with the individual child who is unusually apprehensive or disturbed. Our own feeling is that with proper psychological preparation and establishment of a rapport with the anesthesiologists, and with limited separation of the child from parents (up to the induction or including parents during the induction), the majority of children do not need preoperative sedation. But some—up to 20% of all children—do.

If a patient is to undergo repeated painful procedures, is known to be very apprehensive, or is too young to benefit from verbal reassurance, a mild tranquilizer can be ordered in advance and given at home before the child comes to the hospital. When indicated, oral premedication with triclofos (80 mg/kg mixed in a flavored solution to conceal its bad taste)[46] or diazepam suspension (0.2–0.4 mg/kg) has been found useful.[6] An adequate time interval (1–2 hr) must be allowed for the full effect of the drugs. If drying agents are specifically indicated, oral atropine or glycopyrrolate (0.02 mg/kg) can be used. Intramuscular injections should be avoided whenever possible for routine premedication in children. Walters et al.[61] have shown in a prospective double-blind study that oral and intramuscular premedication can be equally effective in producing a cooperative and drowsy patient at anesthetic induction.

PREINDUCTION AGENTS

If preoperative sedation is not used routinely in ambulatory patients, the anesthesiologist must be prepared to handle the occasional uncooperative or extremely frightened child by using a preinduction agent. This is especially important if an inhaled induction has been planned.

The use of preinduction agents is becoming increasingly popular in pediatric anesthesia.[62,63] *Preinduction anesthesia* refers to the use of such drugs as ketamine or other rapidly acting medications as a form of last-minute premedication. The selection of a particular drug and dose should ensure a rapid onset of sedation (3–10 min) with minimal or no prolongation of recovery. Even the possibility of a slightly prolonged recovery is a small price to pay for avoiding the potential psychological trauma of a stormy induction.[64] Table 4-3 indicates the relationships of the various induction techniques.

Several preinduction techniques claim to achieve cooperation of children during inhaled induction of anesthesia. Rectal administration of methohexital has gained wide acceptance since the early reports of its successful use by Goresky and Steward.[65] Following a dose of 25 mg/kg (10% solution), most children fall asleep within 6 to 11 minutes. This onset time makes the technique useful in achieving enough sedation to peacefully separate an upset child from his or her parents, but too long to be really practical in a child who decides to refuse an inhaled (mask) induction at the last minute.

Low-dose (2 mg/kg) intramuscular ketamine has been found to be an acceptable preinduction agent in young children who do not cooperate with other methods of induction.[63] The onset time is short (2–3 min). In a recent study comparing recovery and discharge time following ketamine preinduction to pure inhaled anesthesia in young children undergoing brief surgical procedures, the recovery time was not prolonged. Even though the total discharge time was statistically longer when ketamine was used, the actual delay was less than 15 minutes. There were no emergence or postanesthetic reactions.[63] These recovery characteristics are much more appropriate for the ambulatory patient than those traditionally observed when a full IM induction dose of ketamine (5–10 mg/kg) is used.

Transmucosal administration of short-acting narcotics is also an effective way of producing preoperative sedation in pediatric patients. Only a few analgesics have thus far been evaluated. Although successful use of an oral transmucosal fentanyl "lollipop" (15–20 µg/kg)[66] as well as nasal sufentanil (1.5–3 µg/kg)[62] has been reported, much additional experience is still needed before the ultimate place of these approaches is firmly established. A recent study suggests that oral

TABLE 4-3. Pediatric Induction Techniques

Technique	Onset	Recovery
Premedication	Slow	Prolonged
Preinduction	Rapid	Variable
Induction	Immediate	Prompt

transmucosal fentanyl may be more useful in the management of postoperative pain in patients admitted to the hospital following operations associated with a great deal of pain than it is for preoperative sedation of ambulatory patients.[67] Intranasal administration of midazolam (0.2 mg/kg) also has been reported to produce anxiolysis and sedation in preschool children with a rapid onset (5–10 min) and no evidence of delayed recovery.[68] Unlike intranasal sufentanil, there was no concern about decreased ventilatory compliance during induction, even in the presence of nitrous oxide.

PREOPERATIVE PLAYROOM

In order to reduce the anxiety of the child without the aid of pharmacologic adjuncts, other techniques have been employed. One is the use of the preoperative holding area as a playroom. This area is usually adjacent to the operating rooms and is decorated in a style that makes the child feel at ease (Fig. 4-4). It is important that children be kept occupied while waiting for surgery. Bright colors on the walls; pictures of cartoon characters; toys, doll houses, coloring books, puzzles, and childrens' furniture all are incorporated so that the children identify the surroundings more with a friendly home or school atmosphere than with the often strange, threatening, sterile environment of a hospital or operating room. In a mixed facility, the play area can be incorporated into the general waiting room and is designed to accommodate healthy, unmedicated children and their parents up to the time of induction of anesthesia. The playroom is always su-

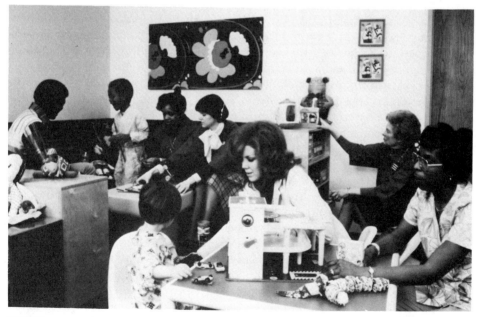

FIGURE 4-4. Unmedicated children must be kept busy while waiting for surgery. The playroom is staffed by volunteers.

pervised by a member of the hospital staff as well as volunteers who may answer questions from the child or parents or, in the absence of the latter, may act as a surrogate. Children are brought from the playroom to the operating room or induction room in a variety of ways, such as in the anesthesiologist's arms, in a red wagon, on a stretcher, or walking alongside the anesthesiologist. In some institutions, such as CNMC, the parent frequently accompanies the child to an induction room.

PARENTAL PRESENCE DURING INDUCTION

For a preschool child (ages two–six), it is very difficult to understand why the parents, who have accompanied him through all the preoperative preparation and orientation, should have to abandon him when the "big moment" arrives. Most of us are aware of the screaming and resistance that often occurs when a young child is taken away from his or her parents for surgery. Traditionally, this unpleasant situation has been avoided by using heavy doses of premedication preoperatively. With that, the anesthetic state is in effect initiated in the parent's presence and the anxiety of separation is minimized.

In ambulatory surgery patients, although it is desirable to avoid routine heavy premedication regimens, it is still essential that the goal of premedication (to make the child sedated or cause sleep before separation from the parents) not be sacrificed. One way of achieving that goal is to allow one or both parents to stay with the child during induction of anesthesia.[69]

Although for many anesthesiologists this may sound untraditional, it is becoming more accepted by others.[50,69–71] Indeed, some anesthesiologists feel that the presence of an intelligent, supportive parent during induction of anesthesia may be the best available substitute for premedication. It is largely because we encourage parents to be with their children during induction at CNMC that our use of pharmacologic sedation is minimal, especially for outpatients.

The majority of children scheduled for elective surgery at CNMC are unmedicated. They have anesthesia for elective surgery induced in one of the four induction rooms after coming to a preinduction play area. Both the play area and the induction rooms are located within the general operating room area, but outside the area limited to those operating room personnel who are properly attired. As a result, parents, volunteers, and staff may walk between playroom and induction rooms without changing into operating room apparel.

The parents are welcome to stay with their child during the induction of anesthesia and usually do. Other participants are at least one anesthesiologist and some other individual who can assist the anesthesiologist and/or escort the parents to the proper location following induction. This individual can be another anesthesiologist, an anesthesia aid, a surgeon, a volunteer, or an operating room nurse. We have had few problems with this concept, except that preschool children are usually more apprehensive and less cooperative than children of school age. Since induction of anesthesia is performed outside the operating room, only healthy children presenting for elective surgical procedures should be considered. Infants under one to one and one-half years of age are rarely suitable candidates.

The method of induction can vary according to the preference of the anesthesiologist and the needs of the child. Intravenous thiopental sodium (4–6 mg/kg), intramuscular ketamine (2–3 mg/kg), or rectal methohexital (25 mg/kg) have all been used satisfactorily. Unless there are specially equipped induction rooms or portable anesthesia machines, the use of an inhalational induction technique may not be possible. In all cases, however, equipment for airway management and resuscitation drugs must be immediately available.

There are nonetheless many possible reasons why the anesthesiologist may prefer not to have the parents present during anesthesia induction. The anesthesiologist may feel uncomfortable being "watched" by the parents. What if something goes wrong? Can the parents be critical? Furthermore, there is always the question of dividing one's attention between the child and parents. An anxious parent may make the child more upset. However, experience shows that these are not common problems.[71] Parent selection and education are very important. Those who are invited to watch their child's induction must be told precisely what to expect and should have an escort to take them back to the waiting area as soon as the child is asleep. Parents must agree to leave the induction area at any moment if so asked by the anesthesiologist. Unduly anxious or hysterical parents should not be encouraged in the induction area, since they can contribute to similar anxiety in their children. Anesthesia induction occurs in the operation room when

> Children are less than one to one and one-half years of age
> There is a serious preexisting illness
> Emergency surgery is scheduled
> An adolescent child does not choose to have his or her parents present
> Parents are unduly anxious about their participation in the experience
> Premedication is considered desirable

Although there are no tightly controlled research studies, most physicians and parents are enthusiastic and find this approach very satisfactory in reducing the anxiety due to separation.

One of the major factors limiting more frequent participation of parents during anesthesia induction in many institutions is the necessity to have specially equipped areas outside the operating room where anesthesia induction can be safely performed with the parents present. This possibility should be very carefully studied by anyone involved in planning or redesigning an operating room suite.

ANESTHETIC AGENTS AND TECHNIQUES
Despite the current popularity of ambulatory surgery, there is still no agreement among major pediatric centers as to what is the best way to prepare the child or

ensure a smooth induction and rapid and comfortable recovery without compromising safety. This remains a continuing challenge for the individual anesthesiologist. Smooth induction of anesthesia in the awake, unmedicated child is probably the most difficult aspect of pediatric short-stay surgery. Realizing that no single approach can be effective for all children in all situations, the anesthesiologist must be familiar with, and have confidence in, many methods of induction. The choice of an agent or technique can then be tailored to fit the needs of the individual child and not made merely because it is the routine choice in a particular institution or is the only method with which the anesthesiologist is comfortable.

INHALATIONAL INDUCTION

The greatest advantage of using inhalational induction in pediatric anesthesia is its apparent simplicity. If the same agents are also used to maintain surgical anesthesia, recovery is usually prompt following most brief outpatient procedures. Successful inhalational induction, however, mandates the child's cooperation and acceptance, especially in unpremedicated outpatients. Beyond perhaps the first year of life, this can very rarely be expected until the child is at least three or four years old, when verbal communication becomes easier. Even at that age, induction by mask is not always acceptable to the fully awake child. Pediatric anesthesiologists have over the years devised many ingenious techniques to reduce the anxiety associated with gas induction and have met with variable degrees of success. These include the following:

1. Elimination of the mask. An N_2O/O_2 mixture is blown over the child's face while he or she is distracted with a story or a song; then halothane is gradually added to the mixture (the anesthesiologist can make believe the new smell is that of candy, perfume, jet fuel, paint, etc.).

2. Use of transparent masks. Since we no longer use explosive agents, there is absolutely no need to use the traditional black conductive rubber mask. A variety of clear face masks are now available in pediatric sizes, and these should be used.

3. Use of "food flavors." As an additional method for getting the child to accept the mask near his or her face, some anesthesiologists paint the inside of the mask with a flavor or a smell of the child's choice. The child may find the smell interesting, and by allowing him or her to choose a pleasant flavor, the child becomes an active participant in the induction technique.

4. Letting the child sit up during the induction (Fig. 4-5). This is less frightening and often more acceptable to the child than being forced to lie down. The child can be given the choice to sit on the operating table or the anesthesiologist's lap. It is often less frightening to the child if the back instrument table is covered and the anesthesiologist

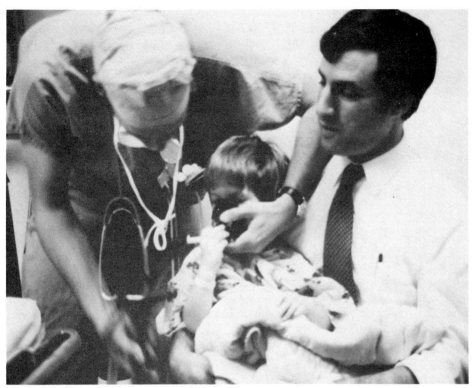

FIGURE 4-5. A parent's presence, security blanket, sitting position, and allowing the child to hold his or her mask all contribute to a smooth inhalational induction in the unmedicated pediatric patient.

and assistant do not wear a mask during induction. Children are used to looking at people's faces, not just their eyes.

INHALATIONAL ANESTHETICS

Nitrous Oxide

Nitrous oxide is the most commonly used inhalational agent. It has the great advantage of being practically odorless, which makes it most suitable for starting a gas induction in the unpremedicated pediatric patient. If nitrous oxide is administered in a high inspired concentration (75%–80%) *initially,* induction is rapid and pleasant, and the child is encouraged to continue with the mask induction. Unfortunately, nitrous oxide has a limited potency (MAC > 100%), and for this reason, it is usually supplemented with either potent inhalational agents or intravenous anesthetics.

Halothane

Halothane is the most commonly used potent inhalational agent in pediatric anesthesia. For the ambulatory surgery patient it offers the advantage of a rapid, smooth induction, either by direct inhalation (with nitrous oxide) or following a sleep dose of an intravenous agent.[72] Use of high inspired concentrations initially (up to 3%) will speed induction; however, this should be reduced quickly to the usual maintenance range of 0.5% to 2%. Hypotension and circulatory depression observed with halothane are dose-dependent and are especially profound in the young, fasting infant.[73]

Recovery after brief halothane anesthesia is usually rapid and uneventful. Nausea and vomiting are not common. With prolonged administration of halothane, however, recovery time is longer. Although there is a tendency to avoid repeated use of halothane in adult outpatient anesthesia for fear of sensitizing the liver and possibly inducing hepatic necrosis with future exposure, it is generally believed that this is rarely a problem in the preadolescent child.[50]

Enflurane

Enflurane is still not as widely used as halothane in pediatric outpatient anesthesia despite physical characteristics (low blood/gas solubility coefficient) that suggest a slightly more rapid induction and recovery. Studies that compared enflurane to halothane as the sole anesthetic agent showed that induction times were comparable, but that enflurane was associated with a higher incidence of hiccough and breath holding.[74] Following brief anesthetics, the rate of recovery of patients from enflurane anesthesia, as measured by return of eyelash reflex and swallowing, was significantly faster than that of patients who received halothane. However, full recovery times were comparable, and children anesthetized with either agent were ready to leave the recovery room at the same time. In other studies of children who received a narcotic premedication or barbiturate induction, the induction times with enflurane were found to be either longer[75] or shorter but associated with more complications[57] than that of halothane. There was no significant difference in the length of stay in the recovery room or return to normal activities at home. Enflurane is less likely than halothane to sensitize the myocardium to the effects of catecholamines.[76] This makes enflurane more compatible with the use of topical vasoconstrictor drugs (Table 4-4).

TABLE 4-4. Dose (ED_{50}) of Epinephrine That Produced Three or More PVCs[76]

Agent	Dose (μg/kg)
Halothane*	2.11 (± 0.15)
Halothane/lidocaine[†]	3.69 (± 0.42)
Enflurane	10.9 (± 8.9)
Isoflurane	6.72 (± 0.66)

*Karl et al. subsequently showed that children tolerate higher doses of subcutaneous epinephrine during halothane anesthesia. At least 10 μg/kg of epinephrine infiltration may be used safely in normocarbic and hypocarbic pediatric patients without congenital heart disease.
[†]It is our practice to limit the volume of subcutaneous lidocaine 1% with epinephrine 1:200,000 to a maximum of 0.5 ml/kg. This volume contains the equivalent of 5 mg lidocaine + 2.5 μg epinephrine per kilogram of body weight.
SOURCE: Johnston et al.[76]

Isoflurane

Isoflurane possesses many characteristics that make it an interesting possibility for use in pediatric outpatient anesthesia.[78] It has a low blood/gas solubility coefficient, which should make induction of anesthesia and postoperative recovery more rapid than with other inhalational agents. Isoflurane is a very stable compound, with less than 0.2% of the drug metabolized in the body and the remainder excreted through the lungs. Thus, in the absence of significant metabolites, rapid recovery should be expected with minimal sequelae.

Kingston compared halothane and isoflurane in 40 unpremedicated children one to six years of age who were scheduled for outpatient surgical procedures.[79] Both agents were administered at predetermined rates until comparable end-expired concentrations of the agents were reached. Induction time as well as the time taken before tracheal intubation was possible were protracted in patients given isoflurane. Clinically, the rate of early postoperative recovery compares favorably with either halothane or enflurane. The return to normal status at home may be slightly more rapid than that of either of the other agents.[80]

Isoflurane may not yet be the ideal agent for induction of anesthesia in pediatric patients. Isoflurane has a more pungent smell than halothane and tends to provoke more excitement, breath holding, coughing, and laryngospasm than halothane during induction. This can be somewhat modified by starting the induction with a 60% to 70% concentration of N_2O for two minutes and then gradually introducing the isoflurane vapor in small (0.25%) increments. In an older child, a sleep dose of intravenous thiopental can improve the acceptance of the agent.

Limitations of Mask Inductions

In the unpremedicated child, induction with a mask mandates the patient's acceptance and cooperation (whether spontaneous or induced). Failure to achieve such cooperation and to get the mask close to the child's face without a struggle is not uncommon (Fig. 4-6). Some anesthesiologists, realizing the unpleasantness of such a situation, decide to get the whole thing over with as quickly as possible by holding the child down and forcing the mask over his or her face with a high concentration of halothane, promptly "smothering" the child to sleep. The struggling child will usually fall asleep quickly, while the anesthesiologist puts the blame on the stubborn child who refused to cooperate. If this type of induction is done repeatedly (and it is), the surgical team tends to become insensitive and regards it as the normal induction technique. By the end of the surgical procedure, everyone has probably forgotten how distasteful the experience was. Everyone, that is, except the child.

Although there are not many well-controlled long-term studies of the consequences of forced mask inductions, careful questioning of children or adults who still remember those horrible moments will reveal many unpleasant or even nightmarish memories that are often passed from generation to generation, consciously or unconsciously, adding a very significant element to the apprehension of anesthesia.

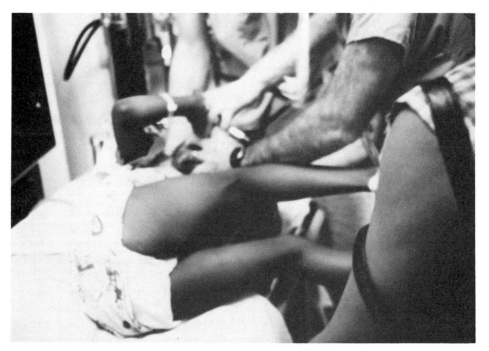

FIGURE 4-6. In up to 20% of cases, mask induction may not be acceptable to unpremedicated children. An alternate induction method must be employed.

NONINHALATIONAL INDUCTION AGENTS AND TECHNIQUES

The major disadvantage of using any noninhalational induction agent in pediatric ambulatory surgery patients is the possibility of prolonging the recovery period. However, with careful selection of agents and use of the minimal single dose necessary to simply induce sleep, some authors have found that the total recovery time is not significantly prolonged.[6,65] The following section is a brief review of the current indications and use of these agents in pediatric outpatient anesthesia.

Intravenous Induction

Intravenous induction is the method of choice in most older children for the same reasons it has become the standard in adults. It ensures a rapid, pleasant induction with minimal struggling and no unpleasant memories of a suffocating mask or a smelly gas. The approach for young children is different from that for adults (Fig. 4-7). The drug should be injected directly in a vein on the dorsum of the hand, usually through a 25-gauge butterfly needle. An intravenous infusion need not be started prior to the drug injection. The real limitation to the more frequent use of intravenous induction in children is the anesthesiologist. No one enjoys injections, but (except in the case of a child who has a definite severe phobia about needles, which can quickly be assessed by his or her reaction to the blood test) most older children will accept intravenous induction if the pro-

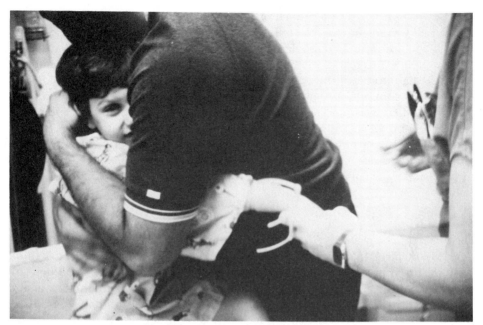

FIGURE 4-7. Concealed IV induction in a child.

posal is made to them in a confident, supportive way. The idea of going to sleep quickly with a "scratch" or a "pinch" in the hand rather than having to breathe the "smelly" gas is more likely to generate acceptance than if the same alternatives are presented as "blowing a balloon" versus "getting a shot." With a little practice on the part of the anesthesiologist, a small injection with a tiny concealed needle is barely felt and is much less painful than deep intramuscular injections (shots).

The age at which intravenous induction is considered practical in children varies considerably among anesthesiologists. For an experienced and skilled anesthesiologist, any child over six months of age with visible veins is an appropriate candidate (especially if mask induction is not accepted). Infants under six months of age, however, are rarely appropriate candidates for noninhalational techniques because of the higher risk of postoperative respiratory depression and the possibility of more prolonged recovery.

Thiopental Sodium

Thiopental sodium (2.5% solution) is the most commonly used induction agent for adult outpatient anesthesia. In a dose of 4 to 5 mg/kg body weight, it is equally suitable for the pediatric outpatient. There is a wide variation, however, in the pediatric patient's response to intravenous thiopental, and the response of each child during induction must be carefully monitored and used to determine the individual dose requirement. Healthy, unpremedicated children may require relatively large doses of thiopental (5 to 6 mg/kg) in order to ensure smooth and rapid transition to general inhalational anesthesia.[81] When Steward[6] compared the recovery times in children following intravenous thiopental induction with those of children who had inhalational induction, he found that after 30 minutes there was no difference in the recovery score between the two groups. Children who had barbiturate induction, however, tended to be sleepier and required more airway support for the first 15 minutes of the recovery period. Steward also found that there was no difference in the eventual return to a "bright and alert" status and normal appetite at home following discharge. Repeated doses of thiopental should be avoided, because they can prolong recovery. Diazepam and opiate narcotics also can have an exaggerated depressant effect if taken in the early postoperative period following the use of intravenous thiopental for induction.[82]

Methohexital
For the ambulatory surgery patient, methohexital (1.5 to 2 mg/kg) offers the distinct advantage of a significantly shorter recovery than an equivalent dose of thiopental.[83] The duration of unconsciousness is similar after a single small dose of either agent. However, since metabolic breakdown products of methohexital are eliminated three times faster than those of thiopental,[84] the time required for complete psychomotor recovery is shorter. This is particularly true after large or repeated doses. When used in a 1% solution, methohexital has a lower tissue toxicity than thiopental following inadvertent subcutaneous infiltration or intraarterial injection. Induction with methohexital is followed by an appreciable incidence of involuntary muscle movements and episodes of hiccough and coughing, which can at times be very troublesome. This can be minimized somewhat by injecting the drug slowly and using a small total dose. A severe burning sensation often develops along the course of the injected vein. This is particularly undesirable in children, because it promotes hand movement and can dislodge the needle from the vein. Pain can be minimized by mixing a very small amount of lidocaine with the methohexital (1 mg/ml). Methohexital has been reported to induce epileptiform convulsions in susceptible patients.[85] Despite these disadvantages, many still consider methohexital the intravenous barbiturate of choice when rapid recovery and early ambulation are required in the outpatient.[82,84]

Etomidate
Etomidate, a nonbarbiturate hypnotic agent, has been used extensively for intravenous induction of anesthesia in Europe. When used in an intravenous dose of 0.2 mg/kg in children, etomidate produces sleep rapidly and safely, with negligible side-effects on the cardiovascular system and little respiratory depression.[86]

Pain is common following injection with etomidate and, unlike with methohexital, is not prevented by adding lidocaine to the solution. Myoclonia is also seen following the use of this drug. Using an analgesic agent (e.g., fentanyl as premedication or with induction of anesthesia) can reduce these problems. Some authors, however, find that the etomidate and fentanyl technique is associated with a greater frequency of nausea and vomiting, which would make early discharge from the ambulatory facility difficult.[87]

Propofol
Propofol is a new short-acting intravenous anesthetic with high lipid solubility, short elimination half-life, and inactive metabolites. The drug is formulated as an aqueous emulsion for intravenous use. When compared to thiopental, it has been shown to result in a more rapid recovery and return to normal neuropsychological function in adults.[88] Early studies with propofol in children indicate that it results in smooth induction with a low incidence of side-effects and similar recovery characteristics to thiopental.[89] When a dose of 2.5 mg/kg was injected in the dorsum of the hand in unpremedicated children, pain on injection and excitatory effects were noted more frequently than when thiopental (5 mg/kg) was used.[90] Pain on injection can be minimized by using the large antecubital veins for injection.[91] More studies are needed to establish the usefulness of propofol as an induction agent in pediatric ambulatory patients.

Intramuscular Induction
Intramuscular injections do not require the high degree of skill needed for intravenous induction in a struggling child. However, deep intramuscular injections are definitely more painful, and they are one of the main reasons children dislike needles and shots. Routine use of intramuscular injections for induction of anesthesia or for premedication is therefore undesirable. However, in certain situations when a struggling child cannot be managed by intravenous induction owing to lack of accessible veins (or experience on the part of the anesthesiologist), a small sedating intramuscular dose of ketamine or methohexital may be the most humane way to induce anesthesia.

The potential for prolonged recovery and emergence delirium makes ketamine undesirable for routine use in ambulatory surgery patients. There is virtually no rational indication for its intravenous use in these children. If it must be used intramuscularly, a small sedating dose (2 to 3 mg/kg) is injected into the deltoid muscle. This should provide satisfactory conditions for a mask induction within four to seven minutes. Atropine (0.02 mg/kg) may be simultaneously injected to reduce the excessive secretions that can lead to airway irritation. This technique is most applicable for the one- to five-year-old group. When ketamine is used in this manner and followed by a thiopental, nitrous oxide, oxygen relaxant technique, the recovery time is prolonged only slightly.[58] When patients are administered a low dose of ketamine as an induction agent, hallucinations and nightmares do not appear to be a problem. Krantz reported no instances of unpleasant dreams or emergence phenomena following administration of 2 to 2.5 mg/kg of ketamine IM used for very brief (<5 min) outpatient procedures in children. Recovery time averaged 13 ± 7.6 minutes, which is satisfactory for outpatient anesthesia.[92]

Another choice for an intramuscular induction agent is methohexital, usually as a 5% solution. A dose of 6 mg/kg injected deep in the muscle has been reported to induce sleep in less than 5 minutes in patients from one to three years of age.[93] When only a single injection was used, recovery was rapid and complete. At the Children's Hospital of Michigan, methohexital sodium (3.5% in distilled water) has been used in a dose of 7.7 mg/kg given deep IM in the anterolateral thigh in more than 25,000 cases. Parents are allowed to hold the child on their lap during the injection and until the eyelids close. The incidence of hiccoughs was less than 8%, and clonic movements for 10 seconds' duration were seen in one patient. Although the injection is painful, no local reactions or subsequent soreness at the injection site was reported.* Intramuscular methohexital sedation (10 mg/kg) has been successfully used in children undergoing CT scans.[94] Onset time was just over 3 minutes, and children were arousable with stimulation in 40 to 50 minutes.

Rectal Induction

Rectally administered anesthetics fell out of favor in the early 1970s because of the long duration of action and the unpredictable absorption of the agents that were given by that route (e.g., thiopental). This method is now being "rediscovered" as an easy, minimally invasive technique for anesthesia induction in very young children.

The use of methohexital is the main reason why rectal induction is again in vogue. Used as a 10% solution in a dose of 25 mg/kg, most children fall asleep in 6 to 11 minutes, and even in outpatients, this dose did not significantly delay immediate and late recovery after short surgical procedures when compared to intravenous thiopental.[65] Occasionally, the onset of sleep may be delayed for up to 20 minutes, and very rarely the child may not fall asleep at all. If the child is at least drowsy, inhalational induction would be readily acceptable. Otherwise, one may have to either repeat the rectal injection (with the risk of prolonged recovery) or use a different induction technique. Rectal methohexital is most suitable for children one to three years of age who would not cooperate with mask induction and have no visible veins for easy intravenous access.[95] The older child would probably be more upset and psychologically traumatized by introducing the drug in his or her rectum than by an intravenous injection.

Kallar studied the effect of 1%, 5%, and 10% concentrations of rectal methohexital (15 mg/kg) on induction time in ambulatory surgery pediatric patients ages one to five years. The shortest induction time was observed with the 1% solution (mean 6.3 min). Failures (cases in which the patient was not asleep after administration of rectal methohexital) were observed with the 5% solution (five patients) and with the 10% solution (four patients). No failures were seen with 1% methohexital. Expulsion or defecation was observed in just under 5% of patients who received the 5% or 10% rectal solutions, but none was observed when the 1% solution was used.†

Other workers also have shown that more dilute solutions may be used. Forbes and Vandewalker reported that the administration of 25 mg/kg of methohexital as a 2% solution results in a significantly higher plasma concentration than when a 10% solution is used.[96] Khalil et al.[97] found that 25 mg/kg of methohexital given as a 1% solution and placed in the sigmoid area was associated with a faster

---

*Jewell MR: Personal communication, 1984.
†Kallar SK: Personal communication, 1984.

onset of sleep (5.9 ± 1.3 min) and 100% success rate and lower incidence of defecation when compared to 2% or 10% solutions. Rectal aspiration of the residual drug after sleep did not affect recovery time. Kestin et al.,[98] on the other hand, found that 45% of an administered dose of methohexital can be recovered by aspiration after loss of consciousness, leading to significantly faster clinical recovery from anesthesia. Recent studies indicate that oxygen desaturation commonly occurs following induction with rectal methohexital.[99] Airway resuscitative equipment, including oxygen, must be immediately available to treat any airway obstruction or respiratory depression. Needless to say, the anesthesiologist must remain in attendance after the drug is administered. Other side-effects include hiccough (9%), involuntary movements, and soiling (9%). The parents must be forewarned about the latter and appropriately protected if they are holding the child during induction.

INTRAOPERATIVE USE OF NARCOTICS

Narcotics can be used in outpatients to maintain anesthesia (with nitrous oxide/oxygen relaxants) as a part of a balanced technique or to supplement a "light" inhalational technique. By reducing the amount of potent inhalational or intravenous agents needed (and absorbed in fat for later release), narcotics may actually contribute to more rapid awakening.[100,101] The residual analgesia may eliminate or reduce the need for further potent pain medication during the recovery period.

When compared with a pure inhalation technique, the intraoperative adjunctive use of narcotics has been reported not to delay discharge home.[52] With psychomotor testing, however, patients who received inhalation anesthetics were found to perform significantly better at 30 to 59 minutes postoperatively than those who received narcotics.[102] After 1 hour, scores were essentially the same for both groups. This finding suggests that narcotics should not be administered to patients who must be discharged within 1 hour of anesthesia.

For ambulatory surgical procedures it is generally advisable to avoid the use of long-acting drugs such as morphine. The currently available short-acting narcotic analgesics such as fentanyl or alfentanil, used in appropriate doses, may be particularly suited for ambulatory patients because of their rapid onset, short duration of action, and fast recovery.

Few studies on the use of these drugs in ambulatory children are currently available. Hannallah and coworkers[103] reported no delay in discharge time when fentanyl (1–2 μg/kg, IV) was used to treat postorchiopexy pain in children. In a similar study of children recovering from circumcision, however, Broadman et al.[104] found that children who did not complain of pain or had their pain controlled by a regional block and therefore did not receive fentanyl in the postoperative period had a significantly shorter discharge time when compared to those who did. Although some recent work suggests that infants and young children seem to tolerate larger doses of fentanyl than adults without displaying significant postoperative ventilatory depression,[105] clinical experience with this approach in pediatric ambulatory patients is still limited.

Alfentanil, the new short-acting derivative of fentanyl, appears to offer some clinically significant advantages as an anesthetic supplement during outpatient anesthesia. Youngberg and coworkers[106] have shown that a group of children who received an initial intravenous bolus of alfentanil (35 μg/kg) at induction, followed by intermittent doses (10 μg/kg) at intervals of 12 to 15 minutes, had a significantly shorter recovery time than a similar group who received halothane for surgical procedures of short duration. Pediatric ambulatory patients who received alfentanil had a significantly lower incidence and severity of pain in the recovery room.

Casey and coworkers[107] have recently compared the safety and efficacy of alfentanil to halothane in children undergoing adenoidectomies on an ambulatory basis. The initial bolus of alfentanil (50 μg/kg) produced brief, intense analgesia. Subsequent infusion requirements of alfentanil ranged from 0.5–3 μg/kg per minute of surgery. The extubation time was 9 minutes in patients anesthetized with halothane and 7 minutes in patients given alfentanil. The recovery time was 8 minutes in patients anesthetized with halothane and 13 minutes in patients given alfentanil. Postoperative narcotics were required in 25% of patients given halothane and 10% of patients given alfentanil. That study demonstrated that alfentanil is a suitable anesthetic for ambulatory surgery in children and does not prolong recovery and discharge time when compared to halothane.

USE OF MUSCLE RELAXANTS

The intelligent use of muscle relaxants is not only safe in ambulatory surgical anesthesia, but, if used as a part of a "balanced" technique, can actually reduce the need for higher concentrations of potent anesthetics and help promote promptness of recovery and early discharge.

Succinylcholine

Succinylcholine is most often used to facilitate endotracheal intubation without the need for an excessive depth of inhalational anesthesia. This is particularly advantageous in outpatients and in young infants who do not tolerate deep halothane anesthesia. Succinylcholine can be used intravenously in a dose of 1 mg/kg (2 mg/kg for infants under two years of age) or intramuscularly (4 mg/kg).

Succinylcholine should be combined with, or preceded by, atropine (0.02 mg/kg) when used for pediatric patients to avoid excessive bradycardia, which might otherwise follow even a single injection. Succinylcholine also can be used in repeated doses (preceded by atropine) or as an infusion for prolonged relaxation; however, this is not generally recommended in young children, because the larger doses required and the extremely variable response of small infants to succinylcholine can lead to the development of phase II block.[108]

Muscle pains, with or without excessive fasciculation, can follow rapid intravenous injection of succinylcholine in older children. This is particularly evident with the early ambulation typical of ambulatory surgery. Muscle pain can be avoided by injecting a small dose of *d*-tubocurarine (0.05 mg/kg) two to three minutes before succinylcholine. Because of curare's antagonistic effect, the dose of succinylcholine must be increased by 70% to ensure adequate relaxation. Muscle pains are seldom a problem in younger children,[109] and pretreatment is not generally recommended before the age of six to eight years.

Another potential problem in using succinylcholine in outpatients is the rare possibility of prolonged apnea in children with abnormal pseudocholinesterase.[110] The prolonged paralysis (up to six hours with the homozygous variety) can disrupt a busy schedule but is very simple to treat once the diagnosis is confirmed (with a nerve stimulator). Adequate ventilation (and sedation) must be continued until full muscle power returns. Hospital admission is usually recommended. Blood samples from the child and family should be drawn for analysis and confirmation of the type of the disorder at a later date.

Nondepolarizing Relaxants

Although profound muscle relaxation is seldom, if ever, needed in the type of cases commonly performed on an outpatient basis, a nondepolarizing relaxant/nitrous oxide anesthetic technique supplemented with a small dose of inhalational agent as necessary can be used as a part of a "balanced" technique.[111] This can be especially useful in children in whom anesthesia was induced with a long-acting agent such as a rectal barbiturate or intramuscular ketamine or in young infants who may manifest profound cardiovascular depression if a potent inhalational agent is used as the sole anesthetic. The currently available intermediate-acting nondepolarizing muscle relaxants such as vecuronium (0.1 mg/kg)[112] or atracurium (0.5 mg/kg)[113] have made this approach popular, even for short (less than 30 minutes) surgical procedures. It is absolutely essential to ensure complete reversal at the end of surgery.[114] With careful attention to dosage and the use of a nerve stimulator to ensure an adequate reversal dose of neostigmine (0.07 mg/kg) or edrophonium (1 mg/kg) with atropine (0.02 mg/kg) or glycopyrrolate (0.01 mg/kg), this should not be a problem. The remote possibility of "recurarization" that can result from hypothermia, acidosis, and so forth is not likely in the healthy outpatient undergoing uncomplicated surgery. It should be understood that the preceding statements and dosages apply to the healthy child. Special consideration must be given to the variable response of premature and mature infants to the nondepolarizing muscle relaxants, especially vecuronium.

ENDOTRACHEAL INTUBATION

Outpatient anesthesia per se is not a contraindication for using an endotracheal tube. At many centers, large numbers of pediatric ambulatory surgery patients have been intubated without serious complications. The endotracheal tube size selected should enable full expansion of both lungs and normal inflation while allowing a definite leak with pressure of 20 to 25 cm H_2O (Table 4-5). The indications and techniques of endotracheal intubation are the same as for inpatients.

TABLE 4-5. Recommended Tracheal Tube Sizes by Age

Age	Internal Diameter (mm)	
Premature (2.5 kg)	2.5	
Term newborn	3.0	
6 mos	3.5	Noncuffed
12 mos	4.0	
18–24 mos	4.5	
4 yrs	5.0–5.5	
6 yrs	5.5–6.0	
8 yrs	6.0–6.5	
10 yrs	6.5	
12 yrs	7.0	Cuffed
14 yrs	7.5	
Adult	8.0–9.5	

NOTE: Children of the same age vary in size; occasionally, a size 0.5-mm ID smaller or larger may be required. Cuffs are generally not used with tube size smaller than 5.5 mm. When using a cuffed tube, select a size 0.5-mm ID smaller. General formula for children over 2 years:

$$\text{Tube size mm ID} = \frac{\text{Age (yrs)}}{4} + 4.5$$

There is a tendency, however, to avoid "routine" intubations in outpatients for the following reasons:

1. Many outpatient procedures are of short duration and do not involve body cavities, so intubation may not be indicated.
2. Intubation of the trachea for convenience may unnecessarily complicate the anesthetic. In seeking to achieve good intubating conditions, one may come dangerously close to overdosage if halothane alone is used,[115] or a muscle relaxant may be administered that would otherwise not be needed.
3. There is a definite incidence of trauma to the larynx secondary to intubation that varies according to the skills of the anesthesiologist and size of the endotracheal tube.
4. There is a tendency to delay oral fluid intake for at least one hour in patients who are intubated because of the possibility of laryngeal incompetence following extubation[116] or the presence of a sore throat.
5. The most feared risk associated with the use of an endotracheal tube in ambulatory surgery patients is the possibility that the child may develop postintubation croup during recovery and especially after discharge from the hospital. However, with careful technique and the use of small implant-tested tubes with a leak, the incidence should be very small (<1%).[117] Of special importance is the time at which "significant"

croup develops. Most patients develop symptoms within one hour of extubation; thus many centers allow pediatric patients whose tracheas have been intubated to be discharged after one hour has passed.[6] In our unit, children who are intubated do not meet routine discharge criteria until three hours have elapsed from the time of extubation. This is an arbitrary duration, based on what we believe to be an adequate period of observation to detect possible airway problems. These children can be discharged earlier if the anesthesiologist reexamines the child, detects no signs of airway obstruction, and personally discharges the child. In any case, parents must be advised to observe and report to a previously designated physician or service any respiratory difficulty that may develop after discharge.

PEDIATRIC ANESTHESIA BREATHING SYSTEMS
The choice of a special breathing system for use in pediatric patients varies among individual practitioners. Currently, the usual decision is between a modification of the T-piece or a circle absorption system. Each has its advantages and limitations, and provided one understands the performance characteristics of the system, either can be used safely for the pediatric outpatient.

The T-Piece
The Jackson Rees modification of the original T-piece and all the Bain-type coaxial systems have the same performance characteristics. The greatest advantages of the T-piece are its light weight, simplicity, and the convenience of a long fresh gas flow (FGF) tubing. In the absence of an absorber, changes in the inspired concentration of agents can be readily achieved by changing the dialed concentration on the machine. There are two ways to use the T-piece:

1. As a nonrebreathing system, with high FGF ($2\frac{1}{2} \times$ minute volume). This formula is generally recommended with spontaneous respiration.
2. As a partial rebreathing system, with low FGF. This method (also referred to as *controlled rebreathing*) requires a large minute volume to allow adequate CO_2 elimination. This can be predictably achieved only by controlling ventilation. The recommended FGF and minute ventilation[118] are
   a. FGF:
      <30 kg: 1000 ml + 100 ml/kg
      >30 kg: 2000 ml + 50 mg/kg
   b. Minute ventilation $\geq 2 \times$ FGF

Because of the need for a higher FGF (especially with spontaneous respiration), the T-piece is not usually used for older children (over five years or 20 kg body weight).

The Circle Absorption System

The advantages of the circle system include fresh gas economy, heat and moisture retention, and ease of scavenging. Its potential for use in all age groups eliminates the need for special pediatric systems. This can be extremely convenient in an outpatient facility that has a mixture of adult and pediatric patients.

The two major disadvantages of the circle system in pediatric anesthesia are its high resistance and large dead space. In young children, these can be easily overcome by controlling ventilation and using circle tubing that has minimal dead space at the Y-connection.

MONITORING OF PEDIATRIC PATIENTS

Safe conduct of anesthesia requires the anesthesiologist to maintain continuous vigilance. In the management of the anesthetized child, this can be greatly assisted by using a variety of monitoring devices. Some of them are common to all age groups, while others are of special value in the pediatric patient.

The minimum of monitoring aids for any pediatric patient undergoing general anesthesia include

1. A precordial (or esophageal) stethoscope. As correctly stated by Smith, the stethoscope is the most important of all monitoring devices in pediatric anesthesia and should be used throughout all procedures in which general anesthesia is used. It allows continuous monitoring of heart rate and rhythm, volume of heart sounds, and rate and depth of respiration.[50]
2. Blood pressure measurement. In the pediatric patient, the Doppler ultrasonic flowmeter or an automatic oscillometric device is a valuable adjunct to traditional blood pressure monitoring. Use of the correct size cuff is important in children. The width of the cuff should be approximately two-thirds of the length of the upper arm. If the cuff is too narrow, one will get a falsely high reading, whereas too wide a cuff will result in a falsely low reading.
3. Temperature monitoring. Special attention must be paid to temperature changes in pediatric anesthesia. Hypothermia is a constant threat to infants and can lead to delayed recovery and metabolic acidosis. Protective measures such as warm operating rooms, insulation of the extremities, heating blankets, and infrared lights should be used in small infants. Malignant hyperthermia, on the other hand, is a rare but potentially fatal complication if certain triggering agents are used in susceptible patients. For these reasons, body temperature must be continuously monitored under anesthesia. For most outpatient procedures, an external axillary thermister probe properly positioned near the axillary artery is most convenient and can be reused with no elaborate sterilization. Alternatively, liquid crystal strips can be used to display changes in skin temperature.[119]

4. Electrocardiogram (ECG). Although regarded as a vital monitoring device in adult anesthesia, the ECG is really the least valuable monitoring device in healthy pediatric patients.[50] In the absence of ischemic cardiac disease, its main value is to differentiate arrhythmias already detected by a precordial stethoscope. It is worthwhile to emphasize that a normal tracing may persist for minutes in spite of severe hypotension caused by high concentrations of potent inhalational agents, and it is important to avoid the potential false confidence conveyed by observing a normal tracing.

Oxygenation and ventilation must be continually monitored during anesthesia. An inspired oxygen concentration monitor is a standard safety feature on anesthesia machines. Oxygen saturation monitors are required as standard monitors. The use of an end-tidal carbon dioxide monitor or a similar device is encouraged to confirm correct placement of an endotracheal tube. Other monitors should be employed as needed. The amount of blood loss (expressed as a percentage of blood volume) should be measured in such procedures as adenoidectomy. A nerve stimulator can be used to avoid overdosage of muscle relaxants and to determine the degree of neuromuscular recovery at the termination of surgery. Arterial blood gas measurements are usually not needed in outpatient practice. However, if there is a serious reason to question the adequacy of oxygenation, ventilation, or acid-base status of a patient, arterial sampling is indicated.

PERIOPERATIVE FLUID MANAGEMENT

The need for routine administration of intravenous fluids during outpatient anesthesia for children is controversial. The guidelines for the elective use of conscious sedation, deep sedation, and general anesthesia in pediatric patients that were published in 1985 by the Section on Anesthesiology of the American Academy of Pediatrics originally stated that "patients receiving ambulatory general anesthesia shall have an intravenous line in place."[120] One year later, the guidelines were modified as follows: "Patients receiving ambulatory general anesthesia shall have an intravenous line in place or have immediately available a person skilled in establishing intravenous infusions in pediatric patients."[121]

By definition, ambulatory surgery anesthesia is administered to healthy children undergoing uncomplicated surgical procedures that do not involve major blood loss or translocations of body fluid compartments. Many believe that if the procedure is of short duration and the anesthetic technique is one that ensures rapid recovery and return of normal appetite with minimal nausea and vomiting, these children do not really require infusion of fluids.[122] However, especially if fluids are not administered intravenously, the period of preoperative starvation should be minimized to avoid possible dehydration and hypoglycemia.[123] Although in many centers children over one year of age are usually not allowed solid food on the day of surgery, they are offered clear liquids up to four hours prior to surgery.

TABLE 4-6. Maintenance Fluid Therapy

Child's Weight (kg)	Basic Hourly Rate (ml)
<10	wt $\times$ 4
10–20	(wt $\times$ 2) + 20
>20	wt + 40

NOTE: During the first hour of surgery, up to four times the basic hourly rate may be administered as a hydrating solution.
SOURCE: Oh.[126]

Intravenous fluid therapy during and after surgery, usually 5% dextrose in 0.3 normal saline (Table 4-6), is specifically indicated in the following circumstances:

1. Longer operations (over 30–60 min), which are more likely to result in delayed return of normal appetite.
2. Procedures known to be associated with a high incidence of postoperative nausea and vomiting, such as strabismus surgery,[124] orchidopexy, and otoplasty. Not only should children undergoing these procedures have their preoperative fluid deficit replaced during surgery, but the anticipated continuing postoperative deficit should be considered when an hourly intravenous fluid rate is calculated. In this way there is less risk of dehydration if nausea and vomiting occur following discharge. By ensuring adequate parenteral hydration, less emphasis need be placed in requiring the child to retain oral fluids postoperatively before the stomach can tolerate them. Forcing oral fluids prematurely often results in more persistent nausea and vomiting. In the absence of cardiovascular, respiratory, or renal pathology, the maximum tolerance level for fluids is high and the risk of overloading the child is minimal.[125] In the event that persistent vomiting occurs, the intravenous fluid should be changed to normal saline or Ringer's lactate. Continued use of solutions that contain 0.25% or 0.30% saline may result in severe hyponatremia if they are used to replace losses secondary to protracted vomiting.
3. Procedures that are associated with intraoperative blood loss or that have the potential for postoperative bleeding (e.g., adenoidectomy or tonsillectomy).
4. Young children who have been fasting for a prolonged period of time because they did not receive fluids as ordered or because a delay in the operative schedule extended the NPO period.
5. Children who develop excessive cardiovascular depression and hypotension when potent inhalational agents are administered and who need rapid injection of fluids to restore normal cardiovascular function.
6. Situations in which it is deemed desirable to have a readily available route for administration of intraoperative or postoperative narcotics

for pain relief or for administration of antibiotics as prophylaxis against subacute bacterial endocarditis for children with heart disease.

Many anesthesiologists, on the other hand, prefer to have an infusion started in every child having surgery to guarantee a ready route for emergency administration of drugs. Apart from the extra expense, the time involved, and often the need for an extra pair of hands to begin the infusion, there is no real objection to this practice unless it is carried too far, for example, repeated attempts at venipuncture in a healthy, well-hydrated, chubby child who has been admitted for a brief, uncomplicated procedure.[50] It is reassuring to remember that the two emergency drugs that are likely to be needed in the healthy day-surgery child are succinylcholine and atropine. In the absence of an infusion or visible veins, these two drugs are rapidly effective when administered intramuscularly (in a dose twice that used for intravenous administration).

POSTOPERATIVE ANALGESIA

Successful management of ambulatory surgery anesthesia requires that the anesthesiologist carefully evaluate and manage the child's need for postoperative pain relief. The need for analgesics depends on the nature of surgery and the pain threshold of the patient. It does not depend on whether or not the child is an outpatient or an inpatient.[46] Although many young children do extremely well postoperatively with minimal amounts of oral analgesics or none whatsoever, many others experience pain and require an appropriate dose of a more potent analgesic. Every child deserves individual consideration! It is unfortunate that we still observe many anesthesiologists and surgeons who believe that "children don't experience pain" and deny an appropriate dose of a narcotic to a child who is in pain because "in their own experience," this procedure "usually" does not warrant it or for fear of slightly delaying discharge home.

By definition, procedures that require multiple or frequent use of potent parenteral narcotics are not appropriate for ambulatory surgery. For the more typical pediatric outpatient procedures, postoperative pain or discomfort can be managed by one or a combination of the following.

Mild Analgesics

For infants under six months of age, a combination of care and nursing (or a bottle) is all that is usually needed following a procedure that is not associated with severe pain. Child-parent reunion should be allowed as soon as the child is awake.

For older infants and young children, aspirin and acetaminophen (Tylenol) are the drugs most commonly used for relief of mild pain in the postoperative period. They are usually adequate for treating pain from integumental structures such as bones, joints, muscles, and teeth but inadequate for treating visceral pain. Aspirin, which is known to interfere with platelet aggregation, is best avoided following procedures that can be associated with bleeding, such as adenoidectomy, tonsillectomy, and circumcision. Acetaminophen can be used either orally or rectally in a dose of 60 mg (1 grain) per year of age. At CNMC, Tylenol Children's Elixir is the drug most frequently used at home following discharge.

For more persistent, moderately severe pain, codeine can be used in combination with acetaminophen. Tylenol with Codeine Elixir contains 120 mg acetaminophen and 12 mg codeine per 5 ml. The recommended dose is 5 ml for children 3 to 6 years and 10 ml for the 7 to 12 age group. The analgesic action of codeine is much weaker than that of morphine, and it is less likely to produce nausea and vomiting. These factors, and the absence of respiratory depression in the normal dose range, make it a very useful oral analgesic for the outpatient.

Potent Narcotic Analgesics

The use of potent narcotics in the pediatric ambulatory surgery patient deserves special consideration. It is well known that all narcotics given in the perioperative period may contribute significantly to postoperative drowsiness, nausea and vomiting, and delay in discharge home. However, it is also desirable that the postoperative period be as free of pain and discomfort for the child as possible. Many popular surgical procedures performed on an outpatient basis such as orchidopexy, circumcision, adenoidectomy, and herniotomy[127] are frequently associated with postoperative pain. Such pain, if untreated, may in itself delay full recovery, discourage ambulation, and increase morbidity by producing nausea and vomiting.[127,128]

The choice of the individual drug is usually a matter of individual judgment. Drugs such as morphine and meperidine are generally thought to have too long an action for outpatient use. Although their action can be reversed by antagonists such as naloxone, reversal results in the immediate onset of pain and discomfort. Thus a better approach is the use of a short-acting narcotic analgesic such as fentanyl. Intravenous use allows more accurate titration of the dose to the individual child and avoids the use of "standard" dosages based on weight that may lead to a relative overdose. Fentanyl up to a dose of 2 μg/kg is our drug of choice for intravenous use. Meperidine (0.5 mg/kg) and codeine (1–1.5 mg/kg) can be used intramuscularly if an intravenous route is not established. In some units, codeine is used intramuscularly in doses as large as 1.5 mg/kg of body weight, with a maximum of 60 mg.[6]

Regional Analgesia for Postoperative Pain

Although unsupplemented regional anesthesia is not popular in pediatric patients, many simple blocks can be combined with light general anesthesia to provide excellent postoperative pain relief and early ambulation with minimal or no need for narcotics.

For the purpose of pain relief, a block can be performed at the end of surgery to obtain the maximum duration of analgesia in the postoperative period. For shorter procedures (< 60 min), however, and with the availability of longer-acting local anesthetics (e.g., bupivacaine), there may be yet another advantage in placing the block before surgery starts but after the child is asleep. This would help reduce the requirement for general anesthetic agents during surgery, which may result in a more rapid recovery, early discharge, return of normal appetite, and less nausea and vomiting.[127]

The types of blocks that can be safely used in the pediatric ambulatory surgery patient are limited only by the skill and interest of the individual anesthesiologist. Generally, the techniques chosen should be simple and expedient to perform, have minimal or no side-effects, and not interfere with the motor function and early ambulation of the child. Although manufacturers of bupivacaine do not recommend using it in children younger than 12 years, the drug has been used extensively in pediatric anesthesia and offers the distinct advantage of a long duration of action. Many types of nerve blocks can be used in conjunction with general anesthesia in children. The ones more widely used in pediatric ambulatory surgery patients are discussed in the following sections.[129,130]

Ilioinguinal and Iliohypogastric Nerve Block
This simple block produces effective postoperative pain relief following outpatient hernia repair in children.[127] It also can be used for other procedures requiring an inguinal incision, such as hydrocelectomy and orchiopexy.[103]

The ilioinguinal nerve runs between the transverse and internal oblique muscles. The iliohypogastric nerve runs superficial to the inguinal muscles close to the anterior superior ililac spine. Both nerves can easily be blocked by infiltration of the abdominal wall in the area medial to the anterosuperior iliac spine[127] (Fig. 4-8). A 25-gauge needle is used to puncture the skin 1 cm medial to and 1 cm inferior to the anterosuperior iliac spine, just above the inguinal ligament. Three fan-shaped injections are made as the needle is withdrawn, plus a subcutaneous wheal. If the block is performed at the completion of surgery, the area to be infiltrated may be approached through the lateral edge of the groin incision.

Shandling and Steward[127] used 0.5% bupivacaine in a dose of up to 2 mg/kg with 1:200,000 epinephrine to perform the block in 81 children undergoing elective inguinal herniotomy. The blocks were performed following the induction of

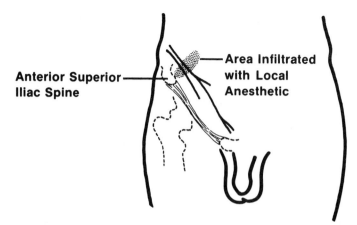

FIGURE 4-8. Ilioinguinal and iliohypogastric nerve blocks are performed by infiltrating the abdominal wall muscle medial to the anterior superior iliac spine.

general anesthesia and before the start of surgery. The time required for the surgeon to complete the block was approximately 60 seconds. Only 3 of the 81 children who received the block required extra analgesics in the PACU, compared with 74 of 75 control patients who were given codeine (1.5 mg/kg IM) in the postanesthetic recovery area. At home, analgesics were given by the parents to 32 of 75 children in the control group and to 24 of 81 children who had received the nerve block. A quicker return to a bright and alert status and to normal activity was seen in a significantly greater number of children with the nerve block. Both groups had a similar incidence of nausea and vomiting. The only observed complication was a transient motor block of the femoral nerve that resulted in a short-lived difficulty with walking in three patients. This probably occurred because the local anesthetic solution had reached the femoral nerve by tracking within fascial planes. In a study performed at our institution, we used a more dilute bupivacaine solution (0.25%) to perform the block and noted no such complication.[103] In that study, which involved children undergoing orchiopexy on an outpatient basis, the blocks were performed by the surgeon before closing the incision. This study scored the postoperative pain and discomfort of the children using an objective pain scale and compared children receiving regional nerve blocks, caudal blocks, and no blocks. Both groups of patients receiving blocks showed significantly better postoperative pain relief than the unblocked patients.[103]

When a 2-mg/kg dose of bupivacaine was used to perform the block in a recent study, the mean peak plasma level was 1.35 ± 0.35 μg/ml, well below the potentially toxic level of 4 μg/ml. Maximum plasma bupivacaine concentrations were observed between 10 and 40 minutes following block placement.[131]

A simple approach to blocking the ilioinguinal and iliohypogastric nerves in the inguinal canal has been recently described. Casey et al.[132] found that simple irrigation of the hernia wound prior to surgical closure with 0.25 to 0.5 ml/kg of a solution of 0.25% bupivacaine was as effective as the previously described method. This so-called instillation block presumably works by blocking the nerve bundles and branches that are exposed during the surgical dissection of the hernia sac.

Nerve Blocks of the Penis

Block of the dorsal nerves of the penis provides effective analgesia for hypospadias repair and circumcision, both of which are commonly performed in pediatric ambulatory patients. The distal two-thirds of the penis is innervated by the dorsal nerves, which are bilateral and adjacent to the midline (Fig. 4-9). They are distal twigs of the pudenal nerves, which arise from the sacral plexus (S2–4). At the base of the penis, they divide into multiple filaments that encircle the shaft before reaching the glans. They are covered by Buck's fascia and lie alongside the paired dorsal arteries and single vein of the penis, as well as midline structures. The base and proximal part of the penis are innervated by the genitofemoral and ilioinguinal nerves.

Two techniques have been described for placing a penile block. Broadman et al.[104] used the subcutaneous ring block, consisting of subcutaneous infiltration

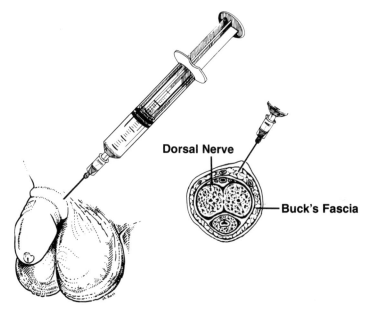

FIGURE 4-9. Ring block of the penis. Note the position of the needle superficial to Buck's fascia.

with 0.25% bupivacaine (see Fig. 4-9). The second method, dorsal penile nerve block, involves injection at the 10:30 and 1:30 positions of 1 to 2 ml of local anesthetic deep to Buck's fascia, either in one or two injections for each of the paired nerves.[133] This was found to provide good analgesia in 96% of cases. In a more recent study, dorsal nerve block was found to provide good pain relief following circumcision, which tended to be of shorter duration than that resulting from caudal block.[134] Children who received a nerve block, however, micturated and stood unaided earlier and had a lower incidence of vomiting than those who received a caudal block. Epinephrine-containing solutions must never be used to block the penis because it is an end-organ and vasoconstriction may seriously compromise circulation to that organ.

Topical lidocaine also has been successfully employed to produce penile analgesia following circumcision in children. In two recent studies, the use of lidocaine spray, ointment, or jelly was found effective in reducing pain and avoiding the need for postoperative analgesics.[135,136] Lidocaine jelly also proved an effective after-hospital treatment for such pain.

Caudal Block for Postoperative Analgesia
Caudal analgesia is the most useful and popular pediatric regional block used today by pediatric anesthesiologists. It is simple to perform and easily adaptable to ambulatory anesthesia practice. Sacral segment procedures such as circumcision, hypospadias repair, anal surgery, and club foot repair are common indications for caudal blocks at CNMC. In these cases, the caudal block greatly re-

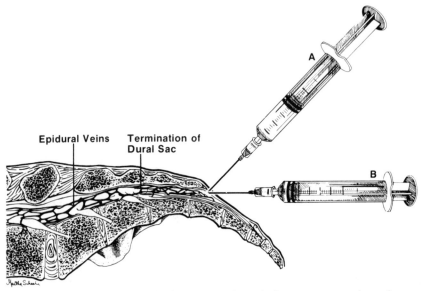

FIGURE 4-10. **A** and **B** placement and advancement through the sacrococcygeal membrane. Note that the bevel is facing anterior to avoid intraosseous introduction. (SOURCE: LM Broadman.[129] Used with permission.)

duces the risk of reflex laryngeal spasm in response to surgical stimulation and may, therefore, remove the need for endotracheal intubation.

The sacral hiatus, which is situated at the lower end of the sacrum, is extremely easy to identify in infants and young children. Its existence is due to the nonfusion of the fifth sacral vertebral arch. The large bony processes on each side are called the *cornua*. The coccyx lies immediately caudal to the sacral hiatus. The hiatus is covered by the sacrococcygeal membrane (Fig. 4-10). In infants and prepubertal children, these landmarks are easily palpable or even visible through the skin because of the absence of the large sacral pad of fat that usually develops at puberty.

The dural and arachnoid sacs may extend to the third or fourth sacral vertebra in infants. In addition, the sacral hiatus is relatively more cephalad in infants; thus the distance between the sacral hiatus and the end of the dural sac is relatively short.

The lateral position is most often employed to perform a caudal block in children. To identify the sacral hiatus, one begins by palpating the tip of the coccyx (lowest bony part of the spine). With the left index finger applying firm pressure to identify the coccyx, one moves the finger gently from side to side and proceeds in a cephalad direction. The first double bony protuberances encountered are the two cornua of the sacrum that define the sacral hiatus. The cornua should be marked either mentally or with a skin-marking pen.

After careful skin preparation, the sacral hiatus is again identified using firm pressure with the left index finger. Asepsis is maintained either by gloving or by palpating the skin through a sterile alcohol swab (Fig. 4-11). The caudal space is

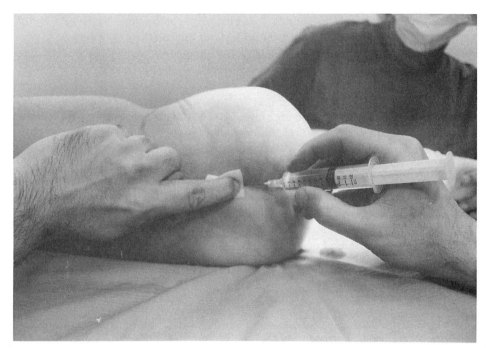

FIGURE 4-11. Strict aseptic techniques are essential. Either a no-touch method as shown or gloving is acceptable.

entered using a short (1-in) 23-gauge needle that has been attached to a syringe containing the appropriate volume of local anesthetic solution. The needle must be placed exactly in the midline and inserted at a 60-degree angle to the coronal plane, perpendicular to all other planes. As the needle is advanced, the bevel should be facing anteriorly to minimize the chance of piercing the anterior sacral wall (the most common reason for aspirating blood). A distinct pop is felt as the sacrococcygeal membrane is pierced. The angle of the needle is then lowered to 20 degrees and advanced an additional 2 to 3 mm to make sure that all the bevel surface is in the caudal space. Further advancement of the needle is not necessary and will increase the chances of dural puncture. After repeatedly demonstrating the absence of blood or CSF following attempts at aspiration, the appropriate amount of local anesthetic is injected and the child is placed in a supine position.

In patients less than four years of age, the caudal space also may be entered by inserting the needle through the cartilaginous back of the third or fourth sacral vertebral arch. This approach is particularly useful in the rare instances when the sacral hiatus is difficult to identify. To avoid dural puncture with this approach, the needle must remain perpendicular to the skin in all planes and should not be advanced any more than absolutely necessary.

Three important variables determine the quality, duration, and extent of a caudal block. These are the volume, total dose, and concentration of the drug. There is currently no general agreement, however, on whether age or weight is the better criterion for achieving the desired level of analgesia in children.

Schulte-Steinberg and Rahlfs examined the statistical significance of age, weight, and height on dose requirements for caudal anesthesia.[137] They found the pattern of spread to be highly predictable in children and further determined that it relates very nicely to age. Using 1% lidocaine or 0.25% bupivacaine solutions, they found that a volume of approximately 0.1 ml per segment per year of age was effective in prepubertal children. The relationship between age and dose requirement is strictly linear, and there is a high degree of correlation up to the age of 12 years.

Takasaki and colleagues[138] studied the dose requirements for caudal anesthesia in a large series of infants and children. They believed that for patients ranging in age from newborn to seven years, segmental dose requirements correlated better with body weight than with age. Using 1% lidocaine with epinephrine 1:200,000, they recommend calculating the volume of local anesthetic needed per segment as follows:

Milliliters per segment = 0.056 × body weight (kg)

In clinical practice, we find the most workable formula is that suggested by Armitage.[139] Using the desired local anesthetic solution, Armitage maintains that a volume of 0.5 ml/kg will result in an adequate sacral block. A dose of 1 ml/kg is used to block the lower thoracic nerves, and 1.25 ml/kg to reach the midthoracic region. The total dosage should always be checked to ensure that it is within the acceptable safe dose of the drug.

Eyres et al.[140] measured plasma bupivacaine concentrations following caudal injection of 3 mg/kg of 0.25% bupivacaine solution in 45 children whose ages ranged from 4 months to 12 years. They found mean blood levels ranging from 1.2 to 1.4 µg/ml, which are well below the limits to projected toxic levels in adults.

The results of using different bupivacaine concentrations on the quality of a caudal block have been recently studied. Broadman et al.[141] found that 0.3% and 0.375% bupivacaine solutions did not offer any advantage over the standard 0.25% concentration. Wolf et al.,[142] on the other hand, reported that a 0.125% bupivacaine solution (0.75 ml/kg) produced the same quality and duration of postoperative analgesic as a 0.25% concentration. Moreover, the more dilute solution resulted in less motor blockade.

The duration of caudal analgesia in children has been studied by recording the time that elapsed before the block level began to recede by at least two spinal segments.[143] When bupivacaine alone was used, that time was two hours; if an epinephrine-containing solution was used, it was slightly longer. Bromage also noted that the total duration of action in the lower sacral segments was considerably longer than the time that elapsed before the beginning of recession.[143] This observation correlates well with clinical experience, where bupivacaine caudal analgesia, as judged by the time elapsing before the child requires supplemental analgesia, may persist for more than five hours.[144]

Caudal blocks in children are usually combined with a light general anesthetic. When short surgical procedures (<1 hr) are performed, the duration of postoperative analgesia is not affected by placement of the block before or after surgery.[145] The former approach is preferred because it reduces the intraoperative need for potent inhalation agents and still ensures excellent postoperative pain relief.

The duration of postoperative analgesia following a caudal block can be substantially prolonged by using preservative-free morphine. In a controlled study involving 22 children, Jensen found that the duration of pain relief was substantially longer with caudal morphine (range 10 to 36 hr) than with bupivacaine (range 4 to 8 hr).[146] Although there were no complications in these patients, the author cautions that there may be a risk of respiratory depression after epidural morphine. He recommends that no child should be permitted to leave the hospital within 24 hours of receiving a caudal block with morphine. More recently, Krane and coworkers[147] reported good pain relief in a study comparing caudal morphine, caudal bupivacaine, and intravenous morphine for postoperative pain relief following genitourinary or lower extremity orthopedic surgery. Krane also reported delayed respiratory depression requiring naloxone infusion in a two-year-old boy who received a caudal dose of 0.1 mg/kg of preservative-free morphine.[148] We therefore continue to avoid and cannot recommend the use of caudal narcotics in our ambulatory patients.

Although clinical experience with pediatric caudal block is quite extensive, it has not been until recently that reports of large series have been published. Broadman and coworkers[149] reported no complications or toxic reactions associated with caudal blocks in a prospective study of 1154 children. The authors stressed that the key to the safety of the procedure is knowledge of the anatomy in children, meticulous attention to detail in site selection and preparation, and careful aspiration before drug injection. Dalens found no major complications or neurologic sequelae as well as good patient and parental acceptance in 750 consecutive patients.[150]

The possibility of intraosseous injection must always be considered when performing caudal blocks in children. The cancellous mass of sacral bone is covered by a wafer-thin, brittle layer of cortex that can be damaged easily. Intraosseous penetration is suggested by the appearance of a gritty aspirate in a small volume of apparently pure blood following aspiration. This complication is best avoided by inserting the needle in the line of the sacral canal, avoiding excessive force, and keeping the bevel of the needle directed anteriorly so that it slides over rather than penetrates the anterior plate of the sacrum.

Intravenous injection can be prevented by repeated gentle aspiration following each needle movement. Use of excessive force while attempting aspiration may fail to show blood if the suction force results in collapse of the vein. In our experience, most bloody aspirates are due to intraosseous injection rather than intravenous placement of the needle. In either case, it is our practice to reposition the needle and inject serially 0.5 ml of the solution with reaspiration until blood staining is slight or lacking. Matsumiya and coworkers[151] have recently reported a case of cardiovascular collapse in an infant after caudal anesthesia with a lidocaine-epinephrine solution. They attributed the problem to an inadvertent intravascular injection. Although other factors may have played a role in that case (e.g., hypoventilation and/or overdose of halothane), such reports heighten our awareness of the possibility of such occurrences.[152]

INTRAVENOUS REGIONAL ANESTHESIA

Although it is possible to employ intravenous regional anesthesia on the lower extremity as well as the upper, there are no reports of lower extremity intravenous regional anesthesia in the pediatric patient. It has, however, often been employed in the upper extremity in children for the setting of simple forearm fractures.[153]

With the patient supine, a double pneumatic tourniquet of appropriate size is placed on the affected extremity. A 20- to 22-gauge plastic cannula (or 19- to 25-gauge butterfly needle) is inserted into a vein close to the operative site. The extremity is elevated for three minutes or exsanguinated with an Esmarch bandage and the proximal cuff is inflated to approximately 50 mmHg above the measured systolic pressure. Then 4 mg/kg of 0.5% lidocaine without preservative is injected. Anesthesia is expected in three to five minutes. Bupivacaine should not be selected for this technique because of the severe cardiovascular complications associated with its use.[154]

Most procedures performed under these techniques have lasted less than 15 minutes, and tourniquet pain was not encountered. Tourniquet pain may be abolished by inflating the distal tourniquet, which should be in an anesthetic area, and then deflating the proximal tourniquet. Staged cuff deflation is recommended following procedures lasting less than 30 minutes.

SURFACE ANESTHESIA
Skin

A topical anesthetic agent can be of great value in performing painful peripheral procedures in children. Many attempts have been made to compound a formulation of local anesthetics that will produce effective anesthesia when applied topically to intact skin. When mixed in equal amounts, the solid pure bases of lidocaine and prilocaine constitute a eutectic mixture of local anesthetics (EMLA) that forms an oil at temperatures greater than 16°C. This mixture has been tested in Europe on adults and premedicated children and in the United States on unpremedicated pediatric outpatients to produce skin analgesia before venipuncture.[155,156]

To become fully effective, an EMLA requires very careful application. After an appropriate amount (2.5 g) is applied over a preselected vein, an occlusive dressing must be applied and left undisturbed for 60 minutes.

Although an EMLA does alleviate the physical pain associated with venipuncture, it does not address the emotional component of anticipating pain that children associate with venipuncture. In a recent study, an EMLA was no more effective in this regard than the standard intradermal injection of lidocaine.[155] The ultimate place of EMLAs in pediatric ambulatory anesthesia remains to be established.

Mucous Membranes

Topical anesthesia may be applied to the nose and nasopharynx before passage of a nasotracheal tube to reduce response to an oral airway in the pharynx or before passage of an endotracheal tube. Topical anesthesia is a great help during diagnostic or operative bronchoscopy. The dose of lidocaine for topical spray on the trachea should not exceed 2 mg/kg. If the calculated volume of the 4% solution is too small, a more dilute formulation should be selected.

Topical anesthesia also may be useful in cystoscopic procedures. An aqueous jelly applied to the urethra often enables one to use very light supplemental general anesthesia. Other uses for topical anesthesia include the removal of foreign bodies from the eyes (0.5% proparacaine) and shrinkage of the nasal turbinates (4% cocaine).

LOCAL INFILTRATION

Whether employed by surgeon or anesthesiologist, local infiltration anesthesia probably has a greater potential in pediatric ambulatory surgery than is currently appreciated. In addition to its usefulness for suturing lacerations and for other minor procedures, local anesthesia may be the best technique for performing superficial procedures in older children.

Two agents have been the primary agents used for infiltration anesthesia and seem equally effective. One may use a total of 10 mg/kg of 0.5% or 1.0% procaine or a total of 5 mg/kg of 0.25% lidocaine with some margin of safety.

Because of its vasoconstrictive effect, the addition of epinephrine would increase the permissible amount of anesthetic. However, its introduction would involve the danger of exceeding the safe limit set for epinephrine unless the solutions were limited to a strength of 1:400,000. Consequently, epinephrine is not used at CNMC when the injection is purely for analgesia. If the epinephrine is infiltrated for the purpose of reducing bleeding, as in plastic surgery, the total allowable dose is considered to be 10 µg/kg if the child is receiving halothane and is not hypercarbic.

RECOVERY AND DISCHARGE CRITERIA

The key to understanding the reasoning behind the selection or avoidance of certain anesthetic agents and techniques in ambulatory surgery is related to recovery. Rapid recovery and early ambulation are major objectives in pediatric ambulatory surgery. When dealing with pediatric outpatients, we must guarantee safe discharge not only from the recovery room but also from the hospital.[157] In our institution, all children recover from anesthesia in the same recovery area. Ambulatory patients are then transferred to a special short-stay recovery unit (SSRU).

In order to provide uniform care and to ensure a complete legal record, some institutions have developed discharge criteria. Unlike a scoring system, all criteria should be met. At CNMC, criteria for discharge from the hospital are

> Appropriateness and stability of vital signs
> Ability to swallow oral fluids and cough or demonstrate a gag reflex
> Ability to ambulate consistent with developmental age level
> Absence of nausea, vomiting, and dizziness, preferably including ability to retain oral fluids
> Absence of respiratory distress
> A state of consciousness appropriate to developmental level

Endotracheal extubation performed within three hours of the time of discharge and depressant medication received within two hours are other factors that need to be considered. Although the intervals noted here are arbitrary, they direct our attention to two potential areas of concern within a time frame when complications might occur.

ROLE OF THE PARENT IN THE RECOVERY PERIOD
Postanesthesia Care Unit (PACU)
Many parents want to be with their child as soon as the operation is terminated. In addition to confirming that the child has indeed survived the procedure, the parents believe that the child will relate to them better than to other unfamiliar faces at a time when anxiety could result from separation. Unfortunately, most PACUs are not large enough or planned properly to allow parents to participate in this aspect of care. In addition, many PACU nurses believe that early parent participation at this level may be detrimental to the care of the child and perhaps that of other children as well. Parent participation in recovery of handicapped children has proved useful in our institution in selected cases. These especially include deaf, blind, and retarded children whose ability to communicate with anyone other than the parent is compromised. In any case, parents should not have access to the PACU until the child's vital signs have stabilized, airway obstruction is no longer a threat, and the child is awakening. They should be told in advance that their role is to provide support for their child. They should stay at the child's bedside, should not walk around the room, and should not inquire about other children in the room. The parent must understand that should the child's condition deteriorate or for any reason it seems prudent to request them to leave the unit at any time they will do so promptly and without argument. It is important that they know they are not required to stay and should feel at liberty to leave the room if they feel uncomfortable.

Short-Stay Recovery Unit (SSRU)
Parents are encouraged to or may even be required to participate in the child's care in the SSRU (Fig. 4-12). Parents can care for and hold, cuddle, and feed the

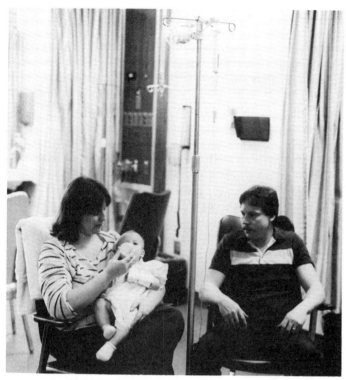

FIGURE 4-12. Parents participate in the child's care in the short-stay unit at CNMC.

child, and their involvement may reduce the need for a very high nurse/patient ratio. The rules and regulations of parent participation in the SSRU should be provided in advance. An example of the issues which should be addressed can be found in "Forms and Policies."

Discharge Home

As noted by Steward,[6] "every child, whatever his or her age, must have an escort home. The journey preferably should be by private car or taxicab, and the escort should be provided with written instructions as to the home care of the child and be provided with a telephone number to call for further advice or to report complications. Such service is essential in the outpatient unit." In addition to counseling the parent of each child about postoperative care, most units have designed handouts that specify the care to be provided and the signs that might herald a complication. For convenience, the handout is usually limited to postoperative instructions for one specific operative procedure. An example of such a pamphlet for patients who undergo inguinal herniorrhaphy can be found in "Forms and Policies."

COMPLICATIONS AND ADMISSIONS
Complications
Aside from pain, the most difficult common complication to prevent or treat is protracted vomiting, which is most commonly associated with tonsillectomy and adenoidectomy[100] and with strabismus surgery.[124,158,159] Vomiting is twice as common following operations that last over 20 minutes as in shorter procedures.[4] In one study of postoperative vomiting in children,[160] it was noted that vomiting occurred less frequently in children less than three years of age but above this age varied between 42% and 51% until puberty. Although factors other than age also influenced the frequency with which postoperative vomiting occurred, a major factor was related to the operative procedure[160] (Table 4-7).

In our institution, frequency of vomiting in intubated, unmedicated children receiving nitrous oxide–halothane anesthesia for strabismus surgery was reported to be as high as 85%.[124] Although treatment with an antiemetic agent is fraught with other potential dangers such as sedation and hypotension, the prophylactic or therapeutic use of droperidol (75 µg/kg IV 30 min before the end of surgery) was found to be highly effective in reducing the frequency and severity of vomiting in children following strabismus surgery.[124] On average, patients who vomited and received droperidol, as well as those who did not, were unable to meet discharge criteria for six hours after discontinuation of the anesthetic agent and admission to the recovery room. Although this is a long recovery for an ambulatory surgical procedure, untreated patients cannot be discharged any earlier because of persistent vomiting; furthermore, they are also more uncomfortable. Lerman et al.[161] found that the same dose of droperidol (75 µg/kg) given at induction of anesthesia but before manipulation of the eye reduced the incidence of vomiting predischarge from 47% to 10% without prolonging either the recovery time or the time before discharge from the hospital.

Droperidol (0.075 µg/kg) also was found to be more effective than lidocaine (1.5

TABLE 4-7. Vomiting Related to Procedures or Surgical Specialty

Procedure	No. of Patients	No. and Percentage of Patients Who Vomited		Average Number of Vomiting Episodes per Patient
Squint	33	25	(76%)	1.82
Hernia	92	50	(54%)	1.71
T&A	89	52	(58%)	1.57
Orchidopexy	64	37	(58%)	1.44
Plastic	145	71	(49%)	1.22
Hypospadias	24	11	(46%)	1.21
Circumcision	49	20	(41%)	1.20

SOURCE: Based on Rowley MP, Brown TCK: Postoperative vomiting in children. Anaesth Intensive Care 10: 309–313, 1982.

mg/kg) in reducing the incidence of vomiting in unpremedicated strabismus patients.[162] Good response also has been reported when intravenous metoclopramide (0.15 mg/kg) was used as an antiemetic immediately following anesthesia for eye muscle surgery in pediatric ambulatory patients.[163] Brown and coworkers compared low-dose droperidol 20 μg/kg IV with droperidol 75 μg/kg IV for prevention of vomiting after pediatric strabismus surgery.[164] Droperidol-treated patients vomited less (35%) than a control group (53%). There was no difference between droperidol 75 μg and droperidol 20 μg on the incidence of vomiting. Brown and colleagues recommend suctioning of gastric contents at the conclusion of surgery, complete replacement of preoperative fluid deficits, avoidance of narcotics, and low-dose droperidol (20 μg/kg) intravenously.

In our institution, severe vomiting also has been observed following orchidopexy performed on an outpatient basis. Interestingly enough, this is the one procedure noted by Cloud et al.[122] to require the use of oral narcotic agents for pain relief in the posthospitalization period. Strabismus surgery and orchidopexy are examples of severe vomiting. Vomiting may be a major problem even after relatively short, uncomplicated procedures. Some patients may vomit repeatedly after oral fluids are offered. As a result, it is frequently judicious to maintain an intravenous infusion until oral fluids are tolerated. The rate of infusion should be increased to account for fluid losses. Replacement for vomiting should be done with normal saline or Ringer's lactate. Droperidol has been used successfully in doses as low as 5 μg/kg in patients with persistent vomiting following procedures other than strabismus surgery or orchidopexy.[165]

Admissions

Complications that result in *admission* of the patient to a hospital are usually the same types of problems discussed previously but with either greater frequency or severity. Less than 1% of the patients operated on in our unit require admission. The most common reasons for admission of the patients operated on at CNMC are shown in Table 4-8.

TABLE 4-8. Reasons for Admission to the Hospital from the Short-Stay Recovery Unit

Reason	No.	%
Protracted vomiting	30	33
Croup	8	9
Family request	6	7
Fever	6	7
Bleeding	3	3
Complicated surgery	15	17
Sleepiness	2	2
Others	20	22
TOTAL	90	100

SOURCE: From Patel and Hannallah.[166]

TABLE 4-9. Postdischarge Complications Reported by Parents of 4998 Pediatric Ambulatory Patients.

Complications	No. of Patients	Percentage
Vomiting (frequency):		
1–2	359	7.2%
3–4	64	1.2%
4	24	0.5%
Vomiting (total)	447	8.9%
Cough	324	6.5%
Sleepiness	297	5.9%
Sore throat	257	5.1%
Fever	235	4.7%
Hoarseness/mild croup	168	3.4%
	——	——
TOTAL	1728	34.5%

SOURCE: From Patel and Hannallah.[166]

FOLLOW-UP

Telephone or mail questionnaires are necessary to determine the frequency of posthospitalization problems. A large percentage of parents report that their child continues to have an upset stomach, dizziness, and so forth after returning home (Table 4-9). Fortunately, most of the complications reported are mild[4,12,167] and require no treatment. A questionnaire should be designed not only to detect problems in the child, but also to determine whether the parents were satisfied with the care received and, if not, to request suggestions for improvement (see the section on Forms and Policies at the end of the book). A small percentage of parents respond that they would prefer to have the child hospitalized if they had it to do over again.[4,167] Some of the reasons for this have been noted previously in the section on disadvantages. Early (1971) studies by Davenport[12] reported this percentage was 9.2%; and in Ahlgren's, 8.0%.[19] This relatively high percentage of dissatisfaction or apprehension rarely occurs in adult ambulatory settings and seems to relate to the parent's desire to have a longer period of observation and care for the child in the hospital and a fear of potential complications at home.

Any ambulatory surgery unit should collect and analyze data for trends that might lead to correction of deficiencies and eventually to improvement in patient care. Design and modification of policy are better done by prospective review of audits than by reacting to mishaps. This leads to more uniform, safe care and minimizes medicolegal actions.

REFERENCES

1. Nicoll JH: The surgery of infancy. Br Med J 2: 753, 1909
2. Herzfeld G: Hernia in infancy. Am J Surg 39: 422, 1938

3. Striker TW: Results of Anesthesia Survey, American Academy of Pediatrics, Section on Anesthesia. Presented at meetings of American Academy of Pediatrics, 1979

4. Steward DJ: Experience with an outpatient anesthesia service for children. Anesth Analg 52: 877, 1973

5. Othersen HB, Clatworthy HW: Outpatient herniorrhaphy for infants. Am J Dis Child 116: 78, 1968

6. Steward DJ: Outpatient pediatric anesthesia. Anesthesiology 43: 268, 1975

7. Steward DJ: Psychological considerations in the pediatric patient. In Guerra F, Aldrete JA (eds): Emotional and Psychological Responses to Anesthesia and Surgery. New York, Grune & Stratton, 1980

8. Steward DJ: Anaesthesia for day-care surgery: A symposium: IV. Anaesthesia for paediatric outpatients. Can Anaesth Soc J 27: 412, 1980

9. Davenport HT, Werry JS: The effect of general anesthesia, surgery and hospitalization upon the behavior of children. Am J Orthopsychiatry 5: 806, 1970

10. O'Donovan TR: Ambulatory Surgical Centers—Development and Management. Germantown, Md., Aspen Systems, 1976

11. Cohen DD, Dillon JB: Anesthesia for Outpatient Surgery. Springfield, Ill., Charles C. Thomas, 1970

12. Davenport HT, Shaw CP, Robinson GC: Day surgery for children. Can Med Assoc J 105: 498, 1971

13. Rigg JRA, Dunn GL, Cameron GS: Paediatric outpatient surgery under general anaesthesia. Anaesth Intensive Care 8: 451, 1980

14. Berry FA: The child with the runny nose. In Berry FA (ed): Anesthetic Management of Difficult and Routine Pediatric Patients, pp 349–367. New York, Churchill-Livingstone, 1986

15. Tait AR, Knight PR: Intraoperative respiratory complications in patients with upper respiratory tract infections. Can J Anaesth 34: 300, 1987

16. McGill WA, Coveler LA, Epstein BS: Subacute upper respiratory infection in small children. Anesth Analg 58: 331, 1979

17. Tait AR, Knight PR: The effects of general anesthesia on upper respiratory tract infections in children. Anesthesiology 67: 930, 1987

18. DeSoto H, Patel RI, Soliman IE, Hannallah RS: Changes in oxygen saturation following general anesthesia in children with upper respiratory infection signs and symptoms undergoing otolaryngological procedures. Anesthesiology 68: 276, 1988

19. Ahlgren EN, Bennett EJ, Stephen CR: Outpatient pediatric anesthesiology: A case series. Anesth Analg 50: 402, 1971

20. Johnson GG: Day care surgery for infants and children. Can Anaesth Soc J 30: 553, 1983

21. Bryan MH, Hardie MJ, Reilly BJ, et al: Pulmonary function studies during the first year of life in infants recovering from the respiratory distress syndrome. Pediatrics 52: 169, 1973

22. Steward DJ: Pre-term infants are more prone to complications following minor surgery than are term infants. Anesthesiology 56: 304, 1982

23. Liu LMP, Coté CJ, Goudsouzian NG, et al: Life-threatening apnea in infants recovering from anesthesia. Anesthesiology 59: 506, 1983

24. Welborn LG, Ramirez N, Oh TH, Ruttimann UE, Fink R, Guzzetta P, Epstein BS: Postanesthetic apnea and periodic breathing in infants. Anesthesiology 65: 656, 1986

25. Welborn LG, DeSoto H, Hannallah RS, et al: The use of caffeine in the control of postanesthetic apnea in former premature infants. Anesthesiology 68: 796, 1988

26. Kurth CD, Spitzer AR, Broennle AM, Downes JJ: Postoperative apnea in preterm infants. Anesthesiology 66: 483, 1987

27. Mestad PH, Glenski JA, Binda, Jr, RE: When is outpatient surgery safe in preterm infants? Anesthesiology 69: 744, 1988

28. Tetzlaff JE, Annand DW, Pudimat MA, Nicodemus HF: Post-operative apnea in a full-term infant. Anesthesiology 69: 426, 1988

29. Coté CJ: At what post-gestational age in a previously premature infant would it be safe to anesthetize a child as an outpatient? Soc Pediatr Anesth Newsletter 2(1): 2, 1989

30. Welborn LG, Hannallah RS, Fink R, Ruttimann UE, Hicks JM: High-dose caffeine suppresses postoperative apnea in former preterm infants. Anesthesiology 71: 342, 1989
31. Downes JJ: At what post-gestational age in a previously premature infant would it be safe to anesthetize a child as an outpatient? Soc Pediatr Anesth Newsletter 2(1): 9, 1989
32. Newburger JW, Rosenthal A, Williams RG, et al: Noninvasive tests in the initial evaluation of heart murmurs in children. N Engl J Med 308: 61, 1983
33. American Heart Association (AHA) Committee Report: Prevention of bacterial endocarditis. Circulation 70: 1123A, 1984
34. Surgicenter: A new idea for one day surgery. Residents Staff Phys 15: 65, 1973
35. Medical Society of the District of Columbia and National Capital Medical Foundation, Inc.: Position Statement on Ambulatory Surgery, October 23, 1978. Washington, November 1980
36. Chiang TM, Sukis AE, Ross DE: Tonsillectomy performed on an outpatient basis: Report of a series of 40,000 cases performed without a death. Arch Otolaryngol 88: 307, 1968
37. Maniglia AJ, Kushner H, Cozzi L: Adenotonsillectomy: A safe outpatient procedure. Arch Otolaryngol Head Neck Surg 115: 92, 1989
38. Jensen BH, Wernberg M, Adersen M: Preoperative starvation and blood glucose concentrations in children undergoing inpatient and outpatient anesthesia. Br J Anaesth 54: 1071, 1982
39. Splinter WM, Stewart JA, Muir JG: The effect of preoperative apple juice on gastric contents, thirst and hunger in children. Can J Anaesth 36: 55, 1989
40. Coté CJ: NPO after midnight for children—a reappraisal. Anesthesiology 72: 589, 1990
41. Goudsouzian N, Coté CJ, Lui LMP, Dedrick DF: The dose-response effects of oral cimetidine on gastric pH and volume in children. Anesthesiology 55: 533, 1981
42. Goudsouzian NG, Young ET: The efficacy of ranitidine in children. Acta Anaesthesiol Scand 31: 387, 1987
43. Henderson JM, Spence DG, Clarke WN, Bonn GG, Noel LP: Sodium citrate in paediatric outpatients. Can J Anaesth 34: 560, 1987
44. Sagel SS, Evens RG, Forrest JV, et al: Efficacy of routine screening and lateral chest radiographs in a hospital-based population. N Engl J Med 291: 1001, 1974
45. Sane SM, Worsing RA, Wiens CW, et al: Value of preoperative chest x-ray examinations in children. Pediatrics 60: 669, 1977
46. Berry FA: Pediatric outpatient anesthesia. In Hershey SG (ed): ASA Refresher Courses in Anesthesiology, Vol 10, pp 17–26. Philadelphia, J.B. Lippincott, 1982
47. Rosen DA, Rosen KR, Hannallah RS: Preoperative characteristics which influence the child's response to induction of anesthesia. Anesthesiology 63: A462, 1985
48. Stein SB: A Hospital Story. New York, Walker, 1983
49. Sewall K: Preoperative medication for children. Surg Clin North Am 50: 775, 1970
50. Smith RM: Anesthesia for Infants and Children, 4th ed. St. Louis, CV Mosby, 1980
51. Desjardins R, Ansara S, Charest J: Preanesthetic medication in paediatric day-care surgery. Can Anaesth Soc J 28: 141, 1981
52. Brustowicz RM, Nelson DA, Betts EK, et al: Efficacy of oral premedication for pediatric outpatient surgery. Anesthesiology 60: 475, 1984
53. Rita L, Cox JM, Seleny FL, et al: Ketamine hydrochloride for pediatric premedication: I. Comparison with pentazocine. Anesth Analg 53: 375, 1974
54. Rita L, Seleny FL: Pediatric outpatient premedication: Premedication versus no premedication and the choice of anesthetic agents. Anesthesiol Rev 1: 9, 1974
55. Shah CP, Robinson GC, Kinnis C, et al: Day care surgery for children: A controlled study of medical complications and parental attitudes. Med Care 10: 437, 1972
56. Van der Walt JH, Nicholas B, Bentley M, Tomkins DP: Oral premedication in children. Anaesth Intensive Care 15: 151, 1987
57. Booker PD, Chapman DH: Premedication in children undergoing day-care surgery. Br J Anaesth 51: 1083, 1979
58. Ryhanen P, Kangas T, Rantakyla S: Premedication for outpatient adenoidectomy: Comparison between ketamine and pethidine. Laryngoscope 90: 494, 1980
59. Rita L, Seleny FL, Mazurek A, Rabins S: Intramuscular midazolam for pediatric pre-anesthetic sedation: A double-blind controlled study with morphine. Anesthesiology 63: 528, 1985

60. Taylor MB, Vince PR, Hatch DJ: Intramuscular midazolam premedication in small children: A comparison with papaveretum and hyoscine. Anaesthesia 41: 21, 1986
61. Nicolson SC, Betts EK, Jobes DR, Chirstianson LA, Walters JW, Mayes KR, Korevaar WC: Comparison of oral and intramuscular preanesthetic medication for pediatric inpatient surgery. Anesthesiology 71: 8, 1989
62. Henderson JM, Brodsky DA, Fisher DM, Brett CM, Hertzka RE: Pre-induction of anesthesia in pediatric patients with nasally administered sufentanil. Anesthesiology 68: 671, 1988
63. Hannallah RS, Patel RI: Low-dose intramuscular ketamine for anesthesia pre-induction in young children undergoing brief outpatient procedure. Anesthesiology 70: 598, 1989
64. Clark AJM, Hurting AB: Premedication with meperidine and atropine does not prolong recovery to street fitness after outpatient surgery. Can Anaesth Soc J 28: 390, 1981
65. Goresky GV, Steward DJ: Rectal methohexitone for induction of anaesthesia in children. Can Anaesth Soc J 26: 213, 1979
66. Strisand JB, Hague B, Van Vreeswijk H, Ho GH, Pace NL, Clissold M, Nelson P, East KA, Stanley TO, Stanley TH: Oral transmucosal fentanyl premedication in children. Anesth Analg 66: S170, 1987
67. Nelson PS, Streisand JB, Mulder SM, Pace NL, Stanley TH: Comparison of oral transmucosal fentanyl citrate and an oral solution of meperidine, diazepam and atropine for premedication in children. Anesthesiology 70: 616, 1989
68. Wilton NCT, Leigh J, Rosen DR, Pandit UA: Pre-anesthetic sedation of preschool children using intranasal midazolam. Anesthesiology 69: 972, 1988
69. Hannallah RS, Rosales JK: Experience with parents' presence during anaesthesia induction in children. Can Anaesth Soc J 30: 286, 1983
70. Schulman J, Foley JM, Vernon TA, et al: A study of the effect of the mother's presence during anesthesia induction. Pediatrics 39: 111, 1967
71. Hannallah RS, Abramowitz MD, Oh TH, et al: Residents' attitude towards parents' presence during anesthesia induction in children: Does experience make a difference? Anesthesiology 60: 598, 1984
72. Schmidt KF, Garfield JM, Korten K: The pharmacology of agents used in outpatient anesthesia. Int Anesthesiol Clin 14: 15, 1976
73. Diaz JH, Lockhart CH: Is halothane really safe in infancy? (abstr). Anesthesiology 51: S313, 1979
74. Hoyal RHA, Prys-Roberts C, Simpson PJ: Enflurane in outpatient dental anaesthesia. Br J Anaesth 52: 219, 1980
75. Steward DJ: A trial of enflurane for pediatric outpatient anaesthesia. Can Anaesth Soc J 24: 603, 1977
76. Johnston RR, Eger EI II, Wilson C: A comparative interaction of epinephrine with enflurane, isoflurane, and halothane in man. Anesth Analg 55: 709, 1976
77. Karl HW, Swedlow DB, Lee KW, et al: Epinephrine-halothane interaction in children. Anesthesiology 58: 142, 1983
78. Wade JG, Stevens WC: Isoflurane: An anesthetic for the eighties? Anesth Analg 60: 666, 1981
79. Kingston HGG: Halothane and isoflurane anesthesia in pediatric outpatients. Anesth Analg 65: 181, 1986
80. Steward DJ: Isoflurane for pediatric outpatients (abstr). Can Anaesth Soc J 28: 500, 1981
81. Jonmarker C, Westrin P, Larsson S, Warner O: Thiopental requirements for induction of anesthesia in children. Anesthesiology 67: 104, 1987
82. Dundee JW: Intravenous Anesthetic Agents. Chicago, Year Book Medical Publishers, 1979
83. Kortilla K, Linnoila M, Ertama P, et al: Recovery and simulated driving after intravenous anesthesia with thiopental, methohexital, propanidid, or alphadione. Anesthesiology 43: 291, 1975
84. Hudson RJ, Stanski DR, Burch PG: Pharmacokinetics of methohexital and thiopental in surgical patients. Anesthesiology 59: 215, 1983
85. Rockoff MA, Goudsouzian NG: Seizures induced by methohexital and thiopental in surgical patients. Anesthesiology 59: 215, 1983
86. Kay B: A clinical assessment of the use of etomidate in children. Br J Anaesth 48: 207, 1976

87. Craig J, Cooper GM, Sear JW: Recovery from day-care anesthesia: Comparison between methohexitone, Althesin and etomidate. Br J Anaesth 54: 447, 1982

88. Johnston R, Noseworthy T, Anderson B, Konopad E, Grace M: Propofol versus thiopental for outpatient anesthesia. Anesthesiology 67: 431, 1987

89. Valtonen M, Iisalo E, Kanto J, Tikkanen J: Comparison between propofol and thiopentone for induction of anesthesia in children. Anaesthesia 43: 696, 1988

90. Meursing AEE, Bell B, Lobatto R, Erdmann W: A comparison of propofol with thiopentone for induction of anesthesia in unpremedicated children. Anesthesiology 69: A741, 1988

91. Hannallah RS, Baker SB, Casey WF, McGill WA, Broadman LM, Norden JM: Induction dose of propofol in unpremedicated children. Anesth Analg 70: S143, 1990

92. Krantz EM: Low-dose intramuscular ketamine and hyaluronidase for induction of anesthesia in non-premedicated children. S Afr Med J 58: 161, 1980

93. Khazzam A, Karkas A: Intramuscular methohexital as a sole pediatric anesthetic-analgesic agent. Anesth Analg 51: 895, 1972

94. Varner PD, Ebert JP, McKay RD, Nail CS: Methohexital sedation of children undergoing CT scan. Anesth Analg 64: 643, 1985.

95. Hannallah RS, Abramowitz MD, McGill WA, Epstein BS: Rectal methohexitone induction in pediatric outpatients: Physostigmine does not enhance recovery. Can Anaesth Soc J 32: 231, 1985

96. Forbes RB, Vandewalker GE: Comparison of 2 and 10 percent rectal methohexitone for induction of anaesthesia in children. Can J Anaesth 35: 345, 1988

97. Khalil SN, Nuutinen LS, Rawal N, Jimenez PA, Marcus MA, Haaren EV, Fallon KD, Stanley TH: Sigmoidorectal methohexital as an induction agent for general anesthesia in children. Anesth Analg 70: 645, 1990

98. Kestin IG, McIlvaine WB, Lockhart CH, Kestin KJ, Jones MA: Rectal methohexital for induction of anesthesia in children with and without rectal aspiration after sleep. Anesth Analg 67: 1102, 1988

99. Voss S, Rockoff M, Brustowicz R, Caceras A: Oxygen saturation in children following administration of rectal methohexital. Anesth Analg 67: S247, 1988

100. Esptein BS, Levy ML, Thein MH, et al: Evaluation of fentanyl as an adjunct to thiopental–nitrous oxide–oxygen anesthesia for short surgical procedures. Anesthesiol Rev 2: 24, 1975

101. Haley S, Edelist G, Urbach G: Comparison of alfentanil, fentanyl and enflurane as supplements to general anesthesia for outpatient gynaecologic surgery. Can J Anaesth 35: 570, 1988

102. Enright AC, Pace-Florida A: Recovery from anesthesia in outpatients: A comparison of narcotic and inhalational techniques. Can Anaesth Soc J 24: 618, 1977

103. Hannallah RS, Broadman LM, Belman AB, et al: Comparison of ilioinguinal/iliohypogastric block for control of postorchiopexy pain in pediatric ambulatory surgery. Anesthesiology 66: 832, 1987

104. Broadman LM, Hannallah RS, Belman AB, et al: Postcircumcision analgesia: A prospective evaluation of subcutaneous ring block of the penis. Anesthesiology 67: 399, 1987

105. Hertzka RE, Gauntlett IS, Fisher DM, Spellman MJ: Fentanyl-induced ventilatory depression: Effects of age. Anesthesiology 70: 213, 1989

106. Youngberg JA, Subaiya C, Graybar GB, et al: Alfentanil for day-stay surgery in children: An evaluation (abstr). Anesth Analg 63: 284, 1984

107. Casey WF, Woodford RA, Martin WJ, Baker SB, Hannallah RS: Comparison of alfentanil and halothane for pediatric ENT surgery. Anesth Analg 70: S52, 1990

108. Goudsouzian NG, Liu LMP: The neuromuscular response of infants to a continuous infusion of succinylcholine. Anesthesiology 60: 97, 1984

109. Bush GH, Roth F: Muscle pains after suxamethonium chloride in children. Br J Anaesth 33: 151, 1961

110. Putnam LP: Pseudocholinesterase deficiency: An additional preoperative consideration in outpatient diagnostic procedures. South Med J 70: 831, 1977

111. Urbach GM, Edelist G: An evaluation of the anesthetic techniques used in an outpatient unit. Can Anaesth Soc J 24: 401, 1977

112. Ferres CJ, Crean PM, Kirakhur RK: An evaluation of Org NC 45 (vecuronium) in paediatric anaesthesia. Anaesthesia 38: 943, 1983

113. Goudsouzian NG, Liu LMP, Coté CJ, et al: Safety and efficacy of atracurium in adolescents and children anesthetized with halothane. Anesthesiology 59: 459, 1983

114. Blitt C: Nitrous-narcotic-relaxant anesthesia vs. volatile anesthesia in the adult surgical outpatient. In Brown BR (ed): Outpatient Anesthesia: Contemporary Anesthesia Practice. Philadelphia, FA Davis, 1978

115. Smith RM: Endotracheal intubation. In Anesthesia for Infants and Children, 4th ed. St. Louis, CV Mosby, 1980

116. Tomlin PJ, Howarth FH, Robinson JS: Postoperative atelectasis and laryngeal incompetence. Lancet 1: 1402, 1968

117. Koka BV, Jeon IS, Andre JM, et al: Postintubation croup in children. Anesth Analg 56: 501, 1977

118. Rose DK, Byrick RJ, Froese AB: Carbon dioxide elimination during spontaneous ventilation with a modified Mapleson D system: Studies in a lung model. Can Anaesth Soc J 25: 353, 1978

119. Casey WF, Broadman LM, Rice LJ, Daily M: Comparison of liquid crystal skin temperature probe and axillary thermistor probe in measuring core temperature trends during anaesthesia in pediatric patients. Can J Anaesth 36: S62, 1989

120. American Academy of Pediatrics: Guidelines for the elective use of conscious sedation, deep sedation and general anesthesia in pediatric patients. Pediatrics 76: 317, 1985

121. American Academy of Pediatrics: Guidelines for the elective use of conscious sedation, deep sedation and general anesthesia in pediatric patients. Pediatrics 77: 754, 1986

122. Cloud DT, Reed WA, Ford JL, et al: The surgicenter: A fresh concept in outpatient pediatric surgery. J Pediatr Surg 7: 206, 1972

123. Graham IFM: Preoperative starvation and plasma glucose concentrations in children undergoing outpatient anaesthesia. Br J Anaesth 51: 161, 1979

124. Abramowitz MD, Oh TH, Epstein BS, et al: The antiemetic effect of droperidol following outpatient strabismus surgery in children. Anesthesiology 59: 579, 1983

125. Berry FA: Pediatric anesthesia for the practitioner-fluid balance. ASA Refresher Course Lecture Outline No. 221. 1976.

126. Oh TH: Formula for calculating fluid maintence requirements (Letter). Anesthesiology 53: 351, 1980

127. Shandling B, Steward DJ: Regional analgesia for postoperative pain in pediatric outpatient surgery. J Pediatr Surg 15: 477, 1980

128. Anderson R: Pain as a major cause of postoperative nausea. Can Anaesth Soc J 23: 366, 1976

129. Broadman LM: Regional anesthesia for the pediatric outpatient. Anesth Clin North Am 5: 53, 1987

130. Rice LJ, Broadman LM, Hannallah RS: Regional anesthesia in pediatric patients. Adv Anaesth 6: 291, 1989

131. Epstein RH, Larijani GE, Wolfson PJ, Ala-Kokko TI, Boerner TF: Plasma bupivacaine concentrations following ilioinguinal-iliohypogastric nerve blockade in children. Anesthesiology 69: 773, 1988

132. Casey W, Rice L, Hannallah RS, et al: A comparison between bupivacaine instillation versus ilioinguinal/iliohypogastric nerve block for postoperative analgesia following inguinal herniorrhaphy in children. Anesthesiology 72: 637, 1990

133. Soliman MG, Tremblay NA: Nerve block of the penis for postoperative pain relief in children. Anesth Analg 57: 495, 1978

134. Vater M, Wandless J: Caudal or dorsal nerve block? A comparison of two local anesthetic techniques for postoperative analgesia following day case circumcision. Acta Anaesthesiol Scand 29: 175, 1985

135. Tree-Trakarn T, Pirayavaraporn S: Postoperative pain relief for circumcision in children: Comparison among morphine, nerve block and topical analgesia. Anesthesiology 62: 519, 1985

136. Tree-Trakarn T, Pirayavaraporn S, Lertakyamanee J: Topical anesthesia for relief of post-circumcision pain. Anesthesiology 67: 395, 1987

137. Schulte-Steinberg O, Rahlfs VM: Spread of extradural analgesia following caudal injection in children: A statistical study. Br J Anaesth 49: 1027, 1977

138. Takasaki M, Dohi S, Kawabata Y, et al: Dosage of lidocaine for caudal anesthesia in infants and children. Anesthesiology 47: 527, 1977
139. Armitage EN: Regional anaesthesia in paediatrics. Clin Anaesth 3: 553, 1985
140. Eyres RL, Oppenheim R, Brown TCK: Plasma bupivacaine concentrations in children during caudal epidural analgesia. Anaesth Intensive Care 11: 20, 1983
141. Broadman LM, Hannallah RS, Norrie WC, et al: Caudal block in pediatric outpatient surgery: A comparison of three different bupivacaine concentrations. Anesth Analg 66: S19, 1987
142. Wolf AR, Valley RD, Fear DW, Roy WL, Lerman J: Bupivacaine for caudal analgesia in infants and children: The optimal effective concentration. Anesthesiology 69: 102, 1988
143. Bromage PR: Aging and epidural dose requirements. Br J Anaesth 41: 1016, 1969
144. Warner MA, Kunkel SE, Offord KO, et al: The effects of age, epinephrine, and operative site on duration of caudal analgesia in pediatric patients. Anesth Analg 66: 995, 1987
145. Rice LJ, Pudimat MA, Hannallah RS: Timing of caudal block placement in relation to surgery does not affect duration of postoperative analgesia in paediatric ambulatory patients. Can J Anaesth 37: 429, 1990
146. Jensen BH: Caudal block for post-operative pain relief in children after genital operations: A comparison between bupivacaine and morphine. Acta Anaesthesiol Scand 25: 373, 1981
147. Krane EJ, Jacobson LE, Lynn AM, et al: Caudal morphine for postoperative analgesia in children: A comparison with caudal bupivacaine and intravenous morphine. Anesth Analg 66: 647, 1988
148. Krane EJ: Delayed respiratory depression in a child after caudal epidural morphine. Anesth Analg 67: 79, 1988
149. Broadman LM, Hannallah RS, Norden J, et al: Kiddie caudals: Experience with 1154 consecutive cases without complications. Anesth Analg 66: S18, 1987
150. Dalens B, Hasnaoni A: Caudal anesthesia in pediatric surgery: Success rate and adverse effects in 750 consecutive patients. Anesth Analg 68: 83, 1989
151. Matsumiya N, Dohi S, Takarashi H, et al: Cardiovascular collapse in an infant after caudal anesthesia with a lidocaine-epinephrine solution. Anesth Analg 65: 1074, 1986
152. Rice LJ, Broadman LM: Caudal anesthesia and cardiovascular collapse in an infant. Anesth Analg 66: 694, 1987
153. Gingrich TF: Intravenous regional anesthesia of the upper extremity in children. JAMA 200: 135, 1967
154. Yaster M, Maxwell LG: Pediatric regional anesthesia. Anesthesiology 70: 324, 1989
155. Soliman IE, Broadman LM, Hannallah RS, et al: Analgesic effects of eutectic mixture of local anesthetic (EMLA) vs. intradermal lidocaine infiltration prior to venous cannulation in children. Anesthesiology 68: 804, 1988
156. Broadman LM, Soliman IE, Hannallah RS, et al: Evaluation of EMLA (eutectic mixture of local anesthetics) for topical analgesia in children. Anesth Analg 67: S21, 1988
157. Epstein BS: Recovery from anesthesia. Anesthesiology 43: 285, 1975
158. Weinstock SM, Flynn JJ: Brief hospital admission for pediatric strabismus surgery. Am J Ophthalmol 80: 525, 1975
159. Hadaway BG, Ingram AM, Traynor MJ: Day care surgery in strabismus in children. Trans Ophthalmol Soc UK 97: 23, 1977
160. Rowley MP, Brown TCK: Postoperative vomiting in children. Anaesth Intensive Care 10: 309, 1982
161. Lerman J, Eutis S, Smith DR: Effects of droperidol pretreatment on postanesthetic vomiting in children undergoing strabismus surgery. Anesthesiology 65: 322, 1986
162. Christensen S, Farrow Gillespie A, Lerman J: Incidence of emesis and postanesthetic recovery after strabismus surgery in children: A comparison of droperidol and lidocaine. Anesthesiology 70: 251, 1989
163. Broadman LM, Cerruzi W, Patane PS, Hannallah RS, Ruttimann U, Friendly D: Metoclopramide reduces the incidence of vomiting following strabismus surgery in children. Anesthesiology 72: 245, 1990
164. Brown, RE, James DJ, Grey Weaver R, et al. Low-dose droperidol versus standard-dose dro-

peridol for prevention of vomiting after pediatric strabismus surgery. Anesth Analg 70: 537, 1990
165. Rita L, Goodarzi M, Seleny F: Effect of low-dose droperidol on postoperative vomiting in children. Can Anaesth Soc J 28: 259, 1981
166. Patel RI, Hannallah RS: Anesthetic complications following pediatric ambulatory surgery: A 3-year study. Anesthesiology 69: 1009, 1988
167. Ahlgren EW: Pediatric outpatient anesthesia. Am J Dis Child 126: 36, 1973

Adult and Geriatric Patients

5

JEFFREY L. APFELBAUM, SURINDER K. KALLAR, BERNARD V. WETCHLER

The American Hospital Association recently reported that from 1981 through 1988 the number of ambulatory surgical procedures performed in hospitals increased by more than 120%. During this same period, the surgical volume of inpatients suffered a substantial decrease. Like the demand for hospital-based ambulatory surgery, the market for freestanding ambulatory surgery centers has boomed, with nearly 1000 such Medicare-participating centers in the United States in 1989. With the proliferation of such facilities and the challenge they pose for the administration of anesthesia, anesthesiologists have been forced to re-evaluate the traditional approaches to anesthesia care for adult and geriatric patients. In this chapter we will examine some of the challenges presented by adult and geriatric patients who require anesthesia for ambulatory surgical procedures, beginning with preparation, both psychological and physiological. We next consider various agents for premedication and the conditions under which their effects are optimal, followed by choice of anesthetic technique, including a discussion of intravenous and inhalational agents for the administration of general anesthesia. We then present a discussion of the conscious sedation technique and conclude with a review of the problem adult patient and the geriatric patient.

PSYCHOLOGICAL PREPARATION

The anesthetic management of the surgical outpatient often begins several days prior to the date of surgery during the patient's visit for preanesthetic assessment and evaluation. It is at this time that the anesthesiologist can begin to allay the patient's natural fear of losing consciousness. What may seem like a minor,

197

straightforward procedure to the physician is often perceived as an impending catastrophe by the patient. Several studies have shown that up to 85% of patients are either anxious or afraid prior to surgery.[1-3] Some studies have suggested that adult women are more likely than adult men to be anxious before surgery[2]; others have found no correlation between age or sex differences and levels of preoperative anxieties.[4,5] Egbert and coworkers found an average of nearly 60% of patients who are anxious before surgery, with the highest levels of anxiety noted in patients scheduled for cancer surgery. The importance of preoperative anxiety cannot be minimized because of the patient's ambulatory status.[6,7] In fact, Levy and Weintraub have stated that the ambulatory patient is frequently more apprehensive about the anesthetic, which is perceived as major, than about the surgery, which is often minor and certainly not life-threatening.[8]

Particularly in the ambulatory setting, the psychological component of preoperative preparation can often be provided during the patient's interview with the anesthesiologist. In a classic study, Egbert and coworkers found that a preoperative visit by an anesthesiologist was more effective than a barbiturate in reducing anxiety.[4] In this study, more patients who received an informative preoperative interview without medication were calm compared with those who received medication alone but no interview (Table 5-1). In 1977, Leigh and coworkers reported that anxiety levels in adult patients who had received a preoperative visit from an anesthesiologist were significantly lower than anxiety levels in patients who received no visit at all.[9] Furthermore, these investigators found that the preoperative visit was more effective in decreasing preoperative anxiety levels than a booklet given to the patients the day before surgery. Although a pamphlet was specifically designed to reassure patients about anesthesia, these authors concluded that the dissemination of paperwork was not a substitute for a proper preoperative visit and interview.

Levy and Weintraub recommended that the anesthesiologist have a frank discussion with the patient in which the anesthetic, monitoring, and potential side effects are reviewed well in advance of the day of surgery.[8] They concluded that the intelligent, well-informed patient will understand and accept the rationale of foregoing traditional methods of providing premedication.

Design considerations in modern ambulatory surgery facilities should create an ambiance that is warm, relaxing, pleasant, and nonthreatening for patients and their families.[10] For example, providing the patient with an attractive waiting

TABLE 5-1. Reducing Patient Anxiety: Comparison of Preoperative Visit and Intramuscular Pentobarbital (2 mg/kg)

	Anxious (%)	Calm (%)
Control group	58	35
Pentobarbital	61	48
Preoperative visit	40	65
Preoperative visit and pentobarbital	38	71

SOURCE: Adapted from Egbert et al.[4]

room with reading material, television, and games for children and limiting separation time from family or friends help the unpremedicated patient remain calm.[11,12] Unfortunately, psychological preoperative preparation cannot "cure" all fears. The very apprehensive patient will likely benefit to some degree from preoperative psychological preparation and may well be a candidate for supplementary pharmacologic relief of anxiety. Indeed, several studies have recently suggested that a preoperative visit with the anesthesiologist in lieu of premedication may actually increase preoperative anxiety.[13-15] Pharmacologic intervention to allay preoperative apprehension may include a variety of medications, most notably the barbiturates, phenothiazines, benzodiazepines, antihistamines, and opioids.

PREMEDICATION

The decision to utilize pharmacologic premedication and the subsequent choice of a specific agent are based on a tradition[16] usually influenced by one's training, clinical experience, and personal biases. Modern ambulatory surgery and anesthesia are a break from tradition; we must now consider tailoring both our psychologic and pharmacologic preoperative preparations to fit the concentrated perioperative care that the outpatient receives. Much of the rationale for traditional preoperative medication is derived from experiences with pungent inhalational agents (i.e., diethyl ether, cyclopropane) to induce anesthesia in hospitalized patients. With the explosive growth of ambulatory surgery and the extraordinary advances in the field of pharmacology, we must now choose medications, dosages, and routes of administration for our patients that are practical and convenient but do not prolong length of stay in the postanesthesia care unit (PACU).

Pharmacologic preoperative preparation should never be routine. The appropriate medication or medications can be selected only after the psychological and physiologic condition of the patient has been evaluated so that specific needs can be determined. Standaert has said, "Everyone involved with therapeutic agents, patient, physician, medical chemist, wants a magic bullet, a drug that does exactly what is expected of it and nothing else."[17] What is needed is a drug that has a rapid onset, a predictable duration of action, a specific site of action, and no postoperative side-effects. Unfortunately, no such "magic bullet" exists. Our goals for preoperative pharmacologic preparation vary tremendously from patient to patient (Table 5-2). The armamentarium to meet these goals includes anticholinergics, barbiturates, benzodiazepines, phenothiazines, antihistamines, butyrophenones, opioids, antacids, and H_2 receptor antagonists.

Anticholinergics

Anticholinergic medications have evolved as a component in preoperative pharmacologic preparation because of their antisialagogic and vagolytic actions.[18] When very irritant anesthetics were in vogue (e.g., diethyl ether), it was customary to treat patients with anticholinergics to minimize the reactions evoked by these anesthetic agents. Secretions often accumulated near the glottis and provoked

TABLE 5-2. Objectives of Treatment with Preoperative Medications

Anxiolysis

Amnesia

Sedation

Analgesia

Anticholinergic effects:
  Antisialagogue
  Vagolytic

Prophylaxis:
  Acid aspiration
  Postoperative emesis
  Allergy
  Infection

coughing or even laryngospasm. Inhalational anesthetics currently used are considerably less irritating, and routine anticholinergic premedication is no longer essential. Furthermore, drying mucous membranes by means of anticholinergics is believed to contribute to postoperative sore throat and complaints of dry mouth.[19] The lung's cleaning mechanisms may be inhibited as tracheobronchial secretions decrease and thicken and mucociliary flow is slowed. This may be particularly problematic in the elderly patient whose baseline salivary gland production is markedly decreased. Although no longer recommended "as a matter of routine," anticholinergics may, of course, be administered as indicated (e.g., to control secretions secondary to airway insertion during light mask anesthesia or to inhibit further secretions if a difficult intubation develops).

With regard to the vagolytic action of anticholinergics, the blocking of vagal reflexes during anesthesia requires larger doses than those generally administered in traditional premedication. Vagal reflexes are usually best treated by intravenous administration of an appropriate anticholinergic if and when they occur. Some anesthesiologists prefer to administer atropine or glycopyrrolate intravenously just prior to the anticipated bradycardic stimulus.[20] Of the three commonly used anticholinergics, atropine is more likely to cause an increase in the heart rate than glycopyrrolate or scopolamine[21] (Table 5-3). For routine intramuscular premedication, the effect of atropine is less predictable; it has been

TABLE 5-3. Comparative Effects of Anticholinergic Premedication

	Atropine	Glycopyrrolate	Scopolamine
Increased heart rate	+ + +	+ +	+
Antisialagogue	+	+ +	+ + +
Sedation	+	0	+ + +

NOTE: 0 = no effect; + = small effect; + + = moderate effect; + + + = large effect.
SOURCE: Adapted from Stoelting RK[39].

shown to augment tachycardia and increase the incidence of cardiac dysrhythmias that occur during endotracheal intubation.[22]

Some anesthesiologists administer glycopyrrolate, a quaternary ammonium compound, to provide prolonged antisecretory effects with less tachycardia and central nervous system excitement. Despite these potential advantages, the more prolonged and intense drying effect limits its use for short procedures.[23,24]

Scopolamine is eight to ten times more potent than atropine in its action on the central nervous system and significantly less potent than atropine in its peripheral autonomic effects.[25] Recent studies with transdermally administered scopolamine patches (1.5 mg per 72 hours) indicate that it may be a useful premedicant in patients with a history of motion sickness because of its sedative, antisialagogue, and antiemetic effects.[26]

Unfortunately, excessive doses of scopolamine or atropine may cause central nervous system toxicity, the so-called central anticholinergic syndrome.[27] Because of differences in potency, this syndrome is most likely to occur after the administration of scopolamine, but it can occur after large doses of atropine. The symptoms of central nervous system toxicity resulting from anticholinergic medications include delirium, restlessness, confusion, and rarely, obtundation. Elderly patients appear to be especially susceptible to this syndrome.[28] Obviously, these side-effects are particularly problematic in the ambulatory surgery population; some investigators have suggested that physostigmine may be effective in reversing "mild" episodes of this syndrome.[29,30]

Sedative-Hypnotics and Tranquilizers

The most commonly used sedative-hypnotic premedicants include the barbiturates and the benzodiazepines. In general, sedative-hypnotics produce a dose-dependent depression of the central nervous system; small doses will produce anxiolysis, while increasing doses will result in sedation, hypnosis, and eventually the induction of general anesthesia (Fig. 5-1). This section will focus on the use of these drugs in smaller doses (i.e., as premedicants).

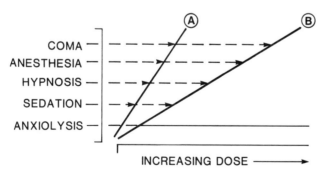

FIGURE 5-1. Spectrum of central nervous system activity. Sedative-hypnotic compounds produce a dose-dependent spectrum of CNS depression. In this schematic, drug A might represent a barbiturate (e.g., pentobarbital), whereas drug B might represent a benzodiazepine (e.g., diazepam). (SOURCE: White PF: Pharmacologic and clinical aspects of preoperative medication. Anesth Anal 65: 963, 1968.)

Barbiturates

The use of secobarbital and pentobarbital for preoperative pharmacologic preparation is a time-tested practice with a long record of safety. Advantages of these drugs include inexpensive cost, sedation, minimal cardiac respiratory depression, rarity of nausea and vomiting, and good effect after either oral or parenteral administration.[31] Unfortunately, the long duration of these drugs and their slow elimination from the body make them poor choices as premedicants for the surgical outpatient.[32] Other disadvantages include lack of analgesia, disorientation (particularly for patients in pain), and the absence of a specific pharmacologic antagonist. Barbiturates should be avoided in patients with a history of acute intermittent porphyria because they may exacerbate this disease.

Benzodiazepines

In recent years, the use of barbiturate premedication has declined dramatically, while the use of benzodiazepine premedication has increased. Comparative studies have suggested that benzodiazepines are more effective in providing anxiolysis and amnesia and are associated with higher patient acceptance than barbiturates.[33-35] Benzodiazepines allay anxiety by depression of the limbic system and amygdalae, where fear, anxiety, and aggression are generated; there appears to be little or no direct effect on the cerebral cortex. It is postulated that the sedative effect is a result of an enhancement of inhibitory neurotransmission mediated by GABA (gamma aminobutyric acid), while the anxiolytic effect is due to the action of glycine-mediated inhibition of neural pathways in the brainstem.[36,37] When used in premedicant doses, the proposed mechanisms of action of the benzodiazepines describe highly specific receptors that produce anxiolysis, anterograde amnesia, and sedation with relatively little cardiopulmonary depression, nausea, or vomiting. Benzodiazepines have a wide therapeutic index and a low incidence of toxicity.[38] Other than the dose-dependent central nervous system depression characteristic of all sedative-hypnotics, there are few side-effects associated with the use of this class of drugs.[39]

There are, however, some potential hazards associated with the use of benzodiazepines. Occasionally patients may be unduly sensitive to the central nervous system depressive effects of these drugs. This phenomenon has been reported in the elderly or in those patients with severe liver dysfunction after a single oral dose of diazepam resulted in sedation lasting up to four days.[40] Benzodiazepines have no analgesic properties and when given to patients in pain can result in a paradoxical restlessness or even delirium.[41] Severe pain and erratic absorption are commonly noted when diazepam is administered intramuscularly, and phlebitis has been reported frequently at the site of an intravenous injection.[42] The clearance of diazepam from plasma has been shown to be delayed by cimetidine, suggesting the possibility of prolonged sedation when these drugs are used in combination for premedication.[43]

At the present time, there are no clinically available benzodiazepine reversal agents. In some circumstances, a small dose of physostigmine may be effective in reversing prolonged sedation secondary to benzodiazepine-induced central nervous system depression.[44] In the future, flumazenil, a receptor-specific benzodiazepine antagonist, may become available for widespread clinical use.[45–49]

DIAZEPAM. In addition to versatility of administration (parenteral or oral), the superb anxiolytic, amnestic, and sedative properties of diazepam have made it the standard to which other benzodiazepines are compared. Drug levels peak 60 to 90 minutes after oral administration of 5 or 10 mg diazepam, with drowsiness persisting up to 120 minutes.[50,51] Larger doses (20 mg) result in more rapid peaking of drug levels with noticeable clinical effects at 30 to 60 minutes and prolonged residual drowsiness for up to 240 minutes. Absorption of orally administered diazepam may be slowed by the concurrent parenteral administration of atropine or narcotics, but absorption is more rapid with metoclopramide or oral aluminum hydroxide antacid.

Intramuscular administration of diazepam results in less predictable absorption and lower drug levels,[42,51] probably related to the insolubility of diazepam in water and to the lack of a true intramuscular injection. Injections into the buttock are not only painful, but they also produce the least reliable systemic drug level.

When injected intravenously in combination with narcotics, diazepam can cause depression of the respiratory and cardiovascular systems. The recommended dose of intravenous diazepam for surgical outpatients is approximately 0.05 to 0.15 mg/kg. Since patients vary tremendously in their clinical response to this drug, it is often recommended that intravenous diazepam be titrated to clinical effect and be administrated in 1.25- to 2.5-mg increments at intervals of no less than 3 minutes. The intravenous administration of 10 mg diazepam to volunteers resulted in ataxia and a positive Romberg sign (8% of patients) and dizziness (16%) persisting for 60 minutes.[50] Acute recovery following intravenous diazepam (12.5 to 30 mg) appeared essentially complete 90 minutes after administration[52] (Fig 5-2).

The redistribution half-life of diazepam is relatively short, about 2.5 hours. However, a recurrence of drowsiness and an increase in plasma concentration occurs at 6 to 8 hours, probably owing to enterohepatic recirculation. Serum concentration has been shown to increase further when fatty solid foods were consumed 3 hours after diazepam administration.[53] This also may be related to enteric recirculation. Food at 7 hours had a similar but lesser effect; ingestion of water had no effect. It appears likely, therefore, that fatty food intake should be limited in the 7 hours after diazepam administration to avoid resedation, particularly at higher drug doses. The elimination half-life of diazepam is 1.5 days after primarily hepatic metabolism. Twenty-five percent of patients who received diazepam (10 mg) intravenously felt tired for more than 24 hours.[50] Diazepam metabolites, notably desmethyldiazepam, are also pharmacologically active. Plasma levels of desmethyldiazepam have been shown to rise steadily over the 48 hours after intravenous diazepam administration. The effect of diazepam should, therefore, not be considered short-lived; patients should be cautioned that they may feel somewhat sedated several days after a single diazepam administration. Because diazepam is insoluble in water, it is formulated in inorganic solvents such

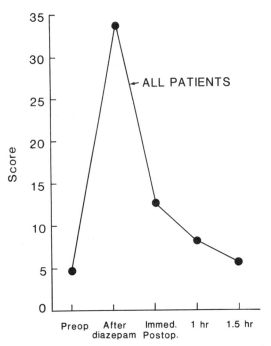

FIGURE 5-2. Time course of patients' performance on psychomotor tests after receiving diazepam preoperatively. (SOURCE: Driscoll et al.[52])

as propylene glycol, a carrier medium that results in pain on injection as well as a high incidence of thrombophlebitis. In one study, the incidence of venous sequelae after diazepam increased with time: 23% after 2 to 3 days and 39% after 7 to 10 days.[54] In Europe, diazepam is available in an oil emulsion as Diazemuls (Kabi Vitrum, Sweden). With this preparation, a lower incidence of pain (1%) and thrombophlebitis (4%) is reported.[55] In the unpremedicated surgical outpatient, the incidence of recall under general anesthesia has been reported to be as high as 9%.[56] Epstein found that when diazepam (0.15 mg/kg, up to a total dose of 5 mg) was given intravenously 2 to 3 minutes prior to anesthesia induction, the incidence of awareness experienced with a balanced anesthetic technique for laparoscopy was significantly reduced. Without diazepam, 4.9% of patients had recall for conversation, 2.1% for extubation, and 0.7% for pain.*

Diazepam (0.25 mg/kg) taken orally significantly decreased preoperative discomfort and apprehension without extending length of stay for outpatients having a variety of surgical procedures.[57] Jansen and coworkers objectively measured postural stability after oral diazepam premedication (0.2 mg/kg). Because patients demonstrated a decreased stability with a tendency to fall, the authors believe patients should not be allowed to walk after taking this dose of oral diazepam.[58]

---

*Epstein BS: Personal communication, 1982.

LORAZEPAM. Lorazepam is a long-acting benzodiazepine available in both intravenous and oral preparations. It is approximately four to ten times as potent as diazepam and has a longer onset and duration of action.[59] When given parenterally, lorazepam can produce amnesia and profound sedation for up to 10 hours. Following oral administration, plasma concentrations of lorazepam persist at therapeutic levels for up to 48 hours. Because of its prolonged sedative and amnesic effects, lorazepam should not be used by any route for premedication in ambulatory surgery patients.

MIDAZOLAM. Midazolam is a water-soluble benzodiazepine with a distribution half-life of only 7.2 minutes and an elimination half-life of approximately 2.5 hours.[60] Its water solubility obviates the need for an inorganic solvent such as propylene glycol, which causes venoirritation and interferes with absorption after intramuscular injection. Midazolam has recently been shown to be four to six times as potent as diazepam.[61] Its rapid onset and short duration of action make it suitable for use in ambulatory surgery.

In one study, sedation and anxiolysis began within 1 to 2 minutes after the intravenous administration of 5 mg midazolam.[62] Drug effect was reported as pleasant by 92% of patients and was acceptable to all. Marked sedation persisted for the entire 30-minute observation period. Anterograde amnesia was present in 96% of patients at 2 minutes after the injection and declined over the ensuing 20 to 40 minutes. Retrograde amnesia was not demonstrated. Recovery times were recorded after a large premedication dose of 5 mg midazolam. Motor performance recovered in 34 minutes, and subjects were fully awake and walked unaided at 73 minutes. As with all benzodiazepines, there was considerable variation in individual patient response.

In extremely anxious patients, intramuscular midazolam may be used as a satisfactory premedicant for the surgical outpatient. Fragen and coworkers compared the effects of midazolam (0.08 mg/kg) and hydroxyzine (1.5 mg/kg) as intramuscular premedicants.[63] Midazolam produced more rapid onset of action, greater anxiolysis for the first hour, greater amnesia, less local irritation, and received a higher overall rating by patients. Drowsiness, greater after midazolam, was neither significant nor prolonged. When midazolam was given intramuscularly, sedative effects began within 15 minutes but wore off between 60 to 90 minutes after injection. In another study, Vinik and colleagues compared midazolam (0.07 mg/kg), hydroxyzine (1.0 mg/kg), and placebo. They found that midazolam and hydroxyzine reduced anxiety more significantly than did placebo, with peak onsets appearing between 30 and 60 minutes after drug administration in both groups.[64] There was significantly less evidence of tissue irritation at the injection site in patients treated with midazolam than in patients treated with hydroxyzine. An oral preparation of midazolam is available in Europe but is not approved for use in the United States.

Other benzodiazepines have been tried as oral premedications. Temazepam is rapidly absorbed and eliminated, with peak plasma levels at 20 to 40 minutes and an elimination half-life of approximately 10 hours.[64,65] Temazepam (20 mg 1 hour before surgery) resulted in satisfactory sedation and anxiolysis in ambulatory surgery patients.[66] Recovery was more rapid than that found after diazepam (10 mg).[67]

Phenothiazines

The phenothiazines (e.g., prochlorperazine) are potent antiemetic drugs. This antiemetic effect is thought to be secondary to inhibition of the chemoreceptor trigger zone. Owing to central depression of the vasomotor reflexes, peripheral adrenergic blockade, and direct vasodilation, the phenothiazines may cause hypotension. Additional side-effects include the occurrence of extrapyramidal signs and cholestatic jaundice. Primarily because of the side-effects and their prolonged duration of action, the phenothiazines are not usually used in the premedication of ambulatory surgery patients.

Antihistamines

Antihistamines, such as diphenhydramine and hydroxyzine, are occasionally used for their sedative and ataractic properties. These medications are responsible for a wide spectrum of pharmacologic activity, including anxiolytic, sedative, analgesic, antihistaminic (H_1-blocker), antiemetic, and antisialagogic properties.

Butyrophenones

Droperidol is the most commonly used butyrophenone. Intravenous or intramuscular administration of droperidol will produce the appearance of sedation, calmness, and tranquility in a patient. Unfortunately, it also may produce dysphoria, restlessness, and a feeling of terror in a small percentage of patients.[68] Such dysphoria has led some patients to refuse their surgical procedures.[69,70] Additional potential side-effects include the development of extrapyramidal signs[71,72] and mild alpha-adrenergic blockade with resultant intraoperative hypotension.

After intravenous administration of 5 mg droperidol, the distribution half-life was 10 minutes and the elimination half-life was 134 minutes.[73] Absorption after intramuscular administration was excellent. However, approximately 86% of the dose was converted to an active metabolite; significant levels of that metabolite were present in plasma for 8 to 12 hours after drug administration. This presence correlates with the observed duration of clinical effect. Korttila and Linnoila evaluated recovery and driving-related skills after intravenous injection of 5 mg droperidol.[74] Clinical recovery as determined by a negative Romberg sign was present after 25 minutes, but drowsiness was still reported at 10 hours by over half the volunteers studied. Tests of coordination and attention remained significantly abnormal at the final 10-hour testing period. The concurrent administration of fentanyl (200 μg) did not affect the results of these tests.

Despite its potential side-effects and long duration of action, droperidol remains a popular premedicant for surgery outpatients because of its potent antiemetic activity. Low-dose droperidol (1.25 to 2.5 mg IV) has been shown to be effective in preventing nausea and vomiting.[75,76] Nevertheless, because of its pronounced side-effect profile and prolonged duration of action, the routine prophylactic use of droperidol is not indicated.

Opioids

Opioids are indicated as premedication when analgesia is needed prior to surgery.[77] For the patient experiencing pain before operation, the administration of narcotic premedication can achieve analgesia or even euphoria. Opioids also have been prescribed for patients before surgery to ameliorate the discomfort that may occur during the administration of a regional or local anesthetic. Long-acting opioids such as meperidine and morphine sulfate are not recommended for premedication in the ambulatory surgery patient because they have been shown to prolong recovery time[78] (Table 5-4).

Fentanyl has recently gained acceptance as the narcotic of choice for premedication in the surgery outpatient. When given intravenously, it has an onset of 2 minutes and a duration of action of 45 minutes.[79] The redistribution half-life is 13.4 minutes; the elimination half-life is 219 minutes. As premedication, fentanyl is most frequently administered intravenously in doses of 1 to 2 $\mu g/kg$ in 25- to 50-μg increments at approximately 1 to 2-minute intervals.

The effect of fentanyl on anxiolysis is extremely controversial. In one study, patients reported a small decrease in anxiety and an increase in sedation after receiving 100 μg fentanyl 1 hour before surgery.[80] However, only 54% of the patients described the effects of fentanyl as pleasant 4 minutes after the injection; at 24 hours after injection, less than 40% of patients reported the premedication as "good to excellent." Other studies have found fentanyl to be no better than placebo.[81,82]

Although the use of opioid premedication in its traditional form has been questioned, intravenous opioid premedication administered just prior to the induction of anesthesia can be advantageous. Epstein and coworkers evaluated a group of patients having elective dilatation and curettage (D&C) or elective termination of pregnancy.[83] Patients were given thiopental, nitrous oxide, and oxygen or thiopental, nitrous oxide, oxygen, and fentanyl. Patients given fentanyl recovered from anesthesia significantly earlier than did those in the other group. In another study, Hunt and colleagues found that the addition of an intravenous fentanyl premedicant resulted in a significant reduction in the incidence of postoperative pain.[84]

Pandit and Kothary compared the use of equianalgesic intravenous premedi-

TABLE 5-4. Relationship Between Premedication and Recovery Time

Type	Number	Recovery Time (min)*
No premedication	1015	179 ± 113
Diazepam	98	168 ± 104
Pentobarbital	25	231 ± 88
Opioids (meperidine and morphine)	388	208 ± 101[†]
Hydroxyzine	92	192 ± 120

*Values are mean ± SD
[†]Differs significantly from patients not receiving any premedication (P<0.001).
SOURCE: Meridy HW.[78] Used with permission.

TABLE 5-5. Recovery Time (minutes)

Premedicant	Orientation	Ambulation	Discharge
Morphine	21.4 ± 6.63	148.4 ± 49.33	210.3 ± 65.84
Meperidine	19.2 ± 6.54	135.2 ± 30.02	187.0 ± 50.87
Fentanyl	19.9 ± 7.41	145.8 ± 51.73	187.9 ± 67.73
Sufentanil	19.7 ± 8.19	134.2 ± 44.05	181.5 ± 62.01
Placebo	20.2 ± 7.69	156.0 ± 54.04	200.0 ± 69.12

NOTE: ANOVA—No significant differences between groups.
SOURCE: From Pandit and Kothary.[85] Used with permission.

cant doses of morphine, meperidine, fentanyl, and sufentanil administered 15 to 30 minutes prior to induction for their effects on anxiety, sedation, ease of anesthetic induction, requirement for postoperative analgesia, and frequency of side-effects.[85] In this study, opioid premedication generally provided more satisfactory induction and maintenance compared with placebo premedication. Interestingly, in this study, opioid premedication did not prolong time to patient discharge, nor did it increase the incidence of postoperative side-effects (Table 5-5).

Antacids and H₂ Antagonists—Patients at Risk for Acid Aspiration Syndrome

Patients at risk of developing acid aspiration syndrome (AAS) have been defined as those with a gastric pH below 2.5 and a gastric volume above 25 ml.[86,87] Morbidity and mortality associated with aspiration vary depending on the volume and the chemical nature of the aspirate.

Ong and colleagues demonstrated that 86% of outpatients presenting for ambulatory surgery and 57% of inpatients have a residual gastric volume greater than 25 ml.[88] Other studies noted that 45% of outpatients and 30% of inpatients were at risk of aspiration,[89] that 76% of pediatric patients had a gastric pH less than 2.5 and a gastric volume in excess of 0.4 ml/kg,[90] and that 75% of obese patients were at increased risk compared to 0% of nonobese patients.[91]

Although the outpatient population at risk is large, the actual incidence of acid aspiration is low. A survey of 181 ambulatory surgery facilities revealed an incidence of aspiration of 1.7 per 10,000 cases during the calendar year 1985.[92] The survey also reported that during 1976–1985, of a total of 266 suspected cases of aspiration, 81 subsequently proved to be definite. Of the total cases, 47% were intubated for the procedure and aspiration occurred most frequently during the induction. Of the 54% that required hospital admission, 27.4% were hospitalized for more than one day; however, no deaths or cases of permanent disability were reported (Table 5-6).

Natof reported only one suspected aspiration in a prospective survey of 32,000 ambulatory procedures.[93] In a later prospective survey of 87,492 procedures, he reported only three aspirations, with an incidence of 0.34 per 10,000 patients.[94] A computerized study from Sweden[95] of 185,358 inpatients reported a mortality of 0.2 per 10,000 cases from acid aspiration, in contrast with a mortality of 40%

TABLE 5-6. Review of Reported Aspirations 1976–1985

	Number	Percent
Total reported	266	100.0
Suspected	185	69.5
Definite	81	30.5
Intubated	126	47.5
Not intubated	140	52.5
Time of aspiration:		
Induction	166	62.5
Maintenance	28	10.6
Emergence	72	26.9
Not hospitalized	122	45.9
Hospitalized	144	54.1
Length of hospitalization:		
1 day	71	49.3
2–3 days	54	37.5
4 or more days	19	13.2
Deaths/disabilities	0	0.0

SOURCE: Kallar SK: Personal communication, 1989.

following confirmed aspiration reported earlier.[96] Of 531 deaths associated with 240,483 anesthetics (2.2 per 10,000) in 1978, Harrison reported only 2 that were caused by vomiting and aspiration.[97]

Patients who are at an increased risk of acid aspiration include those with hiatal hernia, obesity, pregnancy (second and third trimester), peptic ulceration, diabetes mellitus, extreme nervousness, and old age. The incidence of regurgitation has been reported as 7% to 8%,[98] with 8.6% of patients inhaling gastric contents. Regurgitation may be encouraged by the Trendelenburg position, prone position, palpation of the abdomen, and fasciculations after the administration of succinylcholine. Pretreatment with alfentanil abolishes fasciculations due to succinylcholine[99] and prevents any increase in intragastric pressure.[95] Vomiting during anesthesia may be caused by partial respiratory obstruction or an anesthetic that is too light. Insertion of an oropharyngeal airway and strong autonomic stimulation (peritoneal traction and traction on ocular muscles) during light anesthesia also can precipitate vomiting. Although pregnant patients presenting for midtrimester abortions have been considered to be at risk of acid aspiration, Wyner and Cohen found no significant difference in residual gastric volume between pregnant (mean gestational age 15 ± 3 weeks) and nonpregnant outpatients when volume was measured at induction of anesthesia.[100]

Various drug therapies have been suggested to either increase the gastric pH or decrease the volume of gastric juice. Suspension antacids are no longer recommended because they may cause significant pulmonary damage if aspirated. Nonsuspension antacids reduce gastric acidity, but they also increase the gastric fluid volume. Martin and coworkers compared the effect of 15 ml oral Bicitra administered 15 minutes prior to the induction of anesthesia with 300 mg intramuscular cimetidine administered 30 minutes before induction of anesthesia in ambulatory surgery patients.[101] Patients in the Bicitra group had the desired increase in pH but also had an increase in gastric volume. Twenty-six percent of patients in the Bicitra group remained at risk, whereas no patients in the cimetidine group remained at risk. Of patients in the control group, 80% were at risk of aspiration (Tables 5-7 and 5-8).

Cimetidine and ranitidine are competitive H_2-receptor antagonists that inhibit gastric acid secretion.[102] Neither affects acid already in the stomach, so timing of administration and gastric emptying rate are important. Recommended regimens include a preoperative oral dose of 300 mg cimetidine at bedtime and another on the morning of surgery or a combination of an oral and intramuscular dose.[103,104] Oral administration of 150 mg ranitidine the evening before and then again on the morning of surgery decreased the risk of aspiration from 47% to 0% in a study of ambulatory patients.[105] Gonzalez and coworkers demonstrated that oral regimens of either 400 mg cimetidine or 150 mg ranitidine taken 5 hours before induction of anesthesia were both significantly better than placebo at reducing gastric acidity and volume. The percentage of patients at risk of aspiration was reduced from 100% (placebo group) to 46% (cimetidine group) and 15% (ranitidine group).[106] In a subsequent study by Gonzalez and Kallar, both intravenous ranitidine (50 mg) and cimetidine (300 mg) 1 to 1.5 hours before induction of anesthesia significantly ($p < 0.05$) reduced acidity when compared with placebo, but no change in gastric volume was noted.[107]

TABLE 5-7. Gastric pH and Volume with Bicitra, Cimetidine, and Control

	Number of Patients	Volume (ml)		pH (units)		pH > 2.5	
		Mean ± SD*	Range	Mean ± SD*	Range	Number	Percent
Bicitra	15	61.80 ± 25.4	32–114	3.20 ± 1.00	1.43–4.36	11	73.3
Cimetidine	15	12.33 ± 8.5	6–34	6.03 ± 1.06	4.08–7.32	15	100.0
Control	15	44.67 ± 14.1	23–68	1.68 ± 0.30	1.15–2.12	0	0

*Bonferroni t test: All three groups significantly different at $p = 0.05$.
SOURCE: Martin et al.[101]

TABLE 5-8. Distribution of Patients with a pH of 2.5 or Less and a Gastric Volume of 0.4 ml/kg or More

	N	pH < 2.5	Volume > 0.4 ml/kg	pH < 2.5 and Volume > 0.4 ml/kg
Bicitra	15	4	14	4 (26%)
Cimetidine	15	0	1	9 (0%)
Control	15	15	12	12 (80%)

SOURCE: Martin et al.[101] Used with permission.

Although adverse reactions have been reported with both cimetidine and ranitidine, ranitidine is considered superior because of its longer duration of action. Famotidine (Pepcid) 40 mg, a new H_2 antagonist, has been compared with 300 mg ranitidine given 30 to 120 minutes prior to surgery. At equipotent doses, famotidine took longer than ranitidine to achieve a pH of more than 2.5.[108]

Metoclopramide is a dopamine antagonist that increases lower esophageal sphincter tone and stimulates gastric motility. Rao and coworkers have shown that a combination of 300 mg cimetidine and 10 mg metoclopramide PO taken 2 hours before induction of anesthesia significantly reduced gastric volume and increased gastric pH in all patients compared to either cimetidine or metoclopramide alone.[109] Cimetidine 300 mg and metoclopramide 10 mg given intravenously 30 to 90 minutes before the induction of anesthesia has an additive effect in reducing gastric volume and increasing gastric pH[89] (Table 5-9).

Similar results have been demonstrated in pediatric patients. Somori and Kallar administered cimetidine syrup orally to pediatric patients in a dose of 7.5 mg/kg one hour before induction of anesthesia.[110] Patients in the cimetidine group achieved a pH of 5.06 (± 0.35) and a gastric volume of 4.5 ml (± 3.5 ml), whereas the control group had a pH of 1.55 (± 0.09) and a volume of 9.5 ml (± 2.0 ml). A similar effect was seen by Young and coworkers, who administered 2.0 mg/kg ranitidine orally one hour before surgery—ranitidine: pH 5.1 (± 0.5), volume 0.1 ml/kg (± 0.05); control: pH 2.0 (± 0.3), volume 0.31 ml/kg (± 0.07).[111] Sodium citrate (0.4 ml/kg) given orally to pediatric patients 30 minutes prior to surgery has been shown to be as effective as oral cimetidine (10 mg/kg) in increasing gastric pH.[112]

Although drug therapy decreases the number of patients at risk of AAS, it does not eliminate the need for careful anesthetic technique to protect the airway throughout the anesthetic. Whether every patient scheduled for ambulatory surgery should receive prophylaxis against AAS remains a topic for debate. The incidence of aspiration is low (1.7 per 10,000) with a very low mortality; this may be due to the special emphasis placed on preoperative instructions and the thorough questioning of patients about ingestion of food and liquids upon their arrival in the ambulatory surgery center.

TABLE 5-9. Effects of Intravenous Cimetidine and Metoclopramide

Groups	pH	Volume	No. of Patients with pH < 2.5 and Volume > 25 ml
I. Outpatient	2.33 $\pm$ 1.23	29.9 $\pm$ 15.9	9 (4%)
II. Inpatient	2.78 $\pm$ 1.47	23.6 $\pm$ 13.97	6 (30%)
III. Outpatient (300 mg C)	4.76 $\pm$ 1.59*	19.9 $\pm$ 15.21	1 (5%)
IV. Outpatient (C and M)	6.15 $\pm$ 0.71*	11.6 $\pm$ 7.37†	0 (0%)

NOTE: C = cimetidine; M = metoclopramide.
*Compared to pH in groups I and II ($p < 0.05$).
†Compared to volume in group I ($p < 0.05$).
SOURCE: From Katende et al.[89] Used with permission.

Individual ambulatory surgery centers must make their own decisions about which patients receive prophylaxis based on past experiences and estimates of cost-effectiveness, but it seems reasonable that patients at high risk should receive prophylaxis against acid aspiration syndrome.

CHOICE OF ANESTHETIC TECHNIQUES

Local, regional, or general anesthesia may be safely administered to the ambulatory surgery patient. The choice of anesthetic technique should, of course, be determined by surgical requirements, anesthetic considerations, and the patient's physical status and preferences. For example, a healthy young woman who presents for excisional biopsy of a breast mass might well be managed with general anesthesia. If the same patient were to present for arthroscopy of the knee, regional or local anesthesia with monitored anesthesia care (MAC) might be an excellent choice. The octogenarian who requires ophthalmologic surgery may do quite well with peribulbar or retrobulbar block, supplemental sedation, and MAC. Whichever technique is used, the anesthesiologist's approach to the patient is most important. Conversation should be reassuring and upbeat as preparation is made to induce anesthesia. Local and regional anesthetic techniques are discussed in Chapter 6; this section deals with the anesthetic management of the ambulatory surgery patient utilizing parenteral and inhalational techniques.

General Anesthesia

Managing a general anesthetic for the patient undergoing an ambulatory surgical procedure presents unique challenges to the anesthesiologist because the expectations of the outpatient differ significantly from those of the inpatient.[113] The vast majority of outpatients are healthy (ASA physical status 1 and 2); they anticipate a short surgical procedure, rapid recovery, and minimal, if any, perioperative side-effects. Surgical outpatients often expect to return to normal activities within 48 hours of their procedure.

The "compressed" time frame of ambulatory surgery sometimes alters the surgical requirements of a case. The anesthetic management of healthy, normovolemic outpatients should include a rapid induction of surgical anesthesia, maintenance of light but adequate anesthesia throughout the case, and a smooth, prompt recovery to "home readiness" without side-effects. In short, the goal is to anesthetize the patient for the shortest possible time with the lowest concentration of anesthetic compatible with patient safety and surgical need.

The ideal anesthetic technique would allow us to provide rapid, smooth, and pleasant onset of action; intraoperative amnesia, analgesia, and muscle relaxation sufficient to perform surgery; rapid, smooth, and pleasant emergence; and a prompt return to "home readiness" with minimal, if any, side-effects.

The normally minor postoperative morbidities of general anesthesia, including nausea,[113,114] vomiting,[116,117] dizziness,[118] drowsiness,[119] headache,[120] sore throat,[121] amd myalgia,[122] can significantly affect a patient's return to home readiness. Nausea and vomiting, in particular, may significantly prolong time before patient discharge (greater than 50% increase in PACU stay),[114,115] and every effort should be made to minimize these symptoms.

Intravenous Induction Agents

Intravenous agents are popular for the induction of anesthesia because of their ease of administration, rapid onset of action, and high degree of patient acceptance. Unfortunately, there are currently no intravenous induction agents approved or under investigation that fulfill all the criteria for the ideal drug (Table 5-10). Typical induction doses and some of the pharmacokinetic variables of the currently used intravenous induction agents are summarized in Table 5-11.

The use of any of the anesthetic induction agents is absolutely contraindicated when equipment for ventilation and resuscitation is unavailable. Additionally, these agents should be used with great care when difficulties with ventilation are expected to follow the loss of consciousness.

Sodium Thiopental

Despite a long elimination half-life (10 to 12 hr) that can contribute to substantial delay in recovery of psychomotor function (Fig. 5-3), sodium thiopental remains the most popular intravenous induction agent and has become the standard to which newer induction agents are compared. Since its introduction in 1934, so-

---

TABLE 5-10. Properties of an "Ideal" Intravenous Induction Agent

---

I. Physiochemical and pharmacokinetic:
  a. Water soluble
  b. Long shelf life (>1 year)
  c. Stable in solution
  d. Stable on exposure to light (>1 day)
  e. Small volume (±10 ml) required for anesthetic induction
II. Pharmacodynamic:
  a. Small interindividual variation
  b. High therapeutic (safety) index
  c. Onset in one arm-brain circulation time
  d. Short duration of effect
  e. Inactivated by rapid metabolism to inactive, nontoxic metabolites
  f. Rapid, smooth recovery
III. Hypersensitivity:
  a. No anaphylaxis
  b. No histamine release
IV. Side-effects:
  a. No local toxicity (i.e., nonirritating following injection)
  b. No alterations in body organ function, except primary CNS effects:
    1. Central nervous system
    2. Cardiovascular system
    3. Respiratory system
    4. Gastrointestinal system

SOURCE: Modified from Fragen RJ, Avram MJ: Nonopioid intravenous anesthetics. In Barash PG, Cullen BF, Stoelting RK (eds): Clinical Anesthesia. Philadelphia: JB Lippincott, 1989. Used with permission.

TABLE 5-11. Typical Induction Doses and Pharmacokinetic Variables of Intravenous Agents Commonly Used for Induction of General Anesthesia in Ambulatory Surgery Patients

Drug	Induction Dose (mg/kg)*	Distribution Half-Life (min)	Elimination Half-Life (hr)	Clearance (ml/min)	$V_{d,ss}$† (L)
Thiopental	3.0–6.0	2–4 (rapid) 30–60 (slow)	10–12	180–200	100–200
Methohexital	1.0–2.0	5–6	1.5–4	700–900	60–80
Etomidate	0.2–0.4	2–4	1.5–5	800–1400	200–400
Ketamine	0.75–1.5	11–17	2–3	1250–1400	200–250
Midazolam	0.1–0.2	7–15	2–2.5	300–550	70–130
Propofol	1.25–2.5	2–4	1–3	1400–2800	200–500

*Lower dosages are recommended when these drugs are used in combination with narcotic analgesics or when administered to geriatric outpatients.
†$V_{d,ss}$ = volume of distribution, steady state.
SOURCE: White and Shafer.[140] Used with permission.

dium thiopental has been widely used even though the mechanism of its action on the central nervous system has not been fully elucidated. It has been speculated that thiopental depresses polysynaptic responses in the central nervous system, both presynaptically to decrease the release of acetylcholine[123] and postsynaptically to enhance GABA-induced inhibition of central nervous system transmission.[124]

Thiopental is prepared commercially as a sodium salt that is readily soluble in water; prior to administration, it is dissolved to form a 2.5% solution. This highly alkaline solution (pH 10.6) is incompatible for mixture with most other commonly

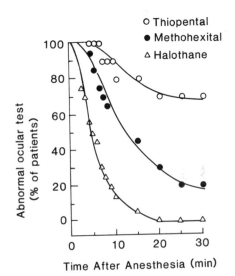

FIGURE 5-3. Percentage of patients with abnormal Maddox wing scores after outpatient operations. (SOURCE: Hannington-Kiff.[132] Used with permission.)

used intravenous medications such as opioids and neuromuscular blocking agents, which are generally acidic in solution. It has recently been determined that despite their high pH, thiopental solutions can support bacterial growth; it is now recommended that unused solutions be discarded within 24 hours of mixture.

When thiopental is administered intravenously, the tissues with a high blood flow per unit volume (e.g., the so-called vessel-rich group—heart, brain, kidney) initially take up most of the blood-borne drug. Thiopental is highly lipophilic and readily crosses the blood-brain barrier. The drug's lipid solubility, pK, and low molecular weight, when combined with high blood flow to the brain, produce a characteristic rapid induction of general anesthesia.

As the blood concentration of thiopental falls below that of the vessel-rich group, redistribution of the drug occurs—initially to muscle and later to fat[125] (Fig. 5-4). It is this redistribution of thiopental from the central compartment (e.g., the vessel-rich group) to the peripheral compartment (e.g., vessel-poor group—muscle, fat, bone) that accounts for the rapid termination of its anesthetic effects.

Nevertheless, the large volume of distribution and long elimination half-life of thiopental can contribute to a slow recovery after large repeated doses. Indeed, Korttila and coworkers have shown that a single large induction dose of thiopental in unpremedicated volunteers resulted in substantially impaired driving skills for at least eight hours.[126] Hemodynamic effects are similar after equipotent doses of thiopental, thiamylal, or methohexital for induction of anesthesia.[127] In healthy, normovolemic patients, thiopental (5 mg/kg IV) produced a transient 10- to 20-mmHg decrease in blood pressure that was offset by a compensatory increase in heart rate of 15 to 20 beats per minute.[128] This dose of thiopental produced minimal direct myocardial depression, although such an effect has been reported at higher doses. Cardiac dysfunction after thiopental is unlikely in the presence of adequate ventilation and oxygenation; in general, barbiturates do not sensitize the myocardium to the effect of catecholamines.

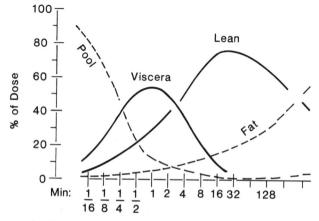

FIGURE 5-4. The uptake of thiopental from body tissues. Note the geometric progression of the time scale. (SOURCE: Price, et al.[125] Used with permission.)

All the ultrashort-acting barbiturates cause respiratory depression. The sensitivity of the respiratory center to carbon dioxide is depressed at all levels of anesthesia. Responsiveness of the peripheral chemoreceptors is more adequately maintained; however, this responsiveness is obliterated at profound depths of anesthesia. After a usual induction dose (3 to 4 mg/kg), tidal volume decreases and the respiratory rate increases.

Extravenous injection of thiopental may cause tissue necrosis because of the solution's alkalinity. The injection of thiopental into an artery can cause serious complications. Following intra-arterial injection, small crystals of thiopental form and cause capillary obstruction. Local release of norepinephrine then causes transient arteriolar spasm. Thrombosis and ischemia may occur, depending on the concentration and volume of the solution injected. Therapy is aimed at dilution of the injected drug, relief of the arterial spasm, and prevention of thrombosis. Infiltration of a local anesthetic drug around the artery may relieve pain and promote further vasodilation. Prevention of thrombosis is achieved by the administration of intravenous heparin. Oral anticoagulant therapy may be continued up to two weeks following the injection. Stellate ganglion or brachial plexus blockade may be performed to obliterate sympathetic vasoconstrictor tone. However, these blocks should not be performed in a patient who has received heparin. The incidence of complications secondary to intra-arterial injections has been substantially reduced with the general use of a 2.5% solution of thiopental rather than a 5% or 10% solution.

Methohexital

Methohexital, an oxybarbiturate with a spectrum of central nervous system activity similar to that of thiopental, is used clinically as a 1% solution with a highly alkaline pH (10.6). Although the distribution half-life and volume of distribution of thiopental and methohexital are similar (Table 5-11), methohexital has a clearance rate three to four times higher than that of thiopental and hence a significantly shorter half-life.[129] In studying the pharmacokinetics of thiopental and methohexital in patients having short surgical procedures, Hudson and coworkers evaluated the following: disposition of a single intravenous bolus of methohexital followed by other agents for the maintenance of anesthesia, comparison of the pharmacokinetics of thiopental and methohexital in surgical patients, and the relative importance of metabolism for the redistribution phase in the recovery process after both intravenous induction agents.[129] Although the kinetics of the distribution phase of thiopental and methohexital appear similar, redistribution is a major factor determining the duration of sedation after a single bolus dose of either drug. The more rapid recovery of complete psychomotor function after methohexital probably results in more rapid metabolism. Hudson and coworkers concluded that methohexital is preferable to thiopental whenever more rapid recovery from anesthesia is desired, particularly after large or repeated doses.

Coordination tests as measured by Vickers showed that patients required 30 to 60 minutes to recover after 1 mg/kg methohexital and 45 to 90 minutes after 2 mg/kg. Patients required 30 to 75 minutes to recover after 2.5 mg/kg thiopental and 105 to 210 minutes after 5 mg/kg. Subjects reported being less sedated and

TABLE 5-12. Recovery Times and Side-Effects When Continuous Infusions of Thiopental, Methohexital, or Etomidate Were Used as Adjuvants to Nitrous Oxide for Outpatient Anesthesia

Hypnotic Group	Dose (mg/min)	Recovery Times* (min)			Postoperative Side-Effects (%)		
		Awake	Oriented	Ambulatory	Nausea	Dizzy	Drowsy
Thiopental	14 ± 4	8 ± 7	12 ± 9	84 ± 9	15	10	50
Methohexital	5 ± 2	2 ± 2[†]	3 ± 2[†]	45 ± 4[†]	10	10	5[†]
Etomidate	2 ± 1	5 ± 3	6 ± 4	67 ± 8	45[†]	5	20

*Mean values ± SD.
[†]Significantly different from thiopental group ($p < 0.05$).
SOURCE: White and Shafer.[140] Used with permission.

mentally more clear after methohexital than after thiopental.[130] Other investigators have similarly found that methohexital was associated with a shorter awakening and recovery time than was thiopental.[131–133] Indeed, because it allows for rapid recovery times and few postoperative side-effects (Table 5-12), several investigators have concluded that methohexital is superior to both thiopental and etomidate for induction of anesthesia in the ambulatory surgery patient.[134,135] However, complete recovery of fine motor skills after methohexital may be as prolonged as after thiopental.[126]

There are some disadvantages to administering methohexital for induction of anesthesia in the outpatient. Respiratory dysfunction including cough and hiccough have been reported in 26% of patients.[136] Tremors, involuntary muscle movements, and pain on injection have been reported in up to 40% of patients. Interestingly, the muscle twitches are not associated with electroencephalographic abnormalities in normal patients. It has been suggested that these side-effects may be minimized by slow injection of a dilute solution of methohexital (0.5%) after administration of a narcotic analgesic (fentanyl 1–2 µg/kg).

Etomidate

Etomidate is a short-acting intravenous induction agent devoid of any analgesic properties. A carboxylated compound containing midazole, it is structurally unrelated to any other intravenous anesthetic agent. The imidazole nucleus renders etomidate water soluble at an acidic pH and highly lipophilic at a physiologic pH. Its mechanism of action is thought to be similar to that of the barbiturates.

The chief advantage of etomidate over other intravenous anesthetic induction agents is that it does not affect hemodynamic stability. When given in an induction dose of 0.2 to 0.4 mg/kg, etomidate does not cause cardiovascular depression or histamine release.[137] There are, however, several disadvantages associated with its use; pain on injection (in up to 50% of patients) and involuntary myoclonic movements (in up to 70% of patients) are two of the major side effects of this drug.[138] Pain has been described as severe enough that patients refuse a second etomidate induction.[139] Involuntary movements can be minimized by administering a benzodiazepine (e.g., midazolam, 0.07 mg/kg, or diazapam, 0.15 mg/kg) and a narcotic (e.g., fentanyl, 1.5 µg/kg), a preinduction intravenous dose of alfentanil (7 µg/kg), or a small intravenous dose (e.g., 25 mg) of lidocaine.[140–143] When etomidate was compared with thiopental, several investigators found a threefold increase in postoperative nausea and vomiting in patients who received etomidate.[135,138] Prophylactic antiemetics are recommended to decrease nausea when etomidate is used for anesthetic induction in outpatients. Additionally, etomidate appears to have a significant effect on the hypothalmic-pituitary axis; a single induction dose of etomidate can produce transient suppression (up to 8 hr) of adrenocortical function.[144]

Ketamine

Ketamine is a rapidly acting phencyclidine derivative that may be used by the intravenous or intramuscular route for induction and maintenance of anesthesia. Ketamine produces a state of dissociative anesthesia, which is characterized by catalepsy, catatonia, amnesia, and analgesia. Although its mechanism of action is unknown, ketamine has been shown to inhibit the effects of excitatory neurotransmitters such as acetylcholine and L-glutamate; additionally, ketamine has been shown to possess intrinsic analgesic properties by binding to the sigma class of opioid receptors.

After intravenous injection of an induction dose of ketamine (1–2 mg/kg), adequate spontaneous ventilation is generally maintained by the patient. Blood pressure and intracranial pressure rise transiently. Accordingly, it has been suggested that ketamine is contraindicated for patients with a history of hypertension, prior cerebral vascular accident, or increased intracranial pressure.

The clinical usefulness of ketamine in the ambulatory surgery setting is limited. It has been associated with postanesthetic confusion, disorientation, bad dreams, hallucinations, and restlessness. Thompson and coworkers compared thiopental and ketamine as induction agents for outpatient anesthesia.[145] Two-thirds of the ketamine patients in this study reported that their unpleasant dreams were frightening. Although the incidence of these unpleasant dreams can be decreased with the administration of diazepam or droperidol, these drugs may further delay the patient's recovery. Patients who have received ketamine should be allowed to recover quietly; if they are disturbed frequently, there is a greater potential for excitement, restlessness, and hallucinations. This contradicts the usual "stir-up" regimen that most ambulatory surgery facilities use to promote early ambulation and discharge. Consequently, ketamine falls far short of the requirements of an ideal ambulatory anesthetic drug and has found little use in the management of adult patients in an ambulatory setting.[146]

Midazolam

The physicochemical properties and pharmacokinetics of midazolam were discussed earlier in the section "Premedication." In this section we will address the role of midazolam as an induction agent for ambulatory surgery.

Induction of anesthesia can be produced by intravenous injection of midazolam over 30 to 60 seconds in doses of 0.2 to 0.35 mg/kg.[147] Unfortunately, when compared with thiopental, midazolam is much slower (50 s versus 110 s) for induction of anesthesia.[36] Several concerns also have been raised about delayed recovery and prolonged, profound amnesia after midazolam.[149,150] Fragen and Caldwell compared midazolam (0.2 mg/kg) with thiopental (4 mg/kg) for induction and maintenance of anesthesia and found significant prolongation to orientation and cognition in the midazolam-induced group.[151] Midazolam produced a profound period of amnesia for 1 to 2 hours postoperatively; important instructions could not be given to patients during that time. However, all patients were awake enough to be discharged from the hospital 200 minutes after the last dose of hypnotic had been administered (Table 5-13).

The use of midazolam as an induction agent in ambulatory surgery is dependent on the length of the surgical procedure and the total dose of midazolam to be administered.[152] For very short outpatient procedures, it may be best not to use midazolam, because not only will patients be drowsy in the postoperative period, but they will be very amnesic and not likely to remember any instructions given to them during that period.

Studies are presently being conducted to determine if flumazenil, a specific benzodiazepine antagonist, can be used to modify the role of midazolam in ambulatory surgery. Flumazenil has been shown to reverse midazolam-induced sedation without producing toxic side-effects.[153] Unfortunately, the duration of action of flumazenil is shorter than that of midazolam; in the ambulatory surgery setting, patient observation must be long enough to preclude the recurrence of significant sedation or profound amnesia after patient discharge.

Propofol

Propofol is a new intravenous anesthetic agent with a unique spectrum of physical-chemical properties and clinical effects. Chemically unrelated to the barbiturates, benzodiazepines, steroids, imidazoles, or eugenols, it is one of a series of alkyl phenols. During investigational trials, it was referred to as "diprofolane" and "disoprofol," but these names have been abandoned in favor of its current generic name *propofol* (chemical structure 2,6-diisopropylphenol).

Propofol is an oily liquid that is virtually insoluble in water. For this reason, it was originally formulated in an aqueous solution in the solubilizing agent Cremophor EL (polyoxyethylated castor oil). However, owing to a high incidence of pain on injection and to the association between Cremophor EL and anaphy-

TABLE 5-13. Time in Minutes for Recovery Characteristics after Thiopental or Midazolam

	Awake	Oriented	Ambulatory	Cognitive
Thiopental (4 mg/kg)	5.7	14.7	52	33
Midazolam (0.2 mg/kg)	14.4*	49.9*	108*	125*
Fentanyl-thiopental	7.3	13.3	65	73
Fentanyl-midazolam	12.0*	37.9*	80	104*

*Significantly different from thiopental-treated group ($p < 0.05$).
SOURCE: Fragen and Caldwell.[151] Used with permission.

lactoid reactions,[154,155] propofol was reformulated in an oil-in-water emulsion containing soybean oil (10%), glycerol (2.25%), and purified egg phosphatide (1.2%). This propofol emulsion is quite similar to Intralipid, a product frequently used for intravenous hyperalimentation. All propofol studies initiated after July of 1983 used this lipid emulsion formulation; the Cremophor EL formulation has never been used in North America and is no longer available for clinical use anywhere in the world.

Propofol is formulated to have a pH of between 7.0 and 8.5 and is physiologically compatible with blood, as well as a number of commonly used intravenous solutions including D_5W, D_5W/LR, LR, $D_5W/.9NS$, $D_5W/.45NS$, and $D_5W/.2NS$. Because of its physiologic pH, accidental perivascular injections should not cause tissue necrosis. Although propofol contains purified egg yolk constituents, it is devoid of protein from egg albumin and should not cause allergic reactions in egg-sensitive individuals.

The pharmacokinetic profile of propofol appears to make it uniquely amenable for use in ambulatory surgery. It is an extremely rapid and short-acting anesthetic agent. Blood concentrations of propofol fall rapidly after a single bolus injection owing to its extensive distribution and rapid elimination (Fig. 5-5). Pharmacokinetic modeling studies of propofol suggest a blood-brain equivalent half-life of only 2 to 3 minutes and a distribution half-life of only 2 to 4 minutes. The total-body clearance rate of propofol has been reported to exceed hepatic blood flow, suggesting extrahepatic sites of drug elimination (e.g., kidney, lungs). When propofol is administered as a single bolus dose, induction of anesthesia is dependent on both the dose and the speed at which the injection is adminis-

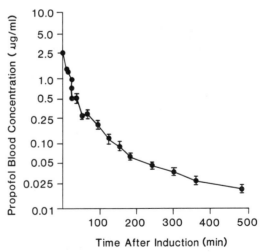

FIGURE 5-5. Blood propofol concentrations in healthy patients following a 2.5-mg/kg IV induction dose. (SOURCE: Cockshott ID: Propofol (Diprivan) pharmacokinetics and metabolism: An overview. Postgrad Med J 61 (Suppl 3): 45, 1985. Used with permission.)

TABLE 5-14. Patient Response after Administration of Propofol, Methohexitone, or Thiopentone

	Propofol	Methohexitone	Thiopentone
Time to open eyes (min)	4.8 ± 0.45	5.6 ± 0.54	9.6 ± 0.74*
Time to repeat date of birth (min)	5.8 ± 0.34	7.2 ± 0.58‡	10.6 ± 0.74*
Sequelae:			
Headache	0	3	7†
Nausea and vomiting	0	3	2
Drowsiness	0	0	7†
Venous problems	0	0	0

NOTE: Crude recovery times (mean ± SEM) and postoperative sequelae (number of patients).
*,†Significance values: propofol *versus* thiopentone: *$p < 0.001$; †$p < 0.01$.
‡Significance values: propofol *versus* methohexitone: $p < 0.05$.
SOURCE: Mackenzie and Grant.[159] Used with permission.

tered.[156] Patients who were given an induction dose of propofol (2.5 mg/kg) predictably lost consciousness in one arm-to-brain circulation time but were able to respond to verbal commands approximately 5.4 minutes later.[158] The induction dose requirement is decreased (1.0–1.75 mg/kg) in the elderly (*i.e.*, patients older than 55 years) and in patients who have been premedicated with CNS depressants (*e.g.*, barbiturates, benzodiazepines, opioids).[157]

Important advantages associated with the use of propofol as an induction agent in ambulatory anesthesia include its extremely rapid elimination and its lower incidence of postoperative side-effects when compared with those of methohexital or thiopental[158–160] (Table 5-14). In one randomized, prospective, double-blind, placebo-controlled crossover trial comparing recovery from induction doses of thiopental or propofol in healthy volunteers, the results were dramatic.[161] Subjects responded to command and were able to sit and stand significantly faster after propofol than after thiopental anesthesia (Table 5-15). The effect of thiopental was more pronounced and the differences in recovery after thiopental or propofol were significant even five hours after induction (Figs. 5-6 and 5-7).

TABLE 5-15. Times (min) to Respond to Command, Sit, and Stand after the Injection of Propofol and Thiopental

	Propofol*	Thiopental*
Response to command	13.9 ± 2.6	18.0 ± 6.2†
Able to sit	17.0 ± 3.3	20.4 ± 5.8†
Able to stand	33.0 ± 6.9	62.0 ± 29.0†

*Mean ± SD.
†$p < 0.05$, propofol vs. thiopental, paired t test.
SOURCE: Korttila et al.[161] Used with permission.

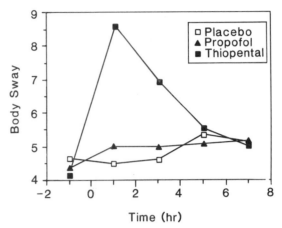

FIGURE 5-6. Mean body sway when standing on a force platform before and 1, 3, 5, and 7 hours after drug injection. (SOURCE: Korttila, et al.[161] Used with permission.)

Disadvantages associated with the use of propofol for induction of anesthesia in outpatients include pain on injection and the possibility of significant cardiovascular depression, particularly when administered to the elderly or debilitated patient. Pain on injection depends on the site of administration (small dorsal hand veins) and is minimized if larger forearm or antecubital veins are used.[162] The use of intravenous lidocaine immediately before propofol injection also may reduce the incidence of pain.[159] Thrombophlebitis after intravenous administration of propofol, unlike of diazepam or of methohexital, does not appear to be a problem. Although many investigators have suggested that the cardiovascular effects of propofol are similar to those of thiopental, others have found that pro-

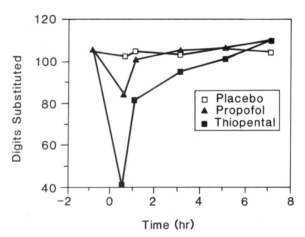

FIGURE 5-7. Mean number of digits substituted in Digit Symbol Substitution Test before and 1/2, 1, 3, 5, and 7 hours after drug injection. (SOURCE: Korttila et al.[161] Used with permission.)

pofol produced greater cardiovascular depression, particularly in the elderly and debilitated.[163–169] When clinically significant cardiovascular depression does occur, it is typically manifested by decreases in arterial blood pressure and cardiac index without a significant change in the heart rate.[170] Most investigators seem to agree that the clinical significance of these hemodynamic changes in young, healthy, normovolemic patients is negligible.[171] Nevertheless, the induction dose of propofol should be individualized and titrated against the patient's response at an appropriate rate of 40 mg every 10 seconds until the clinical signs of anesthesia appear. A lower rate of administration (approximately 20 mg every 10 s) should be used for elderly, debilitated, or hypovolemic patients (physical status 3 and 4).

After induction, propofol anesthesia can be maintained by either repeated bolus injections or continuous infusion. When administered by repeated bolus injections, the timing of the repeat administration (25% to 50% of the induction dose) is determined by the anesthesiologist and is based on the clinical signs of light anesthesia (e.g., movement, tachycardia, hypertension, tearing, and diaphoresis). Clinically, a repeat dose might be expected every 5 to 15 minutes depending on the previous dose, degree of surgical stimulation, and patient variability of response.

Maintenance of anesthesia by intravenous infusion of propofol is generally smoother than with repeated bolus injections since continuous drug administration by infusion avoids the peaks and valleys of blood levels that are associated with changes in the depth of anesthesia. Administration by continuous infusion produces an initial rapid increase in blood propofol concentrations followed by a slow rise to a virtual steady state. When administering propofol by continuous infusion, it is recommended that drop counters, syringe pumps, or volumetric pumps be used to provide controlled infusion rates. Although the rate of administration varies between patients and is somewhat dependent on the use of analgesics and muscle relaxants, infusion rates of 0.1 to 0.2 mg/kg per minute usually provide satisfactory conditions. Some investigators advocate a slightly higher infusion rate of up to 0.3 mg/kg per minute during the first few minutes following induction of anesthesia. This is due to the extremely rapid redistribution of an induction dose of propofol and attempts to ensure that initial blood levels do not fall too rapidly.

In all cases, the infusion rate should be adjusted during surgery according to the clinical response of the patient. A variable infusion technique, rather than a fixed infusion regimen, permits the rate of propofol to be precisely titrated to achieve the desired clinical effect. Ease of control during maintenance of anesthesia has been one of the frequently reported advantages of propofol infusion. Hemodynamic responses are generally quite stable, and it is easy to see changes in an infusion rate quickly reflected in changes in mean arterial blood pressure or heart rate.

Comparisons of propofol and traditional techniques for maintenance of anesthesia are limited. However, preliminary investigations suggest that propofol may offer significant advantages when compared with a conventional thiopental, isoflurane, nitrous oxide, oxygen technique in the management of anesthesia for

TABLE 5-16. Clinical Recovery from Low-Dose Propofol Infusion versus Thiopental-Isoflurane in Patients Undergoing Outpatient Surgery

	Low-Dose Propofol*	Thiopental-Isoflurane*
Patients:		
Age (yrs)	35 ± 2.9	35 ± 1.7
Weight (kg)	70 ± 3.0	63 ± 2.4
Duration of anesthesia (min)[†]	85 ± 12	57 ± 5.2
Clinical recovery (minutes to reach baseline after cessation of N_2O):		
Respond to command[‡]	3.5 ± 0.6	6.1 ± 0.6
Eyes open[†]	4.0 ± 0.7	6.3 ± 0.6
Oriented	5.5 ± 0.8	9.4 ± 1.4
PARS 10	24 ± 6.0	26 ± 3.8
Able to sit	59 ± 5.3	73 ± 6.5
Able to stand	68 ± 6.0	87 ± 8.0
Able to walk	70 ± 7.2	96 ± 9.6
Oral fluids[‡]	61 ± 4.5	130 ± 17
Able to void[‡]	102 ± 15	173 ± 16
"Home ready"[†]	138 ± 18	206 ± 16

*Mean ± SEM.
[†]$p < 0.05$.
[‡]$p < 0.01$ between groups.
SOURCE: Korttila et al.[173] Used with permission.

short ambulatory surgical procedures.[164,172–174] Patients who received propofol demonstrated shorter stays in the PACU and faster times to independent standing,[172] suggesting that the use of propofol may provide faster patient turnaround and less patient expense.[174] In one such study, patients who received propofol were ready to be discharged from the PACU 68 minutes faster than patients who received a conventional thiopental, isoflurane anesthetic technique[173] (Table 5-16).

Inhalational Agents

Patients undergoing anesthesia for ambulatory surgery have needs that differ significantly from those of inpatients. The postoperative goal of "home readiness" places demands on the anesthetic management of these patients that did not exist in the days before ambulatory surgery. This section will highlight some of the clinical and pharmacologic properties of inhalational anesthetics that may affect the clinician's decision to use these agents in the outpatient setting.

Inhalational anesthetics should produce a brain anesthetic concentration sufficient to allow surgery without causing excessive depression of the other vessel-rich organ systems (i.e., heart, liver, kidney). This is accomplished by manipulating a series of partial pressure gradients starting at the source of the inspired anesthetic gas and ending in the brain tissue. Simply put, the inhalational agent is transferred from the anesthesia machine through the breathing system to the alveoli. From the alveoli, the inhalational agent is transferred to the arterial blood

TABLE 5-17. Factors Determining Partial Pressure Gradients Necessary for Establishment of Anesthesia

Transfer of inhaled anesthetic from anesthetic machine to alveoli: 　Inspired partial pressure 　Alveolar ventilation 　Characteristics of anesthetic breathing system
Transfer of inhaled anesthetic from alveoli to arterial blood: 　Blood-gas partition coefficient 　Cardiac output 　Alveolar-to-venous partial pressure difference
Transfer of inhaled anesthetic from arterial blood to brain: 　Brain-blood partition coefficient 　Cerebral blood flow 　Arterial-to-venous partial pressure difference

SOURCE: Adapted from Stoelting RK, Miller RD (eds): Basics of Anesthesia. New York: Churchill-Livingstone, 1984. Used with permission.

and then to the brain and other body tissues. Factors that influence the time needed to reach a given degree of brain tissue saturation with inhalational anesthetics include inspired partial pressure, pulmonary ventilation, characteristics of the breathing system, blood-gas partition coefficient, cardiac output, pulmonary blood flow, brain-blood partition coefficient, brain blood flow, and arterial-to-venous partial pressure differences[175] (Table 5-17). The anesthesiologist can design a plan for the outpatient by combining these facts with some theoretical concepts (e.g., concentration effect, second gas effect, minimum alveolar concentration, overpressurization) about the uptake, distribution, and potency of inhaled agents.

Because of differences in agent solubility, the choice of anesthetic agent can determine the rapidity of induction or emergence from anesthesia. The *blood-gas partition coefficient* is a measure of the inhalational agent's relative solubility in these two phases. Based on their blood-gas partition coefficients, inhalational agents have been traditionally characterized as poorly soluble (N_2O), moderately soluble (isoflurane, enflurane, halothane), or highly soluble (diethyl ether, methoxyflurane). Large amounts of highly soluble anesthetic agents must be dissolved before reaching equilibrium (i.e., brain saturation); much smaller amounts of poorly soluble agents achieve the same effect. In theory, therefore, if all other factors are held constant (e.g., inspired partial pressure, ventilation, blood flow, cardiac output), inhalational agents with low blood-gas partition coefficients (i.e., low solubility) are preferable for ambulatory anesthesia because these agents achieve equilibrium with the brain most rapidly, allowing the quickest induction and emergence.

The *concentration effect* allows the anesthesiologist to more rapidly augment the uptake of inhaled agents that can be administered in high concentrations.[176] Inspired anesthetic concentration influences both the maximum possible alveolar concentration and the rate at which that level can be achieved. For example, the administration of high concentrations of N_2O (greater than 50%) results in an increased uptake because of a concentration action in the alveoli and the augmentation of tracheal inflow (*e.g.*, inspired ventilation).[177]

The *second gas effect* enables the anesthesiologist to alter the rate of uptake of multiple inhaled agents administered simultaneously. The second gas effect reflects the ability of the high-volume uptake of one gas (N_2O) to accelerate the rate of equilibration of a concomitantly administered second gas (a potent agent, *i.e.*, halothane, enflurane, or isoflurane).[177,178] The rapid loss of volume associated with the uptake of N_2O "concentrates" the amount of potent agent actually present in the lung, thereby accelerating the uptake of the second gas.

In 1963, Merkel and Eger described the potency of inhalational anesthetics in terms of *minimum alveolar concentration* (*MAC*).[179] They defined MAC as the minimum alveolar concentration at equilibrium of an anesthetic at 1 atm that is required to abolish movement in 50% of subjects in response to a noxious stimulus (*e.g.*, surgical skin incision). Because the authors defined MAC at equilibrium, FI_{O_2} concentration equals PA_{O_2} concentration, which equals gas concentration at the site of action (*e.g.*, the brain). Since its introduction, MAC has been widely accepted as a definition of anesthetic gas potency for the following reasons:

1. Similar MAC concentrations of all inhaled anesthetics produce equivalent degrees of CNS depression; unlike the so-called clinical signs of anesthesia[180] (*e.g.*, respiratory pattern, pupil size), the concept of MAC applies equally to all inhaled anesthetics.
2. The end point in humans (abolition of movement in response to a surgical incision) is well accepted by clinicians as one of the goals in the administration of an anesthetic.
3. Although the MAC for each agent is different (Table 5-18) and many physiologic and pharmacologic factors may affect MAC (Table 5-19), it is reliably constant and easily reproducible within the species.

MAC values for inhalational anesthetic agents are additive; that is, 0.7 MAC of N_2O plus 0.3 MAC of halothane, enflurane, or isoflurane has the same effect on the brain as 1.0 MAC of any of the potent inhaled agents alone. In order to speed induction (or emergence), anesthesiologists will frequently use high flows of N_2O in conjunction with a potent agent, thereby taking advantage of the principles of

TABLE 5-18. Comparative Potencies of Inhalational Anesthetics

Agent	Minimum Alveolar Concentration (MAC)*
Halothane	0.74%
Isoflurane	1.15%
Enflurane	1.68%
N_2O	104.00%

*30–55-year-old, 37°C, 760 mmHg.

TABLE 5-19. Factors That May Affect MAC

Increase in MAC:
  Young age
  Hyperthermia
  Elevations in CNS catecholamines
  Chronic alcohol abuse

Decrease in MAC:
  Hypothermia
  Decreases in CNS catecholamines
  Acute alcohol intoxication
  Concomitantly administered anesthetic, analgesic, and/or sedative-hypnotic drugs
  Increasing age
  Blood pressure below 40 mmHg
  Pa_{O_2} below 38 mmHg
  Anemia
  Pregnancy
  Lithium
  Local anesthetic

No change in MAC:
  Duration of anesthesia
  Patient gender
  Pa_{CO_2} 15 to 95 mmHg
  Metabolic acidosis/alkalosis
  Thyroid gland dysfunction
  Hyperkalemia
  Hypokalemia
  Anesthetic metabolism

MAC additivity, the second gas effect,[177,178] the concentration effect,[176,177] and the relative insolubility of N_2O.

Overpressure is another technique that can be employed with the potent inhalational agents to speed induction and achieve a more rapid maintenance level of anesthesia in healthy, normovolemic ambulatory surgery patients. High inspired concentrations of the volatile agents are necessary to rapidly drive the partial pressure of these agents in the brain tissue past the level producing anesthesia.[181] The inspired concentration of each potent agent needed to reach 1.0 MAC in the alveoli within several breaths has been determined as follows[182]: halothane, 3.0%; enflurane, 5.7%; and isoflurane, 3.1%. These figures assume that all other determinants of uptake and distribution (*e.g.*, pulmonary ventilation, blood flow, cardiac output) are held constant. Within the limits of safety for each volatile agent, higher inspired concentrations can significantly reduce the time needed to achieve maintenance levels of anesthesia; Torri and coworkers have shown that they could achieve levels of anesthesia sufficient to perform surgery in four minutes with the patient breathing 3.5% enflurane versus two minutes with the patient breathing 5.0% enflurane.[183] To prevent overdosage, overpressure should be applied with extreme care, close observation, and sufficient monitoring.

Nitrous Oxide

Several properties of N_2O have allowed it to become the foundation of most general anesthetics in the ambulatory surgery setting (Table 5-20). Like the other modern inhalational agents, its nonflammability allows this gas to be used in all current operating room environments. N_2O has a pleasant odor that has been described as slightly sweet. Because this gas has no pungency associated with its odor, it is most suitable as an adjunct for starting an inhalational induction in patients who are "afraid of needles," especially unpremedicated children. It is the least soluble of all presently used inhalational anesthetics and theoretically achieves the most rapid equilibration between inspired partial pressure and brain tissue saturation. The speed of induction can be even further enhanced by employing the principles of the concentration effect and the second gas effect. The use of N_2O as a maintenance adjunct can significantly decrease requirements for other anesthetic agents.[185] It appears that N_2O has little or no net depressive effects on the respiratory or circulatory systems.[186] Its slight direct cardiovascular depressant effects are obscured by the sympathetic stimulation the drug produces. Of particular importance in the anesthetic management of ASA physical status 3 and 4 ambulatory surgery patients, the combination of N_2O plus halothane[187] or enflurane[188] appears to produce less depression at a given MAC level than either potent agent alone. In similar studies with isoflurane, Dolan and coworkers found that N_2O combined with isoflurane decreased arterial blood pressure to a lesser extent than isoflurane alone.[189] Although most of the potential disadvantages of N_2O for ambulatory anesthesia are avoidable or of minor consequence, they should, nonetheless, be noted:

1. N_2O has a limited potency (MAC greater than 100%), and for this reason, it is invariably supplemented with either intravenous or potent inhalational anesthetic agents.

2. The potency of N_2O is directly dependent on the altitude at which it is administered; because of the reduced partial pressure of N_2O in high-altitude environ-

TABLE 5-20. Some Properties of the Currently Utilized Inhalational Anesthetics

	N_2O	Halothane	Enflurane	Isoflurane
Molecular weight	44	197.4	184.5	184.5
Vapor pressure (mmHg, 20°C)	Gas	244.1	171.8	239.5
Odor	Sweet	Organic solvent	Ethereal	Ethereal
Pungency	None	None	Moderate	Moderate
Preservative necessary	No	Yes	No	No
Stability:				
Soda lime	Stable	Decomposes	Stable	Stable
Sunlight	Stable	Decomposes	Stable	Stable
Reacts with metal	No	Yes	No	No

ments, 70% N_2O would be less potent in the mountains of Colorado than it would be at sea level.

3. Although the solubility of N_2O is less than that of any currently used potent inhalational agent, it is far greater than that of several other gases (e.g., nitrogen) generally present in the body. Blood passing a nitrogen-filled gas space (e.g., middle ear) within the body can deliver a greater volume of N_2O to that space than the volume of nitrogen it replaces. Consequently, either the pressure within the space or the volume of space will increase when high concentrations of N_2O are administered for any substantial period of time.

4. During the immediate recovery from an N_2O-based general anesthetic (i.e., first 5–10 minutes), the elimination of large volumes of N_2O dilutes both alveolar oxygen[190,191] and carbon dioxide (CO_2),[192] potentially causing "diffusion hypoxemia." The displacement of oxygen by N_2O leads indirectly to a decrease in oxygenation, while the dilution of alveolar CO_2 leads indirectly to hypoxia by decreasing respiratory drive. This phenomenon is generally of little importance to the healthy outpatient,[186] but it explains why many anesthesiologists choose to administer high inspired oxygen concentrations for the first 10 minutes postoperatively to patients with preexisting lung disease or to those ambulatory surgery patients whose ventilatory drive may be pharmacologically depressed.

5. N_2O may be associated with a higher than practical incidence of postoperative nausea and vomiting.[193–195] Recently, several studies have suggested that postoperative nausea and vomiting can significantly delay time to discharge in ambulatory surgery patients.[176,177] Some anesthesiologists have attempted to link these two hypotheses and have gone so far as to advocate eliminating N_2O from the ambulatory surgery anesthesia medication armamentarium. This conclusion has recently been challenged; in a randomized prospective study of over 100 patients undergoing abdominal hysterectomy under isoflurane, N_2O, oxygen anesthesia or isoflurane, oxygen anesthesia, Korttila and coworkers were unable to demonstrate an increase in the incidence or severity of postoperative emetic symptoms in the group receiving N_2O.[196] Despite these potential drawbacks, the ubiquity of N_2O persists; to date, it continues to be the inhalational anesthetic most frequently administered.[197]

Halothane

At room temperature, halothane is a clear, nonflammable liquid with a fruity, nonirritating odor. Of the modern potent agents, it is the least irritating to the airways and is often the drug of choice in the presence of airway pathology.[198] Unlike enflurane or isoflurane, halothane requires the addition of thymol as a preservative to prevent spontaneous oxidative decomposition. Residual thymol in vaporizers after the vaporization of halothane can cause them to malfunction and lead to accidental halothane overdosage.

Halothane is the most commonly used potent inhaled agent in pediatric anesthesia.[199] Its chief advantage for the pediatric ambulatory surgery patient is that it offers a smooth, nonthreatening (*i.e.*, "no needles") mask inhalational induction with the lowest incidence of excitement.[200] Its intermediate blood-gas solubility (2.5) is offset somewhat by its high potency, permitting a rapid induction, particularly when used in combination with N_2O. As with all the potent inhalational agents, overpressure can speed induction but should be employed with extreme caution, since profound cardiovascular depression and hypotension have been reported with halothane overdosage,[201] particularly in the young, fasting infant.[202] Recovery from halothane anesthesia is usually rapid and uneventful, although postoperative shivering,[203] headaches,[204] and nausea and vomiting have been reported and may affect time to discharge to home care.

Halothane has been reported to sensitize the myocardium to both endogenous and exogenous catecholamines.[205] Factors that increase the likelihood of ventricular dysrhythmias include carbon dioxide retention, sensory stimulation during light planes of surgical anesthesia, parenteral atropine administration, and subcutaneous and parenteral epinephrine administration. Compared with enflurane or isoflurane, ventricular dysrhythmias are far more likely during halothane anesthesia,[206,207] especially in women[208] and younger outpatients.[209]

Of the modern potent inhalational anesthetics, halothane is the most susceptible to metabolic degradation. Halothane undergoes both oxidation and dehalogenation to form trifluroacetic acid as well as bromide and chloride free radicals.[210] These metabolites have been implicated in the development of rare but potentially fatal massive hepatic necrosis.[211,212] Although investigators have yet to prove a cause-effect relationship between halothane and massive hepatic necrosis, most anesthesiologists today tend to restrict the use of this drug in ambulatory anesthesia to pediatrics and to adults with airway pathology (e.g.,, heavy smokers, asthmatics, bronchitics).

Enflurane

At room temperature, enflurane is a clear, nonflammable liquid with a pungent ether-like odor. The physical-chemical characteristics and pharmacologic properties of enflurane seem well suited to the needs of ambulatory anesthesia. Its moderately low blood-gas partition coefficient (2.0), combined with its high potency, permits a rapid induction. As with halothane, overpressure to speed induction with enflurane should be used with caution because profound cardiovascular depression has been reported with enflurane overdosage. Enflurane has the lowest tissue-blood coefficient, suggesting a rapid initial recovery from anesthesia.

Unlike halothane, an enflurane, O_2 anesthetic at high enough concentrations can provide muscle relaxation sufficient for most ambulatory surgical procedures.[213-215] Enflurane significantly enhances the effect of many nondepolarizing neuromuscular blockers, including atracurium,[216] *d*-tubocurarine,[217] pancuronium,[217] and vecuronium.[218] Theoretically, using less muscle relaxant intraoperatively should provide additional safety postoperatively[219] and allow for more rapid return to "street fitness" in the ambulatory surgery patient.

Biotransformation and metabolism of enflurane is approximately one-tenth that of halothane.[220] Although an enflurane-associated hepatic necrosis has been suggested, its incidence is extraordinarily low,[221] and most anesthesiologists doubt its occurrence.

One of the potential limitations of enflurane is its pungency. In a study comparing enflurane and halothane supplemented with N_2O and oxygen for 80 children undergoing dental extractions, Hoyal and coworkers demonstrated a higher incidence of hiccoughing and breath holding in the enflurane group, probably related to the drug's strong ether-like odor.[222]

Isoflurane

At room temperature, isoflurane is a clear, nonflammable, volatile liquid with a markedly pungent, ether-like odor. The physical-chemical characteristics and pharmacologic properties of isoflurane make it well suited to the needs of the ambulatory surgery patient.[223] Isoflurane has the lowest blood-gas partition coefficient (1.4) of all the modern potent inhaled agents. Its low solubility combined with a high potency permits a rapid induction of anesthesia alone or in combination with N_2O or intravenous agents. As with halothane and enflurane, overpressure to speed induction could result in transient cardiovascular depression secondary to overdosage; however, such depression is less with isoflurane than with halothane or enflurane because it has a greater cardiovascular margin of safety.[224] Isoflurane does not appear to sensitize the myocardium to the effects of catecholamines and is more compatible with topical vasoconstrictors than is halothane.

In high enough concentrations, isoflurane, like enflurane, can produce profound muscle relaxation.[225] It also can substantially potentiate the effects of many nondepolarizing muscle relaxants, including atracurium,[226] d-tubocurarine,[225] gallamine,[227] pancuronium,[228] and vecuronium.[229] This effect is reversible when isoflurane is withdrawn and allows the anesthesiologist to use lower doses of relaxant intraoperatively.

Isoflurane is a very stable compound that does not appear to be metabolized in the body to any significant degree. Biotransformation of isoflurane is one-tenth to one-hundredth that of the other modern potent inhaled agents. Isoflurane does not undergo reductive metabolism; its limited biotransformation and degradation do not result in the production of chloride or bromide free radicals. To date, isoflurane has not been associated with a postoperative hepatic necrosis syndrome.

The modest pungency of isoflurane may significantly limit its application in clinical practice. Several studies have suggested that because of its pungent smell and irritating effects to the airway, isoflurane tends to provoke more excitement, breathholding, coughing, and laryngospasm than do either enflurane or halothane[230–232] (Table 5-21). Some investigators have suggested that these reflex respiratory responses should limit the use of isoflurane.[232] Other investigators believe that in spite of its limitations, this drug can be used clinically because of its superior flexibility.[233] Others have gone so far as to label isoflurane an "anesthetic for the eighties."[223]

TABLE 5-21. Incidence of Significant Complications (%) with Enflurane, Halothane, or Isoflurane

	Enflurane (n = 43)	Halothane (n = 46)	Isoflurane (n = 35)
Induction:			
Excitement	33	13*	34
Laryngospasm	2	4	23*
Maintenance:			
Coughing	5	0	20*
Emergence:			
Coughing	19	9	40*
Recovery:			
Coughing (total)	14	20	49*

*Different from other groups by chi-square analysis.
SOURCE: Adapted from Fisher et al.[232] Used with permission.

Sevoflurane

At room temperature, sevoflurane is a clear, nonflammable liquid with little or no pungent odor. Many of the physical-chemical characteristics and pharmacologic properties of sevoflurane suggest that it may be well suited to use in ambulatory anesthesia. Sevoflurane is a methyl-isopropyl ether [CH_2F—O = $CH(CF_3)_2$] whose solubility in blood (a blood-gas partition coefficient of 0.6–0.7[234–236]) approaches that of nitrous oxide.[237] The alveolar concentration of sevoflurane rises more rapidly than that of all other currently available inhalational anesthetic agents. Induction of anesthesia with sevoflurane is achieved rapidly and easily; coughing and breath holding are not the problems they are with isoflurane.[238] The MAC of sevoflurane in humans is 1.71% without nitrous oxide and 0.66% with 65% nitrous oxide.[239]

Like other potent inhalational anesthetic agents, sevoflurane is a circulatory and respiratory depressant.[234,238,240–242] Compared with isoflurane, sevoflurane appears to be more "forgiving" to the cardiovascular system; the decrease in blood pressure associated with sevoflurane appears to be less than that seen with isoflurane, heart rate appears to decrease rather than increase,[238] and the arrhythmogenic dose of epinephrine exceeds that found during anesthesia with isoflurane.[243] The effects of sevoflurane on the neuromuscular junction and human electroencephalogram are similar to those exhibited by isoflurane.[244]

Unfortunately, sevoflurane appears to be unstable under both *in vivo* and *in vitro* conditions.[245–248] Although sevoflurane is degraded *in vitro* by soda lime,[245] this degradation does not appear to produce volatile toxic products.[249] *In vivo* degradation of sevoflurane is enhanced by hepatic enzyme induction,[246–248] but studies in enzyme-induced rats with and without hypoxia have been unable to demonstrate hepatic or renal injury.[246–248] Nevertheless, clinical trials with sevoflurane in the United States have been recently suspended.

Desflurane

At room temperature, desflurane is a clear, nonflammable liquid with a "strong" but not pungent odor.[250] Desflurane's physical-chemical properties suggest that it may become the inhalational anesthetic of the future. It is a fluorinated methyl-ethyl ether (CF_2H—O—CFH—CF_3) identical in structure to isoflurane except for the substitution of a fluorine for the chlorine on the alpha ethyl carbon. It is less soluble (blood-gas partition coefficient of 0.42) than sevoflurane or even nitrous oxide. Induction of anesthesia with desflurane appears to be more rapid than with any currently available potent inhalational anesthetic. The MAC of desflurane in humans has recently been determined to be 6.0 ± 0.09.[251,252] In rats, the rate of recovery from anesthesia with desflurane is twice as rapid as with sevoflurane, three to five times that with isoflurane, and five to ten times that with halothane.[253]

The effects of desflurane on the cardiovascular system are similar to those of isoflurane.[254] In pigs, desflurane decreases myocardial contractility, cardiac output, and blood pressure in a dose-dependent fashion while increasing heart rate at all levels of anesthesia. In humans, desflurane produces smaller preincisional hemodynamic changes than does isoflurane while maintaining stable hemodynamics after incision.[255] One study in human volunteers has recently suggested that desflurane, unlike isoflurane, when combined with nitrous oxide, may actually lead to an activation of beta-adrenergic activity as is seen with diethyl-ether.[256] The effects of desflurane on the cardiac response to catecholamines[257] and on the human electroencephalogram[258] are similar to those seen with iso-flurane.

Unlike sevoflurane, desflurane resists both *in vitro*[259] and *in vivo*[260] degradation. Compared with isoflurane in rats, desflurane does not appear to be toxic to either the renal or hepatic organ systems.[261]

Balanced Anesthesia: Nitrous Oxide, Narcotics, Relaxants
Opioids
Opioids are frequently administered to the ambulatory surgery patient to supplement nitrous oxide for maintenance of general anesthesia as part of a nitrous oxide, narcotics, relaxant "balanced" technique. It has been suggested that the use of a nitrous oxide, narcotic, relaxant technique may be particularly well suited to the surgery outpatient because it may permit the maintenance of a lighter level of anesthesia, thereby resulting in a more rapid emergence and awakening. Epstein and coworkers concluded that the use of a narcotic analgesic to supplement a thiopental, nitrous oxide, oxygen anesthetic improved the intraoperative course by helping to provide a smooth, pain-free awakening and recovery from anesthesia.[262] The terms *opioid, narcotic,* and *narcotic analgesic* are used to describe drugs that specifically bind to any of several subspecies of opioid receptors and provide some opioid agonist effect (Table 5-22). Central nervous system effects of opioids include analgesia, drowsiness/sedation, mood alteration, respiratory depression, and emesis.

Analgesia is the primary reason that opioids are administered. There is minimal evidence that opioids affect the peripheral nervous system; most of their effects are mediated by the receptors found in the brain and spinal cord.[263] Unlike local anesthetics, the opioids are selective for painful stimuli, leaving other sensory and motor modalities intact.[264] A patient may be aware of a stimulus but

TABLE 5-22. Interactions of Morphine and Morphine-like Drugs with Opioid Receptors

	Receptor Types		
	Mu	Kappa	Sigma
Effects	Supraspinal analgesia	Spinal analgesia	Dysphoria
	Respiratory depression	Respiratory depression	Hallucinations
	Euphoria	Sedation	Vasomotor stimulation
	Physical dependence	Miosis	
Drugs:			
Morphine	Ag	Ag	0
Buprenorphine	pAg	—	0
Nalorphine	Ant	pAg	Ag
Pentazocine	Ant	Ag	Ag
Butorphanol	0	Ag	Ag
Nalbuphine	pAg/Ant	Ag	Ag
Naloxone	Ant	Ant	Ant

Abbreviations: Ag, agonist; pAg, partial agonist; Ant, antagonist; 0, no interaction.
SOURCE: Hug.[300] Used with permission.

may describe it as minimally painful or not painful at all. The specific mechanisms by which opioids produce analgesia are extremely complex; they involve the modulation of stimuli by an intricate system of receptors in both afferent and efferent pathways.

Pure agonist narcotics (*e.g.,* morphine, meperidine, fentanyl analogues) can produce sedation or even unconsciousness in some patients. Unfortunately, these medications do not reliably produce amnesia; the risk of awareness during surgery is present unless other specific amnesic or sedative-hypnotic drugs are combined with the opioid as part of the anesthetic technique.[265,266] Opioids have been reported to create alterations in mood.[263] Patients in distress have, after the intravenous administration of opioids, reported not only a decrease in pain, but also an increased feeling of well-being, warmth, and even euphoria.[264] In healthy, pain-free individuals, the intravenous administration of opioids may produce feelings of lethargy or fatigue.[267]

All opioid agonists produce a dose-dependent depression of ventilation, primarily through a direct depressant effect on brainstem ventilatory centers. This depression of ventilation is characterized by a significant reduction in sensitivity to carbon dioxide and is reflected by an increase in resting Pa_{CO_2} as well as a rightward displacement of the CO_2 response curve. Additionally, opioids can significantly depress hypoxic ventilatory drive.

Opioids produce nausea and vomiting by direct stimulation of the chemoreceptor trigger zone in the floor of the fourth ventricle of the medulla oblongata. This may reflect the role of opioids as partial dopamine agonists in the chemoreceptor trigger zone. Apomorphine, for example, is a potent emetic and is also the most potent of the opioids at the dopamine receptor.[268] Stimulation of dopamine receptors as a possible explanation for opioid-induced nausea and vomiting is consistent with the efficiency of butyrophenones in counteracting opioid-induced nausea and vomiting.[268,269]

TABLE 5-23. Pharmacokinetic Variables of Narcotic Analgesics Commonly Used in Outpatient Anesthesia

Drug	Relative Potency	Distribution Half-Life (min)	Elimination Half-Life (hr)	Clearance (ml/min)	$V_{d,ss}$ (L)*
Morphine	1	1–3 (rapid) 9–20 (slow)	2–4	800–1400	200–250
Meperidine	0.1	4–17	3–4	700–1200	200–250
Fentanyl	100	1–2 (rapid) 10–15 (slow)	3–4	700–900	200–300
Sufentanil	700	1–3 (rapid) 10–15 (slow)	2–4	600–900	140–200
Alfentanil	15	1–3	1–2	200–500	30–70

*$V_{d,ss}$ = volume of distribution, steady state.
SOURCE: White PF, Shafer AS: Clinical pharmacology and uses of injectable anesthetic and analgesic drugs. In Wetchler BV (ed): Outpatient Anesthesia, Vol 2, p 47. Philadelphia: JB Lippincott, 1988. Used with permission.

For surgical procedures of short duration in ambulatory patients, the ideal narcotic analgesic would have a rapid onset, a short duration of effect, a profound analgesic effect, and minimal side effects (e.g., nausea, vomiting, drowsiness, respiratory depression). Pharmacokinetic variables for the narcotic analgesics currently available for use in ambulatory surgery are presented in Table 5-23. Although longer-acting opioid analgesics (e.g., morphine and meperidine) have been used in ambulatory anesthesia, none is as advantageous as the more potent and shorter-acting narcotic analgesics fentanyl, sufentanil, and alfentanil.

Fentanyl

Fentanyl is a synthetic narcotic analgesic related to the phenylpiperidines. Although it is approximately 100 times as potent as morphine, a single dose of fentanyl administered intravenously has a more rapid onset and shorter duration of action. The pharmacokinetics and pharmacodynamics of fentanyl are very much influenced by its extreme lipid solubility, which readily facilitates its passage across the blood-brain barrier. Fentanyl has proven to be an excellent narcotic analgesic for use in ambulatory anesthesia. Onset of analgesia after intravenous administration is extremely rapid (1–3 min), and duration of analgesia after a single intravenous dose is a relatively short 45 minutes.[270] Intravenous doses of 1 to 2 µg/kg are recommended for the ambulatory surgery patient.

Several studies have demonstrated potential advantages in the use of fentanyl as a narcotic analgesic in ambulatory anesthesia. Hunt and coworkers compared the use of fentanyl (1.7 µg/kg) with halothane as adjuvants to nitrous oxide, oxygen anesthesia in patients undergoing dilatation and curettage.[271] Patients who received fentanyl reported less abdominal pain postoperatively. Pollard compared the clinical differences between an intravenous technique utilizing fentanyl and droperidol and an inhalational technique with isoflurane in surgical procedures lasting less than 30 minutes.[272] The fentanyl, droperidol group had a more rapid recovery to consciousness and orientation and less need for post-operative analgesics. In another study, Goroszenivk and coworkers demonstrated that fentanyl (1–3 μg/kg) decreased the incidence of involuntary movements and hiccoughing when added to a methohexital, nitrous oxide, oxygen anesthetic.[273] The incidence of tachycardia, tachypnea, and hyperventilation is also decreased when fentanyl is administered as part of a standard "balanced" anesthetic technique.

The use of fentanyl is not, however, without problems. A dose of 1.3 μg/kg resulted in depression of the CO_2 response slope comparable in magnitude and duration to that seen after 0.12 mg/kg morphine, with both responses remaining below 80% of control as long as 4 hours after injection.[274] There is also evidence of a recurrence of respiratory depression, accompanied by decreases in Pa_{O_2} and pH and an increase in Pa_{CO_2}. Respiratory depression occurred first at 30 to 60 minutes and again thereafter with wide individual variation. These delayed effects may be due to secretion of fentanyl into gastric juice and reabsorption from the small intestine or to the return of unchanged active fentanyl from peripheral compartments, such as muscle, when increased patient activity caused increased muscle blood flow. The clinician should be aware that somnolence, respiratory depression requiring ventilatory support, and respiratory arrest have occurred up to 4 hours after apparent recovery from fentanyl.[275] However, these respiratory depressant effects are unlikely to occur with the smaller doses (1–2 μg/kg) commonly used for the ambulatory surgery patient.

Truncal and extremity rigidity may occur after fentanyl administration and may be of sufficient severity to interfere with ventilation by bag and mask. Glottic rigidity and glottic closure have been reported to contribute to the inability to ventilate.[276] This problem also has been seen with other narcotic analgesics, including morphine, meperidine, sufentanil, and alfentanil. Rigidity is common with high-dose fentanyl inductions but rare with the lower doses (1–2 μg/kg) given to ambulatory surgery patients. Moderate-dose fentanyl (3.9 μg/kg), however, caused rigidity in 4% of patients undergoing minor gynecologic surgery.[277] For patients who will be intubated, increments of fentanyl may be given after a pretreatment dose of a nondepolarizing muscle relaxant (e.g., 3 mg d-tubocurarine) to minimize the possibility of rigidity. Rigidity also may be treated by small doses of a muscle relaxant such as pancuronium (1 mg) or succinylcholine (10–20 mg). Naloxone is also effective but is not recommended because it can reverse analgesia as well. Other side effects, such as bronchoconstriction and bradycardia, that have been reported with high-dose fentanyl are rarely seen in the ambulatory surgery patient who typically receives one to two μg/kg. We recommend that this dose be administered in 25- to 50-μg increments with 1 to 2 minutes between injections.

Naloxone has been used to reverse other side-effects of the narcotic analgesics, primarily respiratory depression. However, the use of naloxone has sequelae of its own. Analgesia may be terminated. Hypertension, pulmonary edema, ventricular arrhythmias, and cardiac arrest in healthy patients have been reported after naloxone (0.1–0.4 mg).[278] Accordingly, the routine prophylactic use of naloxone after fentanyl administration is not recommended.

Continuous infusion of fentanyl has been studied in ambulatory surgery patients. As expected, the infusion technique minimizes the "peaks and valleys" of plasma drug concentrations, decreasing the total amount of drug required and shortening recovery times. Another advantage of this technique over intermittent bolus injections is the reduction in postoperative side effects. In one study, after a 100-μg loading dose, a 2-μg/ml solution was administered at a rate of 0.1 μg/kg per minute rather than in intermittent 50-μg bolus increments. In this study, the use of such an infusion resulted in a 45% decrease in the total fentanyl dose for a 23-minute procedure. As predicted, with this lower dose, intraoperative motor and cardiovascular side-effects were less frequent and time to awakening decreased by 62%. Additionally, excessive postoperative sedation decreased from 48% to 4% and discharge times were decreased by nearly 30%.

Sufentanil

Sufentanil is a thiamyl analogue of fentanyl; it is the most potent opioid currently available for clinical use and is 5 to 10 times more potent than fentanyl. Theoretically, the greater potency and more rapid onset of action of sufentanil compared with fentanyl intensifies its specific opioid effects while reducing the likelihood and magnitude of side effects. The pharmacokinetics of sufentanil are similar to those of fentanyl, and most pharmacokinetic properties of fentanyl can be applied to sufentanil. The pharmacodynamics of sufentanil are also similar to those of fentanyl; the slightly shorter elimination half-life of sufentanil suggests a slightly shorter duration of action and hence the possibility of less residual postoperative depression.[279] The optimal preinduction dose of sufentanil for short outpatient procedures is 10 to 15 μg intravenously.[280] In one study using healthy human volunteers, Baily and coworkers compared the magnitude and duration of the effect of three equipotent doses of sufentanil and fentanyl on respiration and analgesia.[281] In all cases and at all doses, sufentanil (0.1, 0.2, and 0.4 μg/kg) produced shorter-lasting respiratory depression and longer-lasting analgesia than did fentanyl. Another study compared sufentanil and fentanyl as adjuncts to a thiopental, nitrous oxide, oxygen anesthetic in patients undergoing dilatation and curettage; a higher degree of postoperative analgesia was demonstrated by the sufentanil groups.[282] Two studies have suggested that when sufentanil (as part of a balanced anesthesia technique) was compared with isoflurane, awakening from anesthesia was more rapid in the opioid group.[283,284] In one of these studies, the use of sufentanil was associated with a lower postoperative analgesic requirement and a shorter PACU stay.[284] In the other study, patient discharge times were similar, but the sufentanil-treated group had a significantly higher incidence of nausea and vomiting (45%) than did the isoflurane-treated group (15%).

Alfentanil

Alfentanil is an analogue of fentanyl that is less potent (1/5 to 1/10), has a more rapid onset of action, and a much shorter duration of action than its parent compound.[285,286] The rapid onset of alfentanil is due to its low pK_a, so that 90% of the drug exists in its nonionized form at physiologic pH. The short duration of action of alfentanil is a result of both rapid redistribution to inactive tissue sites and rapid hepatic metabolism. Bovill and coworkers estimated that alfentanil had an extremely rapid redistribution half-life of 11.6 minutes, with an elimination half-life of 94 minutes, considerably shorter than that of fentanyl (219 min).[285] This shorter elimination half-life is the result of increased protein binding, lower lipid solubility, and a much smaller volume of distribution. Since alfentanil is readily available for metabolic clearance, prolongation of drug effect after large or repeated doses is less likely.[287] Unlike with fentanyl, no secondary increases in alfentanil plasma concentrations have been reported.

The small volume of distribution and short elimination half-life of alfentanil preclude significant accumulation of the drug in the body and make alfentanil a useful drug for continuous infusion.[288] The rapid onset (1–2 min) and rapid equilibration between the plasma concentration of alfentanil and its central nervous system receptors also make alfentanil an excellent drug for titration to response.[289] There is excellent correlation between plasma concentrations and central nervous system effect. Because alfentanil does not accumulate in the body and has a short elimination half-life, plasma concentrations can be rapidly altered by manipulating the infusion rate.

Coe and coworkers showed that the use of alfentanil by infusion rather than intermittent bolus resulted in a 33% decrease in total dose and a 15% decrease in time to ambulation with no significant difference in the incidence of respiratory depression or muscular rigidity.[290] In their study, a loading dose of 250 to 500 µg alfentanil was followed by the infusion of a 10-µg/ml solution at a rate of 0.6 to 1.1 µg/kg per minute.

Alfentanil has been used extensively in ambulatory anesthesia as an adjunct to thiopental, methohexital, etomidate, midazolam, propofol, and nitrous oxide without major sequelae. Coe and colleagues have suggested that alfentanil may be a clinically superior intravenous adjuvant for ambulatory general anesthesia.[290] Comparing fentanyl and alfentanil in patients who underwent termination of pregnancy, they found a higher incidence of chest wall rigidity and ventilatory depression in the fentanyl group, a higher incidence of mild bradycardia and moderate hypertension in the alfentanil group, and no significant difference in the incidence of nausea, vomiting, dizziness, or excessive sedation.

Although Kennedy and Ogg[291] detected impaired memory skills following alfentanil when compared with fentanyl, most investigators have noted shorter recovery times with alfentanil than with fentanyl.[292,293] Kay and Venkataraman compared recovery in ambulatory patients undergoing cystoscopy with fentanyl or alfentanil and found no significant difference in time to early recovery of consciousness.[291] However, in Maddox-Wing and digit substitution tests to assess later recovery, the patients who received alfentanil scored consistently better. Kallar and Keenan evaluated recovery time following alfentanil and fentanyl in 43 patients scheduled for termination of pregnancy.[293] The median time to establish alertness was significantly shorter for the alfentanil group (16 min) than for the fentanyl group (25 min). Additionally, the percentage of completely recovered alfentanil patients was significantly greater than the percentage of fentanyl patients at 20 and 30 minutes postoperatively; however, by one hour, PACU recovery scores indicating alertness were the same in both groups. White and coworkers compared recovery time in ambulatory surgery patients who received fentanyl bolus, fentanyl infusion, alfentanil bolus, and alfentanil infusion as an adjuvant to thiopental, nitrous oxide, oxygen anesthesia.[294] The patients who received alfentanil were awake, oriented, and able to walk significantly sooner than the fentanyl-treated patients (Table 5-24). In another study, Raeder and Hole suggested that surgery outpatients were more "functional" on the evening after operation if they had received alfentanil instead of fentanyl during surgery.[295]

When compared to patients treated with isoflurane, enflurane, or halothane, those treated with alfentanil recovered more rapidly after short outpatient arthroscopic, urologic, and gynecologic procedures.[296–298] Zelcer and coworkers recently compared alfentanil with fentanyl to determine which agent best blunted the hemodynamic response to laryngoscopy. They concluded that alfentanil and propofol anesthesia more effectively attenuated the cardiovascular response to laryngoscopy and intubation than fentanyl and propofol and was associated with a rapid recovery without adverse side-effects.[299]

The major disadvantages of alfentanil in ambulatory surgical anesthesia are similar to those of fentanyl and sufentanil (*i.e.*, emetic effects and the potential for producing laryngeal and chest wall rigidity).

Agonist/Antagonist

The limitations and side-effects of traditional opioid and synthetic narcotics have stimulated the search for improved analgesics with fewer undesirable side-effects.[300] From this search have come mixed agonist/antagonist agents, three of which may have clinical application in ambulatory anesthesia: pentazocine, butorphanol, and nalbuphine. A common characteristic of these drugs is a ceiling on the analgesia and respiratory depression produced with increasing doses; although this limits their value as anesthetic agents, it affords them greater safety as adjuvants in the outpatient setting. These drugs tend to produce less nausea and vomiting in patients with a history of emesis after other narcotics, but analgesic-producing doses of these drugs often result in excessive sedation, thereby severely limiting their effectiveness in ambulatory anesthesia.

Pentazocine (20–30 mg) is equipotent to morphine (10 mg). At higher doses, dysphoria and psychotomimetic effects are intolerable to most patients. Pentazocine antagonizes the analgesia of opioid narcotics that might be administered later. It should be avoided in patients with a history of coronary artery disease because of its tendency to raise heart rate and systemic, pulmonary artery, and left ventricular end-diastolic pressures, as well as cardiac work and presumably cardiac oxygen utilization.

Butorphanol is more potent with fewer psychotomimetic and cardiodepressive effects than pentazocine. Butorphanol (2–3 mg) is equipotent to morphine (10 mg). Fine and Finestone compared discharge time from the PACU and incidence of postoperative sedation in a series of outpatients undergoing cystoscopy who had received fentanyl (3 µg/kg), butorphanol (60 µg/kg), or nalbuphine (300 µg/kg).[301] Fentanyl-treated patients had the shortest time to awakening with no admissions to the hospital; one patient in the nalbuphine-treated group and

TABLE 5-24. Postoperative Recovery Times and Side Effects after the Use of Either Fentanyl or Alfentanil as an Adjuvant to Nitrous Oxide

Groups	Recovery Times (min)*				Side-Effects (%)			
	Awake	Oriented	Ambulatory		Nausea	Vomiting	Dizziness	Drowsiness
Fentanyl bolus (FB)	5.2 ± 0.9	7.7 ± 1.1	67 ± 5		60	48	52	36
Fentanyl infusion (FI)	$3.7 \pm 0.8^{\dagger}$	6.1 ± 1.2	55 ± 5		68	60	24	28
Alfentanil bolus (AB)	$2.5 \pm 0.3^{\ddagger}$	$3.5 \pm 0.4^{\ddagger}$	$48 \pm 4^{\ddagger}$		52	36	24	16
Alfentanil infusion (AI)	$1.2 \pm 0.1^{\dagger,\ddagger}$	$2.6 \pm 0.3^{\dagger,\ddagger}$	$41 \pm 3^{\dagger,\ddagger}$		68	60	28	$8^{\ddagger}$

*Mean values $\pm$ SEM.
†AI or FI group significantly different from AB or FB group ($p<0.05$), respectively.
‡AB or AI group significantly different from FB or FI group ($p<0.05$), respectively.
SOURCE: From White et al.[294] Used with permission.

three patients in the butorphanol-treated group required admission to the hospital because of excessive postoperative sedation. In another study, Wetchler and coworkers examined recovery parameters in patients who had received preinduction intravenous doses of butorphanol (20–40 µg/kg) or fentanyl (2 µg/kg).[302] Although butorphanol (20 µg/kg) appeared to be as suitable as fentanyl (2 µg/kg) for use as a preinduction intravenous narcotic adjuvant, patients treated with butorphanol (40 µg/kg) experienced a higher incidence and duration of nausea and dizziness, as well as a significantly prolonged time to discharge from the PACU.

Nalbuphine is structurally related to the mu agonist oxymorphone and the antagonist naloxone. It provides its analgesic effect at the kappa receptor as well as the mu receptor. It is equipotent to morphine sulfate at analgesic doses (10 mg) and has a similar onset, peak, and duration of action. However, like all other agonist/antagonists, nalbuphine demonstrates a ceiling effect on analgesia and respiratory depression at higher doses. Since it has virtually no effect at the sigma receptor, nalbuphine produces far fewer psychotomimetic side effects than other agonist/antagonist drugs.

Garfield and coworkers recently compared nalbuphine (300 and 500 µg/kg) with fentanyl (1.5 µg/kg) as adjunctive analgesics to a thiopental, nitrous oxide, oxygen anesthetic in patients undergoing outpatient gynecologic procedures. They found a significantly longer recovery phase for both the nalbuphine-treated groups and a higher incidence of postoperative anxiety in the group treated with the higher nalbuphine dose.[303] In response to specifically directed questions, nearly 40% of the nalbuphine-treated patients reported "bad" dreams during their perioperative experience. Although this side-effect deserves further investigation, it clearly limits the effectiveness of nalbuphine in the ambulatory surgery patient.

Narcotics by Alternate Delivery Systems
Because of its high tissue solubility and potency, fentanyl may be suitable for alternate delivery systems. Fentanyl's stability, resistance to heat, and high solubility in various chemical matrices suggest that it could be incorporated into a nonthreatening, psychologically appealing delivery system. At the present time, both candy lollipops and transdermal patches are under investigation as possible delivery devices.[304–306] Wetchler also has completed a study that examines the possible administration of transnasal butorphanol for postoperative pain relief in ambulatory surgery patients.*

Neuromuscular Blocking Agents
General anesthesia has been defined as the triad of amnesia, analgesia, and muscle relaxation. Deep levels of anesthesia with diethyl ether provided all components of the triad without compromising patient safety. Unfortunately, modern inhalational anesthetics do not provide profound muscle relaxation unless dangerously high and potentially toxic concentrations are administered. The intro-

*Wetchler BV: Personal communication, 1989.

duction of muscle relaxants to clinical anesthesia has revolutionized the practice of general anesthesia. Intravenous muscle relaxants now permit optimal surgical conditions to be achieved with smaller doses of intravenous sedative-hypnotic agents and analgesics and with lower concentrations of inhalational agents than might otherwise be required. Since the patient can be maintained at lighter levels of general anesthesia, more rapid recovery to the preanesthetic state can occur, and theoretically, fewer drug-induced side effects will be observed. This phenomenon is extremely important in the ambulatory anesthesia arena where rapid, clearheaded emergence results in earlier patient discharge from the facility.[307]

Many short outpatient operations require no neuromuscular blocking agents, others may require an ultrashort-acting agent only to facilitate endotracheal intubation, and still other procedures may require a neuromuscular blocking agent to provide profound muscle relaxation during an entire operation. Although the ideal muscle relaxant for ambulatory surgery has yet to be discovered, many clinicians would agree with its clinical profile as summarized in Table 5-25. Except for extraordinarily unusual circumstances, the long-acting neuromuscular blocking agents are inappropriate for use in the surgery outpatient; the balance of this section will discuss the pharmacology and clinical use of succinylcholine, atracurium, vecuronium, and mivacurium in ambulatory anesthesia.

Succinylcholine

Succinylcholine is a depolarizing muscle relaxant that has a rapid onset and a short duration of action. It may be used as a bolus to facilitate endotracheal intubation or as an infusion to provide a short period of profound muscle relaxation during the surgical procedure. The short duration of action of succinylcholine is related to its rapid breakdown by plasma cholinesterase. Some patients may be receiving anticholinesterase drugs (i.e., for the treatment of glaucoma), which can decrease the activity of pseudocholinesterase and thereby prolong the action of succinylcholine. Organophosphate insecticides have this same effect. There is also a genetic variant that produces an atypical form of the cholinesterase enzyme. This atypical enzyme hydrolyzes succinylcholine and other esters (e.g., local anesthetics) at markedly reduced rates. Patients with decreased pseudocholinesterase activity may have prolonged paralysis after receiving succinyl-

TABLE 5-25. Characteristics of the Ideal Neuromuscular Blocking Agent
for Use in Ambulatory Surgery

Nondepolarizing mechanics of action

Rapid, predictable onset of action

Short, predictable duration of action

Rapid, predictable recovery

Spontaneous degradation to inactive, nontoxic metabolites

Noncumulative action

No side effects

Easy, predictable reversibility

choline. Consequently, the anesthesiologist must exercise extreme caution when administering this drug to any patient who gives a personal or family history of suspicious respiratory problems during anesthesia or in the PACU. Should prolonged succinylcholine apnea occur, ventilatory support must be provided until the effects of the drug have dissipated. However, unless sedation is also provided, the paralyzed patient will be awake and aware of the problem.

For the healthy ambulatory surgery patient, the occurrence of postoperative skeletal muscle aches and pains is a significant drawback to the use of succinylcholine. Myalgia may occur up to the fourth postoperative day and may be more painful than the surgery itself. Churchill-Davidson first drew attention to the muscle pains experienced by patients following the administration of succinylcholine in 1954.[308] Pain is most frequently reported in the neck and shoulder muscles and may be mild to severe. Churchill-Davidson found the incidence and severity of myalgia significantly greater in outpatients (66%) than in inpatients (13.9%).

Myalgia has been associated with the fasciculations seen after succinylcholine administration.[308–310] These contractions of the muscle fiber of a motor unit can be explained by prejunctional activation of the motor nerve by succinylcholine. Despite the association between myalgia and fasciculations, there is no correlation between the development of postoperative pain and the intensity of the fasciculations. In fact, postoperative myalgia can occur in patients receiving succinylcholine who do not exhibit fasciculation. Myalgia often develops or worsens after discharge from the ambulatory surgery facility.[309]

Pretreatment with a variety of drugs has been reported to lessen and even eliminate myalgia following succinylcholine (Tables 5-26 and 5-27). Perry and Wetchler evaluated the effects of varying pretreatment regimens on outpatients undergoing short oral surgery procedures.[311] Regardless of which method of pretreatment was used, moderate to severe complaints of myalgia were never less than 8% (d-tubocurarine pretreatment) in any group. These investigators also noted that the optimum time for succinylcholine administration following d-tubocurarine pretreatment was 2 minutes. Other investigators have suggested that gallamine (20 mg) or metocurine (1 mg) also may be useful as pretreatment to minimize postoperative myalgia; pancuronium seems to decrease fasciculations but not prevent myalgia.[312,313] Sosis and coworkers have recently shown that d-tubocurarine is a more effective defasciculant than atracurium, but postanesthesia myalgia was significantly less in those patients pretreated with atracurium (0.025 mg/kg).[314] In the healthy outpatient undergoing an elective surgical procedure, onset time of skeletal muscle relaxation is usually less important than minimizing postoperative muscle pain. Consequently, nondepolarizing muscle relaxants are given routinely in many centers prior to succinylcholine to decrease the incidence of fasciculation and postoperative myalgia[315] or have become the relaxants of choice for procedures lasting longer than 20 to 25 minutes.

Other pretreatment techniques have been evaluated. Fahmy and colleagues reported that pretreatment with 0.05 mg/kg diazepam was superior to pretreatment with d-tubocurarine in preventing postsuccinylcholine myalgia.[316] Other investigators have not found diazepam useful.[317] Baraka reported on pretreat-

TABLE 5-26. The Incidence and Severity of Fasciculations

N = 25/Group*	0	+1	+2	+3
Diazepam, 0.05 mg/kg, followed by SCh in 5 minutes	3	7	9	6
dTc, 0.05 mg/kg, followed by SCh in 5 minutes	22	3	0	0
dTc, 0.05 mg/kg, followed by SCh when "eyelids heavy"	13	5	2	5
SCh, 1.5 mg/kg	1	5	9	10
SCh "self-taming"	1	9	8	7
Calcium gluconate, 1000 mg, followed by SCh in 1 minute	4	4	6	11

*0, no fasciculation; +1, fine movement of face and fingers; +2, medium movement of face, fingers, and chest muscles; +3, coarse movement of face, fingers, toes, chest, and abdominal muscles; SCh, succinylcholine; dTc, d-tubocurarine.

ment with a small dose (10 mg) of succinylcholine itself; he found that this "self-taming" dose reduced the incidence of muscle pains.[318] However, other investigators found that although the incidence and severity of fasciculations were decreased by a pretreatment dose of succinylcholine, it had no effect on postoperative myalgia.[319,320] Shrivastava and coworkers administered 10 ml 10% calcium gluconate prior to the administration of succinylcholine and reported a significant decrease in the incidence of postoperative myalgia.[321] Administering succinylcholine by infusion (0.1%) rather than as a 1-mg/kg bolus has been shown to reduce the incidence of myalgia from 68% to 30%.[309]

Succinylcholine usage also has been associated with a transient rise in serum potassium level and occasionally with signs of muscle injury such as a rise in serum creatine phosphokinase level and myoglobinemia. Other side-effects include postoperative sore throat and hoarseness, even in the absence of endotracheal intubation.[309]

Despite the many potential problems associated with the use of succinylcho-

TABLE 5-27. The Incidence and Severity of Postanesthesia Myalgia

N = 25/Group*	None	Slight	Moderate or Severe	Severe (%)
Diazepam, 0.05 mg/kg, followed in 5 minutes by SCh	15	1	9	36%
dTc, 0.05 mg/kg, followed in 5 minutes by SCh	21	2	2	8%
dTc, 0.05 mg/kg, followed by SCh when "eyelids heavy"	21	2	2	8%
SCh, 1.5 mg/kg	17	2	6	25%
SCh "Self-taming"	13	5	7	28%
Calcium gluconate, 1000 mg, followed by SCh in 1 minute	9	7	9	36%

*SCh = succinylcholine; dTc = d-tubocurarine.

TABLE 5-28. Side-Effects Associated with Succinylcholine

Postanesthesia myalgia

Hyperkalemia

Cardiac dysrhythmias

Increased intragastric pressure

Increased intraocular pressure

Phase II block

Prolonged apnea with abnormal pseudocholinesterase

Tachyphylaxis with continuous infusion

Triggering agent for malignant hyperpyrexia

SOURCE: Fragen RJ, Shanks CA: Is there an ideal outpatient muscle relaxant? In Wetchler BV (ed): Outpatient Anesthesia, Vol 2, p 71. Philadelphia: JB Lippincott, 1988. Used with permission.

line (Table 5-28), it remains the muscle relaxant most frequently used in the care of the ambulatory surgery patient. Unfortunately, its use leaves much to be desired.

Atracurium

Atracurium is an interesting example of molecular engineering.[322] It is the result of a deliberate attempt to create a water-soluble neuromuscular blocking agent that undergoes spontaneous metabolism in the human body. This process of spontaneous degradation at body pH and temperature is called *Hofmann elimination* and is only one of the three methods of atracurium inactivation. The other two methods of atracurium degradation are *ester hydrolysis* and *organ elimination*.[323] The relative dominance of each pathway in humans is unknown. The metabolites of atracurium are devoid of neuromuscular blocking activity and hemodynamic effects in the clinical dose range. Extremely high concentrations of its main metabolite, laudanosine, are thought to produce central nervous system toxicity in animals; however, it is important to note that no such toxicity has been demonstrated in humans.[324] Atracurium should be refrigerated to prevent spontaneous degradation from occurring, although it can be stored at operating room temperature for up to 14 days without significant loss of potency.

Basta and coworkers reported that a 2.0-mg/kg dose of atracurium produced 95% neuromuscular blockade with an onset time of 4 minutes, spontaneous recovery to 95% of control of first twitch height in 44 minutes, and a recovery index (return from 25% to 75% of control of first twitch height) of 12 minutes.[325] Stirt and coworkers considered atracurium an acceptable alternative to succinylcholine when speed of intubation was not critical.[326] Intubating conditions were compared at 2.5 minutes following administration of atracurium (0.4 or 0.5 mg/kg) and 1 minute after succinylcholine (1 mg/kg). Excellent or good intubating conditions were noted in 67% of patients who received 0.4 mg/kg and 90% of patients who received 0.5 mg/kg atracurium compared to 100% of those patients who received succinylcholine. Patients who received 0.5 mg/kg atracurium compared favorably to the succinylcholine group with regard to the level of neuromuscular blockade, but speed of onset was four times faster in the succinyl-choline group. Although the recommended intubating dose of 0.4 to 0.5 mg/kg produces intubating conditions more rapidly (2.5–3.0 min), atracurium's duration of action (50–70 min for 95% spontaneous recovery) may be too long for some shorter ambulatory surgical procedures. However, when an even longer period of muscle relaxation is desired, atracurium may be administered by a continuous infusion beginning at a rate of 6 μg/kg per minute.[327] As with all continuous intravenous drug infusions in ambulatory anesthesia, atracurium should be titrated to clinical effect, that is, to maintain neuromuscular blockade at a 90% to 95% level.

In contrast to the longer-acting nondepolarizing neuromuscular blocking agents, once recovery has begun after atracurium, the recovery index appears to be independent of the administered dose. With repeated doses, there appears to be little or no cumulative effect. Atracurium is particularly advantageous for use in patients with renal or hepatic compromise because its metabolism proceeds independently of both organ systems. It is, however, important to remember that all factors that classically prolong the effect of nondepolarizing neuromuscular blocking agents (e.g., hypothermia, acidosis, and concurrent administration of potent inhalational anesthetics) will similarly affect the duration of action of atracurium.

The volatile anesthetics potentiate atracurium (20%) as well as vecuronium (20%–40%). Enflurane (1.25 MAC) potentiates both these muscle relaxants more than do either halothane or isoflurane.[328,329]

In an effort to shorten the time between initial administration of atracurium and intubation of the trachea, some individuals have suggested increasing the initial atracurium dose. An ED_{95} dose of atracurium produces essentially no cardiovascular effects, but rapid bolus doses in excess of 0.5 to 0.6 mg/kg should be avoided because they have been associated with histamine release and subsequent hypotension. These effects can be minimized by giving the bolus slowly[330] and virtually eliminated by not exceeding an ED_{95} dose.

An alternate method for shortening the time to intubation after atracurium injection involves the application of the *priming principle*.[331] This technique consists of a subclinical priming dose of atracurium (0.05–0.075 mg/kg) followed in approximately 2.5 minutes by the induction dose of anesthetic and immediately thereafter by a second dose of atracurium (0.25–0.3 mg/kg). Adequate intubating conditions are usually achieved in 70 to 120 seconds. Wetchler and Perry studied 25 patients and found excellent (22) to good (3) intubating conditions with a pretreatment atracurium dose of 0.075 mg/kg followed by 0.3 mg/kg in 2.5 minutes. Intubation was performed 2 minutes after the 0.3-mg/kg dose.[332] Interestingly, no patient in the atracurium group complained of postoperative myalgia. Whenever using the priming principle, it is important to remember that there is considerable patient variability and sensitivity to the priming dose.[333] The longer one waits after the priming dose, the more likely symptoms of muscle weakness will occur. These symptoms include diplopia, difficulty in swallowing, difficulty in speaking, and even difficulty in breathing. Patients should be warned in advance that they may experience these symptoms just prior to the induction of general anesthesia.

Vecuronium

Vecuronium is a monoquaternary analogue of pancuronium. This simple change in the molecular structure increases its lipid solubility and substantially decreases (95%) its vagolytic properties. Vecuronium has a high specificity for the neuromuscular junction, is virtually devoid of sympathetic and vagal blocking effects, and does not release histamine. The virtual absence of autonomic side effects, although usually advantageous, has led to vecuronium's association with bradycardia and asystole in situations in which vagotonic, beta-blocking, or calcium channel-blocking drugs are given without opposition.[334] Vecuronium is unique among depolarizing neuromuscular blocking agents in its dependence on hepatic metabolism.[335] Patients with a moderate to severe degree of hepatic dysfunction generally display prolongation of drug effect.[336] Vecuronium is unstable in solution and is supplied as a lyophilized powder that must be dissolved in sterile water before use. Unused vecuronium should be discarded within 24 hours of reconstitution.

Krieg and coworkers reported that administration of vecuronium in a dose equal to its ED_{95} (0.05 mg/kg) resulted in an onset time of approximately 4 minutes.[337] Lennon and colleagues suggested that giving doses three or five times the ED_{95} shortened onset time to 2.8 and 1.1 minutes, respectively.[338] Other than prolongation of neuromuscular blockade, vecuronium has no clinically important side-effects in doses up to six times its ED_{95}.[339] Unfortunately, prolongation of neuromuscular blockade generally prohibits the use of high doses (greater than two times the ED_{95}) of vecuronium in the ambulatory surgery facility. As with atracurium, the time to intubation of the trachea after administration of vecuronium can be shortened. A subclinical priming dose of vecuronium (0.01–0.015 mg/kg) should be followed in approximately 2.5 minutes by the induction of general anesthesia and immediately thereafter by the larger dose of vecuronium (0.04–0.05 mg/kg). For longer ambulatory procedures, vecuronium may be administered by continuous infusion, initiated at a rate of 1 µg/kg per minute and titrated to clinical effect in order to maintain a 90% to 95% neuromuscular blockade.

Zahl and Apfelbaum examined the occurrence, location, and severity of postoperative myalgia when vecuronium was used in lieu of succinylcholine during laparoscopy.[340] Surprisingly, data analysis failed to demonstrate that the substitution of vecuronium for succinylcholine lowered the incidence or severity of postoperative myalgia. Laparoscopy without the use of any muscle relaxant (i.e., local anesthesia) carries with it a relatively high incidence of postoperative myalgia.

Mivacurium

Mivacurium is a short-acting nondepolarizing bis-benzylisoquinolinium muscle relaxant that has been under clinical investigation since 1985. It undergoes rapid hydrolysis by plasma cholinesterase at approximately 90% of the rate of succinylcholine hydrolysis.[341] The vast majority of mivacurium is hydrolized to inactive metabolites. The ED_{95} dose of 0.1 mg/kg produces maximum blockade in approximately 4 minutes with sponataneous recovery to 95% of control of the first twitch height in approximately 25 minutes. The recommended dose of 0.2 to 0.25

mg/kg for intubation shortens time to maximum blockade to approximately 2 minutes; spontaneous recovery to 95% of control of the first twitch height takes approximately 30 minutes.[342] The recovery index of mivacurium is stable at 6.6 to 7.0 minutes over the dose range of 0.1 to 0.25 mg/kg. Intubation doses of mivacurium have approximately twice the duration of doses of succinylcholine and approximately half those of atracurium or vecuronium.[343] Recovery from mivacurium seems more predictable and shorter than recovery from succinylcholine when infusions over similar periods are compared and similar depression of neuromuscular blockade is maintained.[343] Ali and coworkers have suggested that continuous infusion of mivacurium may be especially useful where rapid spontaneous recovery from neuromuscular blockade at the end of surgery is desirable. Continuous infusion of mivacurium should be initiated at a rate of 10.0 μg/kg per minute and adjusted to maintain 90% to 95% twitch suppression.

A potential disadvantage of mivacurium is its weak histamine-releasing properties. These can be minimized by avoiding overdosages and administering bolus doses very slowly (75–90 s).

Org 9426*
Org 9426 (under clinical investigation since 1989) is an intermediate–acting (similar to vecuronium in length of action), nondepolarizing monoquaternary compound. The ED_{95} dose (0.3 mg/kg) produces maximum blockade more rapidly than vecuronium. There is a virtual absence of autonomic side effects and no release of histamine. Org 9426 is stable in solution and is supplied in liquid form.

COMMON QUESTIONS ABOUT AMBULATORY ANESTHESIA
1. Does any one general anesthetic agent or technique dominate the subspecialty of ambulatory anesthesia?
Currently, no agent or technique allows us to provide ideal anesthetic conditions for ambulatory surgery. Unless special circumstances require or exclude a specific technique, many anesthesiologists combine the advantages of several types of drugs (intravenous induction agents, narcotics, potent inhaled agents, N_2O); this approach typically requires smaller amounts of each agent.

2. Can potent inhaled agents be used during termination of pregnancy?
During termination of pregnancy procedures, greater blood loss has been associated with the use of potent inhalational agents than with N_2O, narcotic-based techniques.[344,345] Collins and coworkers compared a halothane technique with an intravenous alfentanil technique in 66 unpremedicated patients and found a mean blood loss that was nearly 2½ times greater in the halothane group (213 vs. 90 ml).[346] However, Sidhu and Cullen have suggested that length of procedure and concentration of inhalational agent affect blood loss more than specific choice of inhalational agent; they compared low-dose enflurane (1.0% inspired)

*David Savage Memorial Interface Symposium, London, 1990.

plus 66% N_2O in oxygen with fentanyl plus 66% N_2O in oxygen and were unable to demonstrate a greater blood loss with the inhalational agent.[347]

3. Do noninhalational inductions affect recovery time?

In one study using cases with similar maintenance techniques, Hannington-Kiff[348] found that when compared with halothane, thiopental or methohexital induction prolonged recovery of extraocular muscle balance (a sign of "street fitness"[4]). Other investigators have reported similar prolongations of recovery in children after induction with rectal methohexital[349] and ketamine.[350]

4. Does choice of potent inhalational agent affect recovery time?

Several investigators have performed recovery comparisons after enflurane and halothane techniques on patients undergoing ambulatory surgical procedures; their work strongly suggests that recovery is faster after enflurane.[351-353] Based on its low blood-gas partition coefficient, we might predict that awakening from isoflurane would be even more rapid than awakening from enflurane; however, Azar and coworkers have shown that awakening times are not significantly different in patients who have undergone short ambulatory procedures with these agents.[354] Interestingly, Korttila and Valanne have demonstrated that lengthy enflurane anesthesia (longer than 90 min) was associated with significantly slower recovery than shorter enflurane anesthesia (less than 40 min).[355] With isoflurane, the rapidity of recovery did not depend on the duration of anesthesia. This work strongly suggests that isoflurane may be the inhalational anesthetic of choice when compared with enflurane in patients undergoing ambulatory procedures lasting longer than 90 minutes.

5. Do outpatients recover to "street fitness" faster after a balanced anesthetic or an inhaled anesthetic?

In 1977, Enright and Pace-Floridia reported that patients who had received potent inhalational agents for ambulatory surgery were more alert during the early recovery period than patients who had received opioid analgesics as part of a balanced technique.[356] Simpson and coworkers evaluated recovery of mental efficiency in patients receiving either halothane or a balanced technique with fentanyl as a narcotic for short-stay procedures; they reported that patients receiving a balanced technique had higher performance scores initially, but after six hours postoperatively, the differences in "mental efficiency" were negligible.[357] Recently, multiple investigators have compared recovery from fentanyl,[358,359] alfentanil,[296] and sufentanil[283] anesthetics in patients undergoing ambulatory surgery. Although many of these techniques provided satisfactory intraoperative conditions, incidence of nausea and vomiting increased approximately 300% in the narcotic-based group (3.3%–15% isoflurane versus 36%–57% narcotic). Gaskey and coworkers have suggested that the incidence of nausea and vomiting after ambulatory surgery for gynecologic procedures rises directly in proportion to the amount of narcotic administered perioperatively.[360] Nausea and vomiting presently constitute the number one postoperative side-effect in ambulatory surgery departments in the United States; although generally considered only a minor side effect of anesthesia, these symptoms can be stressful and even disabling. Several investigators have suggested that nausea and vomiting can significantly delay recovery to "street fitness,"[358–360] and many advocate reserving the use of narcotic-based anesthetic techniques in ambulatory surgery for those patients who may require postoperative intravenous analgesics.

CONSCIOUS SEDATION TECHNIQUE

Regional, local, or topical anesthesia alone does not block the cardiovascular, biochemical, and hormonal responses to the stress of surgery,[361] nor does it in any way mitigate the very real psychological stresses and aftereffects of an operation or of the anesthetic itself.[362] In many cases, local anesthesia is inadequate because of patient anxiety, poor tolerance of discomfort, poor impulse control, immaturity, mental or emotional retardation, or neurotic disorders. These patients need some degree of sedation or anxiolysis in addition to analgesia.

Since many patients undergoing surgery with regional anesthesia prefer to be asleep or sedated and to have no recollection of the procedure, a variety of adjuncts to local anesthetic techniques have been recommended. These range from a combination of sedatives and analgesics,[363] to subanesthetic infusions of anesthetic agents,[364] to an approach of distraction. Thus there is a recognized need to optimize sedation during regional anesthesia to achieve amnesia and to minimize physiological insult.

Ambulatory anesthesia is not limited to ASA physical status 1 or 2 patients; an increasing number of physical status 3 and elderly patients are presenting for surgery. Some of these patients are unsuitable for outpatient general anesthesia, but surgery can often be performed by supplementing local or regional anesthesia with a combination of hypnotics and analgesics in subanesthetic doses, a technique called *conscious sedation*. The technique is also useful in relieving anxiety during the surgical procedure and enables the patient to remain comfortable on the operating table during long procedures.[365]

Drug selection and dosage to achieve conscious sedation was first addressed by dentists and oral surgeons. Shane described his "intravenous amnesia" technique for ambulatory dental patients in 1966; he used a combination of a narcotic (alphaprodine), an anticholinergic (atropine), an ataractic (hydroxyzine), and a barbiturate (methohexital), all in low incremental doses, with preoperative and intraoperative suggestion.[366] Bennett appears to have been the first to use the phrase *conscious sedation* to describe the use of IV agents to produce a minimally depressed state of consciousness to supplement regional and local anesthesia while maintaining the patient's protective reflexes intact.[367] Since that time, numerous regimens have appeared in the medical and dental literature[368–372] with various combinations of the same drug classes. Bennett[373] and Shane[374] have both written small monographs on conscious sedation and its application to a wide range of patient-management problems in all areas of surgery.

TABLE 5-29. Definitions Proposed by the American Dental Association Council on Dental Education

Analgesia	Diminution or elimination of pain in the conscious patient
Local anesthesia	Elimination of sensations, especially pain, in one part of the body by the topical application or regional injection of a drug
Conscious sedation	Minimally depressed level of consciousness that retains the patient's ability to independently and continuously maintain an airway and respond appropriately to physical stimulation and verbal command, produced by a pharmacologic or nonpharmacologic method, or a combination
General anesthesia (includes deep sedation)	Controlled state of depressed consciousness or unconsciousness, accompanied by partial or complete loss of protective reflexes, including the ability to independently maintain an airway and respond purposefully to physical stimulation or verbal command, produced by a pharmacologic or nonpharmacologic method, or a combination

SOURCE: McCarthy FM et al.[375] Used with permission.

Definitions and Objectives

Definitions of *conscious sedation* and related terms, as proposed by the American Dental Association Council on Dental Education,[375] are listed in Table 5-29. Under conscious sedation, a patient is capable of rational response to commands and is able to maintain airway patency, two necessary criteria. As McCarthy and coworkers have pointed out that since conscious sedation clearly lies on a dose-dependent continuum leading to deep general anesthesia, the critical factor is that cardiac, respiratory, and reflex functions are not altered to the extent of requiring external support.[375] The objectives of conscious sedation have been outlined by Scamman and coworkers as follows[376]:

1. *Maintain adequate sedation with minimal risk.* The patient's ability to communicate verbally is preserved, usual monitoring is employed, and emergency resuscitation equipment is on hand.
2. *Relieve anxiety and produce amnesia.* These objectives are accomplished by means of good preoperative communication and instruction and low levels of visual and auditory stimuli (including concealed instruments and minimal conversation) in the operating room and by keeping the patient warm and covered (preserving the patient's modesty).
3. *Provide relief from pain and other noxious stimuli.* Narcotics are given to supplement local or topical anesthetics and to block pain sensations remote from the operative site.

Conscious sedation is compared with general anesthetic techniques in Table 5-30.

TABLE 5-30. Conscious Sedation versus Unconscious Anesthetic Techniques

Conscious Sedation	Unconscious Techniques (Deep Sedation, General Anesthesia)
Mood altered	Patient unconscious
Patient conscious	Patient unconscious
Patient cooperative	No patient cooperation
Protective reflexes active and intact	Protective reflexes obtunded: Airway may become obstructed Respiratory: hypoxia/hypercapnia Cardiovascular: hypotension or hypertension; bradycardia or tachycardia
Vital signs stable	Vital signs labile
Analgesia may be present	Pain eliminated centrally
Regional analgesia usually required	Regional analgesia not required
Amnesia may be present	Amnesia always present
Prolonged detainment in recovery room not required	Prolonged detainment in recovery room or hospital admission required
Risk of complications very low	Risk of complications high
Postoperative complications infrequent	Postoperative complications not infrequent
Extremely difficult or mentally handicapped patient cannot always be managed	May be only method by which extremely difficult or mentally handicapped patient can be managed

SOURCE: Adapted from Bennett CR.[373] Used with permission.

Patient Selection

The technique must be suited to the individual patient and to the individual surgeon as well as to the specific surgical procedure. While experienced surgeons readily perform laparoscopic tubal sterilizations or breast biopsies using local infiltration anesthesia with conscious sedation, surgical residents are rarely able to perform similar procedures without a general anesthetic. Similarly, an intelligent, mature adult who has been given a thorough explanation of the planned anesthetic, the rationale behind it, and the advantages of it will often readily accept conscious sedation. An uninformed, anxious patient who is facing the stress of surgery and is filled with fear of pain and complications will more frequently choose to be "all the way out."

Monitoring

Because the level of awareness or consciousness is an essential aspect of the technique of conscious sedation, it is also the primary focus of monitoring during surgery. Shane described the importance of establishing "vocal rapport" with the patient prior to the beginning of the surgical procedure.[374] This allows the anesthesiologist to motivate the patient, partially disinhibited by medication, to cooperate during the procedure. An important factor for the success of the conscious sedation technique, this rapport allows the anesthesiologist to take advantage of the patient's distorted time sense and disrupted short-term memory to structure the perception of the surgical procedure. By eliminating the "shock effect" of stimulating events during the procedure, such as the injection of local anesthetic, the insertion of a laparoscope, or the inflation of a tourniquet, the procedure can be made to seem shorter and less stressful. Any expected event is less stimulating than the same event coming as a surprise.

The responsiveness or level of awareness of a patient can best be evaluated by the patient's ability to obey frequent simple commands (e.g., "Take a deep breath") that do not require a verbal response. Speech has been shown to raise the patient's blood pressure by as much as 10% over the baseline.[377] It seems likely that speech also would require a higher general level of arousal than a mere nod or finger movement or the passive obeying of a command. Noninvasive monitoring techniques allow objective measurement of the adequacy of oxygenation and ventilation in patients ventilating spontaneously.

Drug Combinations

Supplemental agents commonly used for conscious sedation include sedative-hypnotics, opioids, and inhalational agents (Table 5-31). Important pharmacokinetic properties of drugs used for conscious sedation include a high clearance rate and a short elimination half-life. This allows blood concentration, and therefore clinical responses, to be altered quickly and minimizes the problem of drug accumulation during surgery and prolonged postoperative recovery.

The newer sedative-hypnotics and analgesics with these properties are midazolam, propofol, and alfentanil. Midazolam is a water-soluble benzodiazepine with rapid onset of action that produces profound sedation, amnesia, and anxiolysis. It causes less pain on injection and less venoirritation than diazepam. Flumazenil (5–15 μg/kg) rapidly and effectively reverses residual sedation and amnesia produced by midazolam.

TABLE 5-31. Supplemental Agents

Sedative-hypnotics:
  Diazepam
  Midazolam
  Thiopental
  Methohexital
  Ketamine
  Propofol
Opioids:
  Fentanyl
  Alfentanil
  Sufentanil
Inhalational agents:
  Nitrous oxide
  Enflurane
  Isoflurane

Propofol is a sedative-hypnotic with a rapid onset and short duration that allows for rapid recovery. Incidence of nausea and vomiting is decreased and a clear-headed postoperative state is common after propofol. Alfentanil is an opioid analgesic that has a very rapid onset of action, allows for rapid recovery, and produces a clear-headed recovery state. The respiratory depression with alfentanil is of short duration compared to that with fentanyl.

Because of the rapid onset of action of these three drugs, the dose should be titrated carefully. With older patients, patients with preexisting hepatic, renal, or cardiac disease, or patients taking other medications, doses should be reduced.

When a benzodiazepine is supplemented with a narcotic analgesic, there is a significant improvement in patient cooperation during the procedure and more profound sedation than with a benzodiazepine alone.[378] In a recent study, Boldy and coworkers compared midazolam with diazepam and pethidine for sedation during endoscopy and found that although midazolam produced better amnesia for the procedure, diazepam and pethidine resulted in less postoperative sedation.[379] The use of potent opioid analgesics (e.g., fentanyl and alfentanil), however, can cause significant hypoxemia in healthy ambulatory patients when administered in combination with midazolam or diazepam; therefore, pulse oximetry and supplemental oxygen are recommended.[380]

Techniques
Different methods of conscious sedation include subanesthetic administration of intermittent boluses of anesthetic agents (supplemental drugs), subanesthetic infusion of anesthetic agents, and subanesthetic inhalation of anesthetic agents.

Subanesthetic Administration of Intermittent Intravenous Boluses
According to Shane, "Conscious sedation is an art not easily learned."[374] The following outline of conscious sedation for a specific procedure (dilatation and evacuation for elective termination of pregnancy) is given as an illustrative example.

The patient is interviewed, examined, and given a thorough step-by-step description of the anesthetic, the operative procedure, and the recovery period. In the operating room, monitors (ECG, blood pressure, precordial stethoscope, oximeter sensor) are applied. Each device and procedure is explained to the patient. A bolus of midazolam (1–3 mg) is injected. The initial dose is based on clinical judgment with consideration of expected length of the procedure, body weight, level of anxiety, and history of narcotic, alcohol, or other drug use or abuse. The patient is asked to indicate verbally or otherwise when some subjective effect of the initial dose is perceived. Then 2 to 3 minutes later 50 to 100 µg fentanyl or 250 to 500 µg alfentanil is administered. An initial dose of methohexital (10–20 mg) is given to produce amnesia (an adequate dose is signaled by divergent pupils or lateral nystagmus[374]) before the paracervical block is performed by the surgeon. Shortly afterward, the patient should be able to obey commands, to breathe deeply, or to acknowledge comfort but is not otherwise responsive to the surroundings. The patient is kept at this subanesthetic level with incremental doses of methohexital (10–20 mg) or 250 µg alfentanil and occasionally 25 to 50 μg fentanyl. Supplementation with a hypnotic or an analgesic is determined by the patient's response to surgical stimulation and by the respiratory rate. Oxygen is administered by means of nasal cannulae. The anesthesiologist speaks to the patient frequently, reassuring, warning of stimulating events, and responding to any evidence of distress or discomfort.

Typically, patients are amnesic for all events beyond the request for a report of the first subjective symptoms of sedation. Occasionally, a patient expresses vague recall of voices or noises or of feeling the cold of the perineal scrub solution, but without distress. On the way to the PACU, many patients express amazement and even disbelief that the operative procedure has been completed.

Modifications of this technique can be expected in the future. For example, a new specific benzodiazepine antagonist, flumazenil, offers the prospect of more readily coordinating the end of anesthetic effects with the end of operation by reversing the hypnotic effects of midazolam.[381] Additionally, propofol (25–50 mg) may replace methohexital. It should be noted that when used for elderly patients, the dose of midazolam must be decreased because it produces prolonged sedation at standard doses[393] and is eliminated more slowly.

Subanesthetic Intravenous Infusion of Anesthetic Agents

The continuous variable-rate intravenous infusion of anesthetic and analgesic drugs is associated with a stable level of analgesia, fewer intraoperative side effects, decreased total dose of the drug, and a shorter recovery time than is the intermittent-bolus technique.[382–384] A subhypnotic dose is infused over a period of 5 to 15 minutes to achieve a sedated state, and this level of sedation is then maintained with a variable-rate infusion. In a recent study, infusions of methohexital or etomidate were found to compare favorably with midazolam for sedation during regional anesthesia.[385] Decreases in oxygen saturation below 95% were more frequent with midazolam than with methohexital and etomidate, but recall of intraoperative events was less frequent after midazolam.

White and coworkers infused midazolam (0.05–0.15 mg/kg) over three to five minutes followed by ketamine (0.25–0.5 mg/kg IV) in outpatients undergoing plastic surgery and found that this combination produced excellent sedation, amnesia, and analgesia during the injection of local anesthetic solutions without significant respiratory depression.[386] Mackenzie and Grant used propofol as a continuous infusion for sedation and noted the advantage of its rapid onset of action, short duration, and rapid recovery.[387] Propofol dosage, particularly in the elderly or debilitated, should be titrated carefully to minimize cardiorespiratory depression. When propofol was compared with midazolam for endoscopic procedures, hypoxemia $SpO_2 < 90\%$) and cardiovascular depression occurred with both, but there was earlier return to "street fitness" in the group of patients receiving propofol.[388]

Subanesthetic Inhalation of Anesthetic Agents

Advantages of inhalational analgesia for sedation are the ease of administration and maintenance and rapid reversibility. The major disadvantage is the need to have a tight-fitting mask to avoid operating room pollution.

Methoxyflurane was used in the past for inhalational sedation[389] but has been abandoned because of the possibility of nephrotoxicity.[390] Nitrous oxide has been widely used in dentistry because of its sweet odor, rapidity of uptake and elimination, its profound analgesic properties,[391] and because it does not depress the cardiovascular or respiratory system. When administered in concentrations greater than 30%, it may cause excitement, nausea, vomiting, and dizziness. Concentrations of 10% to 60% have been used with a variable response.[392] Korttila and coworkers studied psychomotor effects during inhalation of 30% end-tidal nitrous oxide and reported deterioration of eye-hand coordination, impairment of word recall, and impairment in the ability to do arithmetic problems.[393] Patients reported a significant increase in physical and mental sedation and a relief of tension. After cessation of administration, complete recovery to normal function was achieved in 22 minutes.

Subanesthetic concentrations of enflurane can provide analgesia and dose-related amnesia. Abboud and coworkers reported maximum analgesia in obstetric patients without loss of consciousness with a 0.5% inspired enflurane concentration.[394] Isoflurane also has been used for conscious sedation.[395] Isoflurane (0.5%) in oxygen was compared with placebo (oxygen) and with an equipotent concentration of nitrous oxide in oxygen. The majority of patients were acceptably sedated with 0.5% isoflurane in oxygen and preferred it to both the placebo and nitrous oxide in oxygen. Patients met discharge criteria within 20 minutes of the end of the procedure. The duration of isoflurane sedation ranged from 22 to 46 minutes in this study, and it is possible that during longer procedures patients may lose verbal contact. In addition to the pungent odor, side-effects included headache and dizziness. The incidence of these side-effects was lower in the isoflurane group than in the nitrous oxide group.

Applications

Although early applications of conscious sedation techniques originated in the areas of oral surgery and dentistry, the numbers and types of cases that are being managed with this technique are rapidly growing in the ambulatory surgery centers. At the Ambulatory Surgery Center of the Medical College of Virginia, conscious sedation has been used to supplement local or regional anesthesia for removal of external skeletal fixation, removal of percutaneous Kirschner wires, excision of Morton's neuroma, upper extremity surgery under axillary block, knee arthroscopy (in selected patients), laser coninization of the cervix, cervical dilatation and evacuation of the uterus, laparoscopic tubal sterilization, diagnostic dilatation and curettage (D&C), excision of vulvar lesions, removal of arch bars, face lift, rhinoplasty, blepharoplasty, superficial skin tumor excision, myringotomy and drainage tube insertion in adults, iliac crest bone biopsy, breast biopsy, and other procedures as judged appropriate. From 1981 to 1988, more than 7000 operations were performed in the MCV Ambulatory Surgery Center using the conscious sedation technique[396] without any major complications.

When ASA physical status 3 patients are managed in ambulatory surgery centers, they may be at increased risk of complications during and after general anesthesia. However, these patients can be well managed with the conscious sedation technique, which provides patient comfort, acceptable surgical conditions, and minimal postoperative complications necessitating hospital admissions. Another indication for conscious sedation is the patient who fears and vigorously rejects a general anesthetic for whatever reason (e.g., personal or family history of an anesthetic complication).

Morbidity and Mortality

Most of the data on complications of conscious sedation have come from dental practice. The relative lack of data in the anesthetic literature can be attributed to late adoption of this technique by anesthesiologists, but with the increasing trend for ambulatory surgery, the technique continues to gain popularity.

Experience with more than 7000 conscious sedation anesthetics over a period of eight years at the MCV Ambulatory Surgery Center resulted in no deaths or serious complications.[396] Transient but significant hypoxemia (SpO_2 < 90% by digital pulse oximetry) was noted in 28% of patients undergoing elective termination of pregnancy, but no significant clinical sequelae were observed.* Hypoxemia is more commonly observed in unskilled hands, and as expected, the management of the patient improves dramatically as experience is gained with this technique. The use of pulse oximetry appears to reduce the incidence of severe hypoxemia, and it is our practice to provide supplemental nasal oxygen to all the patients receiving conscious sedation.

The low incidence of complications associated with conscious sedation can be attributed to the following factors: (1) proper patient preparation (physical and psychological), (2) proper patient selection, (3) slow titration of small drug increments to produce desired effects, (4) adequate local analgesia, and (5) meticulous intraoperative monitoring.

The potential for serious complications cannot be ignored even though the risk of such from conscious sedation is probably substantially lower than that from general anesthesia. In patients undergoing dental or oral surgery procedures, the only group for whom data are available, the risk of death from intravenous sedation is only 1 in 314,000.[397] Serious complications reported to date include idiosyncratic drug reactions, anaphylaxis, malignant hyperthermia, respiratory depression, airway obstruction, hypoxemia, aspiration of gastric contents, bronchospasm, severe hypertension, and cardiac dysrhythmias.[398]

A review of deaths during first- and second-trimester abortion by the Centers for Disease Control[399] has shown a statistical association between abortion-related maternal mortality and the use of methohexital, a short-acting barbiturate commonly used for conscious sedation. Details of the anesthetic techniques employed were not included in the report, but the deaths were described as complications of anesthesia due to an overdose of methohexital. This report reinforces the conclusion of McCarthy and coworkers that overdose of anesthetic agents used for conscious sedation may lead to the induction of a general anesthetic state followed by respiratory arrest and vasomotor collapse and eventually

*Kallar SK: Personal communication, 1989.

lead to death.[375] To prevent such sequelae, vigilant monitoring, careful titration of drug dose, and administration of oxygen are essential.

Forty reports of apnea and respiratory or cardiac arrest in patients receiving midazolam for sedation for endoscopy and other procedures have been received by the U.S. Food and Drug Administration.[402] These were mostly older patients who were receiving other drugs and had concomitant diseases. Midazolam, in common with other benzodiazepines, is known to potentiate barbiturates and narcotics.[400,401]

Summary
Conscious sedation is useful, practical, and safe. It was originally developed in the offices and clinics of dentists and oral surgeons but is now becoming an important technique in the armamentarium of the anesthesiologist. With the rapidly increasing numbers of ambulatory surgical procedures being performed, its efficiency and adaptability seem certain to make it a significant part of outpatient anesthesia practice. The technique is particularly useful in patients at increased risk of complications from general anesthesia, to supplement local and regional anesthesia, and in those who fear or refuse general anesthesia. Recovery times and complication rates are markedly reduced.

The key factors in successful use of the conscious sedation technique are (1) gradual minute-by-minute titration of anesthetic drugs according to the length of the procedure and degree of surgical stimulation and (2) constant reassurance of and communication with the patient. The anesthesiologist is accustomed to being part of an immediate dose-effect feedback loop, but with conscious sedation, the onset of effect is much slower, and therefore, time must be allowed to observe the effects. Developing the necessary rapport with a patient and maintaining verbal contact throughout the operative procedure seem somewhat esoteric skills to resident anesthesiologists trained in general endotracheal anesthesia; however, although not easily learned, this art is worth the effort.

THE ADULT PROBLEM PATIENT
Ambulatory surgery has changed dramatically from its initial description in 1919 by Waters.[403] It has progressed from the practice of performing a few simple procedures under local anesthesia in a physician's office to the total care of a broad spectrum of surgical patients undergoing hundreds of different procedures under all types of anesthetics.

The explosive growth of ambulatory surgery has created new roles for the anesthesiologist that demand skills in addition to merely "giving a good anesthetic." Suddenly, it is the anesthesiologist who is most involved with the patient's care; we are the physicians who must ensure that the patient is appropriately screened, evaluated, and informed prior to the day of surgery. Indeed, the anesthesiologist-patient relationship that sometimes develops often takes on the quality of primary care.

Most individuals scheduled for ambulatory surgery today are patients of ASA physical status 1 and 2 who are undergoing procedures associated with only minimal bleeding and minor physiologic derangements.[404] However, with the continued growth of the ambulatory anesthesia subspecialty, we are constantly being "pressured" to consider "simple ambulatory surgery" for patients with formidable baseline disease. Particularly in these patients, the preoperative interview and evaluation by a consultant anesthesiologist are critical. In most cases, the physician will be able to identify potential anesthetic problems in advance, determine their cause, and where indicated, initiate appropriate corrective measures. Our goal should be to resolve preoperative problems as far in advance of the proposed date of surgery as possible, thereby minimizing the numbers of both cancellations and complications. Often patients of ASA physical status 3 and 4 may be considered candidates for ambulatory surgery if their systemic diseases are well controlled preoperatively.[405] In large part, the appropriateness of ambulatory surgery for many of our so-called problem patients is determined by the projected postoperative needs and requirements of these patients during their recovery from anesthesia and surgery. We will consider the anesthetic management for five potentially problematic conditions in adult patients: diabetes mellitus, morbid obesity, mitral valve prolapse, substance abuse, and steroid use (being fully aware that other sections of this book address these issues). We feel that other opinions plus repetition may help prevent potential problems in patients who have these conditions.

Diabetes Mellitus

Diabetes mellitus is the most commonly occurring endocrine disease,[406] with a prevalence in the population of between 3% and 6%. In its early stages, diabetes mellitus often goes undetected. A recent review by the National Institutes of Health suggests that approximately 50% of the 8 million diabetics in the United States are completely unaware of their disease.[407]

Diabetes is characterized by a broad spectrum of physiologic and anatomic abnormalities. Although the disease classically presents as benign glycosuria or hyperglycemia, in its most severe form, diabetes mellitus can have a devastating effect on the gross vasculature and microvasculature of the central and peripheral nervous systems, myocardium, skin, kidney, and retina. Often it is the sequelae of diabetes (premature atherosclerosis, cerebrovascular accidents, myocardial infarction, extensive peripheral vascular disease, renal insufficiency, and somatic and/or autonomic neuropathies) and not the diabetes *per se* that make an individual an unacceptable candidate for ambulatory surgery.

Diabetes is generally classified as type I or type II. *Insulin-dependent diabetes mellitus (IDDM)*, or *type I diabetes mellitus*, is controlled with insulin to prevent ketoacidosis in the patient. This form of the disease was previously called *juvenile-onset diabetes. Non-insulin-dependent diabetes mellitus (NIDDM)*, or *type II diabetes mellitus*, does not require insulin for control because patients with this condition are not prone to ketoacidosis. This form of the disease has also been called *adult-onset diabetes.* Type II diabetes may be induced by pregnancy, medications, or dietary indiscretions. Insulin-dependent and non-insulin-dependent diabetes are pathologically and genetically distinct entities[409] (Table 5-32). IDDM probably results from the destruction of pancreatic beta cells by an autoimmune process.[409] NIDDM is thought to be hereditary and is generally characterized by a gradual decrease in beta-cell function with varying degrees of pe-

TABLE 5-32. Classification of Diabetes Mellitus

Names:	Type I	Type II
	Insulin-dependent diabetes mellitus	Non-insulin-dependent diabetes mellitus
		Maturity-onset diabetes mellitus
	Juvenile-onset diabetes mellitus	
Etiology:	?Autoimmune	
	Weak genetic linkage	Strong genetic linkage
Onset:	Generally before age 20 years	Generally after age 20 years
Pathophysiology:	β cells of pancreas hyalinized	Normal pancreatic β cells
	Requires parenteral insulin for survival	Disease often can be controlled by diet and/or oral agents
	Ketoacidosis develops easily	Very rarely suffer ketoacidosis
	High incidence of microangiopathy, myocardial, hypertensive disorders, peripheral vascular disease, retinopathy, nephropathy, and neuropathy	Develop nonketotic acidosis (on oral agents)

SOURCE: Adapted from Loughran and Giesecke.[409] Used with permission.

ripheral insulin resistance. Since diabetes mellitus represents at least two very different disease processes, some investigators have suggested that each type of diabetes mandates its own perioperative management technique.[410] The balance of this section will address the perioperative anesthetic management of persons with IDDM for ambulatory surgery.

Preoperative Assessment

The acceptability of an insulin-dependent diabetic as a candidate for ambulatory surgery is largely dependent on three areas of consideration: (1) the presence or absence of associated conditions, (2) the degree of baseline control of the disease, and (3) the interest and ability to care for the patient postoperatively. The preoperative assessment of a diabetic patient for ambulatory surgery mandates a search for concomitant disease. These patients often present with a multitude of vascular-related problems, any one of which may require perioperative hospitalization. Atherosclerosis often develops prematurely in these patients with a multitude of complications, including cerebrovascular accidents, coronary artery disease, uncontrolled hypertension, renal insufficiency, significant peripheral vascular disease, and autonomic neuropathy. Simple review of a health survey does not suffice in this patient population. The combination of neuropathies and premature atherosclerosis makes this population particularly susceptible to painless myocardial ischemia.[410] In our facility, diabetic patients receive a thorough history and physical examination, electrocardiogram, and a battery of blood work well in advance of the day of surgery. At the present time, the truly "brittle" diabetic whose baseline state is punctuated by profound swings in serum blood sugar from severe hypoglycemia to marked hyperglycemia (with or without attendant ketoacidosis) does not appear to be a satisfactory candidate for ambulatory surgery.[411,412] However, with close collaboration between the patient, anesthesiologist, surgeon, and primary care physician, the ambulatory surgery center may be an ideal setting for well-controlled, informed adult diabetic patients who require minor surgery.

Normalization of Blood Glucose

The goal of intraoperative diabetic management is to prevent hypoglycemia while attempting to achieve levels of blood glucose as nearly normal as possible.[413] Short-term hyperglycemia (400–600 mg/dl) is not likely to produce permanent problems for the diabetic, but even brief periods of hypoglycemia may produce severe and irreversible brain damage.[406] Furthermore, the danger of hypoglycemia may be increased intraoperatively because the usual central nervous system symptoms of disorientation, dizziness, and coma are obscured by general anesthesia.

At the other extreme, several studies have suggested that chronic hyperglycemia with attendant ketoacidosis may lead to lower wound-healing tensile strength and a higher than predicted incidence of wound infection in type I diabetics.[411] No such evidence exists for type II diabetics, nor does any evidence suggest that acute perioperative changes in blood sugar affect wound healing, even in type I diabetics.

The physiologic response of diabetics to major surgery tends to counter tendencies toward hypoglycemia, even in those taking long-acting insulin preparations; most patients show a marked intraoperative increase in blood sugar.[415] Several studies, however, have recently demonstrated little or no increase in blood glucose during minor procedures.[416] For this reason, we tend to administer glucose solutions intraoperatively to all diabetic outpatients, even those undergoing very brief general anesthetics. Whenever indicated, we follow intraoperative blood glucose levels with spot checks using Dextrostix (Ames).

Perioperative Management

The primary objective in the perioperative management of the diabetic ambulatory surgery patient should be to restore the patient's insulin balance to its preoperative state as soon as possible. This seems to be most easily accomplished in patients undergoing minor surgery where there is less endocrinologic stress,[416] a more rapid return to normal daily living patterns (e.g., home and work environments, baseline activity level, and dietary habits), and a greater likelihood that the diabetes will remain under control.

In recent years, a number of protocols have been developed in an attempt to manage glucose and insulin therapy for the inpatient with diabetes during the perioperative period.[417–420] These methods invariably rely on the continuous administration of intravenous glucose and of insulin, either intravenously or subcutaneously, on a continuous or intermittent schedule. Our experience with the outpatient diabetic population has enabled us to effectively manage these patients without the use of minipumps or continuous-infusion insulin.

Two techniques seem to be particularly effective; both depend on appropriate patient selection. Most well-informed, well-motivated IDDM patients with only minimal end-organ disease whose diabetes is well controlled preoperatively can be considered as possible candidates for ambulatory surgery. In our most frequently utilized protocol, once the decision is made to proceed, we preoperatively counsel all diabetic patients scheduled for anesthesia care that there is a chance they will require postoperative hospitalization secondary to their disease. Most of the patients understand that significant postoperative vomiting will probably result in hospital admission until their dietary habits return to .1ormal.

Surgery is scheduled as early in the day as possible. This allows ample time for thorough postoperative assessment with particular regard to the patient's ability to tolerate oral caloric intake. Patients are instructed to eat nothing (i.e., remain NPO) overnight for surgery, to take no insulin at home on the day of surgery, and to be sure that they carry their favorite "sugar fix" with them to the surgery center. (They are instructed to ingest the sugar only if they experience symptoms of hypoglycemia in transit to the surgery center.) Shortly after arrival at the surgery facility, a baseline fasting blood sugar is obtained and an intravenous line with D_5LR is started. After the dextrose-containing solution is begun, one-half the patient's usual NPH insulin dose is administered. We then proceed with surgery, watchful for any signs of hypoglycemia during general anesthesia. These include tachycardia, hypertension, pupillary dilatation, or diaphoresis. Upon the patient's arrival in the PACU, we quickly establish verbal contact with the patient and encourage resumption of oral fluid intake. Shortly after the patient demonstrates a toleration for oral fluids, the intravenous solution is discontinued. When all other criteria for discharge are met, the patient may be escorted home in the presence of a responsible adult who will remain in attendance until the next morning. If any symptoms suggestive of hypoglycemia or hyperglycemia occur, the patient is instructed to notify the physician immediately. Discharge instructions also include resumption of normal diet as soon as possible. If four to six hours after surgery the patient is eating normally and urine or blood glucose determinations are normal, the patient may take the balance of his or her other daily NPH insulin dose. In most cases, the patient will be able to resume normal dietary intake and insulin regimen on the morning after surgery. (Further discussion will be found in Chap. 9, Case 9.)

Our second commonly employed technique for the management of patients with IDDM was developed by Herbert Natof and is referred to as "moving the sun in the sky." (This technique is more fully discussed in Chap. 8.) The patient presents to the ambulatory surgery unit having been NPO since midnight and brings insulin along. An intravenous line is started. After recovering from surgery, the patient is to begin a regular diet schedule and receive his or her usual insulin dose. Rarely are patients unable to resume a normal caloric intake. For the remainder of the day they move their meals closer together. Patients are cautioned, however, that they may be slightly hypoglycemic on the morning after surgery. They should compensate for this by increasing their oral intake.[421]

Several approaches exist to the management of patients with IDDM undergoing ambulatory surgery and anesthesia, but all possess a single theme: IDDM patients can have their surgical procedure performed on an outpatient basis safely if their diabetes is well controlled preoperatively, they are highly motivated to avoid hospitalization, and they are willing to accept considerable responsibility in their own postoperative management.

Morbid Obesity

Morbid obesity is often associated with marked physiologic derangements of the cardiovascular, pulmonary, endocrine, and hepatic systems. Vaughan suggests that obesity enables chronic illness to begin prematurely, progress at an accelerated rate, and become life-threatening more frequently.[422] The biologic, physiologic, psychologic, and technical problems in morbidly obese patients require major anesthetic, nursing, and housekeeping preparation for even the most trivial outpatient operative procedures.

Obesity is determined by the relation of body weight to height. We know of three techniques commonly used to identify "ideal" body weight:

1. Standard life insurance tables
2. Body mass index (BMI) = (weight in kilograms) ÷ (height in meters)^2
3. Broca index: Ideal weight in kilograms = (height in centimeters − 100)

The definition of morbid obesity varies greatly and may include the patient who is 100 lbs above ideal body weight, the patient who is more than two times ideal body weight, or the patient who has a BMI > 30. Several studies have indicated an increase in both morbidity and mortality after surgery in patients who are morbidly obese.[422–426] (Further discussion will be found in Chap. 9, Case 3.)

Preoperative Assessment

In our facility, obese patients are screened well in advance of the day of surgery. Often the end-organ complications of obesity (*e.g.*, cardiovascular, pulmonary, endocrine disorders), not the obesity *per se*, determine a patient's suitability for ambulatory surgery. Cardiac output in the morbidly obese patient may be significantly increased because of increased metabolic demands. Perfusion of added body tissue necessitates increased blood volume. These increases in cardiac output and blood volume strain the heart and eventually lead to the development of a severe cardiomyopathy.

Pulmonary function studies have shown that chest wall compliance, pulmonary parenchymal compliance, and functional residual capacity in the obese are significantly decreased. Of significant note to the anesthesiologist, airway closure can occur even during normal tidal ventilation. Premature airway closure creates a ventilation-perfusion mismatch, which in turn reduces arterial oxygenation. Obese patients often become hypoxemic in the supine position because their abdominal mass pushes the diaphragm higher into the chest, collapsing lung parenchyma even further and producing an even greater ventilation-perfusion mismatch. These effects are invariably enhanced under general anesthesia and can be potentially catastrophic.

In addition to these pulmonary and cardiac abnormalities, morbidly obese patients have a significantly higher incidence of hypertension, atherosclerosis, coronary artery disease, cerebrovascular disease, diabetes mellitus, and hepatic disease. Complete preoperative assessment and perioperative planning for these coexisting medical problems is absolutely essential.

Preoperative Considerations

Preoperative considerations unique to the patient with morbid obesity include the significant risk of aspiration pneumonitis, the physiologic alterations that occur with change of position, and the technical constraints of the patient's size. Several studies have demonstrated a linear increase in intra-abdominal pressure that occurs with increasing body weight. Obese patients also have a significantly higher incidence of hiatal hernia. The gastric secretions in obese patients differ significantly from those of their nonobese counterparts. Obese patients are "set-ups" for Mendelson's syndrome with preinduction gastric pH below 2.5 and gastric volume consistently greater than 25 ml.[422]

Paul and coworkers showed that simply changing the obese patient from the sitting to the supine position resulted in an 11% increase in oxygen consumption, a 35% increase in cardiac output, and a 30% increase in pulmonary artery wedge pressures.[425] In those patients with a history of preexisting cardiac compromise, the acute demand for increased cardiac output in the supine position can lead to pronounced pulmonary congestion and rapid deterioration of Pa_{O_2}. Indeed, there have been a number of case reports in the anesthesia literature of deaths due to the so-called obesity supine death syndrome.[426] These case reports describe a rapid deterioration of cardiac output with subsequent cardiac arrest when morbidly obese patients are moved from the seated position to the supine position.

Technical difficulties with morbidly obese patients abound. These include things as simple as positioning the patient on the operating table, securing an IV line, and identifying anatomic landmarks for regional anesthetic techniques. Even measuring the blood pressure can be a chore, requiring extralarge arm cuffs to prevent artificially elevated blood pressure readings.

Patient Selection

Because of the relatively high incidence of cardiac and pulmonary disorders in obese patients and the markedly increased potential for pulmonary problems intraoperatively, we feel that many patients who meet the criteria for morbid obesity are not suitable candidates for elective surgery on an ambulatory basis. Highly motivated, active morbidly obese patients with no known medical problems can, however, be considered for outpatient anesthesia.[423]

Many overweight (but not morbidly obese) patients also have significant concomitant disease. Overweight patients often require extra care in preoperative evaluation; we find that despite intensive preoperative cardiopulmonary evaluation and preparation, many of these patients are not suitable candidates for ambulatory surgery.

Intraoperative and Postoperative Management

We usually do not premedicate morbidly obese patients. If a patient is particularly anxious, a small amount of an anxiolytic such as diazepam or midazolam is preferable to a drug that may significantly depress ventilation postoperatively. Since uptake and distribution from an "intramuscular" injection given into fatty tissue will be highly variable, we recommend only the oral or intravenous route for premedication in these patients.

Potential airway problems must be considered during the immediate preoperative airway examination. Obese patients often demonstrate a limited range of head and jaw motion. If airway problems are anticipated, awake intubation has been recommended, either under direct vision or by means of fiberoptic laryngoscopy. In our experience, this is only rarely necessary. Because of the previously mentioned risk of aspiration pneumonitis, we prescribe ranitidine or cimetidine to be taken orally the evening before and the morning of surgery. We usually employ a rapid-sequence intravenous induction (after preoxygenation) with thiopental and succinylcholine combined with cricoid pressure to prevent passive gastric regurgitation. Proper head and neck positioning as well as retraction of the soft tissues of the chest wall from the chin and neck help facilitate placement of the endotracheal tube.

There does not seem to be a "best" anesthesia maintenance technique for obese outpatients. Increased biotransformation and metabolism of both halothane and enflurane have been reported in obese patients, but problems due to anesthetic metabolism appear to be extremely rare in cases of short duration. For general anesthesia, we use small doses of narcotics and 100% oxygen, and titrate a potent inhalational agent as indicated. We continuously monitor intraoperative oxygen saturation with a pulse oximeter, and if indicated, we obtain arterial blood gases. The Trendelenburg position will increase pressure against the diaphragm and significantly reduce Pa_{O_2}, so the head-down position should be avoided unless absolutely necessary to facilitate the surgery. Emergence and extubation are managed as they are with any other patient with a "full stomach." Obese patients must demonstrate the ability to protect their airway prior to being extubated.

Proper positioning in the PACU can improve oxygenation. We generally transport the patients to the PACU in a semirecumbent position with the head elevated 30 to 45 degrees. Supplemental oxygen is provided by means of nasal cannula, and pulse oximeter monitoring of oxygen saturation continues throughout the recovery period. We attempt to get morbidly obese patients up and active as soon as possible postoperatively.

Although obesity alone is not a criterion on which to deny access to ambulatory surgical procedures,[423] the condition is associated with other diseases and sequelae that have a significant impact on the suitability of these patients for ambulatory surgery.

Mitral Valve Prolapse

Mitral valve prolapse has been described as today's most frequently diagnosed valvular cardiac abnormality,[427] with prevalence estimates ranging from as little as 0.5% to as much as 21% in otherwise healthy individuals. Although some of the auscultatory findings have been known for over a century, the entity did not begin to take on "epidemic proportions" until the mid-1960s[428,429] when the technical developments of angiography, echocardiography, and phonocardiography permitted its discovery. According to the Framington Heart Study by Savage and coworkers,[430] clinical symptoms may include angina or nonanginal chest pain, palpitations, syncope, dyspnea, or high levels of anxiety; objective findings may include late or holosystolic murmurs with or without a midsystolic click, ST-T interval changes, T-wave inversions, QT prolongation on the electrocardiogram, and a variety of cardiac dysrhythmias.

Mitral valve prolapse has been associated with a number of other conditions, including coronary artery disease[431] and von Willebrand's disease[432] (Table 5-33); the presence of any one condition mandates a search (at least by thorough history and physical examination) for the others. Although the vast majority of patients with mitral valve prolapse are asymptomatic,[431] some of the possible complications of this syndrome, including cardiac dysrhythmias and bacterial endocarditis, are potentially life-threatening. Given the high prevalence of this syndrome, its associated conditions, and the potentially life-threatening complications that can result from it, several issues should be addressed when the anesthesiologist is presented with such a patient for ambulatory surgery:

1. Are any patients with mitral valve prolapse candidates for elective ambulatory surgery? If so, which ones?
2. What anesthetic management techniques should be employed to minimize risks in this population?

TABLE 5-33. Conditions Associated with Mitral Valve Prolapse

High arched palate

Pectus excavatum

Straight thoracic spine

Marfan's syndrome

von Willebrand's disease

Turner's syndrome

Kyphoscoliosis

Rheumatic valvulitis

Atrial septal defect

Idiopathic hypertrophic subaortic stenosis

Congestive cardiomyopathies

Coronary artery disease

Wolff-Parkinson-White preexcitation syndrome

Myocarditis

Coarctation of the aorta

Migraine anxiety neurosis

Autonomic dysfunction

3. Should all patients with mitral valve prolapse receive antibiotic prophylaxis for bacterial endocarditis prior to ambulatory surgery? If not,
   why not? If so, does a single "preferred" regimen exist?

Wynne believes that many patients with the diagnosis are actually "variants of
normal" and that there are two groups of patients with the diagnosis of mitral
valve prolapse.[428] The first consists of completely asymptomatic people in whom
the disorder is primarily an echocardiographic finding. Compared with "healthy"
peers, these individuals have no more arrhythmias, are typically free of most
clinical or laboratory findings, and appear to be at very low risk of complications.
Wynne suggests that "even if these subjects are not truly free of disease, there
appears to be no clinical advantage in separating the trivial from the nonexistent."[428] The second group consists of people who have echocardiographic
evidence of a clinically redundant mitral valve (greater than 5 mm)[423] and have
clinical findings and symptoms specifically related to mitral regurgitation; these
individuals seem to be at significant risk for the life-threatening complications
often associated with mitral valve prolapse.

Preoperative Assessment
Our approach to determining the suitability of patients with mitral valve prolapse
for ambulatory surgery is a rather straightforward one. Asymptomatic, otherwise
healthy patients receive no special preoperative attention but do receive an intraoperative anesthetic plan designed specifically for patients with mitral valve
prolapse (see below). Patients who have symptoms (e.g., angina, palpitations, syncope, shortness of breath, dyspnea on exertion) or signs (electrocardiographic
changes) of significant cardiac dysfunction are evaluated in the same fashion as
any other ASA physical status 3 or 4 candidate for ambulatory surgery; the decision to proceed is based on the degree of the patient's illness and the special
needs of that patient's particular surgical procedure.

Perioperative Management
The choice of anesthetic plan should be based on the pathophysiology of mitral
valve prolapse.[435] Since situations that promote cardiac emptying exaggerate the
degree of valvular prolapse, we avoid conditions that reduce end-diastolic volume by either a decrease in preload or afterload or an increase in myocardial
contractility or heart rate. We keep the patients fully hydrated, maintain their
blood volume, and, whenever possible, avoid the extreme head-up, sitting, or
reverse Trendelenburg position. Spinal or epidural techniques are acceptable
only if adequate precautions to minimize acute volume shifts following sympathetic blockade have been employed. Factors that may increase ventricular irritability (i.e., hypercarbia, hypoxia, electrolyte imbalance) are avoided. Because an
increase in sympathetic activity will increase ventricular irritability, we try to
avoid the release of endogenous or the introduction of exogenous catecholamines. For example, anxious patients with mitral valve prolapse are premedicated, an adequate depth of anesthesia is maintained at particularly stressful
points during the case (i.e., intubation, incision), and drugs that increase heart

rate (*i.e.*, atropine, pancuronium, gallamine, isoflurane, even epinephrine for local vasoconstriction) or anesthetics that promote sympathetic stimulation (*e.g.*, ketamine) are avoided. If cardiac dysrhythmias occur perioperatively, the usual measures should be undertaken to rule out the other common etiologies before mitral valve prolapse is assumed to be the cause.[422] Most dysrhythmias encountered will resolve spontaneously. Beta-blockers have been shown to be the most effective agents for control of many dysrhythmias associated with mitral valve prolapse. Fortunately, the vast majority of patients with mitral valve prolapse have an uneventful anesthetic.[434]

Prophylaxis: When, Why, and What

Bacterial endocarditis is an extremely rare complication of mitral valve prolapse, and the use of antibiotic prophylaxis prior to surgery is extremely controversial.[436] Although the current American Heart Association (AHA) guidelines recommend antibiotic prophylaxis for patients with a diagnosis of mitral valve prolapse with insufficiency undergoing certain procedures[437] (Table 5-34), the AHA cautions that "definitive data to provide guidance in management of patients with mitral valve prolapse are particularly limited. It is clear that in general such patients are at low risk of development of endocarditis, but the risk-benefit ratio of prophylaxis in mitral valve prolapse is uncertain." Many clinicians believe that prophylaxis is not warranted for all patients with mitral valve prolapse. For example, patients with isolated "clicks" do not appear to benefit from antibiotic prophylaxis at all.[438] Our institution follows the current recommendation of several prominent consultants[439,440] as well as the American Heart Association[437] in providing antibiotic prophylaxis only for mitral valve prolapse patients undergoing "susceptible procedures" (Table 5-35), and only if they have mitral valve prolapse with insufficiency or other symptoms.[428] Clearly, no one prophylactic antibiotic regimen exists, since the choice of antibiotic for prophylaxis should be aimed at the most commonly occurring pathogen at the surgical site. However, for the outpatient in need of antibiotic prophylaxis, it is impractical to follow a protocol that recommends IM or IV antibiotics prior to surgery and a subsequent IM or IV dose 8 hours later. Kaye has recently suggested that a single oral 3-g dose of amoxicillin could be used for standard outpatient SBE prophylaxis for oral, genitourinary, and lower gastrointestinal procedures in patients with low-risk cardiac lesions (*i.e.*, mitral valve prolapse without regurgitation).[439] An additional 3-g oral dose at 4 to 6 hours after genitourinary or gastrointestinal procedures would add an additional margin of safety. In the unusual patient who cannot take amoxicillin, parenteral medication could be administered as recommended by the AHA. It is our practice to have the anesthesiologist consult with the patient's internist or cardiologist in advance of the day of surgery to establish an oral regimen whenever possible for the ambulatory surgery patient with mitral valve prolapse. (Further discussion will be found in Chap. 9, Case 8.)

Substance Abuse

The American Psychiatric Association has defined *drug abuse* as a pattern of pathologic drug use that leads to impairment of occupational or social function-

TABLE 5-34. Infective Endocarditis Prophylaxis for Mitral Valve Prolapse with Insufficiency

	Before Procedure			After Procedure		
	Dose	Route	Time	Dose	Route	Time
Dental/respiratory procedure:						
Standard regimen (1 or 2):						
1. Penicillin V	2.0 g	PO	1 hr	1.0 g	PO	1 hr
2. Penicillin G	2-ml units	IV or IM	1/2–1 hr	1-ml units	IV or IM	6 hr
Penicillin-allergic (1 or 2)						
1. Erythromycin	1.0 g	PO	1 hr	500 mg	PO	6 hr
2. Vancomycin	1.0 g	IV (slowly)	1 hr	—	—	—
Gastrointestinal/genitourinary procedure:						
Standard regimen (1 or 2)						
1. Ampicillin and	2.0 g	IV or IM		2.0 mg/kg	IM or IV	8 hr*
Gentamicin	1.5 mg/kg	IV or IM	1/2–1 hr	1.5 mg/kg	IM or IV	8 hr*
Oral regimen (minor repetitive						
procedure: low-risk patient):						
2. Amoxicillin	3.0 g	PO	1 hr	1.5 g	PO	6 hr
Penicillin-allergic						
1. Vancomycin and	1.0 g	IV (slowly)	1 hr	1.0 g	IV (slowly)	8 hr
Gentamicin	1.5 mg/kg	IV or IM	1 hr	1.5 mg/kg	IV or IM	8–12 hr*

*Optional after, and once only.

SOURCE: Adapted from Shulman ST, Amren DP, Bisno AL, et al: Prevention of bacterial endocarditis. Circulation 70: 1123A, 1984, with permission of the American Heart Association, Inc, Dallas, Texas. (Refer to original for additional details regarding which cardiac conditions should receive prophylaxis and for which specific procedures.)

TABLE 5-35. Ambulatory Surgical Procedures for which Endocarditis Prophylaxis Is Indicated

Oral cavity and respiratory tract:
　All dental procedures likely to induce gingival bleeding (not simple adjustment of orthodontic
　　appliances or shedding of deciduous teeth)
　Tonsillectomy or adenoidectomy
　Surgical procedures or biopsy involving respiratory mucosa
　Bronchoscopy, especially with a rigid bronchoscope*
　Incision and drainage of infected tissue
Genitourinary and gastrointestinal tract:
　Cystoscopy
　Prostatic surgery
　Urethral catheterization, especially in the presence of infection
　Urinary tract surgery
　Esophageal dilatation
　Sclerotherapy for esophageal varices
　Upper gastrointestinal tract endoscopy with biopsy
　Colonic endoscopic (i.e., polypectomy) surgery
　Proctosigmoidoscopic biopsy

*The risk with flexible bronchoscopy is low, but the necessity for prophylaxis is not yet defined.
SOURCE: Adapted from Shulman ST, Amren DP, Bisno AL, et al: Prevention of bacterial endocarditis. Circulation 70: 1123A, 1984, with permission of the American Heart Association, Inc., Dallas, Texas. (Refer to original for additional details regarding which cardiac conditions should receive prophylaxis.)

ing and has a minimal duration of 1 month.[441] *Impairment of occupational or social functioning* is liberally defined as work absence, job loss, or social problems with friends or family. The United States Department of Health and Human Services in a National Survey on Drug Abuse found that nearly 30% of individuals surveyed had experimented with cocaine and almost 20% had tried tranquilizers.[442] Drug abuse is a way of life for millions of Americans.[443] It is so prevalent that many anesthesiologists have undoubtedly and unknowingly already administered anesthesia to members of this patient population. Are substance abusers suitable candidates for elective ambulatory surgery? If so, how can they be safely managed?

Preoperative Assessment
In our facility, all patients with a history of drug abuse are carefully evaluated well in advance of the day of surgery. On the day the patient visits the facility, we take additional care to secure all abusable medications as well as our supply of prescription blanks. Chronic drug abuse is associated with a wide variety of serious systemic disorders, including hepatitis, renal insufficiency, cardiomyopathies, thrombocytopenia, endocarditis, septic emboli, and acquired immune deficiency syndrome (AIDS). A history of drug abuse mandates a thorough preoperative history and physical examination. ASA physical status 1 or 2 patients with a history of chronic drug abuse may be acceptable candidates for elective surgery on an ambulatory basis. Because of the increased likelihood of acute untoward cardiovascular responses when one administers an anesthetic to a pa-

tient who has recently abused illicit drugs, we preoperatively counsel these patients and inform them that any sign of recent drug abuse on the day of surgery will result in immediate cancellation of their anesthetic. We tell them no elective surgical procedure "is worth dying for" and encourage their preoperative participation in a rehabilitation program.

Perioperative Management
On the day of surgery, we carefully evaluate the patient for signs of drug abuse or withdrawal (e.g., hyperactivity, disorientation, slurred speech, hallucinations); if the patient appears to be symptom-free, we proceed with our anesthetic plan. Since the personality of the drug abuser is generally not easily distinguished from that of the sociopath, we usually select general anesthesia over major regional anesthesia for these patients. Agonist/antagonist drugs (e.g., butorphanol, nalbuphine) should be avoided because they may precipitate an acute withdrawal syndrome. We avoid narcotics for these patients and prefer to administer an isoflurane-based anesthetic in combination with nitrous oxide and oxygen. Because of the high incidence of hepatitis and AIDS in substance abusers, we recommend increased infection control measures be taken by all facility personnel. For example, disposable materials are used whenever possible and gowns, gloves, caps, and overshoes are recommended for anyone having direct contant with the patient. Although rare, the patient with a history of substance abuse can sometimes be considered a suitable candidate for ambulatory surgery. (Further discussion will be found in Chap. 9, Case 17).

Steroid Use
Reports of intraoperative vascular collapse in patients chronically taking steroid preparations have prompted significant concern on the part of anesthesiologists regarding the risk of perioperative adrenal insufficiency. In dealing with these patients, several issues come to mind:

1. Are patients chronically taking steroids suitable candidates for surgery on an outpatient basis?
2. What is known about the physiologic response to the stress of minor surgery versus major surgery?
3. How much of which types of steroids leads to suppression of the hypothalamic-pituitary-adrenal (HPA) axis?
4. Is there a "preferred" supplementation technique?
5. What are the risks of steroid supplementation?

Most patients chronically taking steroid preparations have serious underlying medical illnesses (e.g., connective-tissue disorders, asthma, renal insufficiency); the decision to schedule the procedure on an ambulatory basis should be the anesthesiologist's and should be based on the particulars of the patient's medical history, physical examination, and proposed surgery. For example, a patient with a history of a kidney transplant on long-term steroid medications scheduled for minor surgery may have the risk of nosocomial infection substantially reduced if the procedure could be performed in an outpatient environment. The physiologic response to the stresss of major surgery (e.g., colectomy) has been shown to be substantially greater than that which occurs following minor surgery (e.g., herniorrhaphy). Good correlation exists between the response of adrenal gland secretion and the duration and severity of surgery,[444] suggesting that patients who undergo minor surgery may not be "maximally" stressed.

A daily regimen of supraphysiologic doses of steroid (greater than 7.5 mg prednisone) suppresses the HPA axis, eventually leading to atrophy of the adrenal glands. Subsequent withdrawal of the exogenous steroid leaves the patient relatively adrenal insufficient and often unprepared for the stress of surgery. Although inhaled and topical steroids are generally not suppressive, several case reports have suggested that they can occasionally block the HPA axis with resultant suppression for as long as 1 year.[445]

Many protocols exist for instituting and tapering steroids in the perioperative period.[444,446] In our facility, for those patients who have regularly taken steroids (more than a single-dose pack) within the 12 months prior to anesthesia and surgery, we generally administer no more than 300 mg hydrocortisone phosphate IV per 70 kg body weight; for minor surgical procedures, we give approximately 100 mg hydrocortisone phosphate per 70 kg. For the patient taking modest daily doses of steroid, we recommend an extra 20-mg dose orally of hydrocortisone on the evening of surgery and resumption of prior therapy on the first postoperative day.

Although rare, there are some potential risks of perioperative steroid supplementation, including fluid retention, acute hypertension, gastrointestinal distress, and osteoporosis. The most common complication described in the literature is abnormal wound healing or postoperative infection. The data, however, are inconclusive, and we generally provide supplementation for all patients who have taken steroids within the past year. (Further discussion will be found in Chap. 9, Case 16.)

THE GERIATRIC PATIENT

In the United States today, more than 50,000 people are older than 100 years of age. In 1980, 20% of our population was aged 55 years or older; that figure will be 30% by the year 2020. Two of the fastest growing age groups are those 75 to 85 years of age and those over 85. Of those who have passed the age of 65, more than one-half will require surgery before they die.[447] These facts, coupled with the growing emphasis on cost containment in the delivery of medical care, will bring greater numbers of elderly patients into the ambulatory setting.

Two factors must be considered in providing anesthesia for the elderly patient: the patient's preexisting diseases and the physiologic changes associated with aging. When dealing with the elderly patient, a primary concern should be to keep hospitalization as brief as possible. A stimulating environment and active efforts by staff to talk to and encourage the patient are significant parts of maintaining preexisting levels of functioning. The elderly patient does remarkably well when given practical information and high levels of interpersonal support by medical staff, family, and visitors.[448] The older patient is less able to cope with a new environment and frequently has fewer psychologic and physiologic defenses to cope with stress. Elderly patients tend to ask fewer questions of physicians and do not like to bother them with questions they feel may not be important. The anesthesiologist should be aware of this attitude, attempt to ascertain the patient's concerns, and provide appropriate information about anesthetic techniques. Over one-half of hospitalized geriatric patients experience some transient confusional state postoperatively. This high incidence can be decreased in the ambulatory surgery geriatric patient because of a quicker return to natural surroundings as well as a significant decrease in the number of medications the patient will be subjected to during the procedure.[448]

The anesthesiologist should do whatever possible to keep elderly patients comfortable and in contact with what has become familiar to them. For example, if their hearing is impaired, we can allow them to come to the ambulatory center with their hearing aids. Friends and relatives should be allowed to be with them in the holding area and should rejoin them postoperatively as soon as possible. In fact, ambulatory surgery itself serves to keep patients in environments familiar to them.

The modifying factors in the acceptability of the geriatric patient for an ambulatory surgical procedure are physiologic age, physical status, surgical procedure, anesthetic technique, and quality of home care.

Preexisting Disease

Many physicians feel that the geriatric patient's postoperative mortality rate is directly proportional to the number and severity of any preexisting diseases.[449,450] Tiret and coworkers prospectively surveyed 198,103 anesthetics; the rate of complications correlated far more closely with the number of medical problems the patient presented with than with the patient's age.[451] Some of the more common disease states of the elderly are listed below. Many of these diseases, although not curable, are amenable to medical therapy and can be controlled; whenever possible, it is important that they be controlled prior to anesthesia and surgery.

    Cardiovascular problems:
        Coronary artery disease
        Hypertension
    Respiratory diseases:
        Chronic obstructive pulmonary disease
        Restrictive disease (often related to arthritis)
    Central nervous system problems:
        Cerebrovascular accidents
        Parkinsonism
        Emotional problems
    Endocrine disease:
        Diabetes mellitus
    Urinary tract problems:
        Prostatism
        Nephrosclerosis

TABLE 5-36. Preanesthetic Conditions*

Condition	No. of Patients	Percent of Total
Hypertension	466	46.6
Arteriosclerotic cardiovascular disease	269	26.9
Myocardial infarction	185	18.5
Cardiomegaly	136	13.6
Congestive heart failure	75	7.5
Angina	64	6.4
Cerebrovascular accidents	58	5.8
Chronic obstructive pulmonary disease	140	14.0
Pulmonary (other)	135	13.5
Diabetes	92	9.2
Renal dysfunction	314	31.4
Liver dysfunction	85	8.5

*Preexisting conditions found by history or examination.
SOURCE: Stephen.[452] Used with permission.

Patients with multiple medical problems who are taking multiple medications require a thorough evaluation before being accepted for an ambulatory surgical procedure. Approximately 75% of patients older than age 70 years have one or more associated diseases. In 1000 patients older than 70 years of age, Stephen encountered multiple preanesthetic problems[452] (Table 5-36). The preoperative ECG was read as being "within normal limits" in less than 25% of the total group of patients. Although the significance of the ECG in reflecting clinical heart disease in the aged patient is of some question, specific abnormalities that have shown clinical correlation include left ventricular hypertrophy, left bundle branch block, intraventricular conduction delay, ST-segment and T-wave changes, and auricular fibrillation.[453]

Cardiovascular Problems
Patients with coronary artery disease are frequently treated with beta-blocking drugs and calcium-channel blockers. If congestive heart failure is part of the clinical picture, these patients may be receiving digitalis and diuretics. During the preoperative visit, the anesthesiologist must determine whether the patient requires any alteration in therapeutic regimen preoperatively.

Patients with hypertension should continue with antihypertensive therapy up to the time of surgery and should resume taking medication as soon as possible in the postoperative period. If their hypertension is poorly controlled, they should be reevaluated by their internist and brought into good control prior to anesthesia and surgery. Inadequately treated hypertensive patients tend to have a decreased blood volume with a smaller intravascular space. With the induction of anesthesia and its attendant expansion of the intravascular space, precipitous decreases in blood pressure may result. Patients who are receiving diuretics as part of their antihypertensive therapy may have a significant total-body deficiency of potassium. All too frequently, serum potassium determinations underestimate this potassium loss.

Respiratory Diseases

Geriatric patients with respiratory diseases should be carefully evaluated in the preoperative period. The importance of a good history and physical examination cannot be overemphasized. Pulmonary function tests should be obtained if they are indicated. A reasonable assessment of respiratory function can be gained with an arterial blood gas study.

Chest physiotherapy and control of chronic pulmonary infection may be required prior to surgery to achieve optimal pulmonary status. The patient who has problems with copious secretions will benefit from physical therapy, whereas the patient whose sputum is yellow (or darker) may have an infection. A preoperative course of pulmonary therapy with bronchodilators, coupled with the administration of a broad-spectrum antibiotic, can reduce the incidence of postoperative pulmonary complications. If a patient has lung disease that will require intensive postoperative care, he or she cannot be considered a candidate for ambulatory surgery.

Central Nervous System

Unfortunately, there is very little that can be done to control central nervous system disorders, but an awareness of them will enable the anesthesiologist to provide a safe anesthetic. The patient with cerebrovascular disease, for example, should be maintained near his or her normal blood pressure and kept relatively normocarbic. The head should be kept in a neutral position, for excessive turning could seriously compromise the vertebral circulation.[454]

The patient with parkinsonism should be allowed to continue taking dopaminergic medication until the time of surgery. The significant therapeutic effect of this drug should not be lost just because the patient is scheduled for surgery. Furthermore, certain drugs (e.g., phenothiazines and butyrophenones) that have an antidopaminergic effect should be avoided.

Endocrine Disease

For the geriatric patient with adult-onset diabetes, surgery presents a particularly stressful situation. Even those with well-controlled diabetes may have problems related to the stress of surgery, fluid and nutritional balance, and normal physical activity. The method required to control the patient's blood sugar is indicative of the extent of the diabetic's problems.

Patients who are controlled by diet alone rarely experience problems after surgery. These patients have (1) a prolonged response from their own insulin secretion, (2) lower fasting blood sugar levels than normal patients, and (3) frequent hypoglycemic episodes. It is this tendency toward hypoglycemia that must most concern the anesthesiologist. Signs of hypoglycemia during general anesthesia include sweating, dilatation of the pupils, tachycardia, and hypertension. Hypoglycemia is also a major concern in patients taking oral hypoglycemic agents (e.g., chlorpropamide).

There are many regimens for managing the insulin-dependent diabetic during and after surgery. Most often, the mode of therapy is chosen in the preoperative period, before the anesthesiologist is involved. It may range from withdrawing the patient from the usual insulin with coverage on a "sliding scale" to keeping the patient on the usual insulin preparation with a preoperative reduction in dosage. In the ambulatory surgery setting, the anesthesiologist may be the one who determines the management of the diabetic patient.

Patients taking oral hypoglycemic drugs are instructed not to take their medication on the morning of surgery; if they are taking an oral hypoglycemic with a reasonably long duration of action (e.g., chlorpropamide), they are told to omit an evening dose. These patients should be scheduled early in the day, receive an intravenous infusion containing dextrose, and resume their usual diet and medications as soon as possible postoperatively.

Insulin-dependent diabetics can be candidates for ambulatory surgery if their diabetes is stable and well controlled and the planned procedure allows them to reestablish their dietary habits soon after surgery. For short procedures, the fear of intraoperative hypoglycemia has prompted some physicians to withhold the patient's insulin until after the surgery. Blood sugar is monitored in these patients, and insulin is administered upon any undue rise in blood sugar.

The insulin-dependent diabetic should be instructed not to take any insulin preparation at home prior to arrival at the facility. Insulin should be brought to the surgery facility where it can be administered after an intravenous infusion has been started.

The more prevalent management approach involves the administration of one-third to one-half of the customary dose of intermediate-acting insulin. An intravenous infusion with dextrose is started simultaneously to counteract any untoward reactions; several studies have demonstrated that when ketosis develops in insulin-dependent diabetics, there is no reactive insulin secretion. The stress of surgery also stimulates catecholamine release, which increases blood sugar. Thus the diabetic with some insulin "on board" is expected to do better with a little extra sugar than one with less sugar and no insulin in his or her system. Additional information on the management of the insulin-dependent diabetic can be found earlier in this chapter, as well as in Chapter 8 and Chapter 9, Case 9.

Urinary Tract Problems

There is little that can be done to control urinary tract problems in the preoperative period. Nephrosclerosis, manifested by elevated blood urea nitrogen, serum creatinine, and urinary protein levels, is a complication of long-term uncontrolled hypertension. Consequently, the anesthesiologist's attention is directed to control of the patient's arterial blood pressure.

Prostatism is another common problem of the elderly. If a patient gives a history consistent with benign prostatic hypertrophy, the anesthesiologist must be concerned about postoperative urinary retention, a common condition in patients with prostatism who have received large intraoperative fluid volumes. Urinary retention may result from bladder distention in the intraoperative period, which causes a loss of detrusor tone in the bladder needed to propel the urine through a partially obstructed urethra. A rational (*i.e.*, conservative) approach to fluid therapy in these patients, coupled with other modes of therapy (*e.g.*, urinary catheterization) to prevent bladder distention, will help to prevent this complication. Patients with prostatism, however, should demonstrate their ability to void prior to their discharge from an ambulatory surgery facility.

The Physiology of Aging

Chronologic age should be neither a consideration nor a deterrent for acceptance to the ambulatory surgery center. A robust, vigorous 80-year-old is a better candidate for ambulatory surgery, for example, than a debilitated 55-year-old. Physiologic age involves both progressive functional changes and the cumulative incidence of disease. Some changes in physiologic function that occur after age 30 are noted in Figure 5-8.

Anatomic Changes

In addition to physiologic changes associated with aging that must be considered, there are also anatomic problems associated with anesthetizing the elderly. A large number of elderly patients are edentulous or have teeth in poor repair. This challenges the anesthesiologist in maintaining an airway by either mask or endotracheal tube. Cervical arthritis often makes it difficult for the patient to extend the neck. Consequently, care must be taken to avoid extension of the neck for long periods of time, since this may compromise circulation in otherwise atherosclerotic vertebral arteries. The skin of the elderly is particularly sensitive to injury from adhesive tape and electrocardiographic monitoring electrodes. Great care must be taken in taping endotracheal tubes and IV lines in place and in removing tape and electrodes to make certain that the dermis is not removed with them. The patient should be allowed to assume a comfortable position on

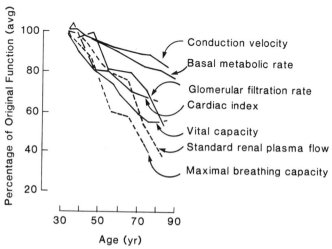

FIGURE 5-8. Changes is physiologic function with age in humans expressed as percentage of mean value at age 30 years. (SOURCE: Miller.[447] Used with permission.)

the operating table, whether for general, regional, or local anesthesia. Those who have stiff joints, contractures, kyphosis, dowager's hump, or arthritis of the spine should be given pillows and padding with no wrinkles underneath.[455] The lithotomy position can be a problem with aging hips and aching backs, and protective upper airway reflexes decrease with age, leaving elderly patients susceptible to bronchial aspiration.[456] There is an increased incidence of hiatal hernia, suggesting that regurgitation and aspiration of gastric contents are more likely in the elderly patient.[450] Manchikanti and coworkers evaluated acid aspiration risk factors in pediatric (6 months–12 years), adult (18–64 years), and geriatric (>65 years) patient groups.[457] In that particular study, the risk of aspiration pneumonitis theoretically was present in all age groups, with children being at greatest risk and geriatric patients at least risk.

Pharmacokinetics

When a drug is administered parenterally, its uptake and redistribution to rapidly equilibrating tissues is relatively unaffected by age. Gastrointestinal absorption, however, is affected by age. There are changes in gastric acidity, intenstinal motility, and intestinal perfusion that decrease the uptake of drugs given by this route. This must be considered when a predictable response to premedicant drugs is desired.

Once the drug has gained access to the circulation, it rapidly equilibrates with the vessel-rich group of tissues. The elderly patient, however, has increased body fat, decreased body mass, and a decreased muscle mass. These changes, coupled with decreases in perfusion, tend to delay redistribution to the more slowly equilibrating tissues, particularly for drugs that are highly lipid-soluble. Thus the half-life of such lipid-soluble drugs is markedly prolonged. Drug metabolism may further be delayed by a reduction in both hepatic perfusion and liver microsomal enzyme activity. The metabolites of these drugs also will be excreted more slowly because of changes in renal function. Drugs that depend on renal excretion for their elimination will thus have more prolonged effects. Consequently, an increase in a drug's half-life is common in the geriatric patient. This can result in the accumulation of a drug following repeated doses.[450,454]

Other factors also have been cited as contributing to the elderly patient's response to drugs. Decreased muscle mass in the elderly permits the anesthesiologist to achieve good muscle relaxation with a lower dose of neuromuscular blocking agent because decreased baseline muscle tone and the decreased number of receptor sites produce an increased drug effect. Another factor is the decreased plasma protein binding of drugs caused by less available plasma protein and a change in the quality of this protein such that drug-binding potential is decreased. The net result of this decrease in protein binding is a marked increase in the free drug available in the blood with access to the receptor sites so that a smaller quantity of drug may produce the desired effect.

The dosage of all anesthetic drugs [induction, inhalation, narcotic, tranquilizer (sedative-hypnotic), and local anesthetic] should be reduced in the elderly, and the rate at which anesthesia is induced should be altered because of the known changes in circulatory and respiratory status.[447] Over the age of 55 years,[482] most

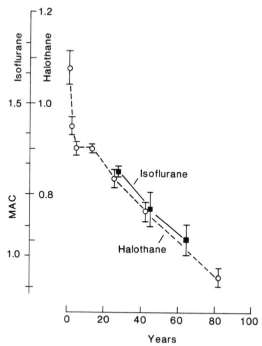

FIGURE 5-9. Minimal alveolar concentration (MAC) for isoflurane and halothane decreases with increasing age. (SOURCE: Quassha AL, et al: Determination and applications of MAC. Anesthesiology 53: 31S, 1980. Used with permission.)

drugs should be reduced by 25% to 30%. There is a MAC decrease of almost 25% in both halothane and isoflurane as patients approach the age of 80 years[481,483] (Figs. 5-9, 5-10, and 5-11).

Dundee and coworkers evaluated 609 unpremedicated patients to assess the influence of patient age on the response to propofol for induction of anesthesia.[484] A reduction in the induction dose required for elderly patients became marked around 60 years. Doses of 2.25 to 2.5 mg/kg were required to induce anesthesia in patients under 60 years, whereas 1.5 to 1.75 mg/kg was adequate in those over 60 years. In a prior study, Dundee and colleagues demonstrated a reduction in thiopental requirements with age for both males and females.[485] Steib and coworkers compared hemodynamic effects of thiopental (2 mg/kg) and propofol (1 mg/kg) for induction of anesthesia in elderly high-risk patients.[486] They noted no significant intragroup or intergroup hemodynamic changes, with the exception of a decrease is diastolic pressure and rate-pressure product after propofol. They concluded that propofol (1 mg/kg) can be used to induce anesthesia in elderly high-risk patients without deleterious cardiovascular effects.

Scott and Stanski confirmed the clinical impression that with increasing age there is a significant decrease in the narcotic dose needed.[487] The dose requirement of fentanyl or alfentanil decreases significantly with increasing age (a 50% decrease from age 20 to 89).

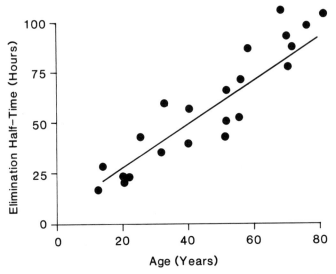

FIGURE 5-10. The duration of the elimination half-time of diazepam from the plasma was measured following the administration of intravenous (0.1 mg/kg) or oral (10 mg) diazepam to normal volunteers between 15 and 82 years of age. There was a linear increase in elimination half-time of diazepam with increasing age. (SOURCE: Adapted from Klotz U, et al.[40] Used with permission.)

The intensity of neuromuscular blockage from intermediate nondepolarizing muscle relaxants (atracurium, vecuronium) is not enhanced significantly by increasing age. Delays in recovery from neuromuscular blockade with *d*-tubocurarine, metocurine, or pancuronium have been attributed to age-related decreases in glomerular filtration rate. Even though vecuronium is partially

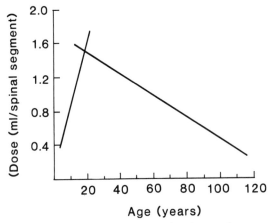

FIGURE 5-11. Epidural segmental dose requirements related to age between 4 and 102 years. SOURCE: Miller.[447] Used with permission.

cleared by the kidney, its neuromuscular effect is not excessively prolonged in the aged when administered within recommended dose range. O'Hara and co-workers compared dose-response curves using single intravenous doses of ve-curonium and detected no differences between younger and older adult patient groups.[488] With atracurium, dose requirements and recovery rates for patients younger than 40 or older than 60 years of age appear to be the same.[489] When muscles are weak from disuse or disease, lesser amounts of muscle relaxants will provide the desired effects.

Medications

The geriatric patient has an altered response to medication caused by changes in absorption, distribution, metabolism, and excretion. There is an increased in-cidence of drug interactions (11.9% at 50 years of age vs. 24.9% after age 80) be-cause of the large number of drugs taken by the elderly.[458]

The elderly have a tendency to become confused and to forget not only what drug they are taking but how much and when the last dose was taken.[447] Am-bulatory surgery facilities should ask elderly patients to bring medications with them to determine what they are and how many of each is being taken. Patients should take any essential medications early on the morning of surgery with some water. Although we try to limit the amount of water to 1 to 2 tablespoons, this can be a problem when someone is taking several essential medications.

Maltby and associates evaluated the effect of 150 ml of water taken orally 2 to 3 hours preoperatively on residual gastric fluid volume and pH.[459] The ingestion of 150 ml of water actually reduced residual gastric volume. The addition of oral ranitidine (150 mg) caused a further reduction in residual gastric volume and also elevated pH. Are we making much ado about nothing in attempting to limit amounts of preoperative fluids? The value of fasting, the optimum duration of fasting, and the possible role of preoperative fluid intake have yet to be defined for elective ambulatory surgery.

Renal Function

Most notable of the physiologic changes of aging is a decrease in tissue elasticity. Elastic changes in the vascular system cause irregular changes in blood flow throughout the body; renal blood flow, for example, is severely affected. By 75 years of age, renal blood flow is decreased by more than 50%. Therefore, glomer-ular filtration decreases, and the distribution of renal blood flow is altered such that a greater proportion of the blood goes to the renal medulla. The geriatric patient is therefore more susceptible than others to renal failure. This change in physiology, however, should not influence one's decision as to whether or not a geriatric patient is a candidate for ambulatory surgery; it is just a part of the aging process.

Pulmonary Function

Geriatric patients who do not have specific lung diseases still have significant changes in pulmonary function. Not only is the elastic recoil of the lung affected by the general changes in tissue elasticity, but the chest wall also becomes stiffer, probably because of arthritic changes in the chest. Pulmonary blood flow also decreases, leading to changes in the ventilation-perfusion ratio. This ratio is also affected by the closing volume and the dead space, both of which increase with age. These changes result in an increase in the alveolar-arterial oxygen tension difference so that arterial oxygen tension decreases. Residual volume and functional residual capacity increase as lung elasticity decreases. Vital capacity and forced expiratory volume are likewise reduced.

Circulatory Function

Decreased elasticity of tissue leads to decreases in vessel compliance and the development of hypertension. Decreases in vessel compliance also can affect autoregulation in various organ systems. When its vasculature is unable to alter pattern of flow, an organism cannot respond well to stress. The decreasing cardiac index and changes in coronary vasculature that occur with age add to this inability to respond well to stress.

Patient Selection

In view of the preceding factors, it may at first seem odd to consider geriatric patients as candidates for ambulatory surgery. However, not all elderly patients have all the problems enumerated above, nor do they all have them to the same degree. Physiologic age is more important than chronologic age. Is the patient in question a young 80 or an old 65? A physiologic profile consisting of past medical history, current level of physical activity, and present physical condition will serve as a better indicator of the patient's ability to tolerate the planned procedure than an evaluation of the patient on age alone.

Of equal importance is the physical capability and emotional maturity of the responsible party who will take the patient home and provide care in the perioperative period. Proper postoperative home care is one of the most important factors in geriatric ambulatory surgery. Family members who are unreliable or not physically able may not be capable of providing such care. Should this be the case, the safety of the patient's postoperative course is in question. Consequently, it is just as important to evaluate the responsible person during the preoperative visit. Is this person able to follow instructions and to do what will be required of him or her? Support services (social worker, home health care, visiting nurse, transportation) should be arranged when necessary in order to provide the geriatric patient with a safe ambulatory surgical experience.

The type of surgery performed is also important. Ambulatory surgery should be limited to procedures that do not require extensive postoperative nursing care. If there is little to be gained from admitting the patient to the hospital and a responsible person is available to care for the patient postoperatively, surgery may be safely performed on an ambulatory basis. The geriatric patient may benefit from having close friends and family members nearby during recovery.

Natof concluded after an extensive evaluation of outpatient procedures at his facility that despite reduced systemic functioning caused by the process of aging and the presence of many systemic pathologies in the elderly, major complications were more likely to be related to the specific type of surgery than to the physical status of the patient or the presence of preexisting medical problems, if these were under control.[460]

For the geriatriac outpatient with multiple problems, consultation with the patient's physician as well as with a responsible family member can play an important role in bringing a properly prepared patient to the facility for surgery and anesthesia. The patient's family physician must understand that he or she is not being asked for "medical clearance" but rather, given this patient's disease processes, will this patient be medically stable and in optimal physical condition on the scheduled day of surgery and anesthesia.

Cataract Surgery

The most common surgical procedure performed on the elderly patient is cataract removal. In 1886 it was shown that early ambulation following cataract extraction caused no unusual ill effects.[461] Although the trend away from inpatient hospitalization toward outpatient care had already started in the early 1980s, changes in Medicare reimbursement have made cataract extraction the most frequently performed procedure in freestanding ambulatory surgery centers.

Anesthesiologists are often expected to manage these procedures; total anesthesia involvement can include the administration of the retrobulbar or peribulbar block by the anesthesiologist. Techniques are well documented in the literature,[462-464] and they are not difficult for an anesthesiologist to master. Who is better trained in administering regional block and more aware of the effects of local anesthetic drugs than an anesthesiologist? In comparing retrobulbar and peribulbar block techniques in 3500 patients, Hamilton noted less discomfort for the patient, a higher incidence of excellent and good block, and a lesser incidence of retrobulbar hemorrhage and brainstem anesthesia following the peribulbar technique.[462] Currently, in the majority of procedures, however, the surgeon performs the block with or without a member of the anesthesia department providing monitored anesthesia care.

Sedation (*i.e.*, midazolam in 0.5-mg IV increments) is best provided 5 to 10 minutes before the block while the patient is observed and monitored (blood pressure, precordial stethoscope, ECG, pulse oximeter). Usually 1 to 2 mg midazolam IV is sufficient to lessen anxiety and limit postprocedure awareness for the block.[466] Some anesthesiologists include a small dose of fentanyl (25–50 μg). Methohexital (0.5 mg/kg IV) is also used for preblock sedation. For the geriatric patient with parkinsonism undergoing ophthalmologic surgery, Stone and DiFazio found that diphenhydramine administered in 25-mg IV increments produced a well-sedated patient with minimal tremor.[467] They did not encounter any oversedation or delirium. Zahl and colleagues noted that alkalinization of local anesthetic solutions (0.4 mEq sodium bicarbonate per 10 ml local anesthesia solution) improved onset time and quality of peribulbar block anesthesia.[468]

Is monitored anesthesia care necessary for cataract surgery? During approximately 1000 cases of intraocular surgery without the involvement of the anesthesia department, Meyers noted a 5.6% incidence of complications that required an anesthesiologist's intervention[469] (Table 5-37). In 300 patients undergoing intraocular surgery with monitored anesthesia care, problems arising were more

TABLE 5-37. Complications after Intraocular Surgery

Number	Complication
40	Marked bradycardia, diaphoresis, nausea, and hypotension
	Additional problems in 14 of these patients:
	2 convulsive seizures
	3 numerous VPCs with runs of bigiminy
	1 third-degree heart block
	1 VPCs with congestive heart failure
	2 multiple APCs
	1 severe parkinsonian tremors
	1 hysteria
	3 anginas
16	Problems without bradycardia:
	2 paroxysmal atrial tachycardias
	1 CO_2 narcosis
	2 grand mal seizures
	1 hysteria
	1 hypotension, nausea
	2 ventricular arrhythmias
	1 unresponsive, airway obstruction
	1 insulin reaction
	5 hypertension > 230/110 mmHg
56	Incidence 5.6%

NOTE: Subjects: Approximately 1000 patients, mean age 68 years, undergoing intraocular surgery without monitored anesthesia care.

numerous but were not severe and were quickly controlled. No surgical procedure had to be canceled; no patient became hysterical or restless. Meyers concluded that patients undergoing ocular surgery without monitored anesthesia care develop a significant number of life-threatening complications that may not be noted unless they are bothersome to the surgeon.

The scenario of either ophthalmologist or anesthesiologist performing the block and leaving the patient unattended is fraught with danger. Numerous complications of retrobulbar block, including brainstem anesthesia with unconsciousness and apnea, grand mal seizures, retrobulbar hemorrhage, and toxic reaction from intravascular injection, have been reported.[470–474] Both Lee and Kwon[475] and Nicoll and coworkers[476] consider shivering as an early warning sign of brainstem anesthesia.

The rare life-threatening central nervous system complications occur within 2 to 40 minutes of injection (mean onset time 8 min). Symptoms may include shivering, loss of consciousness, apnea, hypertension, tachycardia, cranial nerve III and IV palsy, nystagmus, contralateral pupil dilatation and amaurosis, seizures, bradycardia, and cardiac arrest.[476]

Draping, commonly used during cataract surgery, can produce an atmosphere low in oxygen and rich in carbon dioxide. Zeitlin and colleagues measured the partial pressure of carbon dioxide (P_{CO_2}) in the gas mixture under the drapes.[477] Accumulation of CO_2 occurred in all patients, but an oxygen flow of 10 L/min prevented any additional rise of CO_2 levels during the procedure. Reducing oxygen flow below 10 L/min led to increased retention of CO_2 under the drapes. Paper draps, permeable to CO_2 are thus preferable to plastic drapes, which are impermeable to CO_2, for such procedures.

In elderly outpatients undergoing cataract surgery, Kareti and coworkers evaluated factors leading to hospital admission following ambulatory surgery cataract procedures.[478] There was an increased incidence of admission in near octogenarians and patients with prior coronary artery disease. Sustained hypertension in the PACU was another influencing factor leading to hospitalization.

Chung and coworkers evaluated cognitive impairment of mental function in elderly patients following cataract operations performed with retrobulbar block and intravenous sedation.[479] Mental function was assessed preoperatively and at 6 and 24 hours by a Mini-Mental State (MMS) test (Fig. 5-12), a general-purpose cognitive screening test consisting of 11 items and requiring 5 to 10 minutes to administer. The score is a weighted sum of the items; a maximum score is 30 points; a score of 23 points or below is considered evidence of cognitive impairment.

Chung and coworkers demonstrated that cognitive impairment of mental function could occur in patients undergoing cataract surgery with retrobulbar block and intravenous sedation at 6 hours postoperatively; however, function returned to baseline at 24 hours. Patients with a low preoperative MMS score were more likely to experience greater postoperative mental impairment than were patients with higher preoperative MMS scores. Because cataract patients receiving intravenous sedation may have difficulty remembering instructions that are given during the first 6 postoperative hours, advice regarding care of the operative eye, medication, and follow-up appointment should be given to the patient before the operation, preferably in conjunction with written instructions. For the geriatric outpatient, written instructions are a must, and they should be discussed with both the patient and the person responsible for home care.

Except for the anesthesia risk, hospitalization of the average cataract patient is unnecessary. Given the choice of being asleep or awake during surgery, most patients want to be asleep. If carefully questioned, cataract patients usually admit they are afraid of seeing the surgeon operate on the eye; some believe the eye is removed, surgery is performed, and the eye is then replaced. It is important to dispel these fears, discuss the safety of regional block anesthesia, and stress the importance of an early return to a familiar home environment. If presented with the facts in a concerned, nonthreatening manner, the majority of elderly patients willingly enter into cataract extraction under "local anesthesia."

Good patient education is very important in ambulatory cataract surgery. McMahan provides patients and families with preoperative information by way of a video recording that fully explains the procedure from start to finish.[480] Patients are also given written material and detailed instructions about what to expect before, during, and after surgery. The informed geriatric patient is less likely to feel threatened by cataract surgery.

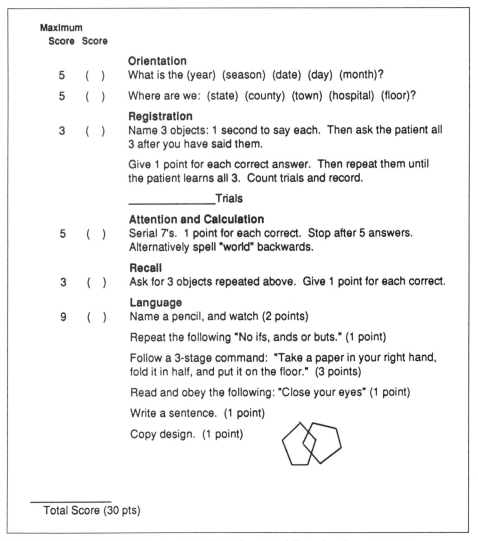

Maximum
Score Score

Orientation
5   (   )   What is the (year) (season) (date) (day) (month)?

5   (   )   Where are we: (state) (county) (town) (hospital) (floor)?

Registration
3   (   )   Name 3 objects: 1 second to say each. Then ask the patient all
                3 after you have said them.

                Give 1 point for each correct answer. Then repeat them until
                the patient learns all 3. Count trials and record.

                _____Trials

Attention and Calculation
5   (   )   Serial 7's. 1 point for each correct. Stop after 5 answers.
                Alternatively spell "world" backwards.

Recall
3   (   )   Ask for 3 objects repeated above. Give 1 point for each correct.

Language
9   (   )   Name a pencil, and watch (2 points)

                Repeat the following "No ifs, ands or buts." (1 point)

                Follow a 3-stage command: "Take a paper in your right hand,
                fold it in half, and put it on the floor." (3 points)

                Read and obey the following: "Close your eyes" (1 point)

                Write a sentence. (1 point)

                Copy design. (1 point)

Total Score (30 pts)

FIGURE 5-12. Mini-Mental State Test. (SOURCE: Chung et al.[479] Used with permission.)

Anesthetic Technique

The superiority of a specific anesthetic technique in the elderly has not been demonstrated. We are aware of surgeons, internists, and anesthesiologists who recommend local or regional anesthesia whenever possible. These opinions are usually based on impressions and on tradition, not on prospective studies.

The consequences of different types of anesthesia are difficult to assess. In a large prospective study (hip surgery) in elderly patients Valentin and coworkers found no difference in long-term survival between patients given general or spinal anesthesia.[490] Psychologic issues and rehabilitation were not addressed. Chung and coworkers demonstrated that mental function in the elderly popu-

TABLE 5-38. Patients Aged 60 Years and Older: Methodist Ambulatory SurgiCare, 1981–1988

Type of Anesthesia	Age (yrs)				
	60–69	70–79	80–89	90 +	Total
Local	3231	2774	1181	140	7326
MAC*	439	342	140	12	933
Regional	688	1083	602	60	2433
Inhalation	1078	518	101	11	1708
TOTALS	5436	4717	2024	223	12,400

*Monitored anesthesia care.

lation was better maintained following spinal anesthesia than after general anesthesia.[491] For certain procedures, regional anesthesia may be a better choice in the elderly, providing less deterioration of mental function, less incidence of postoperative confusion, and a reduced risk of drug interactions.

Methodist Ambulatory SurgiCare (MASC) has taken care of 12,400 patients older than age 60 years between the years 1981 and 1988 (Table 5-38). Of that number 7326 (59%) had their procedure done with local anesthesia (no sedation) administered by the operating physician, whereas 5074 (41%) utilized services of the anesthesia department (monitored anesthesia care, regional, inhalation). There were a total of 153 (1.2%) unanticipated admissions: local, 39 (0.5%); monitored anesthesia care, 27 (2.9%); regional, 8 (0.3%); and inhalation, 79 (4.6%). Leading causes of unanticipated hospitalization are noted in Table 5-39.

TABLE 5-39. Etiology of Direct Hospital Admissions among Patients 60 Years and Older from Methodist Ambulatory SurgiCare, 1981–1988

Problem	No. of Patients
More extensive procedure performed or planned	57
Bleeding	20
No responsible person to provide home care	17
Positive biopsy results	16
Pain	12
Arrhythmias	9
Syncope and weakness	5
Nausea and vomiting	3
Chest pain	3
Hypertension	3
Unable to void	3
Infection control (chills/fever)	3
Reaction to IVP dye or medication	2
	153

TABLE 5-40. Percent of Unanticipated Admissions of Patients Aged 60 Years and Older:
Methodist Ambulatory SurgiCare, 1981–1988

Type of Anesthesia	Patient	Patients Admitted	Percent
Local	7326	39	0.5
MAC*	933	27	2.9
Regional	2433	8	0.3
Inhalation	1708	79	4.6
TOTAL	12,400	153	1.2

*Monitored anesthesia care.

A goal of ambulatory surgery is to return the patient to home care on the same day as surgery has been performed. Tables 5-40 and 5-41 describe the relationship between anesthetic technique in patients older than the age of 60 years and the number of unanticipated admissions.

During this same time frame (1981–1988), MASC took care of slightly over 65,000 patients, and the unanticipated admission rate for this group was 0.8%. The MASC geriatric admission rate (1981–1988) of 1.2% is somewhat higher than this; more significant is the 4.6% admission rate for geriatric patients receiving inhalation anesthesia (Table 5-40). For the overall patient population (1981–1988) at MASC, the admission rate for patients receiving inhalation anesthesia was 1.4%. The type of anesthesia the geriatric patient receives should depend on the surgical procedure, the patient's general health and emotional state, and the comfort level of the anesthesiologist who has considered these factors.

Special Care and Handling
Surgery for the geriatric patient presents a special challenge for all members of the ambulatory surgery team. In today's high-tech society, the geriatric patient

TABLE 5-41. Unanticipated Admissions of Patients 60 Years and Older:
Methodist Ambulatory SurgiCare, 1981–1988

Type of Anesthesia	Age (yrs)				Total
	60–69	70–79	80–89	90 +	
Local	15	20	3	1	39
MAC*	7	18	2	0	27
Regional	3	5	0	0	8
Inhalation	34	36	8	1	79
TOTALS	59	79	13	2	153

*Monitored anesthesia care

must be provided with a lot of "high touch." Geriatric patients should be brought in earlier than usual on the morning of surgery. They take longer to get from the parking area to the facility, longer to register, longer to answer questionnaires, and longer to change their clothes.[492] They require gentle patience; they should not be rushed or made to feel like they are keeping everyone waiting. The elderly show significantly poorer comprehension of consent information.[493] A little extra time is needed for explanations and reassurance.

The geriatric outpatient has other special needs in the ambulatory facility. Chairs that are not too low and that have arm rests are important. Stepstools with handles can be helpful; these allow the geriatric patient to get on and off stretchers in preoperative and postoperative areas. Wheelchairs are an absolute necessity.[494] The older patient is less able to cope with a new environment and frequently has fewer psychological and physiologic defenses to cope with stress. Active efforts by the staff to engage and to relate to the patient are important. Agitation and confusion can occur if the patient is alone in unfamiliar surroundings without adequate interpersonal interaction with staff or a family member.[448]

Ambulatory surgery should be viewed as a potentially positive experience for the geriatric patient because separation from family, friends, and a familiar environment is limited. As anesthesiologists, we must be aware not only of the physiologic and anatomic changes associated with aging that cause us to modify anesthetic management, but also of the specialized care and caring required by the geriatric outpatient. Goethe said, "No skill or art is needed to grow old; the trick is to endure it." And the trick of caring for elderly patients having surgery is to help them endure what must eventually affect all of us.[495]

REFERENCES

1. Ramsey M: A survey of preoperative fear. Anaesthesia 27: 396, 1972
2. Norris W, Baird WLM: Preoperative anxiety: A study of the incidence and aetiology. Br J Anaesth 39: 503, 1967
3. Johnston M: Anxiety in surgical patients. Psychol Med 10: 145, 1980
4. Egbert LD, Battit GE, Turndorf H, Beecher HK: The value of the preoperative visit by an anesthetist. JAMA 185: 553, 1963
5. Lichtor JL, Johanson CE, Mhoon D, Faure EAM, Hassan SZ, Roizen MF: Preoperative anxiety: Does anxiety level the afternoon before surgery predict anxiety level just before surgery? Anesthesiology 67: 595, 1987
6. Lichtor JL, Korttila K, Lane BS, Faure EAM, deWit H, Robert MK, Ward J: The effect of preoperative anxiety and premedication with midazolam on recovery from ambulatory surgery. Anesth Analg 68: S163, 1989
7. Thompson GE, Remington JM, Millman BS, et al: Experiences with outpatient anesthesia. Anesth Analg 52: 881, 1973
8. Levy ML, Weintraub HD: Premedication: Yes or no? In Wetchler BV (ed): Outpatient Anesthesia: Problems in Anesthesia, Vol 2, p 23. Philadelphia: JB Lippincott, 1988
9. Leigh JM, Walker J, Janaganathan P: Effect of preoperative anesthetic visit on anxiety. Br Med J 2: 987, 1977
10. Ring WH, Wong HC. Designing and administering an outpatient facility. In Wetchler BV (ed): Outpatient Anesthesia: Problems in Anesthesia, Vol 2, p 9. Philadelphia, JB Lippincott, 1988
11. Wetchler BV: Anesthesia for outpatients. In Mauldin BC (ed): Ambulatory Surgery: A Guide to Perioperative Nursing Care. New York: Grune & Stratton, 1983

12. Wetchler BV. Anesthesia for outpatient surgery. AORN J 34: 283, 1981
13. Rosenblatt MA, Bradford C, Miller R, Zahl K: A preoperative interview does not lower preoperative anxiety in outpatinets. Anesthesiology 71: A926, 1989
14. Twersky RS, Lewis M, LeBovits AH: Early evaluation of patients in an ambulatory surgical setting: Does it really help? Anesthesiology 71: A1186, 1989
15. Zvara DA, Howie MB, Rubeis MJ, Robinson M, Benson G: The identification of preoperative patient concerns about anesthesia. Anesthesiology 71: A927, 1989
16. Beecher H: Measurement of Subjective Responses—Quantitative Effects of Drugs. New York: Oxford University Press, 1959
17. Standaert FG: Magic bullet, science and medicine. Anesthesiology 63: 577, 1985
18. Mirakhur RK, Dundee JW, Connolly JDR. Studies of drugs given before anaesthesia: Anticholinergic premedicants. Br J Anaesth 51: 339, 1979
19. Clark AJM, Hurtig JB: Premedication with meperidine and atropine does not prolong recovery to street fitness after outpatient surgery. Can Anaesth Soc J 28: 390, 1981
20. Meyers EF, Tomeldan SA: Glycopyrrolate compared with atropine in prevention of the oculocardiac reflex during eye-muscle surgery. Anesthesiology 51: 350, 1979
21. Mirakhur RK: Anticholinergic drugs. Br J Anaesth 51: 671, 1979
22. Fassoulaki A, Kaniaris P: Does atropine premedication affect the cardiovascular response to laryngoscopy and intubation? Br J Anaesth 54: 1065, 1982
23. Wyant GM: Glycopyrrolate methobromide. Can Anaesth Soc J 21: 230, 1974
24. Wyant GM, Kao E: Glycopyrrolate methobromide: Effect on salivary secretion. Can Anaesth Soc J 21: 230, 1974
25. Mikrakhur RK: Anticholinergic drugs. Br J Anaesth 52: 671, 1979
26. Jackson SH, Schmitt L, McGuire J: Transdermal scopolamine as a preanesthetic drug and postoperative antinauseant and antiemetic. Anesthesiology 56: A330, 1982
27. Longo VG: Behavioral and electroencephalographic effects of atropine and related compounds. Pharmacol Rev 18: 965, 1966
28. Smith DS, Orkin FK, Gardner SM, et al: Prolonged sedation in the elderly after intraoperative atropine administration. Anesthesiology 51: 348, 1979
29. Holzgrafe RE, Vondrell JJ, Mintz SM: Reversal of postoperative reactions to scopolamine with physotigmine. Anesth Analg 52: 921, 1973
30. Duvoisin RC, Katz RL: Reversal of central anticholinergic syndrome in man by physostigmine. JAMA 206: 1963, 1968
31. Smith TC, Stephen GW, Zeiger L, et al: Effects of premedicant drugs on respiration and gas exchange in man. Anesthesiology 28: 883, 1967
32. Koch-Weser J. Greenblatt DJ: The archaic barbiturate hypnotics. N Engl J Med 291: 790, 1974
33. Conner JT, Parson N, Katz RL, Wapner S, et al: Evaluation of lorazepam and pentobarbital as surgical premedicants. Clin Pharmacol Ther 19: 24, 1975
34. Heisterkamp DV, Cohen PJ: The effect of intravenous premedication with lorazepam, pentobarbitone, or diazepam on recall. Br J Anaesth 47: 79, 1975
35. Aleniewski MI, Bulas BJ, Maderazo L, Mendoza C: Intramuscular lorazepam versus pentobartibal premedication: A comparison of patient sedation, anxiolysis and recall. Anesth Analg 56: 489, 1977
36. Richter JJ: Current theories about the mechanisms of benzodiazepines and neurolytic drugs. Anesthesiology 54: 66, 1981
37. Study RE, Barker JL: Cellular mechanisms of benzodiazepine action. JAMA 247: 2147, 1982
38. Stoelting RK: Psychological preparation and premedication. In Miller RD (ed): Anesthesia, p 385. New York: Churchill-Livingstone, 1986
39. Stolting RK: Benzodiazepines. In Stoelting RK (ed): Pharmacology and Physiology in Anesthesia Practice, p 227. Philadelphia: JB Lippincott, 1987
40. Klotz U, Avant GR, Hoyumpa A, Schenker S, Wilkinson GR: The effects of age and liver disease on the disposition and elimination of diazepam in adult man. J Clin Invest 55: 347, 1975
41. Houghton, DJ: Use of lorazepam as a premedicant for caesarian section. Br J Anaesth 55: 767, 1983

42. Hillestad L, Hansen T, Melsom H, et al: Diazepam metabolism in normal man. Clin Pharmacol Ther 16: 479, 1974

43. Greenblatt DJ, Abernathy DR, Morse DS, Harmatz JS, Shader RI: Clinical importance of the interaction of diazepam and cimetidine. N Engl J Med 310: 1639, 1984

44. Caldwell CB, Gross JB: Physostigmine reversal of midazolam-induced sedation. Anesthesiology 57: 125, 1982

45. Catoire P, Hort-Legrand C, Vignoli T: Reversal of midazolam by flumazenil: Objective evaluation using evoked potentials. Anesthesiology 71: A117, 1989

46. Breimer LTM, Hennis PJ, Danof M, Bovill JG, Spierdijik J: The EEG effect of flumazenil vs placebo in volunteers. Anesthesiology 71: A122, 1989

47. Breimer LTM, Hennis PJ, Bovill JG, Burm AGL, Vletter A: The pharmacokinetics of flumazenil in volunteers. Anesthesiology 71: A293, 1989

48. Servin F, Bougeois B, Farinotti R, Desmonts JM: Does flumazenil improve recovery after midazolam anesthesia in patients over 80 years? Anesthesiology 71: A299, 1989

49. Philip BK, Hauch MA, Mallampati SR, Simpson TH: Flumazenil for reversal of sedation after midazolam-induced ambulatory general anesthesia. Anesthesiology 71: A301, 1989

50. Baird ES, Hailey DM: Delayed recovery from a sedative: Correlation of the plasma levels of diazepam with clinical effects after oral and intravenous administration. Br J Anaesth 44: 803, 1972

51. Divoll M, Greenblatt DJ, Ochs HR, et al: Absolute bioavailability of oral and intramuscular diazepam: Effects of age and sex. Anesth Analg 62: 1, 1983

52. Driscoll EJ, Smilack ZH, Lightbody PM, et al: Sedation with intravenous diazepam. J Oral Surg 30: 332, 1972

53. Korttila K, Mattila MJ, Linnoila M: Prolonged recovery after diazepam sedation: The influence of food, charcoal ingestion and injection rate on the effects of intravenous diazepam. Br J Anaesth 48: 333, 1976

54. Hegarty JE, Dundee JW: Sequelae after the intravenous injection of three benzodiazepines: Diazepam, lorazepam, and flunitrazepam. Br Med J 2: 1384, 1977

55. Schou Oleson A, Huttel MS: Local reactions to IV diazepam in three different formulations. Br J Anaesth 52: 609, 1980

56. Thompson GE, Remington JM, Millman BS, et al: Experiences with outpatient anesthesia. Anesth Analg 52: 881, 1973

57. Jakobsen H, Hertz JB, Johansen JR, et al: Premedication before day surgery: A double-blind comparison of diazepam and placebo. Br J Anaesth 57: 300, 1985

58. Jansen EC, Wachowiak-Andersen G, Munster-Swendsen J, et al: Postural stability after oral premedication with diazepam. Anesthesiology 63: 557, 1985

59. Dundee JW, McGowan WAW, Lilburn JK, McKay AC, Hegarty JE: Comparison of the actions of diazepam and lorazepam. Br J Anaesth 51: 439, 1979

60. Reves JG, Fragen RJ, Vinik HR, Greenblatt DJ: Midazolam: Pharmacology and uses. Anesthesiology 62: 310, 1985

61. Nuotto E, Korttila K, Lichtor L, Östman P, Rupani G: Sedative effects and recovery after different doses of intravenous midazolam and diazepam. Anesth Analg 68: S214, 1989

62. Conner JT, Katz RL, Pagano RR, et al: RO 21-3981 for intravenous surgical premedication and induction of anesthesia. Anesth Analg 57: 1, 1978

63. Fragen RJ, Funk DI, Avram MJ, et al: Midazolam versus hydroxyzine as intramuscular premedicant. Can Anaesth Soc J 330: 136, 1983

64. Vinik HR, Reves JG, Wright D: Premedication with intramuscular midazolam: A prospective randomized double-blind controlled study. Anesth Analg 61: 933, 1982

65. Beechey APG, Eltringham RJ, Studd C: Temazepam as premedication in day surgery. Anaesthesia 36: 10, 1981

66. Greenwood BK, Bradshaw EG: Preoperative medication for day-case surgery. Br J Anaesth 55: 933, 1983

67. Clark G, Erwin D, Yate P, et al: Temazepam as premedication in elderly patients. Anaesthesia 37: 421, 1982

68. Herr GP, Conner JT, Katz RL, et al: Diazepam and droperidol as IV premedicants. Br J Anaesth 51: 537, 1979
69. Lee CM, Yeakel AE: Patients refusal of surgery following Innovar premedication. Anesth Analg 54: 224, 1975
70. Briggs RM, Ogg MJ: Patient's refusal of surgery following Innovar premedication. Plast Reconstr Surg 51: 158, 1973
71. Rivera VM, Keichian AH, Oliver RE: Persistent parkinsonism following neurolept analgesia. Anesthesiology 42: 635, 1975
72. Patton CM: Rapid induction of acute dyskinesis by droperidol. Anesthesiology 43: 126, 1975
73. Cressman WA, Plostnieks J, Johnson PC: Absorption, metabolism and excretion of droperidol by human subjects following intramuscular and intravenous administration. Anesthesiology 38: 363, 1973
74. Korttila K, Linnoila M: Skills related to driving after intravenous diazepam, flunitrazepam or droperidol. Br J Anaesth 46: 961, 1974
75. Korttila K, Kauste A, Auvinen J: Comparison of domperidone, droperidol, and metoclopramide in the prevention and treatment of nausea and vomiting after balanced general anesthesia. Anesth Analg 58: 396, 1979
76. Santos A, Datta S: Prophylactic use of droperidol for control of nausea and vomiting during spinal anesthesia for cesarean section. Anesth Analg 63: 85, 1984
77. Cohen EN, Beecher HK: Narcotics in preanesthetic medication: A controlled study. JAMA 147: 1664, 1951
78. Meridy HW: Criteria for selection of ambulatory surgical patients and guidelines for anesthetic management: A retrospective study of 1553 cases. Anesth Analg 61: 921, 1982
79. McClain DA, Hug CC: Intravenous fentanyl kinetics. Clin Pharmacol Ther 28: 106, 1980
80. Conner JT, Herr G, Katz RL, et al: Droperidol, fentanyl and morphine for IV surgical premedication. Br J Anaesth 50: 463, 1978
81. Dionne RA: Differential pharmacology of drugs used for intravenous premedication. J Dent Res 63: 842, 1984
82. Morrison JD: Studies of drugs given before anaesthesia: XXII. Phenoperidine and fentanyl, alone and in combination with droperidol. Br J Anaesth 42: 1119, 1970
83. Epstein BS, Levy ML, Thein MH, et al: Evaluation of fentanyl as an adjunct to thiopental–nitrous oxide–oxygen anesthesia for short surgical procedures. Anesth Rev 2(3): 24, 1975
84. Hunt TM, Plantevin OM, Gilbert JR: Morbidity in gynaecological day-case surgery: A comparison of two anaesthetic techniques. Br J Anaesth 51: 785, 1979
85. Pandit SK, Kothary SP: Should we premedicate ambulatory surgical patients? Anesthesiology 65: A352, 1986
86. Teabeaut JR: Aspiration of gastric contents: An experimental study. Am J Pathol 28: 51, 1952
87. Roberts RB, Shirley MA: Reducing the risk of acid aspiration during cesarean section. Anesth Analg 53: 859, 1974
88. Ong BY, Palahniuk RJ, Comming M: Gastric volume in outpatients. Can Anaesth Soc J 25: 36, 1978
89. Katende R, Dimich I, Michula S, et al: The effect of intravenous cimetidine and metoclopramide on gastric pH and volume in outpatients. Anesth Analg 67: S109, 1988
90. Coté CJ, Goudsouzian NG, Liu LMP, et al: Assessment of risk factors related to the acid aspiration syndrome in pediatric patients: Gastric pH and residual volume. Anesthesiology 56: 70, 1982
91. Vaughan RW, Bauer S, Wise L: Volume and pH of gastric juice in obese patients. Anesthesiology 43: 686, 1975
92. Kallar SK: Aspiration pneumonitis: Fact or fiction? In Wetchler BV (ed): Problems in Anesthesia: Outpatient Anesthesia, Vol 2, p 29. Philadelphia, JB Lippincott, 1988
93. Natof HE: Complications. In Wetchler BV (ed): Anesthesia for Ambulatory Surgery, p 344. Philadelphia, JB Lippincott, 1985
94. Natof HE: FASA Special Study I. Alexandria, Va., Federated Ambulatory Surgery Association, 1986

95. Olsson GL, Hallen B, Hambraeus Jonzon K: Aspiration during anesthesia: A computer aided study of 185,358 anaesthetics. Acta Anaesthesiol Scand 30: 84, 1986

96. Morgan JG: Pathophysiology of gastric aspiration: Pulmonary aspiration. Int Anesthesiol Clin 15: 1, 1977

97. Harrison GG: Deaths attributable to anesthesia: A ten-year survey (1967–1976). Br J Anaesth 50: 1041, 1978

98. Blitt DC, Gutman HL, Cohen DD, Weisman H, Dillon JB: Silent regurgitation and aspiration during general anesthesia. Anesth Analg 49: 707, 1970

99. Lindgren L, Saarnivaara L: Increase in intragastric pressure during suxamethonium-induced muscle fasciculations in children: Inhibition by alfentanil. Br J Anaesth 60: 176, 1988

100. Wyner J, Cohen SE: Gastric volume in early pregnancy: Effect of metoclopramide. Anesthesiology 57: 209, 1982

101. Martin CC, Kallar SK, Ciresi SA: The effect of oral Bicitra compared with intramuscular cimetidine on gastric volume and pH in outpatient surgery. Amer Assoc Nurse Anesth J 56(6): 515, 1988

102. Stoelting RK: Gastric fluid pH in patients receiving cimetidine. Anesth Analg 57: 675, 1978

103. Hodgkinson R, Glassenberg R, Joyce TH, Coombs DW, Ostheimer GW, Gibbs CP: Comparison of cimetidine (Tagamet) with antacid for safety and effectiveness in reducing gastric acidity before elective cesarean section. Anesthesiology 59: 86, 1983

104. Weber L, Hirshman CA: Cimetidine for prophylaxis of aspiration pneumonitis: Comparison of intramuscular and oral dosage schedules. Anesth Analg 58: 426, 1979

105. Manchikanti L, Colliver JA, et al: Ranitidine and metoclopramide for prophylaxis of aspiration pneumonitis in elective surgery. Anesth Analg 63: 903, 1984

106. Gonzalez ER, Butler SA, Jones MK, et al: Cimetidine versus ranitidine: Single-dose, oral regimen for reducing gastric acidity and volume in ambulatory surgery patients. Drug Intell Clin Pharm 21: 192, 1987

107. Gonzalez ER, Kallar SK, Dunnavent BW: Single-dose intravenous H_2 blocker prophylaxis of aspiration pneumonitis. Amer Assoc Nurse Anesth J 57: 238, 1989

108. Silverman DG, Jacobs BR, Green AM, et al: Oral H_2-antagonist prophylaxis in the outpatient setting: Ranitidine vs Famotidine. Anesth Analg 68: S263, 1989

109. Rao TLK, Suseeda M, El-Etv AA: Metoclopramide and cimetidine to reduce gastric pH and volume. Anesth Analg 63: 264, 1984

110. Somori GJ, Kallar SK: The effects of cimetidine on gastric pH and volume in pediatric patients in an ambulatory surgical center. Anesthesiology 62: 3A, 1984

111. Young ET, Goudsouzian NG, Shah A: Effect of ranitidine on intragastric pH in children. Anesth Analg 65: S170, 1986

112. Solamki DR, Nicholas DA, Williams KR; Comparative effects of oral sodium citrate and oral cimetidine on gastric pH in pediatric patients. Anesth Analg 65: S147, 1986

113. Ogg TW: Use of anaesthesia: Implications of day-case surgery and anaesthesia. Br Med J 281: 212, 1980

114. Doze VA, Shafer A, White PF: Nausea and vomiting after outpatient anesthesia: Effectiveness of droperidol alone and in combination with metoclopramide. Anesth Analg 66: S41, 1987

115. Metter SE, Kitz DS, Young ML, Baldeck AM, Apfelbaum JL, Lecky JH: Nausea and vomiting after outpatient laparoscopy: Incidence, impact on recovery room stay and cost. Anesth Analg 66: S116, 1987

116. Hackett GH, Harris MNE, Plantevin OM, Pringle DB, Avery AJ: Anaesthesia for outpatient termination of pregnancy. Br J Anaesth 54: 865, 1982

117. White PF, Coe V, Shafer A, Sung M-L: Comparison of alfentanil with fentanyl for outpatient anesthesia. Anesthesiology 64: 99, 1986

118. Tracey JA, Holland AJC, Unger L: Morbidity in minor gynaecological surgery: A comparison of halothane, enflurane and isoflurane. Br J Anaesth 54: 1213, 1982

119. White PF: Continuous infusions of thiopental, methohexital or etomidate as adjuvants to nitrous oxide for outpatient anesthesia. Anesth Analg 63: 282, 1984

120. Fahy A, Marshall M: Postanaesthetic morbidity in outpatients. Br J Anaesth 41: 433, 1969

121. Skacel M, Sengupta P, Plantevin OM: Morbidity after day case laparoscopy: A comparison of two techniques of tracheal anaesthesia. Anaesthesia 41: 537, 1986

122. Collins RM, Docherty PW, Plantevin OM: Postoperative morbidity following gynaecological outpatient laparoscopy: A reappraisal of the service. Anaesthesia 39: 819, 1984

123. Richter J, Waller MB: Effects of pentobarbital on the regulation of acetylcholine content and release in different regions of rat brain. Biochem Pharmacol 26: 609, 1977

124. Fragen RJ, Avram MF: Comparative pharmacology of drugs used for the induction of anesthesia. In Stoelting RK, Barish PG, Gallagher TJ (eds): Advances in Anesthesia, p 103. Chicago: Year Book Medical Publishers 1986

125. Price HL, Kovnat BS, Safer JN, et al: The uptake of thiopental by body tissues and its relation to the duration of narcosis. Clin Pharmacol Ther 1: 16, 1960

126. Korttila K, Linnoila M, Ertama P, Häkkinen S: Recovery and simulated driving after intravenous anesthesia with thiopental, methohexital, propanidid, or alphadione. Anesthesiology 43: 291, 1975

127. Todd MM, Drummond JC, Sang H: The hemodynamic consequences of high-dose methohexital anesthesia in humans. Anesthesiology 61: 495, 1984

128. Filner BF, Karliner JS: Alterations of normal left ventricular performance by general anesthesia. Anesthesiology 45: 610, 1976

129. Hudson RJ, Stanski DR, Burch PG: Pharmacokinetics of methohexital and thiopental in surgical patients. Anesthesiology 59: 215, 1983

130. Vickers MD: The measurement of recovery from anaesthesia. Br J Anaesth 37: 296, 1965

131. Carson IW: Recovery from anaesthesia: A review of methods for evaluation of recovery from anaesthesia. Proc R Soc Med 68: 108, 1975

132. Hannington-Kiff JG: Measurement of recovery from outpatient general anaesthesia with a simple ocular test. Br Med J 3: 132, 1970

133. Elliott CJR, Green R, Howells TH, et al: Recovery after intravenous barbiturate anaesthesia. Lancet 1: 68, 1962

134. Cooper GM: Recovery from anaesthesia. Clin Anaesth 2: 145, 1984

135. White PF: Continuous infusions of thiopental, methohexital, or etomidate as adjuvants to nitrous oxide for outpatient anesthesia. Anesth Analg 63: 282, 1984

136. Dundee JW: Clinical studies of induction agents: VII. A comparison of eight intravenous anaesthetics as main agents for a standard operation. Br J Anaesth 345: 784, 1963

137. Craido A, Maseda J. Novarro E, Escarpa A, Avello F: Induction of anaesthesia with etomidate: Haemodynamic study of 36 patients. Br J Anaesth 52: 803, 1980

138. Fragen RJ, Caldwell N: Comparison of a new formulation of etomidate with thiopental—Side effects and awakening times. Anesthesiology 50: 242, 1979

139. Lees NW, Hendry JGB: Etomidate in urological outpatient anaesthesia. Anaesthesia 32: 592, 1977

140. White PF, Shafer A: Clinical pharmacology and uses of injectable anesthetic and analgesic drugs. In Wetchler BV (ed): Outpatient Anesthesia: Problems in Anesthesia, Vol 2, p 37. Philadelphia: JB Lippincott, 1988

141. Giese JL, Stanley TH, Pace NL: Fentanyl pretreatment reduces side effects associated with etomidate anesthesia induction. Anesthesiology 59: A320, 1983

142. Collin RIW, Drummond GB, Spence AA: Alfentanil supplemented anaesthesia for short procedures: A double-blind study of alfentanil used with etomidate and enflurane for day cases. Anaesthesia 41: 477, 1986

143. Melnick BM, Phitayakorn P, McKenzie R: Abolishing pain on injection of etomidate. Anesthesiology 66: 444, 1987

144. Wagner RL, White PF: Etomidate inhibits adrenocortical function in surgical patients. Anesthesiology 61: 647, 1984

145. Thompson GE, Remington JM, Millman BS, et al: Experiences with outpatient anesthesia. Anesth Analg 52: 881, 1973

146. Wetchler BV: For ambulatory surgery patients, use ketamine with caution. Same-Day Surg 8(1): 11, 1984

147. White PF: Comparative evaluation of intravenous agents for rapid sequence induction—Thiopental, ketamine and midazolam. Anesthesiology 57: 279, 1982
148. Sarnquist FH, Mathers WD, Brock-Utne J, Carr B, Canup C, Brown CR: A bioassay of a water-soluble benzodiazepine against sodium thiopental. Anesthesiology 52: 149, 1980
149. Berggren L, Eriksson I: Midazolam for induction of anaesthesia in outpatients: A comparison with thiopentone. Acta Anaesthesiol Scand 25: 492, 1981
150. Verma R, Ramasubramanian R, Sachar RM: Anesthesia for termination of pregnancy: Midazolam compared with methohexital. Anesth Analg 64: 792, 1985
151. Fragen RJ, Caldwell NJ: Awakening characteristics following anesthesia induction with midazolam for short surgical procedures. Arzneimittelforschung 31: 2261, 1981
152. Fragen RJ: The use of midazolam. Anesth Rev 12: 29, 1986
153. Alon E, Baitella L, Hossli G: Double-blind study of the reversal of midazolam-supplemented general anaesthesia with RO15-1788. Br J Anaesth 59: 455, 1987
154. Clarke RSJ, Dundee JW, Garrett RT, McArdle GK, Sutton JA: Adverse reactions to intravenous anaesthetics. Br J Anaesth 47: 575, 1975
155. Dye D, Watkins J: Suspected anaphylactic reaction to Cremophor EL. Br Med J 280: 1353, 1980
156. Rolly G, Versichelen L, Huyghe L, et al: Effect of speed of injection on induction of anaesthesia using propofol. Br J Anaesth 57: 743, 1985
157. Dundee JW, McCollum JSC, Robinson FP, Halliday NJ: Elderly patients are unduly sensitive to propofol. Anesth Analg 65: S43, 1986
158. Jones DF: Recovery from day-care anaesthesia: Comparison of a further four techniques including the use of the new induction agent diprivan. Br J Anaesth 54: 629, 1982
159. Mackenzie N, Grant IS: Comparison of the new emulsion formulation of propofol with methohexitone and thiopentone for induction of anaesthesia in day cases. Br J Anaesth 57: 725, 1985
160. Doze VA, Westphal LM, White PF: Comparison of propofol with methohexital for outpatient anesthesia. Anesth Analg 65: 1189, 1985
161. Korttila K, Nuotto E, Lichtor JL, Östman P, Apfelbaum J, Rupani G: Recovery and psychomotor effects after brief anesthesia with propofol and thiopental. Anesth Analg 68: S151, 1989
162. McCulloch MJ, Lees NW: Assessment and modification of pain on induction with propofol (Diprivan). Anaesthesia 40: 1117, 1985
163. Youngberg JA, Texitor MS, Smith DE: A comparison of induction and maintenance of anesthesia with propofol to induction with thiopental and maintenance with isoflurane. Anesth Analg 66: S191, 1987
164. Doze VA, White PF: Comparison of propofol with thiopental-isoflurane for induction and maintenance of outpatient anesthesia. Anesthesiology 65: A544, 1986
165. Johnson RG, Anderson BJ, Noseworthy TW: Diprivan versus thiopentone for outpatient surgery. Can Anaesth Soc J 33: S106, 1986
166. Henricksson BA, Carlsson P, Hallen B, et al: Propofol versus thiopentone as anesthetic agents for short operative procedures. Acta Anaesthesiol Scand 31: 63, 1987
167. Dundee JW, McCollum JSC, Milligan KR, et al: Thiopental and propofol as induction agents. Anesthesiology 65: A545, 1986
168. Fahy LT, van Mourik GA, Utting JE: A comparison of the induction characteristics of thiopentone and propofol. Anaesthesia 40: 939, 1985
169. O'Toole DP, Milligan KR, Howe JP, et al: A comparison of propofol and methohexitone as induction agents for day case isoflurane anaesthesia. Anaesthesia 42: 373, 1987
170. Grounds RM, Twigley AJ, Carli F, Whitwam JG, Morgan M: The haemodynamic effects of intravenous induction: Comparison of the effects of thiopentone and propofol. Anaesthesia 40: 735, 1985
171. Apfelbaum JL: The use of Diprivan (propofol) in procedures of one hour or less. Semin Anesth 7(Suppl 1): 21, 1988
172. Cork RC, Scipione P, Vonesh MJ, Magarelli JL, Pittman RG: Propofol infusion vs thiopental/isoflurane for outpatient anesthesia. Anesthesiology 69: A563, 1988
173. Korttila K, Faure E, Apfelbaum JL, Ekdawi M, Prunskis J, Roizen MF: Recovery from propofol

versus thiopental/isoflurane in patients undergoing outpatient anesthesia. Anesthesiology 69: A564, 1988

174. Marais M, Maher M, Wetchler BV, Korttila K, Apfelbaum JL: Reduced demands on recovery room resources with Diprivan compared to thiopental-isoflurane. Anesth Rev 15(5): 23, 1988

175. Eger EI II: Anesthetic Uptake and Action. Baltimore, Williams & Wilkins, 1974

176. Eger EI II: Effect of inspired anesthetic concentration on the rate of rise of alveolar concentration. Anesthesiology 24: 153, 1963

177. Stoelting RK, Eger EI II: An additional explanation for the second gas effect: A concentrating effect. Anesthesiology 30: 273, 1969

178. Epstein RM, Rackow H, Salnitre E, et al: Influence of the concentration effect on the uptake of anesthetic mixtures: The second gas effect. Anesthesiology 25: 364, 1964

179. Merkel G, Eger EI II: A comparative study of halothane and halopropane anesthesia. Anesthesiology 24: 346, 1963

180. Guedel AE: Inhalation Anesthesia: A Fundamental Guide, p 14. New York, Macmillan, 1937

181. Eger, EI II: Isoflurane (Forane). Madison, Wisc. ANAQUEST, 1985

182. Philip JH: Gas Man: Understanding Anesthesia Uptake and Distribution. Menlo Park, Calif., Addison-Wesley, 1984

183. Torri G, Damia G, Fabiani ML, et al: Uptake and elimination of enflurane in man. Br J Anaesth 44: 789, 1972

184. Lichtiger M, Wetchler BV, Philip BK: The adult and geriatric patient. In Wetchler BV (ed): Anesthesia for Ambulatory Surgery, p 193. Philadelphia, JB Lippincott, 1965

185. Saidman LJ, Eger EI II: Effect of nitrous oxide and of narcotic premedication on the alveolar concentration of halothane required for anesthesia. Anesthesiology 25: 302, 1964

186. Eger EI II: A review of the present status of present nitrous oxide. Amer Assoc Nurse Anesth J 54: 1, 1986

187. Bahlman SH, Eger EI II, Smith NT, et al: The cardiovascular effects of nitrous oxide–halothane anesthesia in man. Anesthesiology 35: 274, 1971

188. Smith NT, Calverley RK, Prys-Roberts C, et al: Impact of nitrous oxide on the circulation during enflurane anesthesia in man. Anesthesiology 48: 345, 1978

189. Dolan WM, Stevens WC, Eger EI II, et al: The cardiovascular and respiratory effects of isoflurane-nitrous oxide anesthesia. Can Anaesth Soc J 21: 557, 1974

190. Fink BR: Diffusion anoxia. Anesthesiology 16: 511, 1955

191. Sheffer L, Steffenson JL, Birch AA: Nitrous oxide-induced diffusion hypoxia in patients breathing spontaneously. Anesthesiology 37: 436, 1972

192. Rackow H, Salanitre E, Frumin MH: Dilution of alveolar gases during nitrous oxide excretion in man. J Appl Physiol 16: 723, 1961

193. Eger EI II: Should we not use nitrous oxide? In Eger EI II (ed): Nitrous Oxide, p 339. New York, Elsevier, 1985

194. Palazzo MGA, Strunin L. Anaesthesia and emesis: I. Etiology. Can Anaesth Soc J 31: 178, 1984

195. Burtles R, Peckett BW: Postoperative vomiting: Some factors affecting its incidence. Br J Anaesth 29: 144, 1957

196. Korttila K, Hovorka J, Erkola O: Omission of nitrous oxide does not decrease the incidence or severity of emetic symptoms after isoflurane anesthesia. Anesth Analg 66: S98, 1987

197. Hickey RF, Eger EI II: Circulatory pharmacology of inhaled anesthetics. In Miller RD (ed): Anesthesia, p 656. New York, Churchill-Livingstone, 1986

198. Smith RM (ed): Choice of inhalational anesthetics. In Anesthesia for Infants and Children, p 114. St. Louis, CV Mosby, 1980

199. Hannallah RS: Pediatric outpatient anesthesia. Urol Clin North Am 14: 51, 1987

200. Fisher DM, Robinson S, Brett CM, Perin G, Gregory GA: Comparison of enflurane, halothane and isoflurane for diagnostic and therapeutic procedures in children with malignancies. Anesthesiology 63: 647, 1985

201. McGregor M, Davenport HT, Jegier W, et al: The cardiovascular effects of halothane in normal children. Br J. Anaesth 30: 398, 1958

202. Diaz JH, Lockhart CH: Is halothane really safe in infancy? Anesthesiology 51: S313, 1979

203. Jones HD, McLaren AB: Postoperative shivering and hypoxaemia after halothane, nitrous oxide, oxygen anaesthesia. Br J Anaesth 37: 35, 1965
204. Tyrell MF, Feldman S: Headache following halothane anaesthesia. Br J Anaesth 40: 99, 1968
205. Katz RL, Bigger JT: Cardiac arrhythmias during anesthesia and operation. Anesthesiology 33: 193, 1970
206. Ryder W, Wright PA: Halothane and enflurane in dental anaesthesia. Anaesthesia 36: 492, 1981
207. Johnston RR, Eger EI II, Wilson C: A comparative interaction of epinephrine with enflurane, isoflurane, and halothane in man. Anesth Analg 55: 709, 1976
208. Sigurdsson GH, Lindahl S: Cardiac arrhythmias in intubated children during adenoidectomy: A comparison between enflurane and halothane anesthesia. Acta Anaesthesiol Scand 27: 484, 1983
209. Miller JR, Redish CH, Oehler RC: Factors in arrhythmias during dental outpatient general anesthesia. Anesth Analg 49: 701, 1970
210. Rehder KI, Forbes J, Alter H, Hessler O, Stier A: Biotransformation in man: A quantitative study. Anesthesiology 31: 560, 1967
211. Brody GL, Sweet RB: Halothane anesthesia as a possible cause of massive hepatic necrosis. Anesthesiology 24: 29, 1963
212. Lindenbaum J, Leifer E: Hepatic necrosis associated with halothane anesthesia. N Engl J Med 268: 525, 1963
213. Botty C, Brown B, Stanley V, Stephen CR: Clinical experiences with compound 347, a halogenated anesthetic agent. Anesth Analg 47: 499, 1968
214. Lebowitz MH, Blitt CD, Dillon JB: Clinical investigation of compound 347. Anesth Analg 49: 1, 1970
215. Lebowitz MH, Blitt CD, Walts LF: Depression of twitch response to stimulation of the ulnar nerve during ethrane anesthesia in man. Anesthesiology 33: 52, 1970
216. Ramsey FM, White PA, Stullken EH, Allen LL, Roy RC: Enflurane potentiation of neuromuscular blockade by atracurium. Anesthesiology 57: A225, 1982
217. Fogdall RP, Miller RD: Neuromuscular effects of enflurane, alone and combined with d-tubocurarine, pancuronium, and succinylcholine in man. Anesthesiology 42: 173, 1975
218. Foldes FF, Bencini A, Newton D: Influence of halothane and enflurane on the neuromuscular effects of ORG-Nc 45 in man. Br J Anaesth 52: 64S, 1980
219. Gencarelli PJ, Miller RD, Eger EI II, Newfield P: Decreasing enflurane concentrations and d-tubocurarine neuromuscular blockage. Anesthesiology 56: 192, 1982
220. Eger EI II: Enflurane (Ethrane). Madison, Wisc. ANAQUEST, 1985
221. Lewis JH, Zimmerman HJ, Ishak KIG, et al: Enflurane hepatotoxicity. Ann Intern Med 98: 984, 1983
222. Hoyal RHA, Prys-Roberts C, Simpson PJ: Enflurane in outpatient dental anesthesia. Br J Anaesth 52: 219, 1980
223. Wade JG, Stevens WC: Isoflurane: An anesthetic for the eighties? Anesth Analg 60: 666, 1981
224. Wolfson B, Hetrick WD, Lake CL, Siker ES: Anesthetic indices: Further data. Anesthesiology 48: 187, 1978
225. Miller RD, Eger EI II, Way WL, Stevens WC, Dolan WM: Comparative neuromuscular effects of Forane and halothane alone and in combination with d-tubocurarine in man. Anesthesiology 35: 38, 1971
226. Rupp SM, Fahey MR, Miller RD: Neuromuscular and cardiovascular effects of atracurium during nitrous oxide-fentanyl and nitrous oxide-isoflurane anesthesia. Br J Anaesth 55: 67S, 1983
227. Miller RD, Way WL, Dolar WM, Stevens WC, Eger EI II: Comparative neuromuscular effects of pancuronium, gallamine, and succinylcholine during Forane and halothane anesthesia in man. Anesthesiology 35: 509, 1971
228. Ali HH, Savarese JJ: Monitoring of neuromuscular function. Anesthesiology 45: 216, 1976
229. Rupp SM, Miller RD, Gencarelli PJ: Vecuronium-induced neuromuscular blockade during enflurane, isoflurane, and halothane anesthesia in humans. Anesthesiology 60: 102, 1984

230. Homi J, Konchigeri HN, Eckenhoff JE, Linde HW: A new anesthetic agent: Forane. Preliminary observations in man. Anesth Analg 41: 439, 1972
231. Buffington CW: Clinical evaluation of isoflurane: Reflex actions during isoflurane anesthesia. Can Anaesth Soc J 29: S35, 1982
232. Fisher DM, Robinson S, Brett CM, Perin G, Gregory GA: Comparison of enflurane, halothane and isoflurane for diagnostic and therapeutic procedures in children with malignancies. Anesthesiology 63: 647, 1985
233. Wren WS, McShane AJ, McCarthy JG, Lamont BS, Casey WF, Hannon VM: Isolfurane in paediatric anaesthesia. Anasethesia 40: 315, 1985
234. Wallin RF, Regan BM, Napoli MD, Stern IJ: Sevoflurane: A new inhalational anesthetic agent. Anesth Analg 54: 758, 1975
235. Strum DP, Eger EI II: Partition coefficients for sevoflurane in human blood, saline, and olive oil. Anesth Analg 66: 654, 1987
236. Lerman J, Gregory GA, Eger EI II: Hematocrit and the solubility of volatile anesthetics in blood. Anesth Analg 63: 911, 1984
237. Siebeck R: Uber die Aufname von Stickoxydul in Blut. Scand Arch Physiol 21: 368, 1909
238. Holaday DA, Smith FR: Clinical characteristics and biotransformation of sevoflurane in healthy human volunteers. Anesthesiology 54: 100, 1981
239. Katoh T, Ikeda K: The minimum alveolar concentration (MAC) of sevoflurane in humans. Anesthesiology 66: 301, 1987
240. Manohar M, Parks CM: Porcine systemic and regional organ blood flow during 1.0 and 1.5 minimum alveolar concentrations of sevoflurane anesthesia without and with 50% nitrous oxide. J Pharmacol Exp Ther 231: 640, 1984
241. Doi M, Ikeda K: Respiratory effects of sevoflurane. Anesth Analg 66: 241, 1987
242. Strum DP, Johnson BH, Eger EI II: Stability of sevoflurane in soda lime. Anesthesiology 67: 779, 1987
243. Imamura S, Ikeda K: Comparison of the epinephrine-induced arrhythmogenic effect of sevoflurane with isoflurane and halothane. J Anesth (Japan) 1: 62, 1987
244. Avramov MN, Shingu K, Yoshiteru O, Osawa M, Mori K: Effects of different speeds of induction with sevoflurane on the EEG of man. J Anesth (Japan) 1: 1, 1987
245. Strum DP, Johnson BH, Eger EI II: Stability of sevoflurane in soda lime. Anesthesiology 67: 779, 1987
246. Cook TL, Beppu WJ, Hitt BA, Kosek JC, Mazze RI: Renal effects and metabolism of sevoflurane in Fischer 344 rats: An in-vivo comparison with methoxyflurane. Anesthesiology 43: 70, 1975
247. Cook TL, Beppu WJ, Hitt BA, Kosek JC, Mazze RI: A comparison of renal effects and metabolism of sevoflurane and methoxylflurane in enzyme-induced rats. Anesth Analg 54: 829, 1975
248. Martis L, Lynch S, Napoli MD, Woods EF: Biotransformation of sevoflurane in dogs and rats. Anesth Analg 60: 186, 1981
249. Strum DP, Eger EI II, Johnson BH, Steffey EP, Ferrell LD: Toxicity of sevoflurane in rats. Anesth Analg 66: 769, 1982
250. Eger EI II: Partition coefficients for I-653 in human blood, saline and olive oil. Anesth Analg 66: 971, 1987
251. Rampil IJ, Zwass M, Lockhart S, Eger EI, Johnson BH, Yasuda N, Weiskopf RB: MAC of I-653 in surgical patients. Anesthesiology 71: A269, 1989
252. Jones RM, Cashman JN, Eger EI, Johnson BH, Marshall CA: Kinetics and potency of I-653 in volunteers. Anesthesiology 71: A270, 1989
253. Eger EI II, Johnson BH: Rates of awakening from anesthesia with I-653, halothane, isoflurane, and sevoflurane: A test of the effect of anesthetic concentration and duration in rats. Anesth Analg 66: 977, 1987
254. Weiskopf RB, Holmes MA, Eger EI II, Johnson BH, Rampil IJ, Brown JG: Cardiovascular effects of I-653 in swine. Anesthesiology 69: 303, 1988
255. Rampil IJ, Zwass M, Lockhart S, Eger EI, Johnson BH, Yasuda N, Weiskopf RB: Hemodynamics of I-653 in patients. Anesthesiology 71: A25, 1989
256. Cahalan M, Weiskopf R, Ionescu P, Yasuda N, Eger EI, Rampil I, Lockhart S, Freire B, Caldwell

J, Koblin D, Kelly S, Johnson B, Holmes M: Cardiovascular effects of I-653 in humans. Anesthesiology 71: A26, 1989

257. Weiskopf RB, Eger EI II, Holmes MA, et al: Epinephrine-induced premature ventricular contractions and changes in arterial blood pressure and heart rate during I-653, isoflurane, and halothane anesthesia in swine. Anesthesiology 70: 293, 1989

258. Rampil IJ, Weiskopf RB, Brown JG, et al: I-653 and isoflurane produce similar dose-related changes in the electroencephalogram of pigs. Anesthesiology 69: 298, 1988

259. Eger EI II: Stability of I-653 in soda lime. Anesth Analg 66: 987, 1987

260. Koblin DD, Eger EI II, Johnson BH, Konopka K, Waskell L: I-653 resists degradation in rats. Anesth Analg 67: 534, 1988

261. Eger EI II, Johnson BH, Strum DP, Ferrell LD: Studies of the toxicity if I-653, halothane, and isoflurane in enzyme-induced, hypoxic rats. Anesth Analg 66: 1227, 1987

262. Epstein BS, Levy ML, Thein MH, et al: Evaluation of fentanyl as an adjunct to thiopental–nitrous oxide–oxygen anesthesia for short surgical procedures. Anesth Rev 2(3): 244, 1975

263. Kitahata LM, Collins JG, Robinson CJ: Narcotic effects on the nervous system. In Kitahata LM, Collins JG (eds): Narcotic Analgesics in Anesthesiology, p 57. Baltimore, Williams & Wilkins, 1982

264. Murphy MR: Opioids. In Barash PG, Cullen BF, Stoelting RK (eds): Clinical Anesthesia, p 255. Philadelphia, JB Lippincott, 1989

265. Lowenstein E: Morphine "anesthesia"—A perspective. Anesthesiology 35: 563, 1971

266. Mummaneni N, Rao TLK, Montoya A: Awareness and recall with high-dose fentanyl-oxygen anesthesia. Anesth Analg 59: 948, 1980

267. Lichtor JL, Dohrn C, Faure EAM, Ward J, deWit H: Effectiveness of premedication in anxious patients: Does fentanyl or midazolam allay anxiety? Anesth Analg 68: S165, 1989

268. Stoelting RK: Opioid agonists and antagonists. In Stoelting RK (ed): Pharmacology and Physiology in Anesthetic Practice, p 80. Philadelphia, JB Lippincott, 1987

269. Poler SM, White PF, Margrabe D, Krause B: Nausea and vomiting in outpatients: Use of droperidol prophylaxis. Anesthesiology 71: A134, 1989

270. McClain DA, Hug C: Intravenous fentanyl kinetics. Clin Pharmacol Ther 28: 106, 1980

271. Hunt TM, Plantevin OM, Gilbert JR: Morbidity in gynaecological day-case surgery. Br J Anaesth 51: 785, 1979

272. Pollard J: Clinical evaluation of intravenous vs inhalational anesthesia in the ambulatory surgical unit: A multicenter study. Curr Ther Res 36(4): 617, 1984

273. Goroszeniuk T, Whitwam JG, Morgan M: Use of methohexitone, fentanyl and nitrous oxide for short surgical procedures. Anesthesiology 32: 209, 1977

274. Rigg JRA, Goldsmith CH: Recovery of ventilatory response to carbon dioxide after thiopentone, morphine and fentanyl in man. Can Anaesth Soc J 23: 370, 1976

275. Adams AP, Pybus DA: Delayed respiratory depression after use of fentanyl during anaesthesia. Br Med J 1: 278, 1978

276. Scamman FL: Fentanyl-O_2-N_2O rigidity and pulmonary compliance. Anesth Analg 62:332, 1983

277. White PF: Use of continuous infusion versus intermittent bolus administration of fentanyl or ketamine during outpatient anesthesia. Anesthesiology 59: 294, 1983

278. Taff RH: Pulmonary edema following naloxone administration in a patient without heart disease. Anesthesiology 59: 576, 1983

279. Clark NJ, Meuleman T, Liu W-S, Zwanikken P, Pace NL, Stanley TH: Comparison of sufentanil-N_2O in patients without cardiac disease undergoing general surgery. Anesthesiology 66: 130, 1987

280. White PF, Sung ML, Doze VA: Use of sufentanil in outpatient anesthesia: Determining an optimal preinduction dose. Anesthesiology 63: A202, 1985

281. Bailey PL, Streisand JB, Pace NL, et al: Sufentanil produces shorter lasting respiratory depression and longer lasting analgesia than equipotent doses of fentanyl in human volunteers. Anesthesiology 65: A493, 1986

282. Phitayakoran P, Melnick BM, Vicinie AF: Comparison of continuous sufentanil and fentanyl infusions for outpatient anesthesia. Can J Anaesth 34: 242, 1987

283. Zuurmond WWA, van Leeuwen L: Recovery from sufentanil anaesthesia for outpatient arthroscopy: A comparison with isoflurane. Acta Anaesthesiol Scand 31: 154, 1987

284. Wasudev G, Kambam JR, Hazlehurst WM, et al: Comparative study of sufentanil and isoflurane in outpatient surgery. Anesth Analg 66: S185, 1987

285. Bovill JG, Sebel PS, Blackburn CL, Heykants J: The pharmacokinetics of alfentanil (R39209): A new opioid analgesic. Anesthesiology 57: 439, 1982

286. van Leeuwen L, Deen L: Alfentanil, a new, potent and very short-acting morphinomimetic for minor operative procedures. Anaesthetist 30: 115, 1981

287. Hudson RJ, Stanski DR: Metabolism versus redistribution of fentanyl and alfentanil. Anesthesiology 59: A243, 1983

288. Murphy MR: Opioids. In Barash PG, Cullen BF, Stoelting RK (eds): Clinical Anesthesia, p 270. Philadelphia, JB Lippincott, 1989

289. Scott JC, Ponganis KV, Stanski DR: EEG quantitation of narcotic effect: The comparative pharmacodynamics of fentanyl and alfentanil. Anesthesiology 62: 234, 1985

290. Coe V, Shafer A, White PF: Techniques for administering alfentanil during outpatient anesthesia: A comparison with fentanyl. Anesthesiology 59: A347, 1983

291. Kennedy DJ, Ogg TW: Alfentanil and memory function: A comparison with fentanyl for day case termination of pregnancy. Anaesthesia 40: 537, 1985

292. Kay B, Venkataraman P: Recovery after fentanyl and alfentanil for minor surgery. Br J Anaesth 55: 169S, 1983

293. Kallar SK, Keenen RL: Evaluation and comparison of recovery time from alfentanil and fentanyl for short surgical procedures. Anesthesiology 61: A379, 1984

294. White PF, Coe V, Shafer A, et al: Comparison of alfentanil with fentanyl for outpatient anesthesia. Anesthesiology 64: 99, 1986

295. Raeder JC, Hole A: Outpatient laparoscopy in general anaesthesia with alfentanil and atracurium: A comparison with fentanyl and pancuronium. Acta Anaesthesiol Scand 30: 30, 1986

296. Zuurmond WWA, van Leeuwen L: Alfentanil vs isoflurane for outpatient arthroscopy. Acta Anaesthesiol Scand 30: 329, 1986

297. Short SM, Rutherford CF, Sebel PS: A comparison between isoflurane and alfentanil supplemented anaesthesia for short procedures. Anaesthesia 40: 1160, 1985

298. Jellicoe JA: A comparison of alfentanil, halothane and enflurane for day-case gynaecological surgery. Anaesthesia 40: 810, 1985

299. Zelcer J, Tyers M, White PF, Kennedy JT, Sherman GP: Comparison of alfentanil and fentanyl as adjuvants to propofol and nitrous oxide anesthesia. Anesthesiology 71: A28, 1989

300. Hug CC: New narcotic analgesics and antagonists in anesthesia. Semin Anesth 1: 14, 1982

301. Fine J, Finestone SC: A comparative study of the side-effects of butorphanol, nalbuphine and fentanyl. Anesth Rev 8(9): 13, 1981

302. Wetchler BV, Alexander CP, Shariff MSY, Gaudzels GM: A comparison of recovery in patients receiving fentanyl vs those receiving butorphanol. J Clin Anesth 1(5): 339, 1989

303. Garfield JM, Garfield FB, Philip B, et al: A comparison of clinical and psychologic effects of fentanyl and nalbuphine in ambulatory surgical patients. Anesth Analg 66: 1303, 1987

304. Mock DL, Streisand JB, Hague B, Dzelzkalns RR, Baily PL, Pace NL, Stanely TH: Transmucosal narcotic delivery: An evaluation of fentanyl (lollipop) premedication in man. Anesth Analg 65: S102, 1985

305. Streisand JB, Ashburn MA, LeMaire L, Varvel JR, Stanley TH, Tarver S: Bioavailability and absorption of oral transmucosal fentanyl citrate. Anesthesiology 71: A230, 1989

306. Chauvin M, Srumza P, Levron JC, Assoune P, Falson F: Plasma fentanyl concentration during transdermal delivery. Anesthesiology 71: A717, 1989

307. Herbert M, Healy TEJ, Bourke JB, et al: Profile of recovery after general anesthesia. Br Med J 286: 1539, 1983

308. Churchill-Davidson HC: Suxamethonium (succinylcholine) chloride and muscle pains. Br Med J 74: 209, 1954

309. Capan LM, Bruce DL, Patel KP, et al: Succinylcholine-induced postoperative sore throat. Anesthesiology 59: 202, 1983

310. Hegarty P: Postoperative muscle pains. Br J Anaesth 28: 209, 1956

311. Perry J, Wetchler BV: Outpatient anesthesia: The effects of diazepam pretreatment of succinylcholine on fasciculation or postoperative myalgia. Amer Assoc of Nurse Anesth J 52(1): 48, 1984

312. Blitt CO, Carlson GL, Rolling GO, et al: A comparative evaluation of pretreatment with nondepolarizing neuromuscular blockers prior to the administration of succinylcholine. Anesthesiology 55: 1687 1981

313. Brodsky JB, Brock-Utne JG, Samuels SI: Pancuronium pretreatment and postsuccinylcholine myalgias. Anesthesiology 51: 259, 1979

314. Sosis M, Broad T, Larijani GE, et al: Comparison of atracurium and d-tubocurarine for prevention of succinylcholine myalgia. Anesth Analg 66: 657, 1987

315. Cullen DJ: The effect of pretreatment with nondepolarizing muscle relaxants on the neuromuscular blocking action of succinylcholine. Anesthesiology 35: 572, 1971

316. Fahmy NR, Malek NS, Lappas DG: Diazepam prevents some adverse effects of succinylcholine. Clin Pharmacol Ther 26: 395, 1979

317. Erkola O, Salmenpera M, Tammisto T: Does diazepam pretreatment prevent succinylcholine-induced fasciculations? A double-blind comparison of diazepam and tubocurarine pretreatments. Anesth Analg 59: 943, 1980

318. Baraka A: Self-taming of succinylcholine-induced fasciculations. Anesthesiology 46: 292, 1977

319. Brodsky JB, Brock-Utne JG: Does "self-taming" with succinylcholine prevent postoperative myalgia? Anesthesiology 50: 265, 1979

320. Siler JN, Cook FJ, Ricca J: Does "self-taming" decrease postoperative myalgia in outpatients? Anesthesiology 52: 98, 1980

321. Shrivastava OP, Chatterji S, Kachawa S, et al: Calcium gluconate pretreatment for prevention of succinylcholine-induced myalgia. Anesth Analg 62: 59, 1983

322. Stenlake JB, Waigh RD, Urwin J, et al: Atracurium: Conception and inception. Br J Anaesth 55: 3S, 1983

323. Fisher DM, Canfell PC, Fahey MR, Rosen JI, Rupp SM, Sheiner LB, Miller RD: Elimination of atracurium in humans: Contribution of Hofmann elimination and ester hydrolysis versus organ elimination. Anesthesiology 65: 6, 1986

324. Nigrovic V, Koechel DA: Atracurium: Additional information needed. Anesthesiology 60: 606, 1984

325. Basta SJ, Ali HH, Savarese JJ, et al: Clinical pharmacology of atracurium besylate (BW 33A): A new non-depolarizing muscle relaxant. Anesth Analg 61: 723, 1982

326. Stirt JA, Katz RL, Murray AL: Intubation with atracurium in man. Anesthesiology 59: A266, 1983

327. Shanks CA: Pharmacokinetics of the nondepolarizing neuromuscular relaxants applied to calculation of bolus and infusion dosage regimens. Anesthesiology 64: 72, 1986

328. Rupp SM, McChristian JW, Miller RD: Neuromuscular effects of atracurium during halothane–nitrous oxide and enflurane–nitrous oxide anesthesia in humans. Anesthesiology 63: 16, 1985

329. Rupp SM, Miller RD, Gencarelli PJ: Vecuronium-induced neuromuscular blockade during enflurane, isoflurane and halothane anesthesia in humans. Anesthesiology 60: 102, 1984

330. Scott RP, Savarese JJ, Basta SJ: Clinical pharmacology of atracurium given in a high dose. Br J Anaesth 58: 834, 1986

331. Mehta MP, Choi WW, Gergis SD, Sokoff MD, Adophson AJ: Facilitation of rapid endotracheal intubation with divided doses of nondepolarizing neuromuscular blocking drugs. Anesthesiology 62: 392, 1985

332. Wetchler BV, Perry J: Limiting post-operative myalgia in the outpatient: Succinylcholine versus atracurium. Presented at the Medical College of Virginia Symposium on Anesthesia for Ambulatory Surgery, Williamsburg, Virginia, 1984

333. Glass P, Wilson W, Mace J, Ossey K, Maroof M: Assessment of the optimal priming dose for atracurium, pancuronium and vecuronium to obtain rapid onset muscle relaxation. Anesth Analg 66: S69, 1987

334. Starr NJ, Sethna DH, Estafanous FG: Bradycardia and asystole following the rapid administration of sufentanil with vecuronium. Anesthesiology 64: 521, 1986

335. Bencini AF, Houwertjes MC, Agoston S: Effects of hepatic uptake of vecuronium bromide and

its putative metabolites on their neuromuscular blocking actions in the cat. Br J Anaesth 57: 789, 1985

336. Lebrault C, Berger JL, D'Hollander AA, et al: Pharmacokinetics and pharmacodynamics of vecuronium (ORG NC45) in patients with cirrhosis. Anesthesiology 62: 601, 1985

337. Krieg N, Crul JF, Booij LHDJ: Relative potency of ORG NC45, pancuronium, alcuronium and tubocurarine in anaesthetized man. Br J Anaesth 52: 783, 1980

338. Lennon RL, Olson RA, Gronert GA: Atracurium or vecuronium for rapid sequence endotracheal intubation. Anesthesiology 64: 510, 1986

339. Casson WR, Jones RM: Vecuronium-induced muscular blockade: The effect of increasing dose on the speed of onset. Anaesthesia 41: 354, 1986

340. Zahl K, Apfelbaum JL: Muscle pain occurs after outpatient laparoscopy despite the substitution of vecuronium for succinylcholine. Anesthesiology 70: 408, 1989

341. Savarese JJ, Wastila WB, El-Sayad HA, Scott R, Gargarian M, Beemer G, Basta SJ, Sunder N: Comparative pharmacology of BW B1090U in the rhesus monkey. Anesth Analg 61: A306, 1984

342. Basta SJ, Savarese JJ, Ali HH, et al: The neuromuscular pharmacology of BW B1090U in anesthetized patients. Anesthesiology 63: A318, 1985

343. Ali HH, Savarese JJ, Embree PB, et al: Clinical pharmacology of BW B1090U continuous infusion. Anesthesiology 65: A282, 1986

344. Dolan WM, Eger EI, Margolis AJ: Forane increases bleeding in therapeutic suction abortion. Anesthesiology 36: 96, 1972

345. Cullen BF, Margolis AJ, Eger EI II: The effects of anesthesia and pulmonary ventilation on blood loss during therapeutic abortion. Anesthesiology 32: 108, 1971

346. Collins KM, Plantevin OM, Whitburn RH, Doyle JP. Outpatient termination of pregnancy: Halothane or alfentanil-supplemented anaesthesia. Br J Anaesth 57: 1226, 1985

347. Sidhu MS, Cullen BF: Low-dose enflurane does not increase blood loss during therapeutic abortion. Anesthesiology 57: 127, 1982

348. Hannington-Kiff JG: Measurement of recovery from outpatient general anaesthesia with simple ocular test. Br Med J 3: 132, 1970

349. Goresky GV, Steward DJ: Rectal methohexitone for induction of anesthesia in children. Can Anaesth Soc J 26: 213, 1979

350. Saint Maurice C, Laquenie G, Couturier C, et al: Rectal ketamine in paediatric anaesthesia. Br J Anaesth 51: 573, 1979

351. Stanford JB, Plantevin OM, Gilbert JR: Morbidity after day care gynaecological surgery: Comparison of enflurane with halothane. Br J Anaesth 51: 1143, 1979

352. Govaerts MJM, Sanders M: Induction and recovery with enflurane and halothane in paediatric anaesthesia. Br J Anaesth 47: 877, 1975

353. Padfield A: Recovery after outpatient isoflurane and enflurane anesthesia. Anesth Analg 64: 239, 1985

354. Azar I, Karambelkar DJ, Lear E: Neurologic state and psychomotor function following anesthesia for ambulatory surgery. Anesthesiology 60: 347, 1984

355. Korttila K, Valanne J: Recovery after outpatient isoflurane and enflurane anesthesia. Anesth Analg 64: 239, 1985

356. Enright AC, Pace-Floridia A: Recovery from anaesthesia in outpatients. A comparison of narcotic and inhalational techniques. Can Anaesth Soc J 24: 618, 1977

357. Simpson JEP, Glynn CJ, Cox AG, et al: Comparative study of short-term recovery of mental efficiency after anaesthesia. Br Med J 1: 1560, 1976

358. Rising S, Dodgson MS, Steen PA: Isoflurane vs fentanyl for outpatient laparoscoppy. Acta Anaesthesiol Scand 29: 251, 1985

359. Melnick BM, Chalasani J, Hy NTL: Comparison of enflurane, isoflurane, and continuous fentanyl infusion for outpatient anesthesia. Anesth Rev 11: 36, 1984

360. Gaskey NJ, Ferriero L, Pournaras L, Seecot J: Use of fentanyl markedly increases nausea and vomiting in gynecological short stay patients. Amer Assoc Nurse Anesth J 54: 309, 1986

361. Hempenstall PD, Campbell JPS, Bajurnow AT, et al: Cardiovascular, biochemical, and hormonal responses to intravenous sedation with local analgesia versus general anesthesia in patients undergoing oral surgery. J Oral Maxillofac Surg 44: 441, 1986

362. Blacher RS: General surgery and anesthesia: The emotional experience. In Blacher RS (ed): The Psychological Experience of Surgery, pp 1–25. New York, Wiley, 1987
363. Coniam SW, Roberts BA: Subanaesthetic infusion of althesin during local alangesia. Anaesthesia 36: 532, 1981
364. O'Callaghan AC, Normandale JP: Continuous infusion of diisoprofol (ICI-35868): Comparison with Althesin to covery surgery under local anesthesia. Anesthesia 37: 295, 1982
365. Philip BK: Supplemental medication for ambulatory procedures under regional anesthesia. Anesth Analg 64: 1117, 1985
366. Shane SM: Intravenous amnesia for total dentistry in one sitting. J Oral Surg 24: 27, 1966
367. Bennett CR: Conscious Sedation in Dental Practice, pp 14–22. St. Louis, CV Mosby, 1974
368. Baer SS: Parenteral medication for amnesalgesia in dentistry: A review. NY Dent J 37: 147, 1971
369. Wibby WW: Intravenous amnesia in general dental practice. Anesth Progr 19: 62, 1974
370. Goroszeniuk T, Whitwam JG, Morgan M: Use of methohexitone, fentanyl and nitrous oxide for short surgical procedures. Anaesthesia 32: 209, 1977
371. Dionne RA, Driscoll EJ, Gelfman SS, et al: Cardiovascular and respiratory response to intravenous diazepam, fentanyl, and methohexital in dental outpatients. J Oral Surg 39: 343, 1981
372. Campbell RL, Kallar SK: Dental outpatient anesthesia. Anesth Clin North Am 5: 167, 1987
373. Bennett CR: Conscious Sedation in Dental Practice, 2d ed, pp 12–22. St. Louis, CV Mosby, 1978
374. Shane SM: Conscious Sedation for Ambulatory Surgery, pp 1–11. Baltimore, University Park Press, 1983
375. McCarthy FM, Solomon AL, Jastak JT, et al: Conscious sedation: Benefits and risks. J Am Dental Assoc 109: 46, 1984
376. Scamman FL, Klein SL, Choi WW: Conscious sedation for procedures under local or topical anesthesia. Ann Otol Rhinol Laryngol 94: 21, 1985
377. Lynch JJ: The effects of talking on the blood pressure of hypertensive and normotensive patients. Psychosom Med 43: 25, 1981
378. Boldy DAR, English JSC, et al: Sedation for endoscopy: A comparison between diazepam and diazepam plus pethidine with naloxone reversal. Br J Anaesth 56: 1109, 1984
379. Boldy DAR, Lever LR, et al: Sedation for endoscopy: Midazolam or diazepam and pethidine? Br J Anaesth 61: 698, 1988
380. Tucker MR, Ochs MW, White RP: Arterial blood gas levels after midazolam or diazepam adminstered with or without fentanyl as an intravenous sedative for outpatient surgical procedures. J Oral Maxillofac Surg 44: 688, 1986
381. Alon E, Baitella L, Hossli G: Double-blind study of the reversal of midazolam-supplemented general anaesthesia with Ro 15-1788. Br J Anaesth 59: 455, 1987
382. White PF: Use of continuous infusion versus intermittent bolus administration of fentanyl or ketamine during outpatient anesthesia. Anesthesiology 59: 294, 1983
383. White PF, Coe V, et al: Comparison of alfentanil with fentanyl for outpatient anesthesia. Anesthesiology 64: 99, 1986
384. Seo LT, Mather LE, Cousins MJ: Comparison of the efficacy of chlormethiazole and diazepam and IV sedatives for supplementation of extradural anaesthesia. Br J Anaesth 57: 747, 1985
385. Urquhart ML, White PF: Comparison of sedative infusions during regional anesthesia: Methohexital, etomidate, and midazolam, Anesth Analg 68: 249, 1989
386. White PF, Vasconez LO, et al: Comparison of midazolam and diazepam for sedation during plastic surgery. Plast Reconstr Surg 81: 703, 1988
387. MacKenzie N, Grant IS: Propofol for intravenous sedation. Anaesthesia 42: 3, 1987
388. Patterson KW, Casey PB, et al: Propofol sedation for outpatient endoscopy: A comparison with midazolam. Anesth Analg 68: S222, 1989
389. Edmunds DH, Rosen M: Inhalation sedation for conservative dentistry: A comparison between nitrous oxide and methoxyflurane. Br Dent J 139: 398, 1987
390. Cousins MJ, Mazze RI: Methoxyflurane nephrotoxicity: A study of dose response in man. JAMA 225: 1611, 1973

391. Parbrook GD, Rees GAD, Robertson GS: Relief of postoperative pain: Comparison of a 25% nitrous oxide and oxygen mixture with morphine. Br Med J 2: 480, 1964

392. Dworkin SF, Schubert MM, Chen ACN, et al: Analgesic effects of nitrous oxide with controlled painful stimuli. J Am Dent Assoc 107: 581, 1983

393. Korttila K, Ghoneim MM, Jacobs L, et al: Time course of mental and psychomotor effects of 30% nitrous oxide during inhalation and recovery. Anesthesiology 54: 220, 1981

394. Abboud TK, Shnider SM, Wright RG, et al: Enflurane analgesia in obstetrics. Anesth Analg 60: 133, 1981

395. Rodrigo MRC, Rosenquist JB: Isoflurane for conscious sedation. Anaesthesia 43: 369, 1988

396. Kallar SK, Dunwiddie WC: Unpublished data from Ambulatory Surgery Center Data Base, Medical College of Virginia, 1988

397. Campbell RL: Prevention of complications associated with intravenous sedation and general anesthesia. J Oral Maxillofac Surg 44: 289, 1986

398. Miler JR, Redish CH, Fisch C, Oehler RC: Factors in arrhythmia during dental outpatient general anesthesia. Anesth Analg 49: 701, 1970

399. Centers for Disease Control: Maternal deaths associated with barbiturate anesthetics—New York City. MMWR 35: 579, 1986

400. Tucker MR, Ochs MW, White RPO Jr: Arterial blood gas levels after midazolam or diazepam adminstered with or without fentanyl as an intravenous sedative for outpatient surgical procedures. J Oral Maxillofac Surg 44: 688, 1986

401. Davis PJ, Cook DR: Clinical pharmacokinetics of the newer intravenous anaesthetic agents. Clin Pharmacokinet 11: 18, 1986

402. Food and Drug Administration: Warning reemphasized in midazolam labeling. FDA Drug Bull 27: 5, 1986

403. Waters RM: The Downtown Anesthesia Clinic. Am J Surg 33: 71, 1919

404. Epstein B: Outpatient anesthesia. In Hershey SG (ed): ASA Refresher Courses in Anesthesiology, Vol 2, p 80. Philadelphia, JB Lippincott, 1974

405. Natof HE: Complications associated with ambulatory surgery. JAMA 244: 1116, 1980

406. Miller J, Walts LF: Perioperative management of diabetes mellitus. In Brown BR, Blitt CD, Giesecke AH (eds): Anesthesia and the Patients with Endocrine Disease, p 92. Philadelphia, FA Davis, 1980

407. Harris MI, Hadden WC, Knowler WC, Bennett PH: Prevalence of diabetes and impaired glucose tolerance and plasma glucose levels in the U.S. population aged 20–74 yr. Diabetes 36: 523, 1987

408. Cahill GF Jr, McDevitt HO: Insulin-dependent diabetes mellitus: The initial lesion. N Engl J Med 304: 1454, 1981

409. Loughran PG, Giesecke AH: Diabetes mellitus: Anesthetic considerations. Semin Anesth 3: 207, 1984

410. Roizen MF: Endocrine abnormalities and anesthesia. In Hershey SG (ed): ASA Refresher Courses in Anesthesiology, Vol 12, p 167. Philadelphia, JB Lippincott, 1984

411. Wetchler BV: Outpatient general and spinal anesthesia. Urol Clin North Am 14(1): 31, 1987

412. Orkin FK: Selection. In Wetchler BV (ed): Anesthesia for Ambulatory Surgery, p 95. Philadelphia, JB Lippincott, 1985

413. Ingelfinger FJ: Debates on diabetes. N Engl J Med 296: 1228, 1977

414. Rosen RG, Enquist IF: The healing wound in experimental diabetes. Surgery 50: 525, 1961

415. Sieber FE, Smith DS, Traystman RJ, Wollman H: Glucose: A reevaluation of its intraoperative use. Anesthesiology 67: 72, 1987

416. Doze VA, White PF: Effects of fluid therapy on serum glucose levels in fasted outpatients. Anesthesiology 66: 223, 1987

417. Walts LF, Miller J, Davidson MB, et al: Perioperative management of diabetes mellitus. Anesthesiology 55: 104, 1981

418. Taitelman U, Reece EA, Bessman AM: Insulin in the management of the diabetic surgical patient. JAMA 237: 658, 1977

419. Meyer EJ, Lorenzi M, Bohannon NV, et al: Diabetic management by insulin infusion during surgery. Am J Surg 107: 323, 1979

420. Barnett AH, Robinson MH, Harrison JH, et al: Minipump: Method of diabetic control during minor surgery under general anaesthesia. Br Med J 1: 78, 1980

421. Alexander C, Wong HC: In the real world. In Wetchler BV (ed): Anesthesia for Ambulatory Surgery, p 387. Philadelphia, JB Lippincott, 1985

422. Vaughan RW: Definitions and risks of obesity. In Brown BR Jr (ed): Anesthesia and the Obese Patient, p 107. Philadelphia, FA Davis, 1982

423. Jensen S, Wetchler BV: The obese patient: An acceptable candidate for outpatient anesthesia. J Am Assoc Nurs Anesth 50: 369, 1982

424. Vaughan RW, Bauer S, Wise L: Volume and pH of gastric juice in obese patients. Anesthesiology 43: 686, 1975

425. Paul DR, Hoyt JL,Boutros AR: Cardiovascular and respiratory changes in response to change of posture in the very obese. Anesthesiology 45: 73, 1976

426. Tseuda K, Debrand M, Zeok S, Wright BD, Griffin WO: Obesity supine death syndrome: Reports of two morbidly obese patients. Anesth Analg 58(4): 345, 1979

427. Kowalski SE: Mitral valve prolapse. Can Anaesth Soc J 32(2): 138, 1985

428. Wynne J: Mitral valve prolapse. N Engl J Med 314: 377, 1986

429. Barlow JB, Pocock W, Marchand P, Deany M: The significance of late systolic murmurs. Am Heart J 66: 443, 1963

430. Savage DD, Devereux RB, Garrison RJ, et al: Mitral valve prolapse in the general population: II. Clinical features. The Framingham study. Am Heart J 106: 577, 1983

431. Aranda JM, Befeler B, Lazzara R, Embi A, Machado H: Mitral valve prolapse and coronary artery disease: Clinical hemodynamic and angiographic correlations. Circulation 52: 245, 1975

432. Pickering NJ, Brody JI, Barrett MJU: Von Willebrand syndromes and mitral valve prolapse: Linked mesenchymal dysplasias. N Engl J Med 305: 131, 1981

433. Nishimura RA, McGoon MD, Shub C, Miller FA Jr, Ilstrup DM, Tajik AJ: Echocardiographically documented mitral valve prolapse: Long-term follow-up of 237 patients. N Engl J Med 313: 1305, 1985

434. Twersky RS, Kaplan JA: Junctional rhythm in a patient with mitral valve prolapse. Anesth Analg 65: 975, 1986

435. Krantz EM, Viljoen JF, Schermer R, et al: Mitral valve prolapse. Anesth Analg 59: 379, 1980

436. Legler DC: Uncommon diseases and cardiac anesthesia. In Kaplan JA (ed): Cardiac Anesthesia, 2d ed, p 796. New York, Harcourt Brace Jovanovich, 1987

437. Shulman ST, Amren DP, Bisno AL, et al: Prevention of bacterial endocarditis. Circulation 70: 1123A, 1984

438. Hickey AJ, MacMahon SW, Wilcken DEL: Mitral valve prolapse and bacterial endocarditis: Occurrence in patients with mitral valve prolapse. Arch Intern Med 146: 119, 1986

439. Kaye D: Prophylaxis for infective endocarditis: An update. Ann Intern Med 104: 419, 1986

440. Bergquist EJ, Murphy SA: Prophylactic antibiotics for surgery. Med Clin North Am 71(3): 357, 1987

441. Diagnostic and Statistical Manual of Mental Disorders, 3d ed. Washington, American Psychiatric Association, 1980

442. U.S. Department of Health and Human Services: Main Findings 1982: National Survey on Drug Abuse. Washington, USDHHS, 1983

443. Vaillant GE: Alcoholism and drug dependence. In Nicholi AM Jr (ed): The Harvard Guide to Modern Psychiatry, p 567. Cambridge, Mass., Harvard University Press, 1978

444. Roizen MF: Anesthetic implications of concurrent diseases. In Miller RD (ed): Anesthesia, p 207. New York, Churchill-Livingstone, 1986

445. Rabinowitz IN, Watson W, Farber EM: Topical steroid depression of the hypothalamic-pituitary-adrenal axis in psoriasis vulgaris. Dermatologica 154: 321, 1977

446. Byyny RL: Preventing adrenal insufficiency during surgery. Postgrad Med 67: 219, 1980

447. Miller RD: Anesthesia for the elderly. In Miller RD (ed): Anesthesia, p 1801. New York, Churchill-Livingstone, 1986

448. Vandam LD: To Make the Patient Ready for Anesthesia: Medical Care of the Surgical Patient, 2d ed, pp 231–233. Reading, Mass., Addison-Wesley, 1983

449. Evans TI: Problems in general anesthesia-geriatrics. Aust Fam Physician 6: 339, 1977

450. Janis K: Anesthesia for the geriatric patient. In Hershey SG (ed): ASA Refresher Courses in Anesthesiology. Philadelphia, JB Lippincott, 1979

451. Tiret L, Desmonts JM, Hatton F, et al: Complications associated with anaesthesia: A prospective survey in France. Can Anaesth Soc J 33: 336, 1986

452. Stephen CR: The risk of anesthesia and surgery in the geriatric patient. In Krechel SW (ed): Anesthesia and the Geriatric Patient. Orlando, Fla., Grune & Stratton, 1984

453. Fisch C: Electrogram in the aged: An independent marker of heart disease? Am J Med 70: 4, 1981

454. Lichtiger M, Moya F: Physiologic and pathologic considerations in the geriatric patient. Curr Rev Nurs Anesth 1: 1, 1978

455. Brown LL: Anesthesia in the geriatric patient. Clin Plast Surg. 12: 51, 1985

456. Gibbs CP, Modell JH: Aspiration pneumonitis. In Miller RD (ed): Anesthesia, p 2023. New York, Churchill-Livingstone, 1986

457. Manchikanti L, Colliver JA, Marrero TC, et al: Assessment of age-related acid aspiration risk factors in pediatric, adult, and geriatric patients. Anesth Analg 64: 11, 1985

458. Greenblatt DJ, Sellers EM, Shader RI: Drug disposition in old age. N Engl J Med 306: 1081, 1982

459. Maltry JR, Sutherland AD, Sale JP, et al: Preoperative oral fluids: Is a five-hour fast justified prior to elective surgery? Anesth Analg 65: 1112, 1986

460. Natof HE: Ambulatory surgery: Patients with preexisting medical problems. Ill Med J 166(2): 101, 1984

461. Bruns HD: The ambulant after-treatment of cataract extraction. Trans Am Ophthalmol Soc 14: 476, 1916

462. Hamilton RC: Regional anaesthesia for cataract extraction and intraocular lens implanatation. Reg Anesth 13: 2S, 1988

463. Gills JB, Loyd TL: A technique of retrobulbar block with paralysis of orbicularis oculi. Am Intraocular Implant Soc J 9: 339, 1983

464. Nicoll JMV, Treuren B, Acharya A, et al: Retrobulbar anesthesia: The role of hyaluronidase. Anesth Analg 65: 1324, 1986

465. Hamilton RC: Dual peribulbar block, a safe method of regional anaesthesia for ophthalmic surgery, with improved standards of patient comfort: A report of 3500 administrations. Can J Anaesth 34(3): S117, 1987

466. Donlon JV: Anesthesia for ophthalmic surgery. Curr Rev Clin Anesth 15(9): 114, 1989

467. Stone DJ, DiFazio CA: Sedation for patients with Parkinson's disease undergoing ophthalmologic surgery. Anesthesiology 68: 821, 1988

468. Zahl K, Jordan A, Sorensen B, et al: pH-adjusted lidocaine/bupivacaine mixtures are superior for peribulbar anesthesia. Anesthesiolgy 69: 3A, 1988

469. Meyers EF: Problems during eye surgery under local anesthesia. Anesth Rev 6(7): 23, 1979

470. Chang JL, Gonzalez-Avola E, Larson C, et al: Brainstem anesthesia following retrobulbar block. Anesthesiology 61: 789, 1984

471. Follette JW, LoCascio JA: Bilateral amaurosis following unilateral retrobulbar block. Anesthesiology 63: 237, 1985

472. Wang BC, Bogart BI, Hillman DE, et al: Subarachnoid injection: A potential complication of retrobulbar block. Anesthesiology 69: A369, 1988

473. Rosenblatt RM: Cardiopulmonary arrest after retrobulbar block. Am J. Ophthalmol 90: 425, 1980

474. Rigg JD, James RH: Apnoea after retrobulbar block. Anaesthesia 44: 26, 1989

475. Lee DS, Kwon NJ: Shivering following retrobulbar block. Can J Anaesth 35: 294, 1988

476. Nicoll JMV, Acharya PA, Ahlen K, et al: Central nervous system complications after 6000 retrobulbar blocks. Anesth Analg 66: 1298, 1987

477. Zeitlin GL, Hobin K, Platt J, et al: Accumulation of carbon dioxide during eye surgery. J Clin Anesth 1(4): 262, 1989

478. Kareti RKP, Callahan H, Draper GA: Factors leading to hospital admission of elderly patients following outpatient eye surgery: A medical dilemma. Anesth Analg 68: S144, 1989

479. Chung F, Lavelle PA, McDonald S, et al: Cognitive impairment after neuroleptanalgesia in cataract surgery. Anesth Analg 68: 614, 1989

480. McMahan LB: Ambulatory eye surgery. J Miss State Med Assoc 24(7): 181, 1983

481. Conahan TJ, Williams GD, Apfelbaum JL, et al: Airway heating reduces recovery time in outpatients. Anesthesiology 63: A166, 1985

482. Gregory GA, Eger EI II, Munson ES: The relationship between age and halothane requirement in man. Anesthesiology 30: 488, 1969

483. Stevens WC, Dolan WM, Gibbons RT, et al: Minimum alveolar concentrations (MAC) of isoflurane with and without nitrous oxide in patients of various age. Anesthesiology 42: 197, 1975

484. Dundee JW, Robinson FP, McCollum JSC, et al: Sensitivity to propofol in the elderly. Anaesthesia 41: 482, 1986

485. Dundee JW, Milligan KR, Furness G: Influence of age and gender on induction dose of thiopental. Anesthesiology 67: A662, 1987

486. Steib A, Freys G, Beller JP, et al: Propofol in elderly high risk patients: A comparison of haemodynamic effects with thiopentone during induction of anaesthesia. Anaesthesia 43: 111, 1988

487. Scott JC, Stanski DR: Decreased fentanyl/alfentanil dose requirements with increasing age: A pharmacodynamic basis. Anesthesiology 63: A374, 1985

488. O'Hara DA, Fragen RJ, Shanks CA: The effects of age on the dose-response curves for vecuronium in adults. Anesthesiology 63: 542, 1985

489. d'Hollander AA, Luyckx C, Barvais L, et al: Clinical evaluation of atracurium besylate requirement for a stable muscle relaxation during surgery: Lack of age-related effects. Anesthesiology 59: 237, 1983

490. Valentin N, Lomholt B, Jensen JS, et al: Spinal or general anaesthesia for surgery of the fractured hip? A prospective study of mortality in 578 patients. Br J Anaesth 58: 284, 1986

491. Chung F, Meier R, Lautenschlager E, et al: General or spinal anesthesia: Which is better in the elderly? Anesthesiology 67: 422, 1987

492. Lichtiger M, Wetchler BV, Philip BK: The adult and geriatric patient. In Wetchler BV (ed): Anesthesia for Ambulatory Surgery, p 175. Philadelphia, JB Lippincott, 1985

493. Stanley B, Guido J, Stanley M, et al: The elderly patient and informed consent. JAMA 252: 1302, 1984

494. Crawford FJ: Ambulatory surgery: The elderly patient. AORN J 41: 356, 1985

495. Moore AR: Surgery and the aged. Aust Fam Physician 7: 1045, 1978

Local and Regional Anesthesia

6

BEVERLY K. PHILIP, BENJAMIN G. COVINO

Local anesthesia may be defined as a temporary loss of sensation due to the inhibition of nerve endings in a specific part of the body. Local anesthesia is often performed by a surgeon for relatively minor procedures. *Regional anesthesia* may be defined as the interruption of impulses in specific nerve fibers innervating a larger body area. Regional anesthetic techniques are usually performed by an anesthesiologist for more complex procedures. Local and regional anesthesia have long been used for ambulatory surgery; in 1963 and 1964, 56% of ambulatory procedures at the University of California, Los Angeles were performed by these techniques.[1] Success with local and regional anesthesia for ambulatory patients begins with appropriate preparation. A team of anesthesiologist, surgeon, and nurse who enthusiastically support these techniques for the patient must be assembled. The patient must be psychologically suitable and medically free of contraindications. His or her cooperation must be gained by appropriate education. Local anesthetic drugs must be chosen that are effective in the desired time frame, and anesthetic techniques should be employed that will provide patient and surgeon with satisfactory operative conditions. Premedication and supplemental sedation, both verbal and medicinal, maybe used to augment the block-induced analgesia, but they should not delay discharge. Finally the complications of local and regional anesthesia must be known, avoided when possible, and appropriately treated if they occur.

PREPARATION
Excellent conditions for ambulatory surgery that will satisfy patient, surgeon, and anesthesiologist can be obtained with local and regional anesthesia. To achieve

this optimal outcome, all members of the team must be carefully selected. Also, the inherent limitations of local and regional anesthesia itself must be appreciated.

The anesthesiologist must have the personality and skills to communicate well with patients and be able to gain trust rapidly. He or she must be confident, competent, and gentle. The anesthesiologist also functions as an educator. This has particular importance for regional ambulatory anesthesia, because the prepared patient is better able to cooperate. Information needed by the patient includes the minor discomforts often associated with administration of local or regional anesthesia, such as intradermal injection for skin analgesia, insertion of block needle, or paresthesias. The anesthesiologist also must teach the patient to expect sensations that will not be blocked by the anesthetic, such as pressure and movement, and about the often disquieting sensations of numbness, paralysis, and dissociation of the involved body part. The quality of sensation as it returns and postoperative discomforts also need to be discussed. The anesthesiologist must forewarn about sights, sounds, or smells the awake patient may experience during the course of the surgery. Potential complications of the planned anesthetic technique should be discussed, and the patient should be instructed to call the ambulatory surgery unit if any develop. The anesthesiologist who plans to use regional anesthesia must know and be able to discuss the relative benefits of regional anesthesia in an informative but nonthreatening manner.

This detailed preoperative explanation of expected intraoperative and postoperative sensations should be made before the patient is in the operating room. Preoperative teaching can be completed in a quiet office or waiting area in the ambulatory unit on the day of surgery. Anesthesia screening clinics have been established to which the patient comes either on the day of the preoperative surgical appointment or at some time between the scheduling of surgery and the day of operation. A separate anesthesia evaluation and discussion, before the day of surgery, does allow a more relaxed presentation of the benefits and experiences of regional anesthesia.

It is self-evident that the anesthesiologist who plans to perform local or regional anesthesia for ambulatory procedures must be technically skilled. An ambulatory surgery unit is not the place to learn regional blocks. The anesthesiologist's expertise must include choice of the appropriate technique, anesthetic drug, and, if indicated, appropriate sedation to supplement the block. In summary, satisfactory regional anesthesia for ambulatory surgery requires preoperative education, intraoperative analgesia from proper local anesthetic placement, and possibly intravenous supplementation.

For regional anesthesia to be successful for the ambulatory surgery patient, the surgeon must support it. Surgeons with experience in operating on patients under local or regional anesthesia in ambulatory surgery have enthusiastically recommended this anesthesia to other surgeons for herniorrhaphies, laparoscopies, and anorectal and urologic procedures. Support must begin preoperatively, with the surgeon suggesting and encouraging the use of regional blocks to the patient. At the time of operation, the surgeon should be tolerant of extra time that is sometimes required for the performance of the regional anesthetic procedure and for analgesia to develop fully. Inserting the slower-onset epidural or brachial plexus block early, in a holding area or induction room, can be a decided advantage. Preoperative and intraoperative communication between the surgeon and anesthesiologist about duration and extent of surgery is imperative. Since not all sensations are blocked by regional anesthesia, the surgeon must be gentle with the patient's tissues and use careful surgical technique. The particular challenge of operating on an awake and listening patient also should be appreciated.

The surgical procedure also must be compatible with ambulatory regional anesthesia. The body part involved must be accessible by local or regional block. A related issue is the need for the surgeon often to tailor surgical technique to accommodate the not-total loss of sensation that occurs even with good local or regional blockade. For laparoscopic tubal ligation to be well tolerated by the awake patient, surgeons have advocated the use of nitrous oxide rather than carbon dioxide as the insufflating gas, limiting intraperitoneal gas volume and pressure, using only a moderate Trendelenburg position, and applying local anesthetic solution to the uterine and tubal surfaces before manipulation or fulguration.[2] Enthusiastic participation of the ambulatory surgical nurse is invaluable in teaching, encouraging, and preparing a regional anesthesia patient for the procedure.

Local and regional anesthesia has several specific advantages that recommend it to the patient. Recovery time is significantly shorter. For a variety of ambulatory surgical procedures, recovery after local and regional anesthesia required 136 minutes, as compared to 207 minutes after general anesthesia.[3] For patients undergoing laparoscopic tubal sterilization, recovery time was reduced from 176 minutes under general anesthesia to 103 minutes under lumbar epidural block.[4] The likelihood of postoperative hospital admission is also less. In the same series of various ambulatory procedures,[3] 2.9% of the patients who had general anesthesia required admission, compared to 1.2% of those who had local or regional blockade. Another advantage is the postoperative analgesia that can be provided with numbness limited to the operative site. Surgical complications can be reduced; blood loss after therapeutic abortion is least in the patients receiving local anesthesia. Also, complications specific to procedures, such as pneumothorax with laparoscopy, can be detected earlier in a conscious patient. Avoidance of the discomforts of general anesthesia may be most important to the patient. Sore throat, muscle pains, airway trauma, and dizziness are minimized. In a series of patients receiving lumbar epidural rather than general anesthesia for laparoscopy, the incidence of nausea and vomiting was reduced from 38% to 4%.[4] Also, some patients would rather not "go to sleep." This stems from a curiosity about the surgical experience, from a desire to be aware and retain some control over the situation, or from a strong fear of general anesthesia.

The primary requirement for successful ambulatory anesthesia remains proper patient selection. Regional anesthesia requires ongoing cooperation by the patient; patients must be chosen who are psychologically suitable. Education and preparation of the patient by surgeon and anesthesiologist can be decisive in achieving success. Of 116 appropriately chosen and educated patients, 98% were able to complete laparoscopies under local anesthesia.[5] On the other hand, patients who overreact to minor discomforts or who are severely apprehensive or anxious are better excluded. Mentally retarded patients can be handled successfully under ambulatory regional anesthesia with appropriate sedation. These patients often have medical and surgical problems that suggest the use of local or regional anesthesia, and on the whole, the handicapped patients' needs may be better met by same-day surgery, which allows them to return to their home or institution rapidly. In a recent series of 132 handicapped patients, 53% were able to complete dental restorations without general anesthesia.[6] The young child may not be able to understand enough to cooperate with the insertion of a block and maintenance of regional anesthesia. However, caudal anesthesia applied during the surgical general anesthetic can be successfully used to provide intraoperative and postoperative analgesia even for newborn infants.[7] The elderly patient may be a particularly good candidate for regional anesthesia. Pain sensation is decreased, allowing better tolerance of minor discomforts. The incidence of postdural puncture headache after spinal anesthesia decreases with age. Protective airway reflexes are also attenuated in the elderly,[8] which may increase the possibility of aspiration under general anesthesia.

On the other hand, the older patient is less tolerant of adverse physiologic changes that may occur, such as hypotension, with spinal or epidural anesthesia. Decreased sympathetic nervous system activity and a reduced intravascular volume, due to drugs or decreased fluid intake, combine to increase the incidence of hypotension. The dose of local anesthetic for epidural anesthesia may need to be reduced with age.[9] The duration of spinal anesthesia may be prolonged in the elderly because of decreased blood flow in the vessels surrounding the subarachnoid space and therefore decreased anesthetic removal. Blocks can be more difficult to perform because of intervertebral narrowing and calcification. Drugs for supplemental sedation may generate an unexpectedly large effect owing to decreased liver and kidney function. Elderly individuals are more likely to have cardiovascular, respiratory, or other systemic disease; ASA status 3 older patients can be offered ambulatory regional anesthesia after individual anesthetic consultation if their underlying diseases are stable. However, these patients may be better cared for in a hospital (integrated, separated) unit. The elderly also may have associated problems that will interfere with the success of a regional anesthetic, such as tremors, inability to communicate due to deafness or blindness, and disorders of mentation such as confusion and disorientation.[10] Choosing supplemental medications that are tailored to the elderly patient's particular problem can greatly improve success with regional techniques, such as using diphenhydramine to quiet the tremors associated with parkinsonism.[11] Regional anesthesia is a good choice for the older patient, but it should be used with knowledge and care.

Ambulatory patients receiving local or regional anesthesia must be as carefully evaluated and prepared as those who receive general anesthesia. Preoperative requirements should include a written medical history and physical examination for all patients. Surgery under local anesthesia alone can result in cardiorespiratory complications. Changes in systolic blood pressure of at least 40 mmHg have been recorded in 16% of a series of patients undergoing local anesthesia without anesthesia personnel supervision.[12] Meyers reported that 5.6% of approximately 1000 cataract surgery procedures under local anesthesia generated emergency calls for an anesthesiologist.[10] Prompt and appropriate intervention requires definite knowledge of the patient's underlying physical conditions as documented in the history and physical examination report. Appropriate laboratory evaluations are needed for patients who are receiving intravenous sedation or regional block and are suggested for patients undergoing local anesthesia.

Intraoperative monitoring is essential to the safety of local and regional ambulatory anesthesia. Monitoring begins with the assessment of mental status by verbal communication. This is adequate for minor procedures under purely local anesthesia. For more complex procedures requiring intravenous sedation or more extensive anesthesia or regional blockade, additional monitoring is needed. Audible and visible devices displaying cardiac rhythm and blood pressure should be used. A stethoscope placed on the precordium or at the sternal notch monitors respiration as well. An automated blood pressure device is particularly convenient if the circulating nurse is also responsible for watching the patient. However, if intravenous sedation is necessary to complete the procedure, an anesthesiologist should be present. This individual is specifically trained in the safe dosage and duration of action of anesthetics, sedatives, and analgesics and in the identification and treatment of complications of these agents. He or she is responsible solely for monitoring the effects of drug administration on the patient without being distracted by the need to obtain supplies or assist surgery.

When supplemental medications are provided, the potential problem arises of hypoventilation induced by these respiratory depressant drugs. Monitoring of expired carbon dioxide is therefore indicated as an early detector of underventilation or apnea.[13] For a patient having local or regional anesthesia, a CO_2 gas sampling line can be connected to the face mask or nasal prongs often used to provide supplemental oxygen. Pulse oxygen saturation also should be monitored using oximetry. In one study, 39% of patients in a plastic surgery facility who were receiving clinically appropriate sedation developed saturations of less than 89%.[14] The pulse oximeter can detect hypoxemia from a variety of respiratory and circulatory causes before tissue hypoxia develops and a catastrophic event occurs.[15]

Before any local or regional anesthetic is administered, facilities must be present to support a full resuscitation. "Local anesthesia rooms," which may not have a dedicated anesthesia machine, must have immediate access to equipment able to support ventilation, including a manual resuscitation bag, masks, and oral, nasal, and endotracheal airways. Sources of 100% oxygen and suction are needed, as are intravenous fluids and the equipment to start an infusion. These supplies, plus drugs for cardiopulmonary resuscitation and treatment of convulsions, should be stored together in a well-organized and labeled container, such as a mobile crash cart. This equipment must be inspected regularly and staff familiarized with its use. All patients receiving intravenous sedation or any regional block must have an intravenous access line.[16]

The question is often raised whether ambulatory patients for regional anesthesia should be fasting. Ambulatory surgery patients are at risk for pulmonary sequelae of acid aspiration; 60% of ambulatory surgery patients in one study had gastric aspirates of low pH ($\leq$2.5) and elevated volume ($\geq$25 ml).[17] Cigarette smoking also increases outpatient gastric volume.[18] Surgeons should be aware that excessive amounts of local anesthetic can cause a systemic reaction with convulsions or loss of consciousness, which may result in aspiration. Even without a toxic reaction, the ambulatory regional anesthesia patient can be at risk because of supplemental medications given. The administration of 50% nitrous oxide in oxygen depresses the swallowing response, part of reflex closure of the glottis.[19] The use of 50% nitrous oxide to supplement local anesthesia has been shown to cause laryngeal incompetence and tracheal soiling in 20% of patients.[8] Heavy neuroleptanalgesia has been shown to have the same effect in 100% of patients.[20] Supplemental medications, particularly narcotics, may nauseate the patient or cause vomiting. "Heavy sedation" may well be in fact general anesthesia. The ambulatory regional anesthesia patient is already at risk for aspiration; increasing that potential by adding a full stomach is adding unacceptable additional hazard.

Drug interaction is also an important consideration. Ambulatory surgery patients may be taking medicines that interact or interfere with the administration of regional anesthesia. Anticoagulation with coumadin or heparin is a contraindication to major regional anesthesia (spinal and epidural) because of the risk of epidural hematoma formation and paraplegia. Anticoagulation also should be evaluated cautiously for other blocks with a significant possibility of large vessel puncture, such as brachial plexus anesthesia. Large doses of aspirin also may interfere with coagulation.[21] If major regional block is considered in these patients, bleeding, clotting, and platelet studies should be performed. The safety of performing regional anesthesia for patients on "minidose" heparin anticoagulation is still in some doubt.

Antihypertensive agents with effects on the sympathetic nervous system can alter patient's response to the vasopressors that may be needed for spinal or epidural anesthesia. Rauwolfia alkaloids deplete norepinephrine stores in postganglionic sympathetic nerves, so that hypotension during major regional anesthesia may be more difficult to treat. Guanethidine and alpha-methyldopa sensitize postsynaptic effector sites to norepinephrine. The intraoperative response to direct-acting sympathomimetic drugs such as phenylephrine and methoxamine may therefore be exaggerated and the response to indirect vasopressors such as ephedrine may be attenuated. Treatment of hypertension or coronary artery disease often includes beta-adrenergic antagonist drugs such as propranolol. The usual compensatory mechanisms for intraoperative hypotension may be lost owing to drug effect, resulting in inability to increase myocardial contractility or heart rate and inability to vasoconstrict unblocked segments. Correction of intraoperative hypotension in the presence of these drugs requires increased doses of beta-adrenergic agonist drugs acting through blocked pathways; drugs with significant alpha-adrenergic effect such as metaraminol or phenylephrine should be used if the response is inadequate. Atropine and calcium are also effective. Propanolol and cimetidine can decrease the clearance rate of lidocaine from plasma. Since lidocaine is cleared largely by the liver, this effect is due to either a reduction in cardiac output and hepatic blood flow or to competition for hepatic enzyme systems that degrade lidocaine. Systemic lidocaine effects, particularly toxicity, may be enhanced in patients taking propranolol or cimetidine.

Antidepressant drug therapy also may interact with regional anesthetic administration. Tricyclic antidepressants inhibit norepinephrine uptake at postganglionic neurons in the periphery and within the central nervous system.[21] The patient's response to epinephrine and indirect vasopressors during regional anesthesia may be exaggerated. Monamine oxidase inhibitors (MAOIs) also may precipitate an excessive response to indirect vasopressors; epinephrine and norepinephrine are tolerated because of alternate metabolic pathways.[22] The catastrophic interaction between MAOIs and drugs used for supplemental sedation, particularly meperidine, also must be remembered. Butyrophenone derivatives used for supplementation, such as haloperidol or droperidol, may antagonize L-dopa and exacerbate the symptoms of parkinsonism. Other chronic medications also may interact. In patients receiving cimetidine, diazepam clearance is delayed and sedation increased. Exposure to organophosphate insecticides or to cancer chemotherapeutic drugs such as cyclophosphamide and the nitrogen mustards decreases plasma cholinesterase levels. The patient may experience a prolonged regional block if the anesthetic agent chosen is an ester. Echothiophate eye drops are used to constrict the pupil for glaucoma therapy; decreased plasma pseudocholinesterase levels result from systemic absorption, with a similar clinical result on the duration of ester anesthetic block.

Procedure-specific complications are different under local or regional anesthesia than under general anesthesia. The overall complication rate, however, may be the same. Grimes and coworkers found an incidence of 0.35% for complications after abortion under general anesthesia, with greater risk of uterine perforation, cervical injury, and intraabdominal hemorrhage.[23] Under local anesthesia, the incidence was 0.30% (not statistically different), with increased risk of fever and convulsions. Local and regional blocks themselves do have morbidity. Interscalene block may cause phrenic paralysis, and intercostal block may result in spinal anesthesia. Limb exsanguination, as would be performed for intravenous regional anesthesia, has caused a fatal pulmonary embolus.[24] Furthermore, the use of excessive sedation in conjunction with a local or regional block may interfere with a patient's cooperation and jeopardize the success of the procedure.

Evaluation of recovery from regional anesthesia and criteria for discharge are discussed in Chapter 7.

USE OF PREMEDICATION AND SUPPLEMENTAL SEDATION
General Considerations

Premedication serves to reduce fear and anxiety. In addition, premedication and supplemental sedation can provide analgesia, facilitate venipuncture, prevent postoperative nausea and vomiting, and possibly, provide amnesia. Premedicant and supplemental drugs can improve patient tolerance and acceptance of regional anesthetic techniques, particularly when the patient would rather not be fully awake. However, the use of drugs to premedicate patients for ambulatory regional anesthesia is not without problems. The recovery time from local anesthesia with sedation can be longer than from a general anesthetic, and discharge on the day of surgery may be delayed. Premedicant drugs have their own complications, particularly if an inappropriate drug or dose is given. Premedicant drugs should be carefully tailored to the needs of the patient and requirements of the procedure to produce desired effects while minimizing undesired side-effects.[25] When premedication is not needed for the ambulatory regional anesthesia patient, it should not be used to make the anesthesiologist more comfortable.

Oral medications are preferred by some patients to "another needle." Timing of administration is important. If a premedicant is to be given orally, it should be given early enough to be working by the time anxiety-provoking preparations begin. Oral drugs must therefore be given 1 to 2 hours in advance. Supervised administration of the pill to ensure a limited fluid intake is preferable. The anxious patient who regularly takes a sedative at home may on occasion be permitted to continue his or her chronic medication, with appropriate preoperative instruction. The oral premedication chosen should have a duration of action adequate to continue until insertion of the regional block and surgery, but sufficiently limited neither to interfere with the patient's ability to comprehend postoperative instructions nor to delay resumption of usual activities. Intramuscular premedication is not recommended, since a similarly tardy onset and duration of effect are obtained only after a painful injection well before the procedure.

Premedication also can be given intravenously, shortly before the local or regional anesthetic. This is the preferred route, since it avoids the need for the patient to be in the ambulatory unit for a long time before operation. The patient is not chemically sedated before preparations begin, but medication is given promptly after venipuncture and is soon effective. The patient becomes relaxed and is more prepared for insertion of the regional block. Intravenous sedation should be given in small, incremental doses, and the effect should be titrated carefully. Intravenous premedication can then be continued as intraoperative sedation. Intraoperative supplementation may be given in repeated small doses or as a continuous infusion. Administration by continuous infusion may result in lower total drug dose and fewer side effects. However, close attention is needed for frequent readjustment of dosage and infusion rate in response to changing surgical stimulation. Use of a predetermined continuous infusion rate may result in inappropriate dosing.

Is amnesia an appropriate attribute of ambulatory premedication? Brief amnesia may be useful during painful or lengthy series of local anesthetic injections. Thompson noted that patients who appeared in distress during endoscopy but who did not remember it as unpleasant because of supplemental medication were satisfied with their experience.[26] Drug choice and dosage remain important. It also should be emphasized that a lack of recall of perioperative events may be disturbing to some patients, particularly those who chose regional anesthesia to remain in contact with the proceedings.

Perhaps the most effective and innocuous premedication for ambulatory regional anesthesia is verbal reassurance. Egbert and colleagues reported that the patients who were visited by an anesthesiologist and received an explanation of what was to happen were not drowsy but were subjectively and objectively calm.[27] Many patients facing surgery, particularly those facing minor surgery on the genitourinary tract, are afraid of the procedure, anesthesia, and possible complications. Patients are afraid of the unknown, of general hazards including pain, injury, and death, and of specific hazards such as nausea, vomiting, and loss of consciousness and control. Fear of local or regional anesthesia may stem from a lack of understanding of what is involved. This fear is best combatted by providing knowledge and information.

Verbal reassurance does not end when the block is inserted. Reassurance and explanations must continue throughout the operation so that the regional anesthesia patient remains calm. Need for supplemental medications will thereby be decreased. The patient can be helped to remain calm by limiting surgery-related noise of instruments and loud conversations. Listening to music has been shown to reduce the need for sedatives during procedures under regional anesthesia.[28] Distraction with music through headphones is frequently used in our institution; the patient is requested to bring in tapes of preferred music. Alternatively, the institution may provide a modest assortment of music of different styles. Radio or taped music played over speakers in the operating room is also useful but is less effective, becoming part of the general background clatter.

The ambulatory surgery patient receiving regional rather than general anesthesia must be more in control of anxieties and fears in order to cooperate in making surgery under block successful. The ambulatory regional patient cannot simply accede passively to preparations until consciousness is lost. There is, therefore, more of a need for premedication and supplemental sedation in the regional anesthesia patient. Certain characteristics of regional blocks and their administration and maintenance also recommend the use of supplemental medication. Regional blocks can be painful on insertion and, once in effect, may not be able to obliterate all sensation, particularly from the viscera. Supplemental medication also can help the patient to lie still for relatively long periods of time on a hard operating table. The use of sedation increases the acceptability of regional anesthesia for patients who do not desire to be completely awake in the operating room. In the absence of a general anesthetic, judiciously given premedicants are less likely to delay a patient's discharge. Tables 6-1 and 6-2 provide summaries of approximate drug dosages.

Ataractics
Diazepam
Diazepam is a benzodiazepine widely used for premedication and supplemental sedation. Diazepam is well absorbed orally, and serum drug levels correlate with clinical effect.[29,30] Relaxation and drowsiness are seen 10 to 15 minutes after a 10-mg dose. Diazepam is suitable for oral premedications; 5 mg, or 10 mg for the large or very anxious patient, may be given an hour before the procedure and preparation. Use of larger doses will result in prolonged drowsiness.

TABLE 6-1. Use of Selected Drugs for Premedication and Supplemental Sedation

Class	Drug	Suggested Dose
Ataractics	Diazepam:	
	Oral	0.07–0.15 mg/kg
	IV	0.05–0.15 mg/kg
	Midazolam, IV	0.03–0.15 mg/kg
	Droperidol, IV	8–17 μg/kg
Analgesics	Fentanyl, IV	1–3 μg/kg
	Alfentanil, IV	5–20 μg/kg
Inhalation analgesia	Nitrous oxide	30%–50%
	Enflurane	0.5%
Temporary loss of consciousness	Thiopental, IV	1–4 mg/kg
	Methohexital, IV	0.5–2 mg/kg
	Midazolam, IV	0.2–0.25 mg/kg
	Ketamine, IV	0.5 mg/kg

The intravenous route is preferred for rapid preoperative effect. Diazepam (10 mg) given intravenously resulted in clinical sedation within 2 to 3 minutes. Peak serum drug levels were three times those noted after oral administration.[31] Intravenous doses of diazepam should be decreased accordingly to avoid excessive effect. For premedication and supplemental sedation, diazepam in 2.5-mg increments should be used. It also should be remembered to allow 3 minutes for the drug to take effect before administering more, to avoid oversedation. The total dose of intravenous diazepam should be limited to avoid prolonged effects. Ataxia and dizziness sufficient to delay discharge were present in 8% and 16% of subjects, respectively, 1 hour after administration of 10 mg.[31] After 20 mg, these causes of delayed discharge were present in 40% and 30% of subjects, respectively. Tests of coordination and reaction time were abnormal until 6 hours after 0.15 mg/kg intravenous diazepam.[32] Individual dose response is widely variable, and drug requirement is less in the elderly.

The major drawback of diazepam administered intravenously for supplemental sedation is local pain and phlebitis. A faster rate of injection is associated with

TABLE 6-2. Use of Supplemental Drugs by Continuous Infusion

Drug	Concentration (per ml)	Loading Dose (per kg)	Maintenance (per kg/min)
Alfentanil	10 μg	8 μg	0.5 μg
Fentanyl	2 μg	1.6 μg	0.1 μg
Ketamine	1 mg	0.8 mg	50 μg
Methohexital	1–2 mg	0.5–2 mg	0.15 mg
Midazolam	20–40 μg	60 μg	1 μg
Thiopental	3–5 mg	1–4 mg	0.3 mg

a higher incidence of pain. Flushing the vein vigorously with saline may reduce thrombophlebitis.[33]

Diazepam to supplement regional anesthesia is given by some until slurred speech and drooping eyelids occur. This has resulted in doses averaging 0.31 mg/kg for dental procedures[34] and 0.45 mg/kg for outpatient endoscopies.[26] Korttila and Linnoila studied the effect of 0.30 and 0.45 mg/kg diazepam on skills related to driving.[32] Although a negative Romberg test was achieved after 36 minutes, impairment of coordination and reactive skills persisted until 10 hours. Tests of attention were minimally affected. Narcotics are often given in conjunction with diazepam to supplement sedation; this combination delays the return of normal function. Patients should be cautioned not to drive or operate dangerous machinery for 10 hours after sedation with diazepam and 24 hours after diazepam with long-acting narcotics.[35]

Diazepam is particularly useful as premedication before regional anesthesia, since it has been shown to increase the seizure threshold for lidocaine.[36] This should not be construed as a reason to increase the dose of local anesthetic given. Diazepam should not be given without monitoring respiration. Doses of 0.14 mg/kg intravenously depressed the ventilatory response to CO_2, increased the dead space to tidal volume ratio, and increased Pa_{CO_2}. These effects were present within 1 minute and lasted 25 to 30 minutes.[37] Depression of ventilatory response correlated with drowsiness.

Benzodiazepines such as diazepam can cause amnesia. This effect is least marked after oral premedication. Intravenous diazepam is a more reliable amnesic. Lack of recall after 5 to 10 mg intravenous diazepam developed in 50% and 90% of patients, respectively. The percentage of volunteers who developed amnesia was increased by accelerating the rate of diazepam injection and by increasing the dose.[33] Anterograde amnesia was present at 1 minute, peaked at 2 to 3 minutes, and persisted for approximately 30 minutes. Retrograde amnesia after intravenous diazepam has been variably reported. Diazepam given intravenously may be used to provide brief amnesia in the ambulatory surgery patient receiving regional anesthesia, as for the insertion of the block. Although 10-mg intravenous bolus doses have been studied, the use of 2.5-mg increments is preferred in the ambulatory patient to avoid oversedation. This may limit the amnesia obtained.

Midazolam

Midazolam is a newer benzodiazepine that is approximately twice as potent as diazepam.[38] It is water-soluble and therefore causes minimal pain or phlebitis. The therapeutic effect of midazolam is relatively short, with an elimination half-life of 2 to 3 hours and no evidence of enterohepatic recirculation and recurrence of drowsiness. Large doses, however, will result in prolonged drowsiness. Midazolam is a potent amnesic. After 5 mg, 67% of patients experienced total anterograde amnesia and 93% experienced partial amnesia lasting approximately 20 minutes.[39] Brief amnesia has been reported after doses as low as 2 mg. It should be remembered that some patients become distressed when they cannot recall perioperative events; this effect should be discussed with the patient in advance.[40] For the ambulatory patient, midazolam should be given in 1- to 2-mg increments, titrated slowly to effect. Dose response is variable, and the elderly are more sensitive.

The administration of excessively rapid or large doses will increase the possibility of adverse side-effects, particularly respiratory depression. Respiratory depression is exacerbated by the concomitant administration of narcotics.[41] Cardiorespiratory arrests have been reported in the elderly undergoing endoscopic procedures with sedation including midazolam and often with narcotics. Care must be taken during midazolam sedation that respiration is adequately monitored, with trained and dedicated personnel, and that resuscitative equipment is immediately available.

Various nonspecific benzodiazepine antagonists have been tried. Naloxone (0.4 mg), physostigmine (1–2 mg), and aminophylline (1 mg/kg) have all been used with inconsistent success and with significant side-effects, including nausea, vomiting, changes in blood pressure, and cardiac dysrhythmias. The routine use of any of these nonspecific drugs is not recommended. A specific antagonist has been developed, known as flumazenil.[42] It competitively displaces benzodiazepines at the specific central nervous system receptor site. Reversal can be titrated to achieve the degree desired, and side-effects, such as resurgence of anxiety, are minimal at the doses used after ambulatory anesthesia (0.2–1.0 mg).[43,44] The duration of action of this drug is approximately 1 hour, and the potential for benzodiazepine resedation exists.[45]

Droperidol

Droperidol has been used for many years as a supplement to surgical and diagnostic procedures under local or regional anesthesia. This butyrophenone derivative produces sedation and a sense of detachment. Amnesia is minimal. Droperidol does not significantly affect respiration, although wide individual variation of response occurs.[46] When droperidol is administered with a narcotic, neuroleptanalgesia results. Early enthusiastic use of droperidol alone and in neurolept combinations generated many reports of complications, including prolonged and excessive sedation, hypotension, extrapyramidal symptoms, and apprehension and anxiety despite apparent drowsiness.[47,48] Studies included use of the drug for premedication and for supplementation. Doses given were 2.5 to 10 mg in adults; similar effects were seen at similar doses in children, 0.1 to 0.17 mg/kg.[49] Patients sometimes became anxious, agitated, and confused to the extent that they canceled previously desired elective surgery. The incidence of refusal was 4.7% in a series of 121 military patients for plastic surgery[50] and 0.7% in a series of 1438 private patients scheduled for sterilization or plastic procedures.[51]

Droperidol (2.5 mg/ml) is sold alone and in combination with fentanyl (0.05 mg/ml) as Innovar (Janssen Pharmaceutica, New Brunswick, New Jersey). In general, this combination is not appropriate for premedication or sedation of ambulatory patients undergoing regional anesthesia. The dose of butyrophenone is too large and the effect too long-acting relative to the short-acting analgesic.

Droperidol is a potent antiemetic. Lower doses of 0.005 to 0.017 mg/kg (0.625–1.25 mg in adults) have been shown to be significantly effective in reducing the incidence of postoperative vomiting in adults and children.[52,53] Excessive sedation, extrapyramidal symptoms, or anxiety were not seen. The use of low-dose droperidol can therefore be recommended for the ambulatory local or regional anesthesia patient.

Analgesics
Fentanyl
Fentanyl is a potent narcotic analgesic cogener of meperidine. After intravenous administration, analgesia began within 2 minutes and lasted 30 to 60 minutes.[54] Termination of effect was due to redistribution into blood and peripheral tissues; the redistribution half-life of fentanyl was 13.4 minutes. Of the injected dose, 98.6% was cleared from plasma in 60 minutes. These rapid drug kinetics illustrate why fentanyl has become the narcotic of choice to supplement ambulatory surgery regional anesthesia. Fentanyl does cause respiratory depression that is comparable in magnitude and duration to equianalgesic doses of morphine[55] and which may recur. The routine use of naloxone is not, however, recommended because of reports of pulmonary edema, hypertension, and cardiac arrest occurring in healthy young adults after the administration of as little as 0.08 mg naloxone.[56]

Fentanyl is effective both when given before the insertion of a block and when used to supplement the maintenance of local or regional anesthesia. Increments of 25 to 50 μg fentanyl may be given intravenously to achieve desired analgesia, with an initial dose totaling 50 to 200 μg (1–3 μg/kg). Additional doses may be given in 30 to 60 minutes as clinically indicated. The elderly require reduced drug doses. If an ongoing need for fentanyl supplementation of regional anesthesia is anticipated, the continuous infusion technique may be advantageous.[57]

Alfentanil
The need for an even shorter-acting narcotic resulted in the development of alfentanil. Alfentanil, with approximately ⅕ the potency of the older compound, appears to produce more sedation and briefer respiratory depression but more hypotension and more rigidity. Alfentanil has a shorter redistribution half-life, 11.6 minutes, and a more rapid elimination half-life, 94 minutes,[58,59] and recovery has been consistently rapid if appropriate doses are used.[60] However, larger doses will result in prolonged effect, and delayed respiratory depression appearing in the recovery room has been described.[61]

The pharmacokinetics of alfentanil suggest that it best be used by infusion. To supplement ambulatory local and regional anesthesia, loading bolus(es) of 5 μg/kg followed by an infusion of approximately 0.5 μg/kg per minute may be used. It is important to repeatedly titrate the dose being given to reach the desired effect and avoid relative overdosage.

Other Opioids
The agonist/antagonist opioids nalbuphine and butorphanol have been used in the ambulatory setting, with the intent of avoiding classic opiate side-effects: respiratory depression and vomiting. Butorphanol has a sedative, subjectively

pleasant effect.[62] The duration of both these drugs is long, 3 to 4 hours, and they must be used in limited doses to supplement regional anesthesia for the ambulatory patient.

Some longer-acting classic opioid analgesics have been popular in specific institutions, usually as a holdover from inpatient use. Morphine and meperidine are two such drugs. The use of longer-acting opioids results in a longer duration of sedation and of other side-effects such as nausea and dizziness. Meperidine in particular is not recommended for outpatient use. Intramuscular meperidine is associated with syncope after standing up. Tests of coordination and reaction time remain abnormal 12 hours after the administration of 75 mg meperidine.[35] The use of these longer-acting opioid analgesics should be avoided as premedication or supplementation for the ambulatory regional anesthesia patient.

Inhalation Analgesia
Anesthetic gases and vapors administered at subanesthetic concentrations provide analgesia and sedation. These effects can be used to supplement local and regional anesthesia for the ambulatory surgery patient. Advantages of inhalation over intravenous analgesia are related to the mode of drug administration—ventilation through the lung. These advantages include rapid reversibility and easier maintenance of a constant blood concentration and therefore constant anesthetic effect.[63] A disadvantage is the need to administer the gas or vapor through a tight-fitting mask or mouthpiece to avoid contamination of operating room air. The use of devices to scavenge exhaled gas can minimize pollution.[64] Inhalation analgesia is particularly useful for minor surgery on closed-space infections, which are difficult to block with local anesthetic.[65] Pediatric, adult, and mentally retarded patients are all satisfactory candidates.

Most inhalation anesthetic agents have been used for analgesia. Trichlorethylene and chloroform are no longer commercially available. Diethyl ether and cyclopropane are not recommended for the ambulatory surgery setting because they are flammable. Halothane is not effective for analgesia at subanesthetic concentration.[66] Agents that could be used for inhalation analgesia include nitrous oxide, enflurane, and methoxyflurane.

Methoxyflurane is effective for inhalation analgesia given intermittently at concentrations of 0.2% to 0.5% (1.2–3.1 MAC).[67] However, onset of analgesia and recovery are relatively slow because of high blood solubility. In addition, methoxyflurane is metabolized in part to inorganic fluoride, and serum fluoride levels above 50 $\mu M/l$ have been associated with polyuric renal failure. This level has been reached in patients self-administering methoxyflurane for obstetric analgesia.[68] The use of methoxyflurane analgesia for ambulatory surgery regional anesthesia patients is not recommended because of its slow effect and the possibility of renal damage.

Nitrous oxide has achieved widespread popularity particularly as an adjunct to dental regional anesthesia. Concentrations of 10% to 60% in oxygen are used. Onset of analgesia is rapid, as is termination of the effect once administration ceases.[66] Psychomotor effects also have been studied.[69] During the inhalation of 30% end-tidal nitrous oxide, impairment of word recall, the ability to do arithmetic problems, and eye-hand coordination were seen. Impairment was maximal 7 minutes after beginning inhalation and remained at that level for the half-hour of gas administration. Subjects reported a significant increase in physical and mental sedation and in relief of tension (relaxation). Recovery of normal function was complete 22 minutes after administration ceased. An appropriate period of postanesthetic supervision is necessary for any ambulatory patient after nitrous oxide inhalation.

Subanesthetic concentrations of enflurane also have been used for supplemental analgesia. Enflurane was shown to impair digit memory, audiovisual reaction time, and manual dexterity at concentrations greater than 0.09 MAC (0.15% alveolar).[70] Dose-related amnesia also was seen. At 0.24 MAC enflurane (0.4% alveolar and 0.53% inspired), sufficient drowsiness developed to preclude completing the tests. Abboud and coworkers reported similar maximal levels for effective analgesia without loss of consciousness at approximately 0.5% inspired enflurane or 40% inspired nitrous oxide in obstetric patients.[71] Satisfactory analgesia was reported by 89% and 76% of the parturients for the two agents, respectively; the difference was not significant. Complete amnesia (of delivery) developed in 7% and 10% of patients, respectively. Inhalation analgesia to supplement regional anesthesia may be obtained by using 30% to 40% nitrous oxide or 0.5% enflurane; impairment of psychomotor abilities and sometimes amnesia occur at these doses.

The actual percentage of nitrous oxide reaching the patient, and therefore the level of analgesia obtainable, is very dependent on the method of administration. Lichtenthal and colleagues used the ratio of nitrous oxide concentration delivered to the system to the steady-state end-expiratory concentration as a measure of the efficiency of several delivery systems.[72] Nasal prongs at 7 to 8 L/min delivered only 19% of the preset concentration: administered 50% nitrous oxide reached the patient as 9%. A see-through rebreathing mask, such as might be used during regional anesthesia, delivered 34% of preset concentration; with this device, administered 50% yielded 17% end-expired nitrous oxide. To achieve expired concentration approaching that preset, 95% to 98%, a tight-fitting nonrebreathing mask was needed. The true yield of nitrous oxide from a dental-type nasal mask will depend as well on what fraction of respiration occurs through the nose and on how much nitrous oxide is entrained through the nose during oral respiration.

Patient-controlled self-administration of nitrous oxide or methoxyflurane also has been used to provide supplemental analgesia and sedation. Inhalers are available that will deliver 0.3% to 0.9% methoxyflurane in air,[67] or 50% nitrous oxide in oxygen, either premixed[73] or from tandem cylinders.[65] A supposed safety advantage of these devices is the need for patient cooperation in maintaining a tight mouthpiece or mask seal in order to receive anesthetic.[67,73] This is intended to limit excessive anesthesia, with resultant risks of excitement, vomiting, and aspiration. Such failsafes can, of course, be circumvented, as by propping the inhaler on a pillow. Furthermore, methoxyflurane inhalers are able to deliver concentrations of several times 1 MAC, sufficient to produce surgical anesthesia if inspired continuously. Patient-controlled devices are intended to be safe enough to use without an anesthesiologist present. However, the patient receiving self-administered inhalation analgesia still requires a trained individual in constant attendance; this attendant must terminate or decrease the anesthetic if drowsiness, confusion, or excitement develops. Devices for self-administered inhalation analgesia should not be used in "local rooms" or an ambulatory surgery suite without such precautions.

The degree of analgesia obtained is strongly influenced by the expectation of pain or its relief. Pain threshold and tolerance of electrical tooth pulp stimulation are ordinarily increased with 33% inhaled nitrous oxide.[74] Patients were given suggestions that nitrous oxide causes an enhanced sensitivity and awareness of body sensations; afterwards, pain responses were actually heightened during gas inhalation. On the other hand, establishing an expectation of the analgesic effectiveness of nitrous oxide will reduce perceived pain. More subjective relief and decreased anxiety were obtained using the same 15% to 45% inhaled nitrous oxide when the dental stimulation was performed in a pain-research laboratory rather than in a dental clinic.[75] Anxiety and expectation of pain can be reduced by eliminating stressful environments.

Side-effects of nitrous oxide inhalation analgesia have been reported. Lichtenthal and coworkers reported that concentrations of over 30% sometimes caused excitement.[72] Stewart and colleagues evaluated 50% nitrous oxide in oxygen.[73] They reported a 20.6% incidence of minor side-effects, including nausea or vomiting (5.7%), dizziness or lightheadedness (10.3%), excitement (3.7%), and numbness (0.3%).[73] These authors did not include as complications the 7.6% of patients who became drowsy or fell lightly asleep. Oversedation can, however, eliminate one of the advantages of inhalation analgesia—the preservation of airway reflexes. Twenty percent of patients breathing 50% nitrous oxide in oxygen through a nasal mask aspirated dye placed in the mouth during simulated dental treatment.[8]

Temporary Obtundation of Consciousness
Barbiturates

Regional anesthetic blocks can be painful when administered. Administration may become uncomfortable when multiple injections are needed, as with intercostal nerve blocks. A particularly sensitive operative area may be involved, as with anorectal procedures. Also, a combination of both factors may be present, as with the multiple injections required for facial cosmetic surgery. One technique for alleviating the discomfort of these situations is the administration of intravenous agents that will briefly obtund consciousness and prevent memory.

The barbiturates are well-suited for this purpose. Thiopental induces unconsciousness after 1 to 4 mg/kg is injected slowly. A single bolus of 2.6 mg/kg caused sleep lasting for 120 seconds,[76] during which local or regional anesthesia may be established. Five minutes after injection of this bolus, subjects were able to walk and answer questions. Use of larger doses leads to prolongation of recovery. Thiopental also may be administered as a 0.3% to 0.5% solution, suitable to eliminate awareness during the maintenance of a regional anesthetic.[77] Recovery after a 4-

mg/kg loading dose plus a 428-mg thiopental infusion, given over 21 minutes, required 10 minutes to awakening, 20 minutes to orientation, and 1.9 hours until patients were fit for discharge.

One other barbiturate has gained widespread acceptance in ambulatory anesthesia and is useful to supplement regional blockade. This barbiturate is methohexital. Methohexital is administered in a dose of 0.5 to 2 mg/kg to induce sleep. After a single bolus of 0.88 mg/kg, volunteers slept for 143 seconds. Recovery is more rapid than after thiopental,[76] and after larger or cumulative doses, the relative advantage of methohexital over thiopental became even more pronounced. Methohexital also may be used in a 0.1% to 0.2% solution for continuous infusion to maintain basal narcosis during regional anesthesia. Smaller total doses and speedier recovery would be expected with this mode of administration. With intravenous fentanyl premedication, methohexital is the barbiturate of choice to obtund consciousness and supplement regional anesthesia for ambulatory patients.

Methohexital has been widely used by dentists to supplement regional anesthesia. Narcotic and sedative premedication, usually including diazepam, is employed in conjunction with the barbiturate. A typical combination included 5 to 15 mg diazepam, in increments, until the patient was sedated, then methohexital, in 5- to 10-mg increments, during which the local anesthetic was injected and the procedure performed. Perception of painful tooth stimulation was not abolished under barbiturate sedation, even with the addition of alphaprodine (30 mg).[78] Local analgesia must be used. Patients remained conscious and able to obey commands, but complete amnesia of the injection and procedure were usually reported. Under this combined-drug sedation, significant decreases in cardiac output (21%), cardiac rate (30%), and minute work (28%) were found in volunteers.[78] As would be expected, recovery was prolonged. Performance of the Trieger dot test had recovered to normal by 3 hours, but tests of perceptual and cognitive ability revealed that residual impairment was still present at that time.[79]

Midazolam

Midazolam may be useful to blunt consciousness temporarily during ambulatory surgery regional anethesia. Successful trials of midazolam for premedication and sedation encouraged the evaluation of its use as a short-acting sleep-inducing agent. To produce unconsciousness during the insertion of a regional block, an injection of 0.20 to 0.25 mg/kg midazolam may be necessary. A wide variability in induction dose requirement has been noted.

A dose of 0.1 to 0.15 mg/kg midazolam is effective in achieving basal sedation.[81,82] Drowsiness lasted for 128 minutes in volunteers who received 0.15 mg/kg midazolam. Fifty percent of the subjects lost consciousness with this dose for an average duration of 304 seconds. Apnea occurred in 40% of patients and lasted for 30 seconds. Amnesic effect is significant. After 0.15 mg/kg, 100% of subjects developed anterograde amnesia for 40 minutes; they did not remember standing or walking at 22 minutes.

Propofol

Propofol is an alkylphenol that has been solubilized in an aqueous oil emulsion. Use of propofol as an induction agent for ambulatory general anesthesia has consistently been associated with rapid recovery, clearheadedness, and return to neuropsychologic baseline.[83] Propofol also has been used to supplement regional blockade with intermittent boluses and continuous infusion. A bolus dose of 2.5 mg/kg has been used to produce sleep during regional blockade, followed by repeated injections of approximately one-quarter to one-third the initial dose.[84] Given as an infusion, the maintenance dose of propofol needed was 0.10 mg/kg per minute. To provide basal sedation, propofol bolus and maintenance doses of 0.86 and 0.06 mg/kg per minute, respectively, have been employed.[86] Decreases in blood pressure and heart rate occur with propofol and are even larger in the elderly. Postanesthetic sequelae, notably nausea and vomiting, are uncommon, but during induction, dose-related transient apnea and significant pain on injection can be problematic.

Ketamine

Ketamine is another agent that has been used to blunt consciousness temporarily during administration of regional anesthesia. In a dose of 2 mg/kg IV, ketamine produced excellent sedation for the insertion of intercostal blocks.[87] However, unpleasant emergence reactions are consistently a problem with high doses of ketamine. Delirium, vivid hallucinations, and unpleasant dreams have been reported in up to 40% of patients; symptoms may recur for several weeks. In order to decrease the incidence of these reactions, lower doses of ketamine have been tried.

Bovill and Dundee reported that analgesia persisted up to 40 minutes after ketamine anesthesia had terminated.[88] It also was observed that subanesthetic doses of parenteral ketamine, approximately 0.5 mg/kg, could be used for postoperative analgesia.[89] At this lower dose, analgesia developed within 5 minutes after intramuscular injection and lasted 60 to 90 minutes. Side-effects were experienced by 35% of patients but were of lesser severity. Dizziness, incoordination, blurred vision, and difficulty in communication were most common, but one case of severe agitation also was reported. Patients remained conscious and oriented. Ketamine analgesia is also effective by the oral route, with a longer onset of action, 30 minutes.

On the basis of this subdissociative analgesic effect, ketamine at low doses (0.4–0.5 mg/kg) has been used before administering local anesthesia. In a series of 200 plastic surgery patients, 87% had significant amnesia and no unpleasant memories. An additional 8.5% had unpleasant memories but were cooperative. One patient had unpleasant dreams for 3 days after surgery. It should be noted that this low dose was inadequate for maintenance of the procedure; injection of local or regional anesthesia was required during the period of amnesia.[90]

Various premedications have been tried in order to decrease the incidence of unpleasant emergence reactions. Combinations of droperidol, opiates, and scopolamine have all been shown to decrease emergence delirium and dreams. Benzodiazepines are the most effective, whether given as premedication or at the end of the procedure. This may be due to their ability to generate amnesia.[87] Patient acceptance of ketamine is not related to an observer's report of difficult induction or emergence delirium. Diazepam (5–10 mg) is the agent of choice.[91,92] Patients who received 0.15 mg/kg diazepam with 0.5 mg/kg ketamine for supplementation after regional anesthetic blockade had a similar incidence of dreaming and similar postoperative nursing care needs compared with control patients receiving no supplementation. However, the incidence of visual disturbances remained high. Increasing the dose of diazepam to 30 mg resulted in more postoperative anxiety, confusion, and terrifying dreams, as well as in a need for increased postoperative nursing supervision.

Lorazepam (4 mg) is highly effective by any route of administration in reducing ketamine sequelae and greatly improving patient acceptance. The combination of lorazepam with ketamine led to prolongation of recovery, however, and is not recommended for ambulatory surgery patients.

A chemical derivative of phencyclidine, ketamine also may have significant abuse potential as a hallucinogen. It should be avoided in patients with a history of psychiatric problems. This drug has several additional disadvantages as a supplement for ambulatory regional anesthesia. It is associated with increased postoperative vomiting. Airway reflexes are not consistently preserved, and there is a risk of aspiration.[93] Any drugs used to treat vomiting or emergence symptoms prolong the duration of anesthetic action, making ketamine less suitable for ambulatory surgery patients. Despite the administration of ketamine by low-dose infusion and the selection of appropriate premedication, emergence reactions remain a significant issue. Specific indications should be weighed before ketamine is used for supplementation of ambulatory regional anesthesia.

LOCAL ANESTHETIC DRUGS

Local anesthesia, like many other therapeutic modalities, originated among the natives of South America. In 1860, cocaine was isolated from the leaves of a Peruvian bush *Erythroxylon coca*, but its medicinal use remained obscure until 1884, when Koller reported the use of cocaine for topical anesthesia in ophthalmology. Since that time, numerous topical and injectable anesthetic agents have been introduced, and several may be used for ambulatory anesthesia. Local anesthetic drugs are unique, since they produce a loss of sensation and muscle paralysis in a circumscribed area of the body by a localized effect on peripheral nerve endings or fibers.

Mechanism of Local Anesthesia

Neural excitation depends on depolarization of the nerve membrane from a resting potential of approximately -90 mV to a threshold potential level of approximately -60 mV. Attainment of the threshold potential results in spontaneous and complete nerve depolarization followed by a phase of repolarization that leads to reestablishment of the original resting potential. This entire process occurs within 1 msec, the depolarization phase being completed in 0.3 msec and repolarization requiring 0.7 msec. Nerve conduction requires only that depolarization occur in a localized segment of nerve which, in turn, will activate the adjacent segment such that a self-perpetuating wave of depolarization will proceed along the entire length of the nerve fibers.

The changes in membrane potential during and after nerve excitation are related to changes in permeability of the cell membrane to various electrolytes, particularly sodium and potassium. During depolarization, sodium permeability increases, allowing sodium ions to flow passively from the extracellular space into the cell. Repolarization is associated with a decrease in sodium permeability, which results in a passive efflux of potassium ions from the interior to the exterior of the cell membrane. At the conclusion of the repolarization phase, the sodium-potassium pump actively extrudes sodium from inside the nerve cell and returns potassium to the intracellular space.

Local anesthetic drugs interfere with the initial step in the excitation-conduction process by decreasing the rate and degree of depolarization without altering the resting potential, threshold potential, or repolarization phase.[94] When the degree of depolarization is sufficiently depressed that the threshold potential is not achieved, then a propagated action potential fails to develop and nerve conduction is blocked. Since depolarization is related to an influx of sodium ions from the exterior of the cell, it was logical to assume that local anesthetics depress depolarization by inhibiting sodium conductance across the membrane. Indeed, all local anesthetics tested markedly decrease sodium permeability with minimal effects on potassium flux. Isolation of the biotoxin tetrodotoxin from puffer fish ovaries provided the most convincing evidence for the mechanism of local anesthesia. This substance, which specifically inhibits sodium conductance and nerve depolarization alone, is the most potent local anesthetic substance studied to date in animal models.

In summary, the mechanism of action of local anesthetic agents is related to the following sequence of events:

> Binding of local anesthetic molecules to receptor sites in the nerve membranes
> Reduction in sodium permeability
> Decrease in the rate of depolarization
> Failure to achieve threshold potential level
> Lack of development of a propagated action potential
> Conduction blockade

The receptor site for local anesthetic agents is believed to reside at the nerve membrane. However, the specific receptor location varies according to the type of local anesthetic employed. The conventional agents, such as lidocaine and procaine, are believed to bind at receptor sites located on the inner surface of the nerve membrane. Biotoxins, such as tetrodotoxin and saxitoxin, act at receptor sites located on the external surface of the membrane. Finally, agents such as benzocaine and benzyl alcohol act by penetrating the nerve membrane, causing membrane expansion and a decrease in the diameter of the sodium channel.

Active Form of Local Anesthetic Agents

Most of the clinically useful anesthetic preparations are available in the form of solutions of a salt; lidocaine, for example, is usually prepared as 0.5% to 2.0% solutions of lidocaine hydrochloride. In solution, the salts of these local anesthetic compounds exist as uncharged molecules (B) and as positively charged cations (BH^+). The relative proportion between the uncharged base (B) and charged cation (BH^+) depends on the pK_a of the specific chemical compound and the pH of the solution, that is $pH = pK_a - \log (BH^+/B)$. Since pK_a is constant for any specific compound, the relative proportion of free base and charged cation depends essentially on the pH of the local anesthetic solution ($BH^+ \rightleftharpoons B + H^+$). As the pH of the solution is decreased and H^+ concentration increased, the equilibrium will shift toward the charged cationic form, more cation will be present than free base. Conversely, as the pH is increased and H^+ concentration decreased, the equilibrium will be shifted toward the free-base form and more of the local anesthetic agent will exist in the free-base form. Both the uncharged base form (B) and the charged cationic form (BH^+) of local anesthetic agents are involved in the process of conduction block. The uncharged base form diffuses more easily through the nerve sheath and so is required for optimal penetration, which is reflected clinically in onset of anesthesia. Following diffusion through the epineurium, equilibrium reoccurs between B and BH^+, and the charged cation actually binds to the receptor site in the nerve membrane. Therefore, the cationic form is ultimately responsible for the suppression of electrophysiologic events in peripheral nerve, which is reflected clinically in the profoundness of anesthesia.

Structure-Activity Relationship

Chemical compounds that demonstrate local anesthetic activity usually possess the following chemical arrangement:

Aromatic portion—intermediate chain—amine portion

The agents of clinical importance can be categorized into two distinct chemical groups. Local anesthetics with an ester link between the aromatic portion and the intermediate chain are referred to as *aminoesters* and include procaine, chloroprocaine, and tetracaine. Local anesthetics with an amide link between the aromatic end and the intermediate chain are referred to as *aminoamides* and include lidocaine, mepivacaine, prilocaine, bupivacaine, and etidocaine. The basic differences between the ester and amide compounds reside in the manner in which they are metabolized and their allergic potential. The ester agents are hydrolyzed in plasma by pseudocholinesterase, whereas the amide compounds undergo enzymatic degradation in the liver. *Para*-aminobenzoic acid is one of the metabolites formed from the hydrolysis of ester-like compounds. This substance is capable of inducing allergic reactions in a small percentage of the general population and so is responsible for the allergies reported in association with ester-like local anesthetic agents. The amide, lidocaine-like drugs are not metabolized to *para*-aminobenzoic acid, and reports of allergic phenomena with these agents are extremely rare.

Chemical alterations within a homologous group produce quantitative changes in physicochemical properties such as lipid solubility and protein binding that can alter the anesthetic properties of the compounds (Table 6-3). For example, within the ester series, the addition of a butyl group to the aromatic end of the procaine molecule increases lipid solubility and protein binding and results in tetracaine, a compound that has a greater intrinsic anesthetic potency and longer duration of anesthetic activity. In the amide series, the addition of a butyl group to the amine end of mepivacaine transforms this agent into bupivacaine, a compound that is more lipid soluble, is more highly protein bound, and biologically possesses a greater intrinsic potency and longer duration of action. In the case of lidocaine, substitution of a propyl for an ethyl group at the amine end and addition of an ethyl group to the alpha carbon in the intermediate chain yield etidocaine, which is more lipid soluble, more highly protein bound, and biologically, a local anesthetic agent of greater potency and longer duration.

On the basis of differences in anesthetic potency and duration of action, it is possible to classify the clinically useful injectable local anesthetic compounds into three categories:

> Group I—Agents of low anesthetic potency and short duration of action (procaine and chloroprocaine)
> Group II—Agents of intermediate anesthetic potency and duration of action (lidocaine, mepivacaine, and prilocaine)
> Group III—Agents of high anesthetic potency and long duration of action (tetracaine, bupivacaine, and etidocaine). These are rarely used for ambulatory surgery anesthesia.

Physiologic Disposition of Local Anesthetic Agents

The vascular absorption, tissue distribution, metabolism, and excretion of local anesthetic agents is of particular importance in terms of their potential toxicity.[95] Absorption varies as a function of site of injection, dosage, addition of a vasoconstrictor agent, and specific agents employed. Absorption occurs most rapidly after intercostal nerve blockade, followed by injection into the caudal canal, lumbar epidural space, brachial plexus and sciatic femoral sites, and subcutaneous tissue. For example, the intercostal administration of 400 mg lidocaine without epinephrine results in an average peak venous plasma level of approximately 7 μg/ml, whereas the same dose of lidocaine employed for brachial plexus block yields a mean maximum blood level of approximately 3.5 μg/ml.

The blood level of local anesthetic agents is related to the total dose of drug administered rather than the specific volume or concentration of solution employed. A linear relationship tends to exist between the amount of drug administered and the peak anesthetic blood level. For example, the maximum blood level of lidocaine increases from approximately 1.5 to 4 μg/ml as the total dose administered into the lumbar epidural space is raised from 200 to 600 mg. De-

TABLE 6-3. Chemical Structure and Physicochemical and Anesthetic Properties of Various Local Anesthetic Agents

	Chemical Structure			Lipid Solubility	Protein Binding	pKa	In Vitro Potency	Anesthetic Duration	Onset Time
	Aromatic End	Intermediate Chain	Amine End						
Aminoesters									
Procaine	H_2N-⟨ring⟩	$COOCH_2CH_2-N$	C_2H_5 / C_2H_5	1	5	8.9	1	Short	Slow
2-Chloroprocaine	H_2N-⟨ring, Cl⟩	$COOCH_2CH_2-N$	C_2H_5 / C_2H_5	1	?	9.1	2	Short	Fast
Tetracaine	$H_9C_4-N(H)-$⟨ring⟩	$COOCH_2CH_2-N$	CH_3 / CH_3	80	85	8.6	16	Long	Slow
Aminoamides									
Lidocaine	⟨ring, CH_3, CH_3⟩	$NHCOCH_2-N$	C_2H_5 / C_2H_5	4	65	7.7	4	Moderate	Fast
Prilocaine	⟨ring, CH_3⟩	$NHCOCH-N$ (CH_3)	C_3H_7 / H	1.5	55	7.7	3	Moderate	Fast
Etidocaine	⟨ring, CH_3, CH_3⟩	$NHCOCH-N$ (C_2H_5)	C_2H_5 / C_3H_7	140	95	7.7	16	Long	Fast
Mepivacaine	⟨ring, CH_3, CH_3⟩	$NHCO-$⟨piperidine⟩	CH_3	1	75	7.6	2	Moderate	Fast
Bupivacaine	⟨ring, CH_3, CH_3⟩	$NHCO-$⟨piperidine⟩	C_4H_9	30	95	8.1	16	Long	Moderate

pending on the site of administration, a peak blood level of 0.5 to 2 μg/ml is achieved for each 100 mg lidocaine or mepivacaine injected.

Addition of a vasoconstrictor to local anesthetic solutions decreases the rate of absorption of certain agents from various sites of administration. Epinephrine (1:200,000), 5μg/ml, significantly reduces the peak blood levels of lidocaine and mepivacaine irrespective of the site of administration. Epinephrine decreases the peak blood levels of prilocaine, bupivacaine, and etidocaine achieved after peripheral nerve blocks but has little influence on the absorption of these drugs following lumbar epidural administration. Phenylephrine and norepinephrine (1:20,000) also can reduce local anesthetic absorption, but not as effectively as epinephrine 1:200,000.

The rate and degree of vascular absorption varies among various agents. Lidocaine and mepivacaine are absorbed more rapidly than prilocaine, whereas bupivacaine is absorbed more rapidly than etidocaine. The lower blood levels of prilocaine probably reflect its tendency to produce less vasodilation than lidocaine or mepivacaine. The lower peak blood levels of etidocaine compared to bupivacaine may be related to the greater lipid solubility and uptake by peripheral fat of etidocaine.

Following absorption from injection site, local anesthetic agents distribute throughout total body water. An initial rapid disappearance from blood (alpha phase) occurs, which is related to uptake by rapidly equilibrating tissues, that is, tissues with a high vascular perfusion. A secondary slower disappearance rate (beta phase) reflects distribution to slowly perfused tissue and metabolism and excretion of the compound. The disappearance rate of prilocaine is significantly more rapid than that of lidocaine or mepivacaine. The rate of tissue redistribution for the latter two agents is similar. Although all tissues will take up local anesthetics, the highest concentrations are found in the more highly perfused organs, such as lung and kidney. The greatest percentage of an injected dose of a local anesthetic agent distributes to skeletal muscle because of the large mass of this tissue in the body.

The metabolism of local anesthetic agents varies according to their chemical classification. The ester-like or procaine-like agents undergo hydrolysis in plasma by the enzyme pseudocholinesterase. Chloroprocaine shows the most rapid rate of hydrolysis (4.7 μmol/ml/hr) compared to procaine (1.1 μmol/ml/hr) and tetracaine (0.3 μmol/ml/hr). Less than 2% of unchanged procaine is excreted, whereas approximately 90% of *para*-aminobenzoic acid, which is the primary metabolite of procaine, appears in urine. On the other hand, only 33% of diethylaminoethanol, the other major metabolite of procaine, is excreted unchanged.

The amide-like or lidocaine-like agents undergo enzymatic degradation primarily in the liver. Prilocaine undergoes the most rapid rate of hepatic metabolism. Lidocaine, mepivacaine, and etidocaine are intermediate in terms of rate of degradation, whereas bupivacaine is metabolized most slowly. Some degradation of the amide-like compounds may occur in nonhepatic tissue as indicated by the formation of certain metabolites following the incubation of prilocaine with kidney slices. Complete metabolism for all the amide compounds has not been elucidated. Lidocaine, which has been studied most extensively, undergoes primarily oxidative de-ethylation to monoethylglycinexylidide, followed by a subsequent hydrolysis to hydroxyxylidine. Less than 5% of unchanged amide-like drugs is excreted into the urine. The major portion of an injected dose appears in the form of various metabolites. For example, 73% of lidocaine can be accounted for in human urine by hydroxyxylidine. The renal clearance of the amide agents is inversely related to their protein-binding capacity. Prilocaine, which has a lower protein-binding capacity than lidocaine, has a substantially higher clearance value than lidocaine. Renal clearance also is inversely proportional to the pH of urine, suggesting urinary excretion by nonionic diffusion.

ANESTHETIC TECHNIQUES
On the basis of anatomic considerations, regional anesthesia for the ambulatory surgery patient may be divided into three categories: infiltration, peripheral nerve blockade (minor and major), and central neural blockade (epidural, caudal, and spinal). Since surgical procedures performed on an ambulatory basis are, by definition, relatively brief, the long-acting local anesthetic agents are rarely used for ambulatory surgery anesthesia. Therefore, the following discussion will be limited to the agents of short or moderate duration. The reader is encouraged to refer to any of the standard anesthesia textbooks for a detailed description of the various anesthetic techniques. Surgical indications for the various techniques are summarized in Table 6-4.

TABLE 6-4. Surgical Indications for Ambulatory Anesthetic Technique

Technique	Surgical Indication
Infiltration:	
Extravascular	Any superficial surgical procedure
	Herniorrhaphy
	Laparoscopy
	Endoscopy
	Postoperative analgesia
Intravascular	Orthopedic or plastic hand procedure
	Orthopedic or plastic foot procedure
Peripheral nerve blockade:	
Minor nerve block	Orthopedic or plastic hand procedure
	Orthopedic or plastic foot procedure
Major nerve block	Orthopedic procedures involving arm, hand, leg, foot
	Plastic procedures involving arm, hand, leg, foot
	Vascular procedures on arm or leg
Central neural blocks:	
Epidural and spinal	Orthopedic procedures of lower limbs
	Vascular procedures of lower limbs
	Gynecologic procedures
	Herniorrhaphy
	Hemorrhoidectomy

Infiltration Anesthesia

Infiltration anesthesia involves administration of a local anesthetic agent into an extravascular or intravascular site and subsequent diffusion to nerve endings where excitation is inhibited. Extravascular infiltration anesthesia includes the injection of local anesthetic into or around the operative site, as well as topical administration to mucous membranes or peritoneum. Intravascular infiltration anesthesia consists of the injection of anesthetic drug into the vasculature of a tourniquet-occluded limb such that the drug cannot enter the central circulatory compartment but instead diffuses from the peripheral vascular bed to nonvascular tissue such as nerve endings.

Extravascular Infiltration

In terms of frequency of adequate analgesia, 1% to 2% procaine, 0.5% to 1% lidocaine, 2% chloroprocaine, 0.5% to 1% mepivacaine, and 1% prilocaine are equivalent. Onset of action is almost immediate for all agents following intradermal or subcutaneous administration. Absorption from mucous membranes is almost as rapid as after intravenous injection. However, the various agents can be differentiated according to duration of infiltration anesthesia (Table 6-5). Procaine and chloroprocaine have a short duration, whereas lidocaine, mepivacaine, and prilocaine are agents of moderate duration. Epinephrine may be added to prolong infiltration anesthesia and thereby provide intraoperative and postoperative analgesia. The effect is most pronounced when epinephrine is added to solutions of lidocaine. Epinephrine should be used in concentrations no higher than 1:200,000. Its use is contraindicated in infiltration anesthesia and minor nerve blocks of the hands, feet, and digits in the presence of coronary artery disease and when blood supply to the area is compromised by severe peripheral vascular disease.

The dosage of a local anesthetic required for adequate infiltration anesthesia depends on the extent of the area to be anesthetized and the expected duration of the surgical procedure. It is frequently necessary to anesthetize large surface areas for surgical procedures performed under infiltration techniques. In order not to exceed the maximum dosage limits of the various agents and thus avoid possible toxic reactions, large volumes of dilute anesthetic solutions should be employed. For example, 500 mg with epinephrine is considered the maximum single dose of lidocaine. Surgical procedures involving a large surface area may require the use of 75 to 100 ml of anesthetic solutions. In such a situation, a 0.5% solution of lidocaine with epinephrine should be employed rather than the 1% solution. In most infiltration procedures, 0.5% lidocaine will provide an adequate depth and duration of analgesia.

Arthroscopic knee surgery has been performed using intra-articular local anesthesia.[95a,95b] Both lidocaine (20 ml 1.5% with epinephrine 1:200,000) or bupivacaine (30 ml 0.5% with epinephrine 1:200,000) provide effective anesthesia, with the addition of cutaneous lidocaine infiltration. Intravenous analgesic supplementation is necessary in many patients.

For topical administration to mucous membranes, the permissible dose of local anesthetic does not change. However, higher concentrations are needed, such

TABLE 6-5. Infiltration Anesthesia for Ambulatory Surgery

Agent	Concentration (%)	Plain Solutions			Epinephrine-Containing Solutions		
		Max. Adult Dose (mg)	Max. Dose (mg/kg)	Duration (min)	Max. Adult Dose (mg)	Max. Dose (mg/kg)	Duration (min)
Short duration:							
Procaine							
Chloroprocaine	1–2	800	11	15–30	1000	14	30–90
Moderate duration:							
Lidocaine	0.5–1	300	4	30–60	500	7	120–360
Mepivacaine	0.5–1	300	4	45–90	500	7	120–360
Prilocaine	0.5–1	600	7	30–90	500	Not available	120–360

as 4% lidocaine or 1% tetracaine, for the oronasopharynx and proximal digestive tract. Therefore, only limited volumes may be used.

Infiltration in and around the surgical site at the end of an operation can provide postoperative analgesia. Patient comfort is greatly increased and recovery-room narcotic requirement is decreased. Time to discharge also may be reduced. Extravascular infiltration is effective particularly for anorectal surgery, circumcision, and herniorrhaphy in adults and children. This is one of the indications for a long-acting anesthetic agent in ambulatory anesthesa. Bupivacaine (0.25%), plain or with epinephrine 1:200,000, will provide 3 to 7 hours of pain relief. Maximum recommended adult doses are 175 and 225 mg, respectively.

Intravascular Infiltration (Intravenous Regional)

The essential features of intravascular infiltration are its simplicity and relatively rapid disappearance of analgesia following tourniquet release.[96] The procedure involves the intravascular administration of a local anesthetic agent into a tourniquet-occluded limb. It is imperative that the venous flow from the involved limb be completely obstructed in order to prevent the rapid entrance of local anesthetic drug into the central vascular compartment, which could result in serious toxicity. If properly performed, satisfactory analgesia and muscle relaxation are consistently obtained. Only the fingertips are sometimes not anesthetized.

TOURNIQUET. Both the safety and efficacy of this regional anesthetic procedure depend on the interruption of blood flow to the involved limb. Calibration of the occlusive cuff is of vital importance, since a malfunctioning cuff can lead to inadequate occlusion and potential side-effects due to the rapid introduction of local anesthetic agents into the central circulatory compartment. The tourniquet should be inflated to 300 mmHg or, for higher blood pressures, 100 mmHg above the systolic value. It should remain inflated for at least 15 to 30 minutes, to permit adequate tissue binding of the anesthetic drug. At the conclusion of surgery, intermittent tourniquet release has been advocated as a means of increasing the safety of this procedure. Since peak blood concentrations of local anesthetic agents occur within 30 seconds following cuff deflation, the cyclic deflation/inflation procedure should take place at 10- to 15-second intervals in order to decrease the peak concentrations of local anesthetic drug in the central circulatory compartment. Use of a double pneumatic cuff also has been advocated as an additional safety precaution and as a means of decreasing ischemic pain associated with the tourniquet. For the latter purpose, analgesia is established with the proximal cuff; the distal cuff is then inflated on the anesthetized limb.

PREINJECTION EXSANGUINATION. Exsanguination of the involved limb appears to be of value from a safety and efficacy point of view, since less drug is required to achieve adequate anesthesia if the limb has been exsanguinated prior to injection. Most commonly, the extremity is elevated to ensure gravity drainage and then tightly wrapped, distal to proximal, in an Esmarch bandage. When applied prior to the reduction of fracture, compression by the Esmarch bandage may cause pain. A longer period of gravity drainage (5 min) or a pneumatic splint should be used for exsanguination in these cases instead of the bandage.

INJECTION SITE. The majority of studies of intravenous regional anesthesia have involved surgical procedures on the upper limbs. Injection of local anesthetic into veins at the antecubital fossa should be avoided. High injection pressures there may force anesthetic under the tourniquet and into the systemic circulation. It is considerably more difficult to obtain a satisfactory degree of surgical analgesia with this technique in the lower limbs because of the greater mass of tissue involved. However, short procedures of the foot can be successfully performed under intravenous regional anesthesia without larger amounts of local anesthetic.[97] The tourniquet may be safely applied below the knee with the precaution of avoiding pressure over the superficial peroneal nerve as it runs around the neck of the fibula. The tourniquet then should be applied just below the fibular neck, and extra padding should be applied over the anterior lateral aspect of the leg.

DRUG-RELATED CONSIDERATIONS. Lidocaine has been the agent used most frequently for intravenous regional anesthesia. Prilocaine is also effective and has the potential for less systemic toxicity. Circulating blood levels of 0.5% prilocaine are significantly lower after tourniquet deflation than with equipotent 0.5% lidocaine.[98] More rapid tissue redistribution and hepatic metabolism are believed to be responsible for this difference. Methemoglobin is produced by a metabolic product of prilocaine, o-toluidine, but blood levels of methemoglobin measured after intravenous regional anesthesia with prilocaine remained below levels expected to cause symptoms. Residual analgesia following cuff deflation persists for approximately 5 to 10 minutes with agents such as prilocaine and lidocaine. Thrombophlebitis has been reported after the use of chloroprocaine. With bupivacaine, significant cardiotoxicity can occur and the agent is not recommended for intravenous regional anesthesia.

The concentration and volume of local anesthetic solution influences analgesic adequacy and potential safety of intravascular regional anesthesia. In general, the use of large volumes of more dilute solutions provides the optimum conditions for satisfactory anesthesia and enhanced safety.

Most commonly, 40 ml of a 0.5% solution of lidocaine (200 mg) has been found to produce satisfactory analgesia for the upper arm, which would correspond to a dosage of approximately 3 mg/kg. Since large volumes of local anesthetic solution are required for procedures involving the lower limbs, the use of 75 to 100 ml of a dilute anesthetic solution has been advocated, for example, 0.25% to 0.35% lidocaine (to a 300-mg maximum). Intravascular regional anesthesia is also quite successful in children with 3 to 5 mg/kg of 0.25% to 0.5% lidocaine.

Peripheral Nerve Blockade

Regional anesthetic procedures that involve the inhibition of conduction in nerve fibers of the peripheral nervous system can be classified together under the general category of peripheral nerve blockade.[99] This form of regional anesthesia has been subdivided arbitrarily into minor and major nerve blocks. *Minor nerve blocks* are defined as procedures involving single nerve entities, such as the ulnar or radial nerves at the wrist and the anterior or posterior tibial nerves at the ankle.

Major nerve blocks comprise those procedures in which two or more distinct nerves or a nerve plexus is blocked, for example, brachial plexus blockade.

Minor Nerve Blocks

A classification of the various agents according to their duration of action reveals that procaine and chloroprocaine possess a short duration of anesthetic activity, whereas lidocaine, mepivacaine, and prilocaine are agents of moderate duration (Table 6-6). The duration of both sensory analgesia and motor blockade is prolonged significantly when epinephrine is added to various local anesthetic solutions. As observed for infiltration anesthesia, lidocaine appears to benefit most by the addition of epinephrine.

Major Nerve Blocks

Brachial plexus blockade is the most common major nerve block employed for ambulatory surgical procedures of the upper extremity. A "flooding" technique is frequently employed to achieve satisfactory brachial plexus blockade. This involves the use of large volumes, up to 40 ml, of local anesthetic solution in order to maximize diffusion to the nerve plexus. The axillary approach to the brachial plexus is the safest and simplest to perform. Use of this technique reduces the risk of complications such as pneumothorax, which may become symptomatic after discharge. Interscalene, supraclavicular, and infraclavicular approaches also may be used to achieve somewhat different areas of anesthesia. For children, doses of 0.5 ml/kg may be employed.

ONSET TIME. The onset of complete anesthesia usually requires 10 to 20 minutes for brachial plexus blockade, even with agents such as chloroprocaine and lidocaine, which have a relatively rapid onset of action. However, significant reductions in block onset time have been reported with the addition of sodium bicarbonate to local anesthetic,[100] 1 mEq per 10 ml lidocaine or mepivacaine. Considerable variation in onset time exists based on the technical skill of the anesthesiologist.

TABLE 6-6. Minor Nerve Blocks for Ambulatory Surgery

Agent	Usual Concentration (%)	Plain Solutions			Epinephrine Containing Solutions
		Usual Adult Volume (ml)	Usual Adult Dosage (mg)	Average Duration (min)	Average Duration (min)
Procaine Chloroprocaine	2%	5–20	100–400	15–30	30–60
Lidocaine Mepivacaine Prilocaine	1%	5–20	50–200	60–120	120–180

DURATION OF ANESTHESIA. The greatest duration of anesthesia usually occurs following major nerve blocks (Table 6-7). In general, the agents of moderate duration, such as lidocaine and mepivacaine, produce anesthesia of 2 to 4 hours, whereas short-acting drugs, such as chloroprocaine, will provide 1 to 2 hours of anesthesia. This prolonged duration of effect is due to several factors. In general, a greater dose of local anesthetic agent is used for major nerve blocks as compared with other types of regional anesthetic procedures. In addition, the region of the brachial plexus is poorly vascularized, which results in a slow rate of vascular absorption and a greater uptake of drug by the major nerves. Epinephrine will prolong the duration of most local anesthetic agents employed for major nerve blocks and therefore should be used only when indicated.

Central Neural Blockade
Epidural Anesthesia
Lumbar epidural anesthesia is useful for surgical procedures involving the lower abdomen, pelvis, perineum, and lower extremities.[9] Epidural blockade may be used for laparoscopy with anesthesia to the T4 level, but the patient should be forewarned that shoulder pain will be felt. This referred diaphragmatic irritation can be minimized by modifying the surgical technique, as suggested under "Preparation," above. (The same provisos are applicable for laparoscopy under spinal anesthesia.) For arthroscopy, epidural anesthesia may provide shorter times to ambulation and discharge than general anesthesia, and less postoperative nausea and vomiting.[100a] Caudal anesthesia is usually reserved for pelvic and perineal surgery. In children, caudal epidural anesthesia is most often administered under basal sedation or light general anesthesia to provide postoperative analgesia. Both lumbar and caudal epidural are particularly applicable for use after induction of general anesthesia, since their success does not depend on obtaining paresthesias. Care must be taken to avoid airway obstruction when these blocks are performed in the lateral position under inhalation anesthesia.

VOLUME AND CONCENTRATION OF ANESTHETIC SOLUTIONS. Lumbar epidural administration in adults usually requires the use of 10- to 20-ml volumes to achieve satisfactory analgesic results. Cranial spread occurs more easily than sacral spread following lumbar epidural injections owing in part to negative intrathoracic pressure and to the resistance afforded by the narrowing of the epidural space at the lumbosacral junction. A significant delay in or an absence of analgesia at the first and second sacral segments is frequently observed following lumbar epidural injections. This has been attributed in part to the narrowing of the epidural space at the lumbosacral junction and also to the thickness of spinal roots in this region. Caudal anesthesia usually requires greater amounts of drug (20–30 ml) owing to loss of solution through the anterior sacral foramina and the rapid vascular absorption from this site. Little cranial spread beyond the lumbosacral junction occurs following caudal injections because of the peculiar anatomy of the epidural space in this region. Concentrations of 1.5% to 2.0% lidocaine or mepivacaine, 2% prilocaine, and 2% to 3% chloroprocaine are most commonly employed for lumbar epidural and caudal anesthesias. For children,

TABLE 6-7. Major Nerve Blocks for Ambulatory Surgery

| Agent | Usual Concentration (%) | Plain Solutions | | | | Epinephrine Containing Solutions | | | |
		Usual Adult Volume (ml)	Max. Adult Dose (mg)	Usual Onset (min)	Usual Duration (min)	Usual Adult Volume	Max. Adult Dose	Usual Onset	Usual Duration
Chloroprocaine	2–3	25–40	800	10–20	30–50	30–60	1000	10–20	60–120
Lidocaine	1–1.5	20–30	300	10–20	60–90	30–50	500	10–20	120–140
Mepivacaine	1–1.5	20–30	300	10–20	60–120	30–50	500	10–20	180–300
Prilocaine	1–2	30–50	600	10–20	60–120	Not available			

the recommended dosage for lumbar or caudal epidural anesthesia can be calculated for 1% lidocaine, 1% mepivacaine, and 0.25% bupivacaine by using the formula 0.1 ml per year per segment (± 0.2 ml). The formula is applicable up to the age of 12 in caudal epidural block. For a caudal block, it is often easier to use 0.5 ml/kg of one of these solutions, since this amount will consistently spread to L2–3 and sometimes to T10–11.[101]

PATIENT POSITION. Posture has been demonstrated to influence the quality of epidural analgesia. Larger quantities of anesthetic drug are required to achieve the same dermatomal level in patients in the sitting position than in the horizontal position. Lumbar epidural anesthesia is often performed with the patient in the sitting position in obstetrics to obtain satisfactory perineal analgesia.

AGE AND HEIGHT. Discrepancies exist among studies in which the influence of age and height on epidural anesthesia has been assessed by clinical means, that is, analgesic dermatomal levels, and by radiographic observations. Bromage has reported that dose per segment requirements of epidurally administered anesthetic agents are directly proportional to patient height; dose requirements are directly proportional to patient age until 18 years, then inversely proportional to age after age 18.[9] However, other investigators have failed to demonstrate any correlation in adults between age and height, on the one hand, and the spread of radiopaque material in the epidural space, on the other.

ANESTHETIC AGENT. Lidocaine, mepivacaine, and prilocaine are commonly used for surgical procedures of 1 to 2 hours, whereas chloroprocaine is employed most often for procedures of less than 1 hour (Table 6-8). The use of epinephrine (1:200,000) may significantly prolong the duration of the effects of these agents, and it should be added only when indicated and when adequate time for recovery is available. Onset of epidural anesthesia usually occurs within 5 to 15 minutes following administration of chloroprocaine, lidocaine, mepivacaine, and prilocaine; the addition of sodium bicarbonate may reduce the time needed.[100] Chloroprocaine may provide the shortest recovery times to ambulation and discharge.[101a] Procaine is rarely used for epidural anesthesia because of its slow onset of action.

HEMODYNAMIC CONSIDERATIONS. Interruption of sympathetic impulses can lead to cardiovascular alterations following the establishment of epidural anesthesia. However, since autonomic blockade occurs slowly, cardiovascular changes may not be very marked. On the other hand, profound hypotension may be observed in some patients following the onset of epidural anesthesia. The changes in blood pressure, heart rate, and cardiac output are related to the level of blockade, the amount of drug administered, the specific local anesthetic agent employed, the inclusion of a vasoconstrictor in the anesthetic solution, and the cardiovascular status of the patient.

TABLE 6-8. Epidural Blockade for Ambulatory Surgery

Agent	Usual Concentration (%)	Plain Solutions					Epinephrine-Containing Solutions		
		Usual Adult Volume (ml)	Total Adult Dose (mg)	Usual Onset (min)	Usual Duration (min)	Usual Adult Volume	Max. Adult Dose	Usual Onset	Usual Duration
Chloroprocaine	3	15–25	150–750	5–15	30–60	15–30	150–900	5–15	30–90
Lidocaine	1–2	15–30	150–300	5–15	60–90	15–30	150–500	5–15	60–180
Mepivacaine	1–2	15–30	150–300	5–15	60–120	15–30	150–500	5–15	60–180
Prilocaine	1–3	15–30	150–600	5–15	60–120	Not available			

LEVEL OF BLOCK. The higher the block, the greater the number of sympathetic fibers that are affected, leading to a reduction in vascular tone. Thus peripheral resistance decreases, but a fall in arterial pressure may be prevented by vasoconstriction in unblocked segments. Thus blocks below T5 are seldom associated with marked hypotension. Higher blocks, however, not only prevent compensatory vasoconstriction but also affect the cardiac sympathetic nerves, which arise in the T1–5 segments. At these dermatomal levels of block, a fall in heart rate and cardiac output may occur. The blockade of sympathetic fibers to the heart and the failure to block the vagus nerves can cause vasovagal attacks, which are associated with profound bradycardia and in some patients transient cardiac arrest. This may, in fact, represent the most common cause of profound hypotension following high levels of epidural anesthesia. As the veins forming the capacitance vessels will also be affected by the sympathetic block, venous pooling can occur if the venous return is obstructed by gravity or abdominal tumors including pregnancy. Thus patients are very susceptible to the head-up posture, which causes expansion of the capacitance vessels and can lead to a marked decrease in venous return and cardiac output.

DRUG DOSAGE. Relatively large amounts of local anesthetic drug are required to achieve a satisfactory degree of epidural blockade. The local anesthetic agents are absorbed rapidly, and significant blood levels may be achieved. The absorbed local anesthetic agent may produce systemic effects involving the cardiovascular system. Most local anesthetic agents produce a biphasic effect on the cardiovascular system. For example, it has been shown that blood levels of lidocaine of less than 4 μg/ml following epidural blockade resulted in a slight increase in blood pressure due mainly to an increase in cardiac output. Doses of epidural lidocaine that produce blood levels in excess of 4 μg/ml caused hypotension due in part to the negative inotropic action and the peripheral vasodilator effect of lidocaine.

SPECIFIC AGENTS. Differences in the onset of epidural anesthesia occur as a function of the specific agent employed and the concentration used. In general, local anesthetics commonly used for epidural blockade in ambulatory surgery can be classified as agents of rapid and moderate onset. Chloroprocaine and lidocaine produce a fairly rapid onset of anesthesia, whereas mepivacaine and prilocaine are relatively slower in onset. With all agents there is a tendency for onset to be faster as the concentration is increased. The more rapidly acting agents tend to produce a more profound degree of hypotension due to the more rapid blockade of sympathetic fibers.

ADDITION OF VASOCONSTRICTORS. Epinephrine may be added to local anesthetics intended for epidural use in order to decrease the rate of vascular absorption and prolong the duration of anesthesia. Absorbed epinephrine itself may produce transient cardiovascular alterations. A more profound degree of hypotension has been reported to occur following the use of epinephrine containing local anesthetics for epidural blockade. The absorbed epinephrine is believed to stimulate β_2-adrenergic receptors in all peripheral vascular beds, leading to an enhanced state of vasodilation and a fall in diastolic pressure. The β_1-adrenergic receptor stimulating effect of epinephrine results in an increase in heart rate and cardiac output that will counteract the peripheral vasodilator state to some extent. Although absorbed epinephrine may cause the early cardiovascular changes observed following epidural block, the prolonged hypotension seen with local anesthetics containing epinephrine is probably related to the achievement of a more profound degree of sympathetic blockade.

BLOOD VOLUME STATUS. The cardiovascular alterations described above relate primarily to changes occurring in normovolemic subjects. Cardiovascular depression is more severe and more dangerous following the production of epidural anesthesia in hypovolemic subjects. Epidural anesthesia in mildly hypovolemic volunteers was found to provoke vasovagal attacks associated with profound hypotension and bradycardia. Hypovolemia is usually accompanied by compensatory vasoconstriction that will be abolished by the block, and cardiovascular collapse may ensue.

Spinal Anesthesia

The analgesic properties of subarachnoid blockade may be influenced by a number of factors that can be related to the patient, the anesthetic solution, and anesthetic technique.[102]

PATIENT FACTORS. Patient position during and immediately following subdural administration of a local anesthetic agent will influence the spread of spinal anesthesia. Since hyperbaric anesthetic solutions are commonly used for subarachnoid blocks, the spread in cerebrospinal fluid will be affected by gravity. For example, the patient in a sitting position at the time of injection will experience a lower-level block than the patient who is supine.

A decrease in the spinal fluid capacity of the subarachnoid space will markedly affect the degree of analgesia and the dose requirements for satisfactory spinal anesthesia. Inferior vena cava compression, usually due to pregnancy, is the most common cause of engorgement and distention of the vertebral system, decreasing the capacity of the subarachnoid space for spinal fluid. The dosage requirements for spinal anesthesia are significantly lower in pregnant patients, from midgestation to term, than in nongravid subjects.

ANESTHETIC FACTORS. Relatively few agents are prepared in a form specifically intended for subarachnoid administration (Table 6-9). Lidocaine (5.0%) is the anesthetic of choice for ambulatory surgery patients. Onset of spinal anesthesia is extremely rapid. Isobaric lidocaine (2.0%) also has been used for specific operative situations, such as anorectal surgery, in which it may be advantageous to maintain the patient in a head-down position. Longer-acting agents such as tetracaine or bupivacaine should be used rarely for ambulatory procedures, and only if surgery is scheduled early enough in the day to permit recovery and timely discharge.

TABLE 6-9. Spinal Anesthetic Agents for Ambulatory Surgery

Agent	Usual Concentration (%)	Usual Adult Volume (ml)	Total Adult Dose (mg)	Baricity	Glucose Concentration (%)	Usual Anesthetic Duration (min)
Lidocaine	5	1–2	50–100	Hyperbaric	7.5	45–60
	2	2–3	40–60	Isobaric		60–90
Tetracaine	0.25–1	1–4	5–20	Hyperbaric	5	75–150
	0.1–0.3			Hypobaric		
	0.5			Isobaric		
Bupivacaine	0.5	3–4	15–20	Isobaric		75–150
	0.75	2–3	15–22.5	Hyperbaric	8	

As in other forms of regional anesthesia, vasoconstrictor agents may prolong the duration of spinal anesthesia. The addition of 0.2 to 0.3 mg epinephrine to lidocaine solutions will produce a 50% prolongation of spinal anesthesia for procedures lasting 60 to 90 minutes. An increase in the duration of tetracaine subarachnoid block also has been reported following the addition of epinephrine or phenylephrine, 1 to 5 mg. However, the addition of a vasoconstrictor to spinal anesthetic solutions of tetracaine is not recommended for ambulatory surgery because of the prolonged duration of blockade.

Spinal anasthesia is frequently associated with a fall in systemic blood pressure. The degree of hypotension is related primarily to the extent of the spinal blockade. Subarachnoid blocks that extend to the T10 level are rarely associated with a significant fall in pressure. Extension of block to the T5 dermatomal level usually results in a fall in blood pressure due to a decrease in peripheral vascular resistance that is a direct result of the inhibition of sympathetic outflow below the level of block. Analgesic dermatomal levels above T5 may be associated with a more profound degree of hypotension due to a fall in cardiac output. The decrease in cardiac output may be related, in part, to a decrease in venous return and to the inhibition of sympathetic fibers innervating the heart.

The degree of spinal hypotension may be influenced by patient position. Maintenance of a slight head-up posture following spinal anesthesia usually will lead to a more pronounced fall in blood pressure due to a decrease in venous return. Placement of patients in a slight head-down position will tend to maintain normal venous return so that the degree of hypotension is lessened.

Differences also exist among different agents in terms of spinal hypotension. Lidocaine produces a more rapid onset of block than tetracaine, which usually results in a more profound degree of hypotension. A comparison of tetracaine and bupivacaine indicated that tetracaine caused a significantly greater fall in blood pressure, despite the fact that the level of analgesia produced by the drugs was similar.

Hypovolemia will clearly result in a profound degree of hypotension following spinal anesthesia. Patients should be well hydrated prior to the performance of a subarachnoid block. Hypotension in a normovolemic patient is easily reversed

TABLE 6-10. Spinal Anesthetic Agents for Pediatric Ambulatory Surgery

Agent	Concentration (%)	Dose (mg/kg)
Lidocaine	5	2 (under 3 yrs)
		1 (3–10 yrs)
Tetracaine	1	0.2

by placing the patient in a slight Trendelenburg position or administering either a crystalloid solution or a vasoconstrictor agent such as ephedrine or phenylephrine.

Doses of spinal anesthetic agents suitable for pediatric ambulatory surgery have been determined (Table 6-10). These agents are all hyperbaric and contain glucose, although other formulations could be used. The increased dose requirement for lidocaine spinal anesthesia in infants is due to a higher volume of cerebrospinal fluid relative to body weight.

COMPLICATIONS OF LOCAL AND REGIONAL ANESTHESIA

The potential complications of regional anesthesia include headache, neurologic sequelae, systemic toxicity, and allergic reaction. All may occur in ambulatory surgery patients. With a better understanding of the pathophysiology involved, these complications can often be prevented. If complications do occur, early diagnosis and appropriate treatment should result in a satisfactory outcome.

Headache

Headache is a common postoperative complaint. It may be due to nonanesthetic causes such as dehydration or the psychogenic reactions of tension and depression. Anesthetic causes of headache include postdural puncture and meningeal irritation or infection.

The postdural puncture headache (PDPH) may be of variable intensity. It is described as a dull or aching pressure that begins at the occiput and extends down the neck and over the head to the frontal region. It may be unilateral or generalized. The postdural headache is postural. It occurs, or is at least aggravated, when the patient sits or stands and is relieved upon reclining or with abdominal compression. The PDPH typically begins during the second postoperative day and lasts usually 1 to 4 days. Since headache onset is expected to occur after discharge from the ambulatory unit, it is important to instruct patients to contact the facility if PDPH develops. Symptoms associated with PDPH include nausea and vomiting, dizziness, visual disturbances such as blurred vision and rare abducens palsy, and auditory disturbances such as tinnitus and stuffiness.

The etiology of the pain of PDPH was first proposed by Bier in 1899. The hypothesis is that cerebrospinal fluid (CSF) leaks out through a hole in the dura made by the needle, resulting in a decrease in CSF pressure. With diminishing

CSF pressure, the brain is displaced caudad, with traction on pain-sensitive blood vessels and supporting parts of the dura (falx and tentorium cerebelli). Pain is conducted by way of the trigeminal nerve to the anterior head and by way of the glossopharyngeal, vagus, and upper cervical nerves to the posterior head and neck.

The incidence of headache after spinal anesthesia has been evaluated in many studies. It ranges from 3.5% to 11% in large surgical series, although rates as low as 0.4% have been reported.[102-104] The incidence of PDPH specifically in an ambulatory surgery population is under investigation. An estimation may be gained by examining series of comparable procedures under spinal anesthesia. Burke reported 1.3% headache in 1063 women undergoing laparoscopy.[105] The incidence of PDPH after inguinal hernia repair in men has been reported to be 1.9% to 3.4%.[106,107] Specifically in ambulatory surgery, Mulroy and coworkers reported a PDPH incidence of 5.2% in patients undergoing a variety of procedures.[108] For comparison, the incidence of (nonspinal) headache after general anesthesia is 17% to 26%.[109]

Several factors have been associated with a decreased incidence of PDPH after spinal anesthesia. Factors that decrease the incidence but are not subject to control include male sex and increasing age. However, younger female ambulatory patients can be offered the option of spinal anesthesia with a thorough discussion of advantages and disadvantages. Female surgical patients develop fewer headaches than obstetric patients. Factors under the anesthesiologist's control, and therefore usable for prevention, include needle size and hydration. A decrease in incidence of headache from 41% with a 20-gauge needle to 0.4% with a 26-gauge needle has been demonstrated.[102] In patients who were given fluids (2.5 L/day), the incidence of headache was decreased for all needle sizes. The consistently low incidence of PDPH in modern series of patients undergoing procedures suitable for ambulatory surgery is probably due to increased awareness of the effectiveness of smaller needle size; 25-gauge or 26-gauge needles should be used for spinal anesthesia in ambulatory patients. Needle insertion with the bevel parallel to the longitudinal dural fibers[110] and through a lateral rather than midline approach[111] also may help. Early ambulation has no significant effect on headache occurrence.[104,112,113]

Treatment of PDPH includes bed rest; hydration, intravenous if necessary; increased abdominal pressure by wearing a binder and lying prone; analgesic drugs, from aspirin to narcotics; and the psychological support of reassurance and encouragement.[16] Caffeine may be given orally or as an infusion of caffeine sodium benzoate (500 mg/L). All these therapies are symptomatic. There are, however, treatments that attempt to act on the cause of PDPH—leakage of CSF. Rice and Dabbs first reported the use of epidural placement of saline.[114] Injecting an average of 82 ml through caudal and lumbar catheters, they achieved immediate relief of headache in 99.5% patients. Subsequent studies report 69% to 87.5% success when epidural saline placement was used postpartum for headache prophylaxis, either by continuous infusion or by repeat injections.[115,116] Permanent, immediate cures are thought to be due to inversion of a flap valve preventing further CSF leak. However, epidural saline therapy is often only temporarily successful. Rice and Dabbs reported a 54% recurrence rate. Usubiaga and colleagues[117] demonstrated an increase in CSF and epidural pressures immediately after epidural saline injection. This provided relief of the PDPH, but pressures returned to baseline in 3 to 10 minutes, possibly explaining the transitory effect. Epidural placement of 50 to 100 ml of normal saline without preservative is somewhat successful in preventing PDPH and can be given slowly through the epidural catheter *in situ*. However, a permanent cure for headache may not be achieved with this therapy.

Epidural blood patch (EBP) is another therapy that acts on the cause of PDPH. First described by Gormley,[118] the technique now used at Brigham and Women's Hospital consists of identification of the epidural space at the level at which dural puncture was performed, venipuncture and withdrawal of 10 to 20 ml blood under aseptic conditions, and injection of the blood into the epidural space.[16] Patient tolerance determines the final dose; injection should be terminated if back or radicular pain develops. The patient rests supine for 30 minutes with knees flexed over pillows to decrease the lumbar lordosis, and 1L intravenous crystalloid is given. Limited activity, and particularly avoidance of Valsalva straining,[119] is recommended for the rest of the day to prevent dislodging the clot. EBP is easily performed on an outpatient basis. Relief often occurs immediately or within 24 hours. The success rate for EBP has been reported to be 91% to 100%.[118,120] The mode of action of EBP has been investigated by DiGiovanni and coworkers.[120] They performed epidural injections of autologous blood in goats after dural puncture with a 18-gauge needle. At 24 hours, the goats' epidural space contained intact unorganized blood cells with no fibrous reaction. Fibroblastic activity began at 48 hours and therefore could not play a major role in the immediate relief of headache symptoms. Rather, EBP acts by formation of gelatinous tamponade, which prevents leakage of CSF, allowing the dural tear to undergo normal healing. Subarachnoid pressure studies during EBP show pressures are sustained at 71.4% peak for 15 minutes after completion of the epidural injection.[121] By 3 months after EBP, collagen has been laid down by fibroblasts, with the resulting tissue essentially undistinguishable from underlying dura.[120] Successful epidural anesthesia has been reported 7 to 380 days after EBP.[122,123] Epidural blood placement does not obliterate the epidural space and does not preclude the use of regional block for later surgical or obstetric procedures.

Criteria for use of EBP are that the headache should be identified as PDPH, not migraine or other chronic headache, it should have lasted at least 2 or 3 days, it should be severe enough to interfere with patients' ability to function at daily activities, and conservative therapy should have been ineffective. At the Boston Hospital for Women (one of the predecessors of the present Brigham and Women's Hospital), we examined our need for EBP after spinal anesthesia for obstetric delivery from January 1976 to June 1977.[16] In 1,999 patients, 10% developed headache, but only 0.67% required EBP. We also examined the data for 61 patients who sustained an unintentional dural puncture with a 17-gauge needle during attempted epidural anesthesia. Of these patients, 33% developed PDPH, but only 6.7% required EBP. Based on these data, the majority of PDPH appear to resolve with conservative therapy alone.

Palahniuk and Cumming present additional evidence against the use of pro-phylactic EBP.[124] They evaluated obstetric patients who sustained unintended dural puncture with a 16-gauge Tuohy needle; some were given autologous blood through a correctly placed epidural catheter at the termination of the anesthetic. The incidence of headache was unchanged: 54% for the patients who received epidural blood therapy and 59% for those patients who did not. Loeser and co-workers studied the success rate of EBP in patients with PDPH relative to the time from dural puncture.[125] The patients given EBP within 24 hours of dural puncture had a 29% success rate, whereas those patients who were given EBP after 24 hours had a 96% success rate. The high failure rate of prophylactic EBP may be due to the following factors: (1) blood may not be placed directly over the hole produced by the dural puncture, especially if injected through an epidural catheter, and (2) the pressure and/or volume of leaking CSF may be sufficient to prevent organization of the clot over the dural hole. The use of EBP for headache prevention is not recommended because the prophylactic patch is of limited effectiveness and because the majority of headaches resolve with conservative therapy.

No permanent adverse effects of epidural blood patch have been reported. Transient backache and paresthesias or radicular pain may be experienced. Re-assurance of the patient is essential. The dura may be punctured again during EBP, but the subarachnoid injection of autologous blood (in dogs) was not asso-ciated with neurologic deficits.[126] A major contraindication to the performance of EBP is the presence of infection, either generalized septicemia or local infec-tion in the area of needle insertion. Other major contraindications are preoper-ative coagulopathy and active neurologic disease.

A second class of headaches complicating regional anesthesia is the headache of meningeal inflammation. Aseptic meningitis has been reported after spinal and epidural anesthesia. The headache of aseptic meningitis is severe, general-ized, and nonpostural and may be accompanied by fever, photophobia, and other signs of meningeal irritation. Symptoms appear within several hours of the an-esthetic and last 2 to 4 days. A diagnostic lumbar puncture will reveal clear to slightly cloudy CSF with elevated pressure, increased protein, normal sugar, and leukocytosis—usually polymorphonuclear. Peripheral leukocytosis is also seen. Cultures of the CSF are negative, and no bacteria or pathogens are seen on mi-croscopic examination. Aseptic meningitis has been sporadically reported, but its occurrence is rare. In Dripps and Vandam's series of 10,098 spinals and Lund's series of 10,000 epidurals, none occurred.[127,128] The etiology of this syndrome is uncertain but is thought to include local toxicity due to impurity or overdose of local anesthetic; the introduction of blood, skin, or antiseptic into the subarach-noid space; and the irritative effect of residual detergents used to clean equip-ment or soak ampules of local anesthetic. Therapy for aseptic meningitis is conservative and consists of analgesics and fluids. Recovery is usually complete.

Septic meningitis is another possible cause of headache following spinal an-esthesia. Signs and symptoms of septic meningitis are the same as those of the aseptic variety, but when a diagnostic lumbar puncture is performed, a purulent exudate with decreased sugar content is found; pathogenic organisms, usually cocci or gram-negative rods, are seen on microscopic examination or culture. The incidence of septic meningitis following spinal anesthesia is rare (0.005%). Treatment consists of analgesics, fluids, and appropriate antibiotics.

Neurologic Sequelae

Neurologic complications of regional anesthesia occur primarily associated with spinal and epidural anesthesia. Direct trauma from needle or catheter may injure nerve roots. Sensory rather than motor roots are more often affected, and limited damage occurs over the distribution of the nerve. Needle trauma also may be seen after techniques that elicit paresthesias, such as brachial plexus blocks. Symptoms usually resolve. Injury to the spinal cord itself is accompanied by sharp pain and occasionally loss of consciousness; damage tends to be more extensive and irreversible. Trauma to the bones and ligaments results in backache. Transient backache due to the instrumentation has been reported in 1.6% of patients after epidural and 2.7% of patients after spinal anesthesia.[103,128] Vertebral bodies and intervertebral disks have been penetrated by an anesthetic needle. Direct trauma by needle or catheter can injure blood vessels, usually veins. Significant symptoms may occur if the patient is anticoagulated or has a clotting disorder.

Ischemic injury to the spinal cord is another relatively common cause of neurologic sequelae to regional anesthesia. Ischemia may be caused by arterial hypotension, whether anesthetically induced or accidental.[129] The use of epinephrine in epidural anesthetic solutions may reduce spinal cord circulation. This vasoconstriction is not usually significant in humans unless accompanied by hypotension, arteriosclerosis, or both. Vascular spasm may result in ischemic injury in the absence of actual obstruction. The severity of the ischemic injury is proportional to the distance of the vascular lesion from the spinal cord. Interruption of flow at the level of the aorta or vertebral arteries may lead to complete transverse necrosis of the cord, whereas more distal lesions cause more circumscribed damage. Occlusion of the anterior spinal artery results in a syndrome of motor paralysis with preservation of sensation. With ischemic damage to the anterior two-thirds of the cord, the prognosis for recovery is poor. Posterior spinal artery syndrome is rare and consists of anesthesia below the level of ischemic injury with segmental loss of skin and tendon reflexes.

Compression of the cord may indirectly cause ischemic injury. The resulting neurologic deficit is a function of the severity of the compression, the rapidity of onset of compression, and the function of the compressed tissue. Anesthesia-related causes of ischemic cord compression include epidural abscess and epidural hematoma. Symptoms of epidural abscess include fever and localized back pain and tenderness. Lower extremity root pain, weakness, and flaccid paralysis develop over 1 to 4 days. Peripheral blood cultures may be positive. Epidural abscesses are usually located dorsal to the spinal cord; pus may be aspirated while a diagnostic lumbar puncture is being attempted. Lumbar puncture with manometrics reveals evidence of block; CSF has elevated protein, moderate pleocytosis with lymphocytes, normal glucose, and negative smear and cultures. Epidural abscess is often associated with sepsis or infection elsewhere in the body;

antecedent trauma to the back or chronic debilitation from alcoholism or diabetes are also predisposing factors. The development of an epidural abscess in relation to spinal or epidural anesthesia is rare (<0.0015%). More often, epidural abscesses occur spontaneously, not associated with anesthesia. Treatment is decompression by prompt surgical drainage of the abscess. Recovery may be complete when minimal neurologic deficit has developed and treatment is instituted rapidly, but delays may result in permanent neurologic sequelae.

Epidural hematoma is the second common cause of spinal cord injury from ischemic compression. Epidural hematoma formation is often heralded by sharp pain in the distribution of the affected portion of cord, followed shortly by weakness and flaccid paralysis. Onset is usually sudden and progression to paralysis rapid. Fever does not occur. Lumbar puncture reveals clear fluid, sometimes with elevated protein; medical imaging shows extradural compression. Disseminated intravascular coagulation (DIC) has been reported within 2 hours after second-trimester abortions by dilatation and evacuation; the presumed stimulus is amniotic fluid or placental thromboplastin.[130] These patients should be evaluated carefully, including indicated hematologic tests, before a regional anesthetic is administered for removal of retained products of conception. Hematomas may occur after spinal or epidural anesthesia or after lumbar puncture without anesthesia. Intracranial subdural and intracerebral hematomas have also been reported after spinal anesthesia, possibly related to the decrease in CSF pressure and traction on intracranial blood vessels. Prognosis for recovery of neurologic function is best if surgical decompression with evacuation of the clot is done promptly.

Infection is now a rare cause of neurologic sequelae of regional anesthesia. Extrinsic sources of infection include contaminated equipment or drugs. Aseptic technique with good skin preparation and sterile equipment are necessary. Infection may arise from internal local sources or from elsewhere in the body, transported by the bloodstream or lymphatics. Infections may develop anywhere along the path of the anesthetic needle or catheter. Infections in the spinal cord itself cause localized edema, vascular occlusion, and neuronal destruction, as well as ascending and descending degeneration. Paralysis, sensory deficit, and loss of sphincter control may occur. Prognosis is poor despite antibiotics or decompressive laminectomy.

Exposure to chemical toxic agents is another cause of neurologic sequelae. Neurolytic agents such as alcohol, collodion, hypertonic saline, propylene glycol, and several preservatives, including benzyl alcohol and methyl hydroxybenzoate, have been injected into the epidural and subarachnoid spaces, resulting in temporary or permanent neurologic deficits. Alcohol can be found in antiseptics used for skin cleansing; care should be taken to avoid contamination of equipment with these solutions. Local anesthetic ampules should not be soaked in alcohol because minute cracks in the glass may allow entry of the toxic substance into the solution to be injected. Accidental detergent contamination has also been implicated in the development of neurologic sequelae. Equipment reused for regional anesthesia should be thoroughly rinsed in water before undergoing sterilization.

Excessively high concentrations of some local anesthetics may also be neurotoxic. The hyperosmolality of these solutions is thought to be at fault. Radiopaque contrast materials are also neurotoxic with a 0.22% incidence of sequelae.[129] Complications due to injection of contrast material may be incorrectly ascribed to an ongoing regional anesthesia. Clinical symptoms of chemical neurologic toxicity usually appear as a mild aseptic meningitis. Rarely, a chronic proliferative adhesive arachnoiditis may develop. The specific neurologic deficit depends on the particular location and density of the inflammatory reaction; pain, sensory and motor deficits, and loss of rectal and bladder sphincter control may be seen. Onset of the adhesive arachnoiditis syndrome may be delayed weeks or months, and symptoms are often progressive. Recovery is rare.

Exacerbation of preexisting pathology is a common cause of neurologic sequelae ascribed to regional anesthesia. Preexisting disease may be vascular or neurologic. Vascular pathology may be in the form of anatomic malformations, either congenital or acquired. Embolization of any of the vessels supplying the cord also may cause vascular insufficiency and neurologic deficit. Generalized vascular disease also may predispose to ischemic neurologic injury. Such diseases include atherosclerosis, diabetes mellitus, syphilis, thromboangiitis obliterans, and periarteritis nodosa.

Preexisting neurologic pathology may be aggravated coincident with regional anesthesia. Nerve injury may actually be due to mechanical compression from a prolapsed intervertebral disk, spondylosis, developmental laminar stenosis, or a uterine leiomyoma. Tumor, another cause of neurologic damage, may be first suspected after regional anesthesia. Metastatic epidural tumors causing compressive ischemic injury are the most common, but primary and subdural neoplasma also occur. Neurologic disease affecting the spinal cord, such as multiple sclerosis and tabes dorsalis, may worsen at the time of regional anesthesia, and the deficit may be ascribed to anesthesia. However, stable chronic neurologic disease in itself is not a contraindication to receiving regional anesthesia; the course of such disease is probably not affected by the anesthesia. Informed consent by the patient is, as always, needed.

Extrinsic nonanesthetic factors also may cause neurologic damage during regional anesthesia by means of vascular or direct traumatic mechanisms. Interference of vascular supply to the spinal cord can be a result of surgical section. Causes of direct nerve trauma include improper positioning of the patient on an operating table or in stirrups and the use of retractors. Recovery of function may require several months, but is often complete.

When neurologic injury occurs following regional anesthesia, its cause must be immediately and thoroughly investigated. Anesthesia can often be proved or disproved as the cause of the sequelae. The first step in the differential diagnosis is a complete neurologic examination, followed by diagnostic lumbar puncture unless definite contraindications exist. Medical imaging should be performed if there is evidence of subarachnoid block. The single most important diagnostic test is electromyography. Electromyography can differentiate between intradural and extradural neuropathies; the latter cannot be caused by spinal anesthesia, so the block may be exonerated. Electromyography also can be used to determine the precise level of spinal cord damage and the duration of injury, thereby identifying the lesion as antedating the anesthesia. Marinacci and Courville used electromyography to evaluate 542 patients with neurologic deficit ascribed to spinal anesthesia.[131] They were able to rule out an anesthesia cause in all but four of the cases.

Neurologic sequelae have been reported since the introduction of regional techniques but are rare with modern anesthetic agents. Dripps and Vandam (1954) followed 10,098 spinal anesthesias and found no cases of postanesthetic paralysis.[127] Phillips and coworkers (1969) also reported no cases of major neurologic deficit in their series of 10,440 spinals.[103] These authors also evaluated their patients for minor peripheral nerve symptoms. Dripps and Vandam reported an incidence of 0.7% of areas of numbness or pain in the lower extremities or perineum; most symptoms had resolved by the 6-month postanesthetic evaluation. Phillips and colleagues reported a 0.36% incidence of any symptoms of peripheral nerve injury. Their incidence of persistent peripheral neuropathy after spinal anesthesia was 0.02%.

Epidural anesthesia also has been evaluated for its incidence of neurologic complications. Dawkins reviewed 32,718 lumbar epidural anesthesias and found 0.02% developed permanent and 0.1% transient paralysis.[132] Usubiaga reviewed a separate 780,000 epidural anesthesias.[129] He found that the incidence of major paralytic complication to be 0.01%, of which 13% recovered "almost completely." In two larger subseries totaling 100,000 anesthesias, Usubiaga reported that 0.005% patients developed major neurologic injury; more experienced groups appear to have a lower rate of complication. Caudal epidural anesthesias have a similarly low rate of neurologic sequelae; Dawkins reported 0.005% patients with permanent paralysis and 0.02% with transient paralysis in his review of 22,968 caudal anesthesias.[18]

Neurologic deficits have been reported after regional anesthesia with all modern local anesthetic agents including lidocaine, mepivacaine, bupivacaine, and etidocaine.[133,134] With chloroprocaine, prolonged neurologic deficits have been reported after unintentional subarachnoid injection.[135] Covino and coworkers evaluated the data and suggested that a cause may be the low pH of commercially prepared chloroprocaine, which is 2.167 for the 2% CE solution and 3.126 for the 3% solution.[136] However, low pH in itself is probably not the sole cause of the reported deficits. Ravindran and colleagues showed no sequelae from the subarachnoid placement of pH 3.0 saline.[137] Chloroprocaine, 3.3%, was used by Foldes and McNall in 1952 for spinal anesthesia in 214 patients with no neurologic sequelae; they used a less stable formulation with pH of 4.8.[138] Studies by Gissen and colleagues demonstrated that the combination of low pH (<3.5) and presence of the preservative bisulfite was able to generate the neurologic sequelae seen in the absence of any local anesthetic.[139] Chloroprocaine has been reformulated without bisulfite, and this commercial preparation has been used without neurologic complication.

Recently, there have been reports of moderate to severe back pain after the use of Nesacaine® for ambulatory epidural anesthesia. Fibuch and Opper noted a 40% incidence of localized paralumbar muscle pain and spasm which developed in the PACU following lumbar epidural anesthesia using either 2% or 3% Nesacaine-MPF (Astra Pharmaceutical Products, Incorporated., Westborough, Mass.).[140] Muscle pain lasted for approximately 24 hours postoperatively; before resolving without sequelae all patients required treatment with narcotic analgesics. As summarized in a letter from Astra Pharmaceuticals (W. Spickler, December 1988), there have been no symptoms to suggest neurologic deficits. One possible mechanism is localized muscle tetany caused by calcium chelating action of the preservative disodium EDTA used in this anesthetic formulation. Another possible mechanism is muscle irritation from direct contact with chloroprocaine.[140a] This problem can be minimized by the use of plain lidocaine for direct local infiltration and by incremental administration of the epidural anesthetic drug to avoid injecting large volumes.

Systemic Toxicity
Another of the complications of regional anesthesia is the systemic toxic reaction. These reactions occur when local anesthetic is administered so that the rate of absorption is greater than the rate of destruction. This imbalance can be due to the injection of an excessive dose, either excessive concentration or excessive volume or both. An increased rate of absorption may result from the presence of lacerated veins or normally rich vascularity at the site of injection or from application to mucous membranes or abraded skin. The rate of injection also affects the development of systemic toxicity; a faster rate of injection results in a decreased tolerance to the anesthetic. Toxic reactions may be due to an unintentional intravascular injection, even of a therapeutic dose, because it is the sudden increase in systemic concentration that causes the reaction. Intravenous injection may be accomplished directly, through a needle, or indirectly, as with an epidural catheter, which may find its way into a vein either at the time of initial placement or anytime thereafter. Arterial injection is less likely to cause a toxic reaction, because the longer circuit through the peripheral vascular bed allows time for dilution and ester hydroylsis. However, reverse arterial blood flow has been proposed as another possible cause of systemic toxic reaction. Effects in the cerebral vascular system have been demonstrated after brachial, radial, and femoral intraarterial injection. Systemic toxic reactions also may be due to a decreased rate of detoxification of the local anesthetic. The detoxification rate depends on the chemical composition of the drug, and therefore its mode of metabolism, the functional ability of the detoxifying organ, and the patient's metabolic rate. Other factors that influence the development of a toxic reaction include the effect of concurrent medications, the patient's acid-base balance (acidosis decreases the threshold), general physical status, and variable and unpredictable individual sensitivity.

The signs and symptoms of central nervous systemic toxic reactions occur along a concentration related spectrum.[141] Among the early subjective signs of local anesthetic toxicity, drowsiness is noted first. Patients also may complain of lightheadedness, dizziness, a metallic taste, nausea, tinnitus, circumoral tingling or numbness, or blurred vision. Objectively, confusion, slurred speech, nystagmus, and muscle tremors or twitches can be seen. An inverse relationship exists between the relative potency of local anesthetic agents and the blood levels required to generate toxic symptoms. For lidocaine, a level of 4 µg/ml was the threshold for beginning symptoms. With more potent bupivacaine and etidocaine, toxicity appears in the 2- to 3-µg/ml range.[142] Cortical electroencephalography (EEG) at this stage shows only drowsiness.

Further in the spectrum of toxicity are frank convulsions. Drowsiness proceeds to loss of consciousness, and muscle twitches proceed to generalized tonic-clonic seizures. Ventilation may be impeded by seizure activity, and cyanosis may develop. Pulse and blood pressure may rise as a result of the sympathetic response to hypoxia and hypercarbia, although hypotension sometimes develops due to depressant effects of the local anesthetic. This level of systemic toxicity also has been correlated with lidocaine blood levels. Wikinski and coworkers, using lidocaine for psychiatric shock therapy, found a mean plasma level of 22 µg/ml at the time of convulsion.[130] Usubiaga and colleagues watched the electroencephalogram in human volunteers who were given lidocaine until they convulsed.[141] Slow waves and irregular spiking were seen, which progressed to synchronous epileptiform discharges. Convulsive doses of lidocaine in cats block inhibitory pathways in the cerebral cortex; facilitatory neurons function unopposed, resulting in central nervous system excitation. Subcortical electroencephalograms in experimental animals show that local anesthetics block inhibitory relays, leading to excitation of an epileptogenic focus in the amygdala.[143]

Local anesthetic agents can produce profound effects on the cardiovascular system. The systemic administration of these agents can exert a direct action both on cardiac muscle and on peripheral vascular smooth muscle. In general, the cardiovascular system appears to be more resistant to the effects of local anesthetic agents than the central nervous system. Studies in dogs and sheep have indicated that doses of local anesthetic agents which cause significant cardiovascular effects are approximately three times higher than the dose of these agents which will have distinct effects on the central nervous system.[144,145]

The sequence of cardiovascular events that usually occurs following the systemic administration of local anesthetic agents is as follows: At relatively nontoxic blood levels of these agents, either no change in blood pressure or a slight increase in blood pressure may be observed. The slight increase in blood pressure may be related to a slight increase in cardiac output and heart rate which have been seen in some animal preparations and is believed due to an enhancement of sympathetic activity by these agents. In addition, the direct vasoconstrictor action of local anesthetics on certain peripheral vascular beds at low concentrations may be responsible in part for a slight increase in systemic blood pressure.

As the blood level of local anesthetic approaches toxic concentrations, a fall in blood pressure is usually the first cardiovascular sign. Studies with both the ester and amide agents in intact dogs have demonstrated that the initial hypotension observed is probably not related to peripheral vasodilation and a subsequent decrease in peripheral vascular resistance.[146,147] Rather, initial hypotension appears to be correlated with the negative inotropic action of these agents which results in a decrease in cardiac output and stroke volume. This depression in blood pressure is transient in nature and spontaneously reversible in most patients. However, if the amount of local anesthetic administered is excessive, an irreversible state of cardiovascular depression occurs. Profound peripheral dilation develops due to a direct relaxant effect on vascular smooth muscle. At high concentrations the depressant effect of these agents on the excitability of cardiac tissue will also become evident as a decrease in sinus rate and as AV conduction block. Ultimately, the combined peripheral vasodilation, decreased myocardial contractility and depressant effect on rate and conductivity will lead to cardiac arrest and circulatory collapse.

Most investigations have shown that a general relationship exists between the potency of various agents as local anesthetic drugs and their depressant effect on the cardiovascular system.[146,147] In recent years, there has been some suggestion that the more potent, highly lipid soluble and highly protein bound local anesthetic agents, such as bupivacaine and etidocaine, may be relatively more cardiotoxic than the less potent, less lipid soluble and protein bound local anesthetics such as lidocaine.[148] Several case reports have appeared in the literature in which bupivacaine and etidocaine were associated with rapid and profound cardiovascular depression. These cases differed from the usual cardiovascular depression seen with local anesthetics in several respects. The onset of cardiovascular depression occurred relatively early. In some cases, severe cardiac arrhythmias were observed, and the cardiac depression appeared resistant to various therapeutic modalities. Studies in intact animals to evaluate the relative cardiovascular toxicity of various local anesthetics have been somewhat contradictory. The cardiovascular depression produced by local anesthetic agents appears related to the potency of the various drugs.[146,147] On the other hand, a narrower margin of safety may exist between the dose of bupivacaine or etidocaine to cause CNS toxicity and the dose to cause cardiovascular toxicity, as compared to lidocaine.[149,150] In addition, it has been reported that bupivacaine can induce cardiac arrhythmias in awake animals, whereas no such changes were observed with lidocaine.[151,152]

Changes in acid-base status will alter the potential cardiovascular toxicity of local anesthetic agents. As described previously, hypercarbia and acidosis will decrease the threshold of local anesthetic agents for convulsive activity. Similarly, hypercarbia, acidosis, and hypoxia will tend to increase the cardiodepressant effect of local anesthetic agents. Studies on isolated atrial tissues have shown that hypercarbia, acidosis, and hypoxia will tend to potentiate the negative chronotropic and inotropic action of lidocaine and bupivacaine.[153] It has been postulated that the cardiovascular depression observed with the more potent agents such as bupivacaine may be related in part to the severe acid-base changes that occur following the administration of toxic doses of these agents.

The clinical picture associated with massive local anesthetic overdose is collapse at times without convulsions. Ultimately, death occurs due to respiratory arrest. The incidence of any systemic toxic reaction was 0.2% in one series of 66,366 epidurals.[132] In another series of 93,102 patients receiving a variety of regional anesthetics (epidural, caudal, spinal, and peripheral blocks), the incidence of mild toxic reactions was 0.38% and of convulsions 0.12%.[99]

The best treatment for systemic toxic reactions is prevention. Therefore, aspirate carefully before injecting at any site, inject slowly, and use the optimum dose—minimum concentration and volume—for the desired effect. Ten milliliters of preservative-free normal saline or air can be injected into the epidural space prior to the insertion of a catheter.[154] This may reduce the incidence of blood vessel puncture by the catheter and therefore prevent intravascular anesthetic injection. Large volumes (>3–5 ml) of local anesthetic should not be given as a bolus.[16]

If a patient undergoes a mild reaction, observe him or her closely because the reaction may progress. Administer oxygen by face mask. If a convulsion occurs, ventilation should be assisted with 100% oxygen by bag and mask. Anticonvulsive drugs should be given. Diazepam (5–10 mg) can be given intravenously to terminate lidocaine-induced convulsions and increase the lidocaine seizure threshold.[36] Another choice is thiopental, which is readily available; 50 to 100 mg can be given. Convulsions usually last less than 60 seconds, but if prolonged, succinylcholine and endotracheal intubation may be needed to ensure an adequate airway and oxygenation.

If cardiorespiratory collapse occurs, all the preceding measures may be needed, including ventilation with 100% oxygen and anticonvulsive drug. In addition, the circulation must be supported with fluid and vasopressors. Closed-chest cardiac massage and drugs for resuscitation should be given as indicated. Moore and coworkers have demonstrated the development of profound hypoxia and metabolic and respiratory acidosis within 1 to 3 minutes of the onset of a convulsive toxic reaction, further predisposing the patient to cardiac arrest.[155] Because of the possibility of this full range of reactions, an intravenous line is required before commencing ambulatory regional anesthesia.

Allergic Reactions

The anesthesiologist often must evaluate a patient needing or desiring regional anesthesia who claims to be "allergic" to local anesthetics. True allergic reactions to local anesthetic drugs are rare.[156] It is estimated that 99% of adverse reactions do not involve allergic mechanisms. In order to distinguish whether or not a reaction is allergic, a careful clinical history must be taken first.[157] The patient and attending physician or dentist must be interviewed, and the chart consulted. The exact drug given should be identified, including vasoconstrictors or preservatives, as well as the dosage and route of administration. The time of onset and duration of the reaction and a clear description of the reaction itself and of any treatment given are also needed. Most commonly, adverse reactions incorrectly labeled "allergy" are in fact systemic toxicity due to relative or absolute local anesthetic overdose. Reaction to epinephrine, vasovagal syncope, allergy to other drugs or dental alloys, and surgical orofacial swelling also must be ruled out.

True allergic reactions are mediated primarily by histamine released from mast cells and basophils. Release of histamine can be triggered by any one or combination of four mechanisms. IgE antibodies specific for a local anesthetic may have been produced on previous exposure to the drug; this is anaphylaxis. Activation of the complement system may occur with IgG or IgM antibody-drug interaction or directly by local anesthetic activation of complement C_3. Histamine-releasing cells may be stimulated directly by the local anesthetic; this anaphylactoid reaction is more common in patients with multiple allergies or after repeated exposure to a drug. However, complement-mediated and anaphylactoid pathways of histamine release do not require previous exposure to the offending agent.[156]

Once histamine is released, the clinical syndrome is similar regardless of the trigger. Severity varies according to the individual's susceptibility. Symptoms in the skin are seen first. Erythema of the face, arms, and upper chest appear, due to capillary dilation. Pruritic hives or wheals form secondary to increased capillary permeability. Angioedema of the eyelids is common. Upper airway edema including the larynx can develop, and airway obstruction may occur. Rhinitis and conjunctivitis are also the result of local edema and inflammation. Blood pressure falls, reflecting increased capillary permeability and intravascular hypovolemia. Cardiac dysrhythmias may be caused by local histamine release in the heart as well as histamine-stimulated catecholamine secretion. Patients may complain of abdominal pain and vomiting, caused by hyperperistalsis. Bronchospasm is a potentially severe and life-threatening respiratory complication. Cardiorespiratory collapse can occur immediately and abruptly following drug administration.

An ongoing regional anesthetic may modify the presentation of anaphylaxis caused by another drug given at the same time.[158] Cephalosporin anaphylaxis during spinal anesthesia appeared initially as cardiovascular collapse without respiratory, laryngeal, or cutaneous manifestations. Institution of external cardiac massage led to the appearance of a diffuse rash. Sympathetic blockade due to the spinal anesthetic combined with increased vascular permeability due to the anaphylactic reaction may have generated cardiac arrest by a catastrophic reduction in venous return.

If an allergic reaction occurs, stop the administration of the suspect local anesthetic drug. Epinephrine, 5 µg/kg (0.3–0.5 ml of 1:1000), should be given immediately, subcutaneously or into a muscle or by the intravenous route if the reaction is severe. Epinephrine probably acts by inhibiting degranulation and release of chemical mediators from mast cells and basophils. The antihistamine diphenhydramine (0.5 to 1 mg/kg) also should be given to block unoccupied receptors. Supplemental oxygen should be administered and an endotracheal tube inserted if airway edema is in question. Vascular volume should be maintained by crystalloid or colloid infusion, and vasopressors may be needed. Aminophylline (3 to 5 mg/kg intravenously) is used to treat sustained bronchospasm. Hydrocortisone (100 mg) is also often administered, although its theoretical basis is unclear.

Ester local anesthetics such as benzocaine, procaine and tetracaine are relatively more likely to cause true allergic reactions. These agents are metabolized to *para*-aminobenzoic acid (PABA) and related compounds, which are highly antigenic. Amide local anesthetics such as lidocaine, prilocaine, mepivacaine, and bupivacaine are rarely the cause of allergic reactions; only one case has been well documented, with bupivacaine.[159] Paraben derivatives are frequently present as preservatives in local anesthetic solutions, both in multidose vials and dental cartridges and in numerous over-the-counter preparations. Parabens are structurally similar to *para*-aminobenzoic acid and may cause allergic reactions directly or by cross-sensitization with ester local anesthetics. Cross-reactivity of ester anesthetics also has been reported with *para*-aminobenzoic acid in sunscreens. Patients allergic to procaine may exhibit cross-sensitization with procaine penicillin.[160]

If a patient appears to be allergic to a local anesthetic drug, regional anesthesia probably can safely be given with a preservative-free anesthetic of unrelated structure.[161] If further *in vivo* testing is needed, the intradermal test may be used. Intradermal injection of 0.1 ml local anesthetic is made into the skin of the medial forearm. One percent procaine, 0.5% lidocaine, mepivacaine, or prilocaine, 0.25% tetracaine or bupivacaine, and/or 0.1% methylparaben may be used. Preservative-free normal saline also should be injected intradermally to control for false-positive reactions due to local histamine release from needle trauma or tissue distension. False-positive reactions also may occur because of isolated skin hypersensitivity to procaine and tetracaine, which is unassociated with systemic allergy.[160] If the identity of the offending local anesthetic is not certain, skin testing for drug tolerance should be performed with a preservative-free amide anesthetic. A negative reaction probably indicates safety for use. Patients should be tested at least 1 month after an acute allergic reaction and should not be taking drugs that modify the immune response, such as antihistamines or steroids. A positive reaction consists of a 10-mm or larger wheal appearing within 15 minutes and lasting for at least 30 minutes. Equipment and personnel to support cardiopulmonary resuscitation must be available during intradermal testing, since a systemic reaction may occur.

Intradermal testing was able to demonstrate a lack of reactivity to the suspect local anesthetic drug in up to 92% of patients.[161] Attempts to confirm lack of reactivity by giving increasing intramuscular doses provided no additional information.[157] Testing by intravenous drug challenge carries excessive risk. *In vitro* diagnostic approaches such as IgE inhibition, leukocyte histamine release, and radioallergosorbent tests are currently in use but are expensive and not easily available.[156]

Patients with a strong history of allergies or who need to receive a suspect local anesthetic may be premedicated to attenuate a response. Both H_1- and H_2-receptor antagonists should be used; diphenhydramine (0.5 to 1 mg/kg) and cimetidine (4 to 6 mg/kg) can be given orally. Prednisone (50 mg) has been helpful to attenuate reaction to radiographic contrast media. Prednisone may be given orally every 6 hours for 1 day, with the last dose 1 hour before the procedure.

Local and regional anesthesia can provide optimal conditions for ambulatory surgery. With regional block, intraoperative and postoperative analgesia can be obtained without postanesthetic central depression. With the use of appropriate agents and techniques for anesthesia and supplemental sedation, disadvantages of regional blockade can be minimized and potential complications may be avoided. Ambulatory regional anesthesia can satisfy patient, surgeon, and anesthesiologist.

REFERENCES

1. Cohen DD, Dillon JB: Anesthesia for outpatient surgery. JAMA 196: 98, 1966
2. Penfield AJ: Laparoscopic sterlization under local anesthesia. Obstet Gynecol 49: 725, 1977
3. Meridy HW: Criteria for selection of ambulatory surgery patients and guidelines for anesthetic management: A retrospective study of 1553 cases. Anesth Analg 61: 921, 1982
4. Bridenbaugh LD, Soderstrom RM: Lumbar epidural block anesthesia for outpatient laparoscopy. J Reprod Med 23: 85, 1979
5. Coupland GAE, Townend DM, Martin CJ: Peritoneoscopy use in assessment of intraabdominal malignancy. Surgery 89:645, 1981
6. Indresano AT, Rooney TP: Outpatient management of mentally handicapped patients undergoing dental procedures. J Am Dent Assoc 102: 328, 1981
7. McGown RG: Caudal analgesia in children. Anaesthesia 37: 806, 1982
8. Rubin J, Brock-Utne JG, Greenberg M, et al: Laryngeal incompetence during experimental "relative analgesia" using 50% nitrous oxide in oxygen. Br J Anaesth 49: 1005, 1977
9. Bromage PR: Epidural Analgesia. Philadelphia, WB Saunders, 1978
10. Meyers EF: Problems during eye surgery under local anesthesia. Anesthesiol Rev 6: 23, 1979
11. Stone DJ, DiFazio CA: Sedation for patients with Parkinson's disease undergoing ophthalmologic surgery. Anesthesiology 68: 821, 1988
12. Kitz DS, Aukburg SJ, Lecky JH: It's not "only a local": Hemodynamic and oxygen saturation changes among patients receiving local anesthesia. Anesthesiology 67: A264, 1987
13. Philip JH: Helping the healthy patient survive. In Bennett PB, Watkins WD (eds): Safety Concepts in Perioperative Monitoring, pp 35–43. Boulder, Colo., Ohmeda, 1988
14. Singer R, Thomas PE. Pulse oximeter in the ambulatory aesthetic surgical facility. Plastic Reconstr Surg 82: 111, 1988
15. Tremper KK, Barker SJ: Pulse oximetry. Anesthesiology 70: 98, 1989
16. Philip BK: Complications of regional anesthesia in obstetrics. Regl Anesth 8: 17, 1983
17. Manchikanti L, Marrero TC: Effect of cimetidine and metoclopramide on gastric contents in outpatients. Anesthesiol Rev 10: 9, 1983
18. Wright DJ, Pandya A: Smoking and gastric juice volume in outpatients. Can Anaesth Soc J 26: 328, 1979
19. Nishino T, Takizawa K, Yokokawa N, Hiraga K: Depression of the swallowing reflex during sedation and/or relative analgesia produced by inhalation of 50% nitrous oxide in oxygen. Anesthesiology 67: 995, 1987
20. Brock-Utne JG, Winning TI, Rubin J, et al: Laryngeal incompetence during neuroleptanalgesia in combination with diazepam. Br J Anaesth 48: 699, 1976
21. Cullen BF, Miller MG: Drug interactions and anesthesia: A review. Anesth Analg 58: 413, 1979
22. Davie IT: Specific drug interactions and anesthesia. Anaesthesia 32: 1000, 1977
23. Grimes DA, Schulz KF, Cates W, et al: Local versus general anesthesia: Which is safer for performing suction curettage abortions? Am J Obstet Gynecol 135: 1030, 1979
24. Pollard BJ, Lovelock HA, Jones RM: Fatal pulmonary embolism secondary to limb exsanguination. Anesthesiology 58: 373, 1983
25. Philip BK: Supplemental medication for ambulatory procedures under regional anesthesia. Anesth Analg 64: 1117, 1985
26. Thompson DG, Evans SJ, Murray RS, et al: Patients appreciate premedication for endoscopy. Lancet 2: 469, 1980
27. Egbert LD, Battit GE, Turndorf H, et al: The value of the preoperative visit by an anesthetist. JAMA 185: 533, 1963
28. Walther-Larsen S, Diemar V, Valentin N: Music during regional anesthesia. A reduced need for sedatives. Reg Anesth 13: 69, 1988
29. Divoll M, Greenblatt DJ, Ochs HR, et al: Absolute bioavailability of oral and intramuscular diazepam: Effects of age and sex. Anesth Analg 62: 1, 1983
30. Korttila K, Linnoila M: Absorption and sedative effects of diazepam after oral administration and intramuscular administration into the vastus lateralis muscle and the deltoid muscle. Br J Anaesth 47: 857, 1975

31. Baird ES, Hailey DM: Delayed recovery from a sedative: Correlation of the plasma levels of diazepam with clinical effects after oral and intravenous administration. Br J Anaesth 44: 803, 1972

32. Korttila K, Linnoila M: Recovery and skills related to driving after intravenous sedation: Dose-response relationship with diazepam. Br J Anaesth 47: 457, 1975

33. Korttila K, Mattila MI, Linnoila M: Prolonged recovery after diazepam sedation: The influence of food, charcoal ingestion and injection rate on the effects of intravenous diazepam. Br J Anaesth 48: 333, 1976

34. Gale GD: Recovery from methohexitone, halothane and diazepam. Br J Anaesth 48: 691, 1976

35. Korttila K, Linnoila M: Psychomotor skills related to driving after intramuscular administration of diazepam and meperidine. Anesthesiology 42: 685, 1975

36. deJong RH, Heavner JE: Diazepam prevents and aborts lidocaine convulsions in monkeys. Anesthesiology 41: 226, 1974

37. Gross JB, Smith L, Smith TC: Time course of ventilatory response to carbon dioxide after intravenous diazepam. Anesthesiology 57: 18, 1982

38. Reves JG, Fragen RJ, Vinik HR, Greenblatt DJ: Midazolam: Pharmacology and uses. Anesthesiology 62: 310, 1985

39. Dundee JW, Wilson DB: Amnesic action of midazolam. Anaesthesia 35: 459, 1980

40. Philip BK: Hazards of amnesia after midazolam in ambulatory surgical patients. Anesth Analg 66: 97, 1987

41. Bailey PL, Moll JWB, Pace NL, East KA, Stanely TH: Respiratory effects of midazolam and fentanyl: Potent interaction producing hypoxemia and apnea. Anesthesiology 69: A813, 1988

42. Klotz U, Kanto J: Pharmacokinetics and clinical use of flumazenil (RO 15-1788). Clin Pharmacokinet 14: 1, 1988

43. Rodrigo MRC, Rosenquist JB: The effect of RO 15-1788 (Anexate) on conscious sedation produced with midazolam. Anaesth Intensive Care 15: 185,1987

44. Riishede L, Krogh B, Nielsen JL, Freuchen I, Mikkelsen BO: Reversal of flunitrazepan sedation with flumazenil. Acta Anaesthesiol Scand 32: 433, 1988

45. Philip BK, Hauch MA, Mallampati SR, Simpson TH: Flumazenil for reversal of sedation after midazolam-induced ambulatory general anesthesia. Anesthesiology 71: A301, 1989

46. Prokocimer P, Delavault E, Rey F, et al: Effects of droperidol on respiratory drive in humans. Anesthesiology 59: 113, 1983

47. Ellis FR, Wilson J: An assessment of droperidol as a premedicant. Br J Anaesth 44: 1288, 1972

48. Herr GP, Conner JT, Katz RL, et al: Diazepam and droperidol as IV premedicants. Br J Anaesth 51: 537, 1979

49. Dupre LJ, Stieglitz P: Extrapyramidal syndromes after premedication with droperidol in children. Br J Anaesth 52: 831,1980

50. Briggs RM, Ogg MJ: Patients' refusal of surgery after Innovar premedication. Plast Reconstr Surg 51: 158, 1973

51. Lee CM, Yeakel AE: Patient refusal of surgery following Innovar premedication. Anesth Analg 54: 224, 1975

52. Rita L, Goodarzi M, Seleny F: Effect of low dose droperidol on postoperative vomiting in children. Can Anaesth Soc J 28: 359, 1981

53. Wetchler BV, Collins IS, Jacob L: Antiemetic effects of droperidol on the ambulatory surgery patient. Anesthesiol Rev 9: 23, 1982

54. McClain DA, Hug CC: Intravenous fentanyl kinetics. Clin Pharmacol Ther 28: 106, 1980

55. Rigg JRA, Goldsmith CH: Recovery of ventilatory response to carbon dioxide after thiopental, morphine and fentanyl in man. Can Anaesth Soc J 23: 370, 1976

56. Partridge BL, Ward CF: Pulmonary edema following low-dose naloxone administration. Anesthesiology 65: 709, 1986

57. White PF: Use of continuous infusion versus intermittent bolus administration of fentanyl or ketamine during outpatient anesthesia. Anesthesiology 59: 294, 1983

58. Niemegeers CJE, Janssen PAJ: Alfentanil (R 39209), a particularly short-acting morphine-like narcotic for intravenous use in anaesthesia. Drug Dev Res 1: 83, 1981

59. Bovill JG, Sebel PS, Blackburn CL, Heykants J: The pharmacokinetics of alfentanil (R39209): A new opioid analgesic. Anesthesiology 57: 439, 1982

60. White PF, Coe V, Shafer A, Sung ML: Comparison of alfentanil with fentanil for outpatient procedures. Anesthesiology 64: 99, 1986

61. Jaffe RS, Coalson D: Recurrent respiratory depression after alfentanil administration. Anesthesiology 70: 151, 1989

62. Philip BK, Freiberger D, Gibbs R, Hunt C, Murray E: Butorphanol compared with fentanyl for ambulatory general anesthesia (abstr). Proceedings of the Society for Ambulatory Anesthesia, San Antonio, TX 1989

63. Philip JH: GAS MAN: Understanding Anesthesia Uptake and Distribution. Menlo Park, Calif., Addison-Wesley, 1984

64. Nitka AC, ORiordan EF, Julien RM: A new technique of scavenging exhaled nitrous oxide. Anesthesiology 65: 314, 1986

65. Flomenbaum N, Gallagher EJ, Eagen K, et al: Self-administered nitrous oxide: An adjunct analgesic. JACEP 8: 95, 1979

66. Dundee JW, Moore J: Alterations in response to somatic pain associated with anesthesia: IV. The effect of sub-anaesthetic concentrations of inhalation agents. Br J Anaesth 32: 453, 1960

67. Cohen SE: Inhalation analgesia and anesthesia for vaginal delivery. In Shnider SM, Levinson G (eds): Anesthesia for Obstetrics, pp 121–138. Baltimore, Williams & Wilkins, 1979

68. Maduska LA, Tielens DR: Plasma and cerebrospinal fluid fluoride levels following the obstetrical use of methoxyflurane analgesia. Anesthesiol Rev 3: 40, 1976

69. Korttila K, Ghoneim MM, Jacobs L, et al: Time course of mental and psychomotor effects of 30 percent nitrous oxide during inhalation and recovery. Anesthesiology 54: 220, 1981

70. Cook TL, Smith M, Winter PM, et al: Effect of subanesthetic concentrations of enflurane and halothane on human behavior. Anesth Analg 57: 434, 1978

71. Abboud TK, Shnider SM, Wright RG, et al: Enflurane analgesia in obstetrics. Anesth Analg 60: 133, 1981

72. Lichtenthal P, Philip J, Sloss LJ, et al: Administration of nitrous oxide in normal subjects. Chest 73: 316, 1977

73. Stewart RD, Paris PM, Stoy WA, et al: Patient-controlled inhalational analgesia in prehospital care: A study of side-effects and feasibility. Crit Care Med 11: 851, 1983

74. Dworkin SF, Chen ACN, LeResche L, et al: Cognitive reversal of expected nitrous oxide analgesia for acute pain. Anesth Analg 62: 1073, 1983

75. Dworkin SF, Schubert MM, Chen ACN, et al: Analgesic effects of nitrous oxide with controlled painful stimuli. J Am Dent Assoc 107: 581, 1983

76. Elliott CJR, Green R, Howells TH, et al: Recovery after intravenous barbiturate anesthesia. Lancet 1: 68, 1962

77. White PF, Coe V, Dworsky WA, et al: Disseminated intravascular coagulation following midtrimester abortions. Anesthesiology 58: 99, 1983

78. Everett GB, Allen GD: Simultaneous evaluation of cardiorespiratory and analgesic effects of intravenous analgesia in combination with local anesthesia. J Am Dent Assoc 81: 926, 1970

79. Gelfman SS, Gracely RH, Driscoll EJ, et al: Comparison of recovery tests after intravenous sedation with diazepam-methohexital and diazepam-methohexital and fentanyl. J Oral Surg 37: 391, 1979

80. Reves JG, Corssen G, Holcomb C: Comparison of two benzodiazepines for anesthesia induction: Midazolam and diazepam. Can Anaesth Soc J 25: 211, 1978

81. Conner JT, Katz RL, Pagano RR, et al: RO 21-3981 for intravenous surgical premedication and induction of anesthesia. Anesth Analg 57: 1, 1978

82. Forster A, Gardaz JP, Suter PM, et al: IV midazolam as an induction agent for anaesthesia: A study in volunteers. Br J Anaesth 52: 907, 1980

83. Johnston R, Noseworthy T, Anderson B, Konopad E, Grace M: Propofol versus thiopental for outpatient anesthesia. Anesthesiology 67: 431, 1987

84. MacKenzie N, Grant IS: Comparison of propofol with methohexitone in the provision of anaesthesia for surgery under regional blockade. Br J Anaesth 57: 1167, 1985

85. Jessop E, Grounds RM, Morgan M, Lumley J: Comparison of infusions of propofol and methohexitone to provide light general anaesthesia during surgery under regional blockade. Br J Anaesth 57: 1173, 1985

86. Negus JB, White PF: Use of sedative infusions during local and regional anesthesia: A comparison of midazolam and propofol. Anesthesiology 69: A711, 1988

87. White PF, Way WL, Trevor AJ: Ketamine—Its pharmacology and therapeutic uses. Anesthesiology 56: 119, 1982

88. Bovill JG, Dundee JW: Alterations in response to somatic pain associated with anaesthesia: XX. Ketamine. Br J Anaesth 43: 496, 1971

89. Sadove MS, Shulman M, Hatano S, et al: Analgesic effects of ketamine administered in subdissociative doses. Anesth Analg 50: 452, 1971

90. Vinnick CA: An intravenous dissociation technique for outpatient plastic surgery: Tranquility in the office surgical facility. Plast Reconstr Surg 67: 799, 1981

91. Bovill JG, Sebel PS, Blackburn CL, et al: The pharmacokinetics of alfentanil (R39209): A new opioid analgesic. Anesthesiology 57: 439, 1982

92. Korttila K, Levanen J: Untoward effects of ketamine combined with diazepam for supplementing conduction anaesthesia in young and middle-aged adults. Acta Anaesthesiol Scand 22: 640, 1978

93. Taylor PA, Towey RM: Depression of laryngeal reflexes during ketamine anaesthesia. Br Med J 2: 688, 1971

94. Covino BG, Vassallo HG: Local Anesthetics: Mechanisms of Action and Clinical Use. New York Grune & Stratton, 1976

95. Tucker GT, Mather LE: Clinical pharmacokinetics of local anaesthetics. Clin Pharmacokinet 4: 241, 1979

95a. Dahl MR, Dasta JF, Zuelzer WA, et al: Arthroscopic knee surgery under lidocaine local anesthesia. Anesthesiology 71: A730, 1989

95b. Carnes RS, Butterworth JF, Poehling GS, et al: Safety and efficacy of intraarticular bupivacaine and epinephrine anesthesia for knee arthroscoppy. Anesthesiology 71: A729, 1989

96. D'Amato H, Wielding S (eds): Intravenous regional anesthesia. Acta Anaesthesiol Scand 36(Suppl), 1969

97. Nussbaum LM, Hamelberg W: Intravenous regional anesthesia for surgery on the foot and ankle. Anesthesiology 64: 91, 1986

98. Bader AM, Concepcion M, Hurley RJ, Arthur GR: Comparison of lidocaine and prilocaine for intravenous regional anesthesia. Anesthesiology 69: 409, 1988

99. Moore DC: Administer oxygen first in the treatment of local anesthetic-induced convulsions. Anesthesiology 53: 346, 1980

100. Arthur GR, Covino BG: What's new in local anesthetics. Anesthesiol Clin North Am 6: 357, 1988

100a. Randel GI, Levy L, Kothary SP, et al: Epidural anesthesia is superior to spinal or general for outpatient knee arthroscopy. Anesthesiology 71: A769, 1989

101. Schulte-Steinberg O: Neural blockade for pediatric surgery. In Cousins MJ, Bridenbaugh PO (eds): Neural Blockade in Clinical Anesthesia and Management of Pain. Philadelphia, JB Lippincott, 1980

102. Greene BA: A 26 gauge lumbar puncture needle: Its value in the prophylaxis of headache following spinal analgesia for vaginal delivery. Anesthesiology 11: 464, 1950

103. Phillips OC, Ebner H, Nelson AT, et al: Neurologic complications following spinal anesthesia with lidocaine. Anesthesiology 30: 284, 1969

104. Vandam LD, Dripps RD: Long-term follow-up of patients who received 10,098 spinal anesthetics: Syndrome of decreased intracranial pressure. JAMA 161: 586, 1956

105. Burke RK: Spinal anesthesia for laparoscopy: A review of 1063 cases. J Reprod Med 21: 59, 1978

106. Leaverton GH, Garnjobst W: Comparison of morbidity after spinal and local anesthesia in inguinal hernia repair. Am Surg 38: 591, 1972

107. Urbach KF, Lee WR, Sheely LL et al: Spinal or general anesthesia for inguinal hernia repair? JAMA 190: 25, 1964
108. Mulroy MF, Neal JM, Bridenbaugh LD, Palmen B: Is postspinal headache more frequent in outpatients? Reg Anesth 14(2S): 2, 1989
109. Urbach GM, Edelist G: An evaluation of anaesthetic techniques used in an outpatient unit. Can Anaesth Soc J 24: 401, 1977
110. Mihic DN: Postspinal headache and relationship of needle bevel to longitudinal dural fibers. Reg Anesth 10: 76, 1985
111. Hatfalvi BI; The dynamics of postspinal headache. Headache 17: 64, 1977
112. Carbaat P, van Crevel H: Lumbar puncture headache: Controlled study on the preventive effect of 24 hours' bed rest. Lancet 2: 1131, 1981
113. Jones RJ: The role of recumbency in the prevention and treatment of postspinal headache. Anesth Analg 53: 788, 1974
114. Rice GG, Dabbs CH: The use of peridural and subarachnoid injections of saline solution in the treatment of severe postspinal headache. Anesthesiology 11: 17, 1950
115. Craft JB, Epstein BS, Coakley CS: Prophylaxis of dural-puncture headache with epidural saline. Anesth Analg 52: 228, 1973
116. Crawford SJ: The prevention of headache consequent upon dural puncture. Br J Anaesth 44: 598, 1972
117. Usubiaga JE, Usubiaga LE, Brea LM, et al: Effect of saline injection on epidural and subarachnoid space pressures and relations to post-spinal anesthesia headache. Anesth Analg 46: 293, 1967
118. Gormley JB: Treatment of postspinal headache. Anesthesiology 21: 565, 1960
119. Rao TLK: Temporary relief of postlumbar puncture headache with epidural blood patch. Reg Anesth 10: 191, 1985
120. DiGiovanni AJ, Galbert MW, Wahle WM: Epidural injection of autologous blood for postlumbar-puncture headache. Anesth Analg 51: 226, 1972
121. Bart AJ, Wheeler AS: Comparison of epidural saline and epidural blood placement in the treatment of post-lumbar-puncture headache. Anesthesiology 48: 221, 1978
122. Abouleish E, Wadhwa RK, de la Vega S, et al: Regional anesthesia following epidural blood patch. Anesth Analg 54: 634, 1976
123. Naulty JS, Herold R: Successful epidural anesthesia following epidural blood patch. Anesth Analg 57: 272, 1978
124. Palahniuk RJ, Cumming M: Prophylactic blood patch does not prevent post-lumbar puncture headache. Can Anaesth Soc J 26: 132, 1979
125. Loeser EA, Hill GE, Bennett GM, et al: Time vs. success rate for epidural blood patch. Anesthesiology 49: 147, 1978
126. Ravindran RS, Tasch MD, Baldwin SJ, et al: Subarachnoid injection of autologous blood in dogs is unassociated with neurologic deficit. Anesth Analg 60: 603, 1981
127. Dripps RD, Vandam LD: Long-term follow-up of patients who received 10,098 spinal anesthetics: Failure to discover major neurological sequelae. JAMA 156: 1486, 1954
128. Lund PC: Peridural anesthesia: A review of 10,000 administrations. Acta Anaesthesiol Scand 6: 143, 1962
129. Usubiaga JE: Neurological complications following epidural anesthesia. Intern Anesth Clin 13(2): 1, 1975
130. Wikinski JA, Usubiaga JE, Morales RL, et al: Mechanism of convulsions elicited by local anesthetics. Anesth Analg 49: 504, 1970
131. Marinacci AA, Courville CG: Electromyogram in evaluation of neurological complications of spinal anesthesia. JAMA 168: 1337, 1958
132. Dawkins CJM: An analysis of the complications of extradural and caudal block. Anaesthesia 24: 554, 1969
133. Chloroprocaine Labeling Revised. FDA Drug Bull 10: 23, 1980
134. Ramanathan S, Chalon J, Richards N, et al: Prolonged spinal nerve involvement after epidural anesthesia with etidocaine. Anesth Analg 57: 361, 1978
135. Moore DC, Spierdijk J, vanKleef JD, et al: Chloroprocaine neurotoxicity: Four additional cases. Anesth Analg 61: 155, 1982

136. Covino BG, Marx GF, Finster M, et al: Prolonged sensory/motor deficits following inadvertent spinal anesthesia. Anesth Analg 59: 399, 1980

137. Ravindran RS, Turner M, Miller J: Neurologic effects of subarachnoid injection of 2-chloroprocaine-CE, bupivacaine, and low pH normal saline in dogs. Anesth Analg 61: 279, 1982

138. Foldes FF, McNall PG: 2-Chloroprocaine, a new local anesthetic agent. Anesthesiology 13: 287, 1952

139. Gissen AJ, Datta S, Lambert D: The chloroprocaine controversy: II. Is chloroprocaine neurotoxic? Reg Anesth 9: 135, 1984

140. Fibuch EE, Opper SE: Back pain following epidurally administered Nesacaine-MPF. Anesth Analg 69: 113, 1989

140a. Foster AH, Carlson BM: Myotoxicity of local anesthetics and regeneration of the damaged muscle fibers. Anesth Analg 59: 727, 1980

141. Usubiaga JE, Wikinski J, Ferrero R, et al: Local anesthetic-induced convulsions in man. Anesth Analg 45: 611, 1966

142. Scott DB: Evaluation of the clinical tolerance of local anesthetic agents. Br J Anaesth 47: 328, 1975

143. Warnick JE, Kee RD, Yim GKW: The effects of lidocaine on inhibition in the cerebral cortex. Anesthesiology 34: 327, 1971

144. Liu PL, Feldman HS, Giasi R, et al: Comparative CNS toxicity of lidocaine, etidocaine, bupivacaine and tetracaine in awake dogs following rapid IV administration. Anesth Analg 62: 375, 1983

145. Morishima HO, Pederson H, Finster M, et al: Toxicity of lidocaine in the adult, newborn, and fetal sheep. Anesthesiology 55: 56, 1981

146. Liu P, Feldman HS, Covino BM, et al: Acute cardiovascular toxicity of intravenous amide local anesthetics in anesthetized ventilated dogs. Anesth Analg 61: 317, 1982

147. Liu P, Feldman HS, Covino BM, et al: Acute cardiovascular toxicity of procaine, chloroprocaine and tetracaine in anesthetized ventilated dogs. Reg Anesth 7: 14, 1982

148. Albright GA: Cardiac arrest following regional anesthesia with etidocaine or bupivacaine. Anesthesiology 51: 285, 1979

149. deJong RH, Bonin JD: Deaths from local anesthetic-induced convulsions in mice. Anesth Analg 59: 401, 1980

150. Morishima HO, Pederson H, Finster M, et al: Etidocaine toxocity in the adult, newborn, and fetal sheep. Anesthesiology 58: 342, 1983

151. deJong RH, Ronfeld RA, DeRosa RA: Cardiovascular effects of convulsant and supraconvulsant doses of amide local anesthetics. Anesth Analg 61: 3, 1982

152. Kotelko DM, Shnider SM, Dailey PA, et al: Bupivacaine-induced cardiac arrhythmias in sheep. Anesthesiology 60: 10, 1984

153. Sage D, Feldman H, Arthur GR, et al: Differential sensitivities of mammalian nerve fibers during pregnancy. Anesth Analg 63: 1, 1984

154. Philip BK: Effect of epidural air injection on catheter complications. Regl Anesth 10: 21, 1985

155. Moore DC, Crawford RD, Scurlock JE: Severe hypoxia and acidosis following local anesthetic-induced convulsions. Anesthesiology 53: 259, 1980

156. Stoelting RK: Allergic reactions during anesthesia. Anesth Analg 62: 341, 1983

157. Aldrete JA, O'Higgins JW: Evaluation of patients with history of allergy to local anesthetic drugs. South Med J 64: 1118, 1971

158. Barnett AS, Hirschman CA: Anaphylactic reaction to cephapirin during spinal anesthesia. Anesth Analg 58: 337, 1979

159. Brown DT, Beamish D, Wildsmith JAW: Allergic reaction to an amide local anesthetic. Br J Anaesth 53: 435, 1981

160. Aldrete JA, Johnson DA: Evaluation of intracutaneous testing for investigation of allergy to local anesthetic agents. Anesth Analg 49: 173, 1970

161. Incaudo G, Schatz M, Patterson R, et al: Administration of local anesthetics to patients with a history of prior adverse reaction. J Allergy Clin Immunol 61: 339, 1978

SPINAL ANESTHESIA: IT WORKS
Andrew P. Harris†

Owing to the increasing number of patients presenting for anesthetic management in the ambulatory surgery setting, the issues of optimal anesthesia technique for these patients should be analyzed carefully and critically. Many factors have to be taken into consideration, including some that are not generally considered when treating patients scheduled to be admitted to the hospital following their anesthetic/surgical procedure. Perhaps the primary difference in planning anesthetic management between potential inpatients versus ambulatory surgery patients is that anesthesia for the latter group must be handled expeditiously, with minimal residual postoperative anesthetic effect that may interfere with discharge of the patient from the center following their operative procedure and a short recovery period. Cost containment is becoming increasingly important as well. Whenever planning an anesthetic, potential methods to decrease cost without compromising patient comfort or safety should be considered and implemented if possible.

Alternative forms of anesthesia in the ambulatory surgery setting are general anesthesia, spinal anesthesia, epidural anesthesia (by means of either the lumbar or caudal approach), major nerve blocks, and local infiltration anesthesia. In many cases, ambulatory surgical procedures will be preferentially performed under local infiltration or major nerve blocks if at all possible. If neither of these is acceptable, then the decision lies among general anesthesia, spinal anesthesia, or epidural anesthesia. Given these options, there are several distinct advantages of spinal anesthesia, after taking into account all the preceding considerations. Epidural anesthesia can be considered advantageous as well, but since it involves a long induction time, it is rarely considered useful in busy ambulatory surgery settings unless a separate anesthetic induction area is

utilized for initiating the epidural block. This time constraint is such an overwhelming consideration that spinal anesthesia is usually the only practical major regional anesthetic considered as a reasonable alternative to general anesthesia.

Although there are also potential disadvantages of using spinal anesthesia for ambulatory surgery, methods of dealing with these disadvantages can be incorporated into the practice of spinal anesthesia. By implementing these methods, most of the problems with spinal anesthesia may be minimized or negated. The following discussion of the specific advantages, disadvantages, and methods to minimize the disadvantages of spinal anesthesia for ambulatory surgery can form the basis for each practitioner's decision-making process regarding incorporation of this excellent anesthetic technique into their everyday practice.

Advantages of Spinal Anesthesia

The advantages of spinal anesthesia are outlined in Table SR-1. From the patient's point of view, outstandingly dependable pain relief is characteristic of spinal anesthesia, both intraoperatively and immediately postoperatively. This pain relief is achievable without the impediment of excess central sedation that would be necessary if parenteral narcotics were used to achieve a similar level of pain relief. Sedation can be added, and indeed may be desirable, during the spinal anesthesia, but it is not essential to the technique, as it is with general anesthesia. Some patients fear unconsciousness and a lack of control over their surroundings. For these patients, spinal anesthesia would be more acceptable than general anesthesia.

Postoperative nausea and vomiting, so commonly seen following general anesthesia, are less prevalent following spinal anesthesia.[1] Nausea

*Anesthesiology Report 3(1): 1990. Used with permission.
†Chief, Obstetric and Gynecologic Anesthesia–Johns Hopkins Hospital; Assistant Professor Anesthesiology/Critical Care Medicine and Gynecology/Obstetrics–Johns Hopkins University School of Medicine, Baltimore, Maryland

TABLE SR-1. Advantages of Spinal Anesthesia

To the patient:
  Excellent quality of anesthesia
To the surgeon:
  Good operating conditions
To the facility:
  Efficiency

and vomiting following any anesthetic can be treated, but most agents commonly used as treatment also cause sedation, which may prolong discharge time. Nausea and vomiting, and the inadequate postoperative oral intake that results, are the major reasons for admission to the hospital (for anesthetic reasons) following ambulatory surgery.[2] This alone may provide a major incentive for performing spinal anesthesia.

From the surgeon's point of view, spinal anesthesia can provide optimal operating conditions if properly chosen and performed for the given operative procedure.[3] For example, for perineal or rectal surgery, spinal anesthesia is unsurpassed in providing both good surgical condition and muscle relaxation, unless deep general anesthesia or general anesthesia with profound muscle relaxation is used. Spinal anesthesia for this type of surgery is even preferable to local infiltration analgesia, which frequently requires supplementation with sedatives. Patients also may move during surgery under local infiltration; such movement could interfere with efficient performance of the surgical procedure.

From the hospital's point of view, spinal anesthesia can result in efficiencies of practice in many aspects of the ambulatory surgery patient's care. For the anesthesiologist, spinal anesthesia is less labor-intensive than general anesthesia. One person working alone can more readily handle both the administration of anesthesia and the setting up and cleaning of anesthesia equipment, since less equipment need be cleaned or replaced between cases. Cost is relatively low compared to general anesthesia, where many more disposable supplies must be used due to contamination and reusable equipment must be cleaned. The general anesthetic agents themselves are usually more expensive when compared to commonly available local anesthetics. If muscle relaxants are added to the general anesthetic technique, then the cost is even greater. Even compared to epidural anesthesia,

spinal anesthesia will involve lower costs.

As far as operating room efficiency is concerned, spinal anesthesia can be performed as rapidly as general endotracheal anesthesia in most cases, and certainly more rapidly than the induction of an epidural anesthetic. Even in those cases where spinal anesthesia may take slightly longer to initiate than a general anesthetic, this delay early in the case is more than compensated for at the end of the operative procedure when there is really no need to "emerge" from the spinal anesthetic in the operating room before transfer to the postanesthesia care unit (PACU). In fact, prolonged emergence following general anesthesia may occasionally result in significant delays in transfer from the operating room and interrupt scheduling. Likewise, less time is usually spent transferring care to the PACU staff, since the patient under spinal anesthesia is relatively awake without airway problems and usually is pain-free.

As mentioned above, the use of spinal anesthesia results in higher rates of discharge home on the day of surgery relative to general anesthesia, probably due to the decrease in nausea and vomiting postoperatively. Since smaller amounts of central nervous system sedating medication are used during spinal anesthesia, spinal anesthesia may theoretically also be associated with a more rapid attainment of discharge criteria, although this has not been studied. Epidural anesthesia, although associated with more rapid discharge relative to general anesthesia,[4,5] has not been well studied versus spinal anesthesia in this regard.

Finally, the pain-free emergence following spinal anesthesia provides an advantage to the PACU staff, who need not spend as much time medicating patients for pain in the immediate postoperative period. The relative lack of postoperative pain, combined with a decreased incidence of nausea and vomiting, makes the PACU course significantly smoother for both the nursing personnel and the patient.

Disadvantages of Spinal Anesthesia

The disadvantages of spinal anesthesia are listed in Table 2. Patient initial refusal of spinal anesthesia is the foremost problem and is usually traceable to misconceptions regarding spinal anesthesia, as well as a general lack of education regarding the technique itself. Patients tend to be afraid of a spinal anesthetic. Their fears include (1) a painful needle stick in the back, (2) being left with paralysis or permanent backache, (3) the fear expressed in the PACU when the operative procedure is over but the anesthesia is not (some patients worry whether motor or sensory function will ever return to their legs), and (4) the fear that unless they lie flat or limit their activity for up to a day following a spinal anesthetic, they will risk getting a "spinal headache."

The complication of postdural puncture headache (PDPH) is probably the greatest disadvantage of spinal anesthesia from the anesthesiologist's point of view. Besides being uncomfortable for the patient, it is a complication that will almost always occur after the patient has been discharged home and therefore may require return to the hospital for evaluation. It is also a complication that may even require hospitalization for treatment, even if only for several hours in which an epidural blood patch is performed. Although several factors have been identified as contributing to the risk of PDPH, this complication may occur in any patient regardless of the elegance of the anesthetic procedure.

Backache can occur following spinal anesthesia. Reported incidences range from 21% to 54.9%.[6,7] It should be emphasized, however, that studies that have looked at backache following general versus spinal anesthesia have conflicting results. Some studies have shown similar incidences.[6] At least one recent study has shown a dramatic difference. Backache following spinal anesthesia is thought to result from direct needle trauma of ligamentous and periosteal structures. The backache will usually manifest itself after the patient has been discharged home and therefore may result in readmission to the hospital for follow-up diagnosis or treatment.

Prolonged block is another potential disadvantage of spinal anesthesia, especially when long-acting agents are used. This prolonged block not only affects muscle strength (delaying ambulation), but also sensory and autonomic systems. This may increase PACU stay not only while awaiting ambulation, but also until bladder function and hemodynamic stability have returned. The complete return of somatic sensation is also important, so that self-injury is less likely to occur.

Transient urinary retention certainly can occur following the use of spinal anesthesia. This is usually felt to be the result of disruption of autonomic innervation of the bladder long enough to cause bladder distention and resulting atony. Catheterization may be required and, occasionally, admission to the hospital until urinary retention resolves. Studies that have looked at the incidence of urinary retention following regional versus general anesthesia conclude in general that the incidence is similar.[9] The site of operation and type of surgery are more important factors.

Dealing with the Disadvantages: Making Spinal Anesthesia Work

Spinal anesthesia is a useful technique for ambulatory surgery if certain guidelines and techniques are followed and implemented into everyday practice. These guidelines are based on anal-

TABLE SR-2. Potential Disadvantages of Spinal Anesthesia and Methods to Avoid Them

Disadvantages	Recommendation
High rate of patient refusal	Informative preoperative visit
Spinal headache	Appropriate patient selection, prospective counseling, small-gauge needle
Backache	Adequate local anesthetic infiltration
Prolonged block	Use short-acting agents
Urinary retention	Use short-acting agents, avoid overhydration

ysis of ways to ameliorate each disadvantage of spinal anesthesia.

The patient's fear of the concept of spinal anesthesia can almost always be allayed by a sympathetic preoperative visit, during which spinal anesthesia with sedation is carefully explained. For instance, patients will frequently have a fear of being awake (even if pain-free) during their procedure. In their mind they recall other times, especially the dentist's office, where they have experienced this combination of being awake yet numb and have not enjoyed the experience. Such patients must be assured that sedation will be added when appropriate and that they will be both numb *and* sedated for their procedure. They are likely to readily agree with the anesthetic plan when spinal anesthesia is discussed in this manner. Patients also should be informed preoperatively that the numb feeling will persist into the recovery period. In fact, they can be assured that while they remain numb in the PACU, they will usually experience little or no postoperative pain.

Patients should be counseled that lying flat is not necessary to prevent spinal headache. Several studies have repeatedly indicated that this prophylactic practice, once universally used, is unnecessary.[9-11]

Patient fear regarding residual paralysis, backache, or headache can only be lessened by spending time educating the patient regarding these complications. It should be emphasized to them that paralysis or nerve damage is *exceedingly* rare and may be as common following general anesthesia as following regional anesthesia.[12] Likewise, backache is a complication of general anesthesia as well. Headache should be discussed openly, including how a "spinal headache" would be treated (i.e., bed rest, analgesics, epidural blood patch, and so on) if it occurs.

The risk of PDPH can be lessened. Risk factors associated with increased incidence of PDPH include younger age, female sex (possibly), needle size, bevel type and orientation, midline (versus paramedian) approach, and state of hydration. The smallest-size needle possible should be used. A 27-gauge spinal needle is currently the smallest available disposable needle, and its routine use should be considered, especially in patients at "high risk" for PDPH. The use of 29-gauge needles may further decrease the problem.[1] Attention should be paid to bevel type and orientation.[13] It is also possible that the parame-

dian approach offers an advantage, since that approach has been associated in at least one study with a decreased incidence of PDPH.[14] Finally, the patient should not be allowed to become dehydrated postoperatively.[13]

Appropriate patient selection is important. For example, a person who must return to work as soon as possible following surgery is not an ideal candidate for spinal anesthesia. If regional anesthesia is preferable in such a patient, caudal epidural anesthesia may be the technique of choice, despite the associated longer anesthetic induction time.

If a PDPH does occur, reassurance of the patient and prompt (even if not aggressive) treatment are important. The patient should have received some counseling regarding treatment in the preoperative visit, but if this was not possible, the patient should be seen and counseled as soon as possible following the onset of the headache. The natural course of PDPH should be discussed, and a plan of therapy should be decided on based on the patient's individual needs and ability to follow conservative management. Again, the patient who must return to work should not be treated conservatively for any prolonged time.

Proper selection of anesthetic agent will reduce the incidence of prolonged block. Lidocaine (without epinephrine) should be used for any procedure of 1 hour proposed duration or less. Epinephrine can be added for procedures between 1 and 2 hours in length. The use of tetracaine or bupivacaine is rarely justified, since most ambulatory surgeries are usually scheduled for less than 2 hours. If actual operating time exceeds the proposed posted time, then general anesthesia may become necessary. However, if the reason for the prolonged surgery is a surgical complication, then hospital admission may need to be arranged for surgical indication, and general anesthesia would not be as objectionable if it must be performed in addition to the spinal anesthetic.

Urinary retention and overdistention of the bladder can be partially avoided (1) by using the shorter-acting local anesthetic spinal agents (i.e., lidocaine) whenever possible and (2) by not vigorously hydrating patients prior to the surgical procedure (except when they are pregnant and advanced enough in gestation to be predisposed to vena caval compression). Many anesthesia practitioners vigorously hydrate even young, healthy patients for low spinal anesthesia, a practice that will almost certainly increase the incidence of perioperative urinary catheterization to relieve bladder distention.

Summary

Spinal anesthesia, appropriately chosen and administered, offers many advantages over general anesthesia, and even over epidural anesthesia, for care in ambulatory surgery patients. The disadvantages can be mostly overcome by appropriate modification of technique.

References

1. Dahl JB, Schultz P, Anker-Moller E, et al: Spinal anaesthesia in young patients using a 29-gauge needle: Technical considerations and an evaluation of postoperative complaints compared with general anaesthesia. Br J Anaesth 64: 178, 1990
2. Gold BS, Kitz DS, Lecky JH, et al: Unanticipated admission to the hospital following ambulatory surgery. JAMA 262: 3008, 1989
3. Scarborough RA: Spinal anesthesia from the surgeon's standpoint. JAMA 168: 1324, 1958
4. Bridenbaugh LD: Regional anesthesia for outpatient surgery—A summary of 12 years' experience. Can Anaesth Soc J 30: 548, 1983
5. Bridenbaugh LD, Soderstrom RM: Lumbar epidural block anesthesia for outpatient laparoscopy. J Reprod Med 23: 85, 1979
6. Brown EM, Elman DS: Postoperative backache. Anesth Analg 40: 683, 1961
7. Flaatten H, Raeder J: Forum: Spinal anaesthesia for outpatient surgery. Anaesthesia 40: 1108, 1985
8. Baden JM, Mazze RI: Urinary retention: In Orken SK, Coopeman LH (eds): Complications in Anesthesiology, pp 423–426. Philadelphia, JB Lippincott, 1983
9. Carbaat P, VanCrevel H: Lumbar puncture headache: Controlled study on the preventive effect of 24 hours' bed rest. Lancet 2: 1133, 1981
10. Handler CE, Perkin GD, Smith GD, et al: Posture and lumbar puncture headache a controlled trial in 50 patients. J R Soc Med 75: 404, 1982
11. Jones RJ: The oral recumbency in the prevention and treatment of post-spinal headache. Anesth Analg 53: 788, 1974
12. Schreiner EJ, Lipson SF, Bromage PR, et al: Neurological complications following general anaesthesia. Anaesthesia 38: 226, 1983
13. Moore DC: Regional Block, 4th ed, p 358. Springfield, Ill., Thomas. 1965
14. Mansi ML: Prevention of postpartum, post-spinal headache. JAOA 81: 496, 1982

SPINAL ANESTHESIA: HANDLE WITH CARE
Bernard V. Wetchler

Case Study: A 30-year-old, 6-foot, 175-pound man is scheduled for inguinal herniorrhaphy on an ambulatory surgical basis. At the time of the preanesthesia interview, the patient is given full information about choices of anesthesia (i.e., local, general, spinal, epidural). The patient rejects spinal as a viable alternative because of an approximate 5% incidence of postdural puncture headache.

Case Study: A 32-year-old, gravida 2, para 1 (14 weeks gestation) woman is scheduled for a McDonald's cerclage as an ambulatory patient. At the time of the preanesthesia interview, choice of anesthesia is discussed, with anesthesiolo-gist's preference being either spinal or epidural. The patient rejects spinal but accepts epidural because of the lesser potential for a postdural puncture headache.

At the 1989 New York Post Graduate Assembly, Linda Rice categorized varying types of regional anesthetic techniques for ambulatory surgery into three separate groups: "green light"—perfectly acceptable; "yellow light"—conditionally acceptable; and "red light"—not acceptable. Spinal anesthesia was considered a "yellow light" block. Heading the list of drawbacks to a spinal anesthetic for ambulatory surgery were increased risk of headache, urinary retention, and control over duration of anesthesia.

*Anesthesiology Report 3(1): 1990, with permission.

Headache

Regional anesthesia has been advocated for ambulatory surgical procedures because of perceived advantages in recovery. The use of spinal anesthesia has been questioned, however, because of postdural puncture headache (PDPH). Postdural puncture headache is related to patient age, needle size, and type of needle bevel. Early ambulation as a factor increasing the incidence of PDPH is questionable.

Neal and coworkers evaluated 366 patients undergoing spinal anesthesia for a variety of surgical procedures, both as inpatients and as outpatients.[1] The incidence of PDPH was higher in outpatients (6.6%) than in inpatients (1.4%). Half the PDPH patients required epidural blood patch therapy. No difference was noted between the incidence of PDPH with 22-gauge Greene or 26-gauge Quincke needles, even analyzed according to age. The consistently low incidence of PDPH in modern series of patients undergoing surgical procedures as inpatients has been ascribed to smaller needle size (i.e., 25 or 26 gauge). This may or may not be the case in the ambulatory surgery population; needle bevel (i.e., conical Greene point, which spreads dural fibers, vs. Quincke point, which cuts dural fibers) may be a major factor. Studies are continuing at the Mason Clinic (Seattle, Wash.) evaluating the incidence of headache with regard to needle size and type of bevel. Needle insertion with the bevel parallel to the longitudinal fibers of the dura also may help in eliminating PDPH.[2]

Jones reported that time to ambulation after spinal anesthesia in an inpatient group did not affect the incidence of PDPH.[3] Carbaat and van Crevel described a group of patients (100) who received diagnostic lumbar punctures; 50 patients were discharged to home immediately, whereas 50 were kept at bed rest for 24 hours.[4] The incidence of PDPH was equal in the two groups, although the onset was delayed somewhat in that group that was kept at bed rest. Perz and coworkers reported an 11% incidence of headache in 228 outpatients who had received spinal anesthesia even though they utilized small-gauge needles to offset the greater risk in their young patient group.[5] No headache was reported in any patient over 55 years of age.

Seventeen young, healthy members of an anesthesia department (10 females, 7 males) volunteered to participate in a radioimmunoassay that required a spinal tap be performed prior to the procedure.[6] All blocks were performed with a 25-gauge needle (single tap) between 6:30 and 7:45 A.M., followed by the participants returning to their regular duties in the operating room. Nine of the 17 subjects developed PDPH, 2 severe enough to require epidural blood patch. The authors of the report considered this to be a point for recumbency following spinal tap.

Flaatten and Raeder noted a 37.2% incidence of PDPH in 51 young male outpatients given spinal anesthesia through a 25-gauge needle.[7] In addition, 54.9% complained of backache after surgery. Those patients who developed headache were off work for a significantly longer time than those who did not. Their particularly high incidence of backache may be due to the authors using no local anesthesia for skin and subcutaneous infiltration and the fact that an introducer was used to facilitate placement of the 25-gauge needle.

Randel and coworkers consider epidural anesthesia superior to spinal or general for outpatient knee arthroscopy.[8] The epidural group had significantly faster recovery times than either the spinal or general group; there were significantly more severe headaches (5.2%) in the spinal group versus the epidural (0.0%) or general groups (0.0%); there were no significant differences in the incidence of moderate to severe backaches between the spinal and epidural groups, but they both were significantly higher than the general group.

Where PDPH might be an acceptable complication for an inpatient who anticipates 3 to 4 days of hospitalization, this complication can be considered a serious setback for a young, healthy, active outpatient anticipating a rapid return to work or a resumption of other daily activities. For younger patients (under age 50) who have a higher incidence of headache (slightly greater in females) and who have an urgent need to return to full ambulatory function within 24 hours after their surgical procedure, these patients are far from ideal candidates for spinal anesthesia for an ambulatory surgical procedure.

For those patients who do receive a spinal anesthesia, it is incumbent upon the anesthesiologist and the facility to make careful follow-up contact (telephone) to make certain that no disabling symptoms of headache have developed. If the headache does not respond to bed rest, analgesics, and oral hydration, then this patient will have to return to the hospital for either a course of caffeine IV therapy or an immediate epidural blood patch.

Case Study: A 58-year-old man is scheduled for anal fissurectomy on a ambulatory basis. Following discussion of risks and complications of a variety of anesthetics, the patient chooses a spinal anesthesia. This is a good choice in this age group where the incidence of PDPH is minimal and the side-effects following spinal anesthesia are also considerably less than a general anesthesia.

Urinary Retention

Urinary retention is dependent on age, male gender (prostatic disease), and duration of blockade. Ryan and colleagues compared inguinal herniorrhaphy in outpatients (53) and inpatients (53) performed under a regional anesthesia.[9] Urinary retention requiring catheterization developed in three of the outpatients (a 56-year-old man required catheterization and was hospitalized over night, a 24-year-old woman was catheterized in the postanesthesia care unit, and a 21-year-old man who had voided spontaneously prior to discharge to home care returned to the emergency room requiring catheterization). Of the inpatient herniorrhaphy group, 16 patients developed urinary retention (15 required catheterization). The need for catheterization in the inpatient group was distributed among all ages. The significant difference between the inpatient and outpatient groups was duration of blockade. Long-acting local anesthetic agents (tetracaine, bupivacaine) were used for the inpatient procedures compared to short-acting regional anesthetics (lidocaine) for the outpatients. The authors concluded that duration of regional block was a prime causative factor in urinary retention.

Bridenbaugh reported similar findings in a randomized prospective trial of 200 consecutive obstetric patients who underwent routine vaginal delivery while under continuous caudal anesthesia (63% of patients who received bupivacaine required catheterization, whereas only 22% of patients who received chloroprocaine required catheterization).[10]

The complication of urinary retention requiring catheterization takes on greater significance in the ambulatory surgery setting because it may necessitate an unanticipated hospital admission. Although a single bladder catheterization carries a minimal risk of urinary tract infection, there is associated patient discomfort and additional expense.[11]

Control of Duration

Long-acting local anesthetics that may be acceptable for spinal anesthesia in the inpatient may provide potential problems when used for the ambulatory surgery patient. Drugs such as bupivacaine and tetracaine whose length of action may preclude the patient from ambulating and being transferred from the postanesthesia care unit to home care in less than 6 to 8 hours are not acceptable. This is too long a length of time and is frequently followed by a variety of problems such as orthostatic hypotension and urinary retention.

If one uses lidocaine as the anesthetic drug for spinal anesthesia, its length of action even with epinephrine (120 min) may still be too short for certain ambulatory surgical procedures. If lidocaine is used for a hernia repair and the spinal wears off before the surgeon completes the procedure, there is no problem with the surgeon infiltrating the wound with a longer-acting local anesthetic to conclude the procedure. This would not be necessary if the patient wished a regional anesthetic and the anesthesiologist provided epidural by means of a continuous technique.

Gold and coworkers assessed the feasibility, acceptability, and appropriateness of continuous spinal anesthesia (20-gauge epidural catheter) for elderly (mean age 71 ± 8 yrs) outpatients.[12] Two of 17 patients (12%) had a PDPH, one of whom required an epidural blood patch. Gold and colleagues consider continuous spinal anesthesia to be a feasible and appropriate ambulatory anesthetic technique meriting further investigation (i.e., smaller catheters), especially for the older, medically compromised ambulatory surgery patient.

The Ex-premature Infant

Ex-premature infants are more prone to postoperative apneic episodes if they undergo general anesthesia prior to 46 weeks post-gestational age.[13–15] Regional anesthesia (i.e., spinal) has been advocated as an acceptable alternative. Abajian and coworkers, in an article entitled, "Spinal Anesthesia for Surgery in the High-Risk Infant," stated, "In using spinal anesthesia for surgery in infants, the lumbar puncture is the most difficult part of the technique. Bloody taps are often encountered if the needle is not advanced in the midline. Once this has occurred, it becomes increasingly difficult to locate clear fluid even in adjacent interspaces."[16] Harnik and associates concluded that subarachnoid block with hyperbaric tetracaine for inguinal herniorrhaphy is a satisfactory alternative to general anesthesia for selected premature infants.[17] However, the authors also concluded that it does not change the need for intensive postoperative monitoring. Kataria and colleagues prefer caudal anesthesia when compared to spinal because of a higher success rate (91% vs. 63%) and a longer duration of anesthesia.[18]

Welborn and coworkers prospectively compared the effects of spinal and general anesthesia on the incidence of postoperative apnea, bradycardia, and periodic breathing in former preterm infants.[19] Spinal anesthesia without sedation was not associated with any episodes of life-threatening apnea. Infants who received intraoperative sedation (ketamine) with spinal anesthesia had an extremely high incidence of postoperative apnea. The authors recommend that until larger numbers of patients are studied, postoperative monitoring of these high-risk infants is still recommended following all anesthetic techniques. Postoperative monitoring, to my way of thinking, is best accomplished in a controlled hospital environment.

Conclusion

The role for spinal anesthesia in the ambulatory surgery patient is at best extremely limited. Further study is needed to assess the relative risk-benefit ratio of spinal anesthesia as a technique for the ambulatory surgery patient. Its current application should be reserved for older patients, patients in whom follow-up can be maintained for at least 72 hours, and patients who live close enough to the facility that it is not a marked inconvenience to return for epidural blood patch. For the ambulatory surgery patient, when deciding on a major regional anesthesia, epidural in the majority of situations is a better choice than spinal.

References

1. Neal JM, Bridenbaugh LD, Mulroy MF: Incidence of post dural puncture headache is similar between 22g Greene and 26g Quincke spinal needles. Anesthesiology 71: A678, 1989
2. Mihic DN: Postspinal headache and relationship of needle bevel to longitudinal dural fibers. Reg Anesthesia 10: 76, 1985
3. Jones RJ: The role of recumbency in the prevention and treatment of postspinal headache. Anesth Analg 53: 788, 1974
4. Carbaat P, van Crevel H: Lumbar puncture headache: Controlled study on the preventive effect of 24 hours' bed rest. Lancet 2: 1131, 1981
5. Perz RR, Johnson DL, Shinozaki T: Spinal anesthesia for outpatient surgery. Anesth Analg 67: S1, 1988
6. Coombs DW, Porter JG: Lumbar puncture headache. Lancet 2: 87, 1981
7. Flaatten H, Raeder J: Spinal anesthesia for outpatient surgery. Anaesthesia 40: 1108, 1985
8. Randel GI, Levy L, Kothary SP, et al: Epidural anesthesia is superior to spinal or general for outpatient knee arthroscoppy. Anesthesiology 71: A769, 1987
9. Ryan JA, Adye BA, Jolly PC, et al: Outpatient inguinal herniorrhaphy with both regional and local anesthesia. Am J Surg 148: 313, 1984
10. Bridenbaugh LD: Catheterization after long- and short-acting local anesthetics for continuous caudal block for vaginal delivery. Anesthesiology 46: 357, 1977
11. Ansell J: Some observations on catheter care. J Chron Dis 15: 675, 1962
12. Gold BS, Bogetz MS, Orkin FK, et al: Continuous spinal anesthesia for ambulatory surgery patients. Anesthesiology 71: A722, 1989
13. Steward DJ: Pre-term infants are more prone to complications following minor surgery than are term infants. Anesthesiology 56: 304, 1982
14. Liu LMP, Cote CJ, Goudsouzian NG, et al: Life-threatening apnea in infants recovering from anesthesia. Anesthesiology 59: 506, 1983
15. Welborn LG, Ramirez N, Oh TH, et al: Post-anesthetic apnea and periodic breathing in infants. Anesthesiology 65: 656, 1986
16. Abajian JC, Mellish RWP, Browne AF, et al:

Spinal anesthesia for surgery in the high-risk infant. Anesth Analg 63: 359, 1984

17. Harnik EV, Hoy GR, Potolicchio S, et al: Spinal anesthesia in premature infants recovering from respiratory distress syndrome. Anesthesiology 64: 95, 1986

18. Kataria B, Harnik E, Hoy G: Spinal versus caudal anesthesia in premature infants recovering from respiratory distress syndrome. Anesthesiology 71: A1018, 1989

19. Welborn LG, Rice LJ, Broadman LM, et al: Postoperative apnea in former preterm infants: Prospective comparison of spinal and general anesthesia. Anesthesiology 71: A1025, 1989

Problem Solving in the Postanesthesia Care Unit

7

■ ■

BERNARD V. WETCHLER

Surgery is finished, anesthesia has been discontinued, and the patient now enters the postanesthesia care unit (PACU). If you have not developed a philosophy of care for the ambulatory surgery patient that is different from the way you traditionally manage the hospitalized patient postoperatively, you may find yourself admitting more patients into the hospital than is necessary. In addition, methods of caring for postoperative pain, nausea and vomiting, and fluid intake are not identical. Patients are not recovering from their surgery; wounds take the same length of time to heal regardless of whether the procedure is done on an outpatient or an inpatient basis. Patients are recovering from their anesthesia. Of equal importance to the type and depth of anesthesia the patient has received is the immediate care provided in the PACU.

The patient, responsible person, postanesthesia care nurse, surgeon, and anesthesiologist all play a role in achieving a common goal of early "home readiness" for the patient (Table 7-1). Major roles are played by the anesthesiologist and the PACU nurse. There is no one better qualified than the anesthesiologist to determine when the patient is home ready. In ambulatory surgery, the anesthesiologist can have greater visibility as a physician (evaluation, PACU care) in the eyes of both the patient and the family.

THE FACILITY

Levy and Coakley stressed the need to separate ambulatory patients in the PACU from inpatients because of the psychological and emotional impact that patients who have had more extensive surgical procedures may have on the reactive alert

375

TABLE 7-1. Participants in Achieving Early Home Readiness

Patient:
　　Is motivated to go home
　　Is willing and able to follow instructions

Surgeon:
　　Carries out appropriate scheduling:
　　　　Patient
　　　　Procedure
　　Provides:
　　　　Written discharge instructions
　　　　Prescription for home medications
　　　　Follow-up appointment

PACU Nurse:
　　Monitors vital signs
　　Manages common PACU problems
　　Encourages home readiness
　　Ambulates patient
　　Checks discharge criteria
　　Reviews discharge instructions
　　Evaluates responsible person

Responsible person:
　　Encourages home readiness
　　Takes patient home
　　Provides assistance at home

Anesthesiologist:
　　Makes final preanesthesia patient evaluation
　　Provides appropriate ambulatory anesthesia
　　Treats common PACU problems

outpatient.[1] Separation should start with the preoperative waiting area and proceed into the PACU.

Other disadvantages in mixing outpatients with inpatients are differences in the type, timing, and philosophy of nursing care in dealing with nonsedated outpatients. It is difficult for postanesthesia care nurses trained in inpatient care to adjust their techniques several times a day to accommodate patients returning to hospital beds as well as those returning to their beds at home. If it is not practical to have separate PACUs, then screens should be used to separate an area within the PACU and designate it for ambulatory surgery patients. Grouping ambulatory surgery patients together and having nursing staff work with these patients on a regular basis will minimize problems.

In developing policies and procedures that will determine time spent in the ambulatory surgery PACU, it is best if patients are required to meet specific criteria for discharge rather than simply staying a specific amount of time. At Methodist Ambulatory SurgiCare (MASC) we do not specify absolute times that have to be spent in either of our recovery phases. We rely on a postanesthesia recovery scoring system to determine when our patients can be moved from one phase of recovery to another, and this scoring system plays a part in determining when we consider our patients home ready. If one uses traditional inpatient methods of assigning a minimum stay in the PACU of one or two hours, there can be a great deal of overload in the ambulatory facility because the majority of procedures take less than one hour. Whenever you handle short procedures with quick turnover time between cases, you have the potential to overload your PACU. You cannot tell staff bringing in patients that there will be a delay before a runway is available, that they are in a holding pattern, that they will have to circle the PACU until space is available. The question in this situation is, "How much space is needed?"

For adequate recovery-room space, Brody recommends a ratio of 1.5 recovery stations per operating room if a mix of cases (inpatient and outpatient) is being cared for.[2] If operating rooms are dealing only with short, simple procedures on relatively healthy patients, then four recovery stations (phase 1 and phase 2 combined) are needed per operating room. (These four stations would include space in both phase 1 and phase 2. See Two-Phase Postanesthesia Care Unit p. 379.) Short procedures have comparably short recovery times. Consequently, *flexibility* should be the key word in the postoperative management of ambulatory surgery patients. Build flexibility into your guidelines, but never at the expense of patient safety. Do not etch your PACU length of stay in stone. Do not establish discharge criteria you are unable to follow. Make policies practical for your day-to-day situations.

POSTANESTHESIA SCORING SYSTEMS

The majority of acceptable postanesthesia recovery scoring systems have similarities to the method of evaluation of the newborn proposed by Apgar in 1953 at the 27th Congress of the International Anesthesia Research Society.[3] For any scoring system to be useful, it must be a practical and simple method of evaluating the patient. It also must be easy to remember and be applicable to all postanesthesia situations. In a busy PACU, the assessment of a patient's condition only by the commonly observed physical signs will avoid any added burden on the postanesthesia care personnel. If a scoring system is used, it should not create busy work for the nursing staff and take away from patient care.

By assigning numeric values to parameters indicating patient recovery, progress becomes more obvious than it would if vital signs were merely charted with accompanying nurses notes, such as, "Patient reacting—appears able to go home." In a discussion of a patient's postoperative condition, a numbered system is more easily understood, and it allows physicians and nurses to communicate with a common language. A scoring system is a simple way of providing uniform assessment for all patients and may have added medicolegal value when used in addition to the usual subjective means of assessing a patient's home readiness.

An early scoring system proposed by Carignan and coworkers in 1964 lacked common acceptance because of its complexity.[4] Aldrete and Kroulik devised a postanesthesia recovery scoring system analogous to the Apgar method (Table 7-2). Activity, respiration, circulation, consciousness, and color were assigned numeric scores of 0, 1, or 2, a score of 10 indicating that the patient was in the best possible condition for discharge from the PACU.[5]

TABLE 7-2. Aldrete Scoring System

Postanesthesia Recovery Score	In	15	30	45	Hrs	Out
Activity:						
Able to move voluntarily or on command						
4 extremities	2	2	2	2	2	2
2 extremities	1	1	1	1	1	1
0 extremities	0	0	0	0	0	0
Respiration:						
Able to deep breathe and cough freely	2	2	2	2	2	2
Dyspnea, shallow or limited breathing	1	1	1	1	1	1
Apneic	0	0	0	0	0	0
Circulation:						
Preoperative blood pressure ___ mm						
BP ± 20 mm of preanesthesia level	2	2	2	2	2	2
BP ± 20 to 50 mm of preanesthesia level	1	1	1	1	1	1
BP ± 50 mm of preanesthesia level	0	0	0	0	0	0
Consciousness:						
Fully awake	2	2	2	2	2	2
Arousable on calling	1	1	1	1	1	1
Not responding	0	0	0	0	0	0
Color:						
Normal	2	2	2	2	2	2
Pale, dusky, blotchy, jaundiced, other	1	1	1	1	1	1
Cyanotic	0	0	0	0	0	0

Dismissal Criteria: Total score of 10, plus stable vital signs
A physician's order is required for discharge with lower score.

Total ____

TABLE 7-3. Steward Scoring System

Criterion	Score
Consciousness:	
Awake	2
Responding to stimuli	1
Not responding	0
Airway:	
Coughing on command or crying	2
Maintaining good airway	1
Airway requires maintenance	0
Movement:	
Moving limbs purposefully	2
Nonpurposeful movements	1
Not moving	0
Total	——

SOURCE: Steward DJ.[7] Used with permission.

TABLE 7-4. Robertson Scoring System

Criterion	Score
Consciousness:	
Fully awake; eyes open; conversing	4
Lightly asleep; eyes open intermittently	3
Eyes open on command or in response to name	2
Responding to ear-pinching	1
Not responding	0
Airway:	
Opening mouth or coughing or both, on command	3
No voluntary cough, but airway clear without support	2
Airway obstructed on neck flexion but clear without support on extension	1
Airway obstructed without support	0
Activity:	
Raising one arm on command	2
Nonpurposeful movement	1
Not moving	0
Total	——

SOURCE: Robertson GS et al.[8] Used with permission.

Steward feels a serious limitation of scoring systems is the inclusion of factors such as color, which lacks consistency in interpretation, and blood pressure, which may have little constant relationship to recovery from anesthesia.[4-7] In Steward's modification, only three areas are evaluated (Table 7-3), and these were chosen because they were easily classified into well-recognized stages and demonstrated a series of progressive changes relating to the recovery process and indicating a significant return of protective functions. A total score of 6 indicates a fully recovered patient.

The scoring system of Robertson and coworkers, used to measure arousal from general anesthesia in ambulatory surgery patients, incorporated certain features of the scoring system suggested by Steward[8] (Table 7-4). This system is more cumbersome to use than other systems because several numeric scores are given for the varying parameters. A score of 9 indicates complete recovery to the aware state.

TWO-PHASE POSTANESTHESIA CARE UNIT

Regardless of which scoring system is used, the majority of nonpremedicated patients having short surgical procedures will reach a score indicating early recovery from anesthesia in approximately 30 minutes. We use the Aldrete scoring system, and upon scoring 10, the patient is moved from phase 1 postanesthesia care into phase 2. Our phase 1 PACU has all the usual equipment one expects to find in any recovery area. The majority of our patients ambulate into the operating room, and only at the conclusion of their surgical procedures are they placed on a stretcher for phase 1 PACU care.

In our phase 2 PACU, reclining lounge chairs are used (Fig. 7-1). Here, family members are encouraged to actively engage in attending the patient. We initially set the reclining chair in an almost flat position, and gradually, over a period of approximately 30 minutes, the patient is moved into a sitting position. A patient can progress from a stretcher to a recliner much earlier than to a regular chair. The recliner is more comfortable and can be positioned appropriately if nausea or orthostatic hypotension occur. Patients are usually discharged sooner if their activity is increased to the recliner stage after surgery than if they recover completely on a stretcher or are transferred to a bed.[9]

In the two-phase postanesthesia care room at the North Carolina Memorial Hospital, the first phase is called the *recovery room* and the second phase is called *day op room*. The time spent by patients in the day op room exceeds the time spent in the recovery room. By having a second room, Carolina Memorial has relieved a single recovery room of a tremendous number of patient hours and potential overcrowding.[10]

An ambulatory surgery PACU (phase 1) must be equipped to handle all emergencies. Although ambulatory surgical procedures are not as invasive as procedures performed on hospitalized patients, standards of care must remain the same. The American Society of Anesthesiologists (ASA) Standards for Postanesthesia Care apply to all PACU locations (Appendix 7A). The American Society of

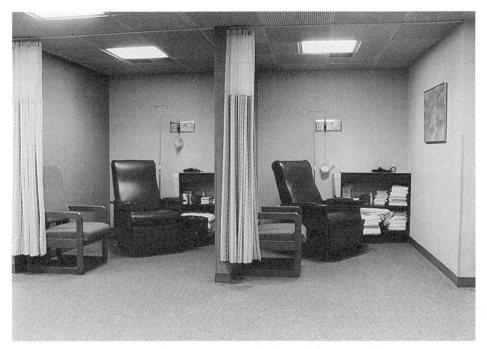

FIGURE 7-1. Phase 2 Postanesthesia Care Unit, Methodist Ambulatory SurgiCare

Post Anesthesia Nurses (ASPAN) has delineated standards for ambulatory surgery nursing practice.

COMPLICATIONS: REASONS FOR ADMISSION

The time interval between admission into the PACU and patient departure with a responsible person will vary depending on the use of premedication, the length or complexity of surgery, anesthetic agents administered, and the severity of common postoperative problems such as drowsiness, dizziness, pain, nausea, and vomiting. Perioperative problems also can be of such a nature and severity that they may result in admission or transfer into the hospital.

During a four-year period at George Washington University Hospital, PACU complications were reviewed in a group of 5516 patients. In order of frequency, these were nausea and vomiting, pain, emergence delirium, bleeding, syncope, hypoventilation, and arrhythmias. During 1988, of a total of 4824 cases, 115 patients (2.4%) were admitted to the hospital. Of those admissions, only 15.65% were considered anesthesia-related, compared to 68.7% related to surgery. The remaining admissions (15.65%) occurred for medical or social reasons.*

At the Phoenix Surgicenter, the hospital transfer rate is approximately 0.2% for all patients, increasing to 0.59% for patients over 65 years of age and to 1.41% for patients who are ASA physical status 3.[11] The most common causes for transfer are bleeding, inadequate pain control, and the need for further elective operations. Meridy reports hospital transfer for 2.44% of patients.[12] Of that number, 0.64% were judged to have complications secondary to anesthesia and 1.8% were judged to have complications secondary to surgery. Of the patients transferred to the hospital, 87% received some form of general anesthesia, whereas 13% received only local anesthesia. Of patients admitted to the hospital because of anesthetic complications, all received a general anesthesia. No single general anesthetic appeared superior to any other in reducing postoperative morbidity.

Laparoscopy is one of the most frequently performed ambulatory surgical procedures. Following laparoscopy, patients have reported weakness (66%), drowsiness (58%), dizziness (42%), vomiting (31%), visual disturbances (15%), and headache (13%) when leaving the PACU.[13] None of the symptoms was severe enough to require admission into the hospital. However, 93% of the patients felt they required an escort home. There were no significant differences in immediate postoperative morbidity among patients who received halothane, enflurane, or fentanyl.

Complications caused by creation of a pneumoperitoneum, although rare, may present as subcutaneous emphysema, pneumothorax, and pneumomediastinum.[14,15] In the PACU, patients may present with palpable subcutaneous crepitus over the upper chest, shoulders, and neck or, in the case of pneumothorax, signs of respiratory embarrassment. A chest radiograph and blood gases should be checked in the PACU. These patients are usually hospitalized for observation and on rare occasion may require insertion of a chest tube.

*Levy M-L: Personal communication, 1989.

At Methodist Ambulatory SurgiCare (MASC), we have taken care of over 85,000 patients through December of 1988. Of that number, 8035 had pelvic laparoscopies, and there were 179 unanticipated (2.2%) hospitalizations. Although higher than our overall unanticipated admission rate of 0.8%, this was not significantly higher than our admission rate for all patients having general anesthesia (1.4%).

Of the 179 unanticipated hospitalizations, 153 were surgically related (more extensive surgery than planned due to pathology found, failed laparoscopy, bleeding, puncture of bowel, bladder, or uterus, or pain). There were 22 anesthesia-related hospitalizations (dysrhythmias, cardiac arrest, syncope, compromised ventilatory status, or vomiting). Four unanticipated hospitalizations were patient-related (refused to go home, cerebral bleed, or hysterical paralysis).

A 41-year-old woman never recovered after her laparoscopic procedure. Within the first 30 minutes in the PACU, she developed signs of a neurologic deficit and was admitted into the hospital. She was appropriately worked up (CT scan) and was diagnosed as having an inoperable massive cerebral bleed from a ruptured congenital A–V malformation. She died nine hours after tubal surgery. Postmortem examination confirmed the radiographic analysis.

Premedication

The anesthesiologist has little control over unexpected length and complexity of surgery, but he or she does have control over premedicant drugs and anesthetic agents administered. The larger the dose and the more long-acting depressant premedication given, the greater is the chance of prolonging recovery with potential for drowsiness, dizziness, hypotension, or vomiting.[16] Meridy retrospectively studied 1553 ambulatory surgery patients and reported that patients who received either meperidine or morphine premedication were discharged 30 minutes later than patients who received no premedication.[12] Scopolamine is not recommended for ambulatory surgery patients because of prolonged residual effects on cognitive performance as compared with atropine.[17] Anesthesiologists differ in opinion as to whether premedication should be used prior to ambulatory surgery. The majority believe that little or no premedication should be given because it may prolong recovery time to the point where the patient may have to be admitted to the hospital,[11] whereas others feel that premedication should be considered a part of good patient care.[18] At George Washington University Hospital, no premedication is used.[19,20] The Phoenix Surgicenter, where over 120,000 patients have been anesthetized since 1970, attributes their patients' rapid recovery following general anesthesia to the absence of using narcotic or sedative premedication.[11]

Some facilities use only belladonna drugs.[21,22] At our facility, where over 10,000 patients are cared for annually and more than 6000 are managed by the anesthesia department, no premedication is more the rule than the exception, atropine alone is used by some anesthesiologists, and sedation is used for selected patients (e.g., a 31-year-old, 50-kg man who is uncooperative and severely handicapped is premedicated with midazolam 0.1 mg/kg IM 30 minutes before the start of the IV induction). Without atropine, patient complaints of dry mouth in the PACU are decreased.[23]

Mackenzie and Bird feel that timolol, a beta-blocker, is effective in reducing situational anxiety without producing sedative effects.[24] Oral timolol (10 mg) taken by patients at home prior to leaving for the ambulatory facility proved to be a useful adjunct in those patients who were particularly anxious. Premedication is fully discussed in Chapter 5.

Pain

Medications given in the PACU must be closely monitored and given in small, immediately effective doses. Intramuscular narcotic analgesic injections for pain control in surgery patients in the PACU is probably more a custom than a well-thought-out process.[25] In patients recovering from anesthesia, analgesics must have a rapid onset in order to alleviate pain promptly, and this is best achieved by the intravenous route. Faster onset and more precise blood levels can be obtained when drugs are given intravenously. When the intramuscular route is used, undertreatment is possible, since drugs may be deposited into subcutaneous rather than muscular tissue.

In general, pain management after ambulatory surgery includes three essential components: potent, rapid-acting intravenous opioid analgesics utilized during the perioperative period to decrease anesthetic requirement and provide effective analgesia in the PACU; long-acting local anesthetic agents administered by infiltration or nerve block to provide for more prolonged analgesia and allow for early ambulation after surgery; and orally administered opioid and nonopioid analgesics to treat pain following discharge from the ambulatory facility.[26]

Postoperative pain and agitation are common PACU problems. Pain can usually be controlled by small doses of intravenous narcotics. Hypoxemia, hypercapnia, distention of the stomach, and urinary retention can result in marked agitation. These problems can be managed easily, however, usually with resolution of the agitated state. The use of a narcotic as a premedicant may delay the first postoperative request for pain medication but usually does not affect the total dose required.[27]

Pain must be treated quickly and effectively. If pain is allowed to linger and become severe before treatment is begun, larger doses of narcotic will be required for relief. Untreated pain will result in nausea and vomiting. In our facility, we have found that fast and effective treatment of pain lessens the amounts of narcotic required and limits postoperative nausea and vomiting.

Postoperative pain control should be started intraoperatively by supplementing inhalation anesthesia with short-acting narcotic analgesics or local/regional block. Patients wake up quickly in the PACU following anesthesia with the currently used inhalation agents and quickly complain of pain. By making appropriate use of short-acting narcotic analgesics or local/regional block intraoperatively, awakening will be smoother and discharge home will occur sooner.

In a group of patients undergoing voluntary interruption of pregnancy or dilatation and curettage (D&C) procedures who were given thiopental, nitrous oxide, and oxygen or thiopental, nitrous oxide, and oxygen with supplemental fentanyl, Epstein and coworkers found a significantly higher incidence of pain and a slightly higher incidence of excitement during recovery in the patients who did not receive fentanyl.[28] Analgesics were required in only 1 of 14 patients in the fentanyl group and in 5 of 25 patients in the nonfentanyl group. Although there was a higher incidence of nausea in the fentanyl group, this group of patients recovered statistically sooner than those who received no narcotic supplementation during anesthesia. In the D&C group in the immediate postoperative period, there was reduction in pain, a shorter time to walk without support and stand with negative Romberg, and less time spent in the PACU. In the first 24-hour postoperative period there was reduction in pain compared to the group that did not receive fentanyl (Table 7-5). Hunt and colleagues added a single dose of fentanyl (75–125 μg) intravenously immediately before induction to a group of ambulatory surgery patients undergoing D&C.[29] The addition of fentanyl significantly reduced the frequency of abdominal pain in the PACU and during the first evening at home, but did not increase the frequency of other postoperative sequelae such as nausea and vomiting.

When comparing types of anesthesia and their effect on recovery following laparoscopic tubal ligation, the use of a longer-acting narcotic, meperidine (1–1.5 mg/kg), instead of fentanyl (2 μg/kg) intraoperatively did not delay recovery from anesthesia or patient discharge. Techniques that provided the best postoperative pain relief, least nausea, and most rapid tolerance of postoperative fluids employed meperidine and epidural anesthesia. Based on observations by the post-anesthesia care nurses, the epidural group had the best scores in every parameter. The study concluded that anesthetic techniques that provide the best pain relief in the first two hours following surgery have a lower incidence of overall morbidity and more rapid recovery.[30]

Sanders and coworkers added alfentanil or halothane to either etomidate or methohexital, nitrous oxide, and oxygen anesthesia for termination of pregnancy.[31] Faster recovery was seen in the patients receiving alfentanil. In both short urologic and gynecologic procedures, patients administered alfentanil recovered more rapidly than patients administered halothane, enflurane, or isoflurane. Late recovery scores as well as subjective feelings of drowsiness and unsteadiness were the same.[32,33]

White and Chang administered intravenous fentanyl (1.5 μg/kg) or meperidine

TABLE 7-5. Advantages of Fentanyl as an Adjunct to Thiopental, Nitrous Oxide, and Oxygen

Operative period:
  Smoother course of anesthesia
  Reduction in dose of thiopental
Immediate postoperative period:
  Reduction in pain
  Shorter time to walk without support, stand with negative Romberg, and to discharge
First 24-hour postoperative period:
  Reduction in pain

SOURCE: Epstein BS et al.[28] Used with permission.

(1 mg/kg) two to five minutes prior to intravenous induction for outpatient dilatation and extraction. Recovery times were decreased in those patients receiving narcotic analgesics as a result of decreased intravenous anesthetic requirement.[34]

The use of regional blocking techniques in pediatric patients as a means of postoperative pain control is discussed in Chapter 4; however, additional comment is appropriate here. Shandling and Steward feel that children over six months of age almost invariably require some postoperative analgesics following inguinal hernia repair.[35] Struggling, crying, and restlessness in the immediate postoperative period may result in bleeding into the wound, resulting in delayed healing. Postoperative vomiting (15%–20%) is more common in pediatric patients than in adults following hernia repair.[36] Fewer analgesics are required in the postanesthesia recovery period in some facilities where narcotic analgesics have been included as part of the anesthetic technique. When regional block supplementation is provided to the patient, there is a decrease in both pain and vomiting during both the recovery period and the first 48 postoperative hours.

Despite the obvious inadequacies of systemic administration of narcotic analgesics, it is still the most frequently used method. Unfortunately, narcotic drugs usually result in incomplete pain control, produce sedation and possible disorientation, and may increase morbidity, especially nausea and vomiting. Bupivacaine is now commonly used to produce nerve blocks for the treatment of postoperative pain. The extended duration of action of this drug may produce postoperative analgesia for 8 to 12 hours.[37]

Besides stressing surgical repair, retching and vomiting can delay discharge from the ambulatory surgery unit. Children who received inguinal blocks (percutaneous infiltration nerve blocks of the ilioinguinal, iliohypogastric, and genitofemoral nerves) at the conclusion of surgery had lower mean combined pain scores (at 1 and 8 hrs) than children in a control (nonblocked) group.[38] The blocked children urinated and ambulated sooner than the control group.

When comparing patients between 1 and 13 years of age who received either caudal analgesia (bupivacaine 0.25%) or an iliohypogastric and ilioinguinal nerve block with skin infiltration (bupivacaine 0.25% with epinephrine 1:200,000), there was no significant difference in the duration or quality of analgesia provided, in the incidence of vomiting, or in the time to first micturation between the two groups.[39] The morbidity associated with the infiltration and nerve block technique is less than for caudal analgesia, and the risks of major neurologic complications are eliminated. The technique is not without its problems, however. If the local anesthetic is injected near the femoral nerve, it may take 3 to 4 hours for quadriceps functions to return. We have never had this problem occur using 0.25% bupivacaine, but it has been reported when 0.5% bupivacaine was used.[35] The pediatric patient can be carried home, but in the adult patient it is wise to wait for this function to return before considering the patient home ready.

In Chapter 4 we refer to the bupivacaine manufacturers' caution about the drug's use in children under the age of 12. I feel, as do Hannallah and Epstein, that sufficient evidence supports bupivacaine as an acceptable local anesthetic drug in the pediatric patient when it is appropriately administered.

Bupivacaine (2 mg/kg) injected percutaneously for ilioinguinal-iliohypogastric nerve blockade in children results in peak plasma venous concentrations below the estimated adult convulsive concentration. It is recommended that a 2-mg/kg dose of bupivacaine (without epinephrine) for ilioinguinal-iliohypogastric nerve blockade not be exceeded and that strong consideration be given to using bupivacaine with epinephrine.[40] Cryoanalgesia of the inguinal nerve alone does not appear to produce significant early postherniorrhaphy pain relief.[41]

Lidocaine aerosol in the surgical wound before skin closure in patients undergoing inguinal hernia repair significantly reduced pain after a single administration compared to untreated patients[42] (Fig. 7-2). Wound healing was normal, and no adverse reactions to lidocaine were reported. Postoperative pain relief provided by simple instillation of bupivacaine (0.25%) into the hernia wound compared with that provided by ilioinguinal/iliohypogastric nerve block was evaluated in pediatric outpatients undergoing inguinal hernia repair.[43] There was no statistically significant difference between the groups with regard to postoperative pain scores, the need for analgesia, the time to reach a recovery score of 10, or the time to discharge from the hospital.

Postoperative morbidity following laparoscopic tubal sterilization is low and primarily related to pain. There is minimal incisional pain, but abdominal discomfort, shoulder pain, and nausea and vomiting frequently delay discharge. The level of discomfort will vary depending on the type of sterilization performed; less pain and cramping occur following cautery compared with Yoon fallopian ring sterilization.[44–46] Infiltration of the mesosalpinx in the area of the Yoon ring

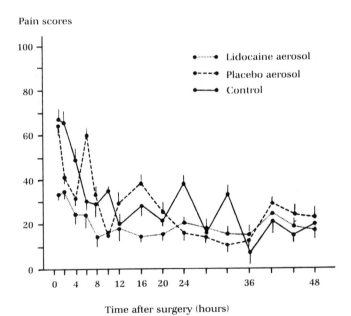

FIGURE 7-2. Pain scores during 48 h after surgery in patients undergoing unilateral hernia repair and treated with lidocaine aerosol or placebo aerosol in the surgical wound and in untreated control patients. SOURCE: Sinclair R, et al.[42] Used with permission.

placement with 0.5% bupivacaine at the conclusion of surgical sterilization significantly decreases patient pain complaints in the PACU.[47,48] Bupivacaine applied to the abdominal wall and fallopian rings did not have a significant effect on lessening postoperative pain.[49]

McGlinchy and coworkers supplemented general anesthesia with regional block of the dorsal nerve of the penis (0.5% bupivacaine) in a group of adult outpatients undergoing circumcision.[50] None of the patients required analgesia in the six hours following surgery, unlike a control group in which all required strong narcotic analgesic supplementation during the recovery stage. Topical anesthesia (lidocaine spray, 10–20 mg of 10%; lidocaine jelly, 0.5–1 ml of 2%; lidocaine ointment, 0.5–1 ml of 5%) has provided postoperative pain relief following pediatric circumcision.[51] The duration of analgesia (four to five hrs) approximated that produced by supplemental dorsal nerve block or intramuscular morphine. Pain relief was comparable with all topical techniques; however, children preferred lidocaine spray if there was need for repeated application. A subsequent study evaluated the efficacy of repeated applications of lidocaine jelly on postcircumcision pain in both children and adults.[52] The pain-free postoperative period was significantly longer in both the children and adult lidocaine groups than in the placebo groups. At home, lidocaine jelly was applied over the wound four times a day. Subcutaneous ring block of the penis with 0.25% bupivacaine is another simple and effective method of providing postcircumcision analgesia without delaying discharge from the hospital.[53]

Caudal block supplementation has been used to limit postoperative pain following not only pediatric circumcision but also hypospadias repair and orchiopexy.[54,55] Caudal block performed with 0.25% bupivacaine containing epinephrine 1:200,000 produces effective postoperative analgesia. There does not appear to be any advantage to using more concentrated solutions.[56] The optimum concentration of a local anesthetic should provide effective analgesia, minimal motor blockade, and few side-effects. Wolf and coworkers noted that 0.0625% bupivacaine was ineffective for caudal analgesia.[57] However, 0.125% bupivacaine (with epinephrine 1:200,000) provided equipotent analgesia and significantly less motor blockade than 0.25% bupivacaine (with epinephrine 1:200,000) for caudal block in infants and children. The volume of local anesthetic solution administered to each child was 0.75 ml/kg.

Knos and coworkers noted a statistically significant difference in pain perception in ambulatory surgery patients undergoing breast biopsy who had 0.5% bupivacaine infiltrated into the wound during the surgical procedure.[58] In the PACU, less narcotic analgesic was used and there was a decrease in nausea and vomiting in the bupivacaine-injected patients. Infiltration of the surgical site had no beneficial effect in decreasing the amount of anesthesia needed as measured by a more rapid return to cognitive ability or by decreasing time in the PACU. Peritonsillar infiltration with 0.25% bupivacaine (with epinephrine 1:200,000) lead to a reduction in blood loss; however, narcotic requirements in milligrams per kilogram over 12 hours postoperatively did not differ between the treated and control groups.[59]

Direct instillation of 50 or 100 mg bupivacaine (0.25%, 0.5%) into the knee joint after arthroscopy provided little analgesia.[60] Plasma levels were all below reported toxic concentrations. Katz and coworkers demonstrated that intraarticular injection of 100 mg bupivacaine is a safe technique, with peak plasma concentrations occurring within the first hour after tourniquet release.[61] Peak plasma levels can be decreased by minimizing total tourniquet inflation times and maximizing the time from bupivacaine injection to tourniquet release. Intraarticular bupivacaine appears to be a safe technique. Further studies are needed to evaluate its effectiveness in postarthroscopy pain control.

Wetchler and coworkers found transnasal butorphanol to be a satisfactory method of controlling moderate to severe pain in ambulatory surgery patients.[62] The initial transnasal dose in the PACU was 0.5 mg; additional butorphanol could be given every 30 minutes. There was no increase in PACU length of stay. In three patients there was a significant discrepancy between number of doses the patients stated they took at home and the amount measured by a Sartorius balance upon return of the medication.

Surgeons may resist injecting local anesthesia during the procedure because they are concerned about the following:

> Hemorrhage into the wound
> Infection
> Reaction to local anesthetic drug
> Numbness that may allow the patient to inflict some type of self-injury

In addition, the surgeon may see no surgical or technical advantages to injecting local anesthesia and may object on the grounds that it will prolong surgery time. Frequently it is necessary to "sell" the surgeon on the basis of the following advantages of regional block supplementation:

> Less pain in the PACU
> Less analgesics needed in the PACU
> Less postoperative minor morbidity
> Earlier home readiness

If anesthesiologists communicate some of these problem-solving techniques to surgeons, patients can be provided with a smoother course in the PACU and the immediate postoperative period at home. Whenever simple regional block can be performed, it should be used—your patients will certainly be appreciative.

PACU Narcotic Analgesics

Although the choice of narcotic analgesic is usually a matter of individual judgment, drugs such as morphine and meperidine are generally thought to have too long an action for outpatient use. Potent narcotic analgesics given in the PACU may contribute significantly to postoperative drowsiness, nausea and vomiting, and delay in discharge home. A delicate balance must be struck in order to provide a postoperative period as free of pain as possible.

At Methodist Ambulatory SurgiCare, pain in both adults and children is managed with a short-acting narcotic analgesic; fentanyl has been our drug of choice. Intravenous fentanyl (0.35 µg/kg) is given at the first sign of discomfort and is repeated at five-minute intervals until pain is controlled. For our pediatric patients, in addition, we administer acetaminophen elixir or an elixir containing acetaminophen (120 mg) plus codeine (12 mg) in 5 ml of solution (5 ml for children between the ages of 3 and 6 years and 10 ml for children between the ages of 7 and 12 years). Our pediatric patients are returned to parent care as soon as they are awake.

At the Children's National Medical Center (Washington, D.C.), a combination of child-parent reunion and nursing (or a bottle) is all that is usually needed following a procedure not associated with severe pain for infants younger than six months of age. For older infants and young children, acetaminophen (60 mg per year of age, orally or rectally) is one of the drugs most commonly given for relief of mild pain in the PACU. Intravenous fentanyl (up to a dose of 2 µg/kg) is the drug of choice for more severe pain. Meperidine (0.5 mg/kg) and codeine (1–1.5 mg/kg) can be used intramuscularly if an intravenous route is not established (see Chap. 4).

Establishing a PACU policy for pain management (acceptable narcotic, route of administration, and so on) eliminates problems that may occur when each physician orders different postoperative pain medications for his or her patients. Without a policy, surgeons and anesthesiologists who are used to working in an inpatient environment might order morphine or meperidine in substantial intramuscular dosages for postoperative pain. One must be careful that this does not happen because of the long-acting effects of these drugs.

Oral analgesics ordered by the surgeon as take-home medications also can be used in the PACU once the patient has taken fluids and shows no signs of nausea or vomiting. Ambulatory surgery facilities should establish a minimum length of time prior to discharge that patients must be observed in the PACU following administration of any depressant medication.

Nausea and Vomiting

Nausea (30%) and emesis (20%) are the most common complications occurring in the PACU at the Phoenix Surgicenter.[11] Contributing factors are pain, narcotic analgesic drugs, sudden movement or position changes, history of motion sickness, hypotension, obesity, and site of surgical procedure. For example, laparoscopic surgery performed around the time of menses resulted in a fourfold increase in the incidence of nausea and vomiting.[63]

Emesis was the most common single complication in the PACU following ambulatory surgery in 977 pediatric patients and was of sufficient severity in 1.7% of the patients to require overnight hospitalization.[21] Jensen and Wetchler have found that ambulatory surgery patients who experienced emesis at some point in their postoperative recovery tended to be heavier than those who experienced no emetic symptoms.[64]

Anderson and Crohg established a relationship between postoperative pain and the frequency of nausea in the early postoperative period.[65] Although the study was not done on an ambulatory surgery population, its implications are significant for outpatients. Complete pain relief without simultaneous relief of nausea was unusual. Patients who had inadequate pain relief and continued to have nausea after the first analgesic injection (50% of the patients) were relieved of both complaints after a supplementary dose of an opiate. Only 10% of patients complained of postoperative nausea without accompanying pain. Nausea often accompanies pain in the postoperative period and can be relieved in 80% of cases when pain relief is achieved by the intravenous use of opiates.

A major problem following ambulatory surgery anesthesia is nausea and vomiting. Admission to the hospital can result not only from uncontrolled nausea and vomiting, but also from prolonged somnolence following treatment with potent antiemetics. A history of motion sickness or nausea and vomiting following prior anesthetics obtained during the preanesthesia interview should alert the anesthesiologist to use antiemetic therapy intraoperatively. Benzquinamide (Emete-con), trimethobenzamide HCL (Tigan), and prochlorperazine (Compazine) have all been tried for the control of postanesthetic nausea and vomiting with limited success.[66]

Cohen and coworkers noted limited effectiveness of prophylactic low-dose droperidol when compared to metoclopramide in patients undergoing outpatient anesthesia.[67] A lack of antiemetic effect was noted for metoclopramide, but these patients were able to sit and walk and were ready for discharge sooner than control or droperidol groups. A combination of droperidol (0.5–1.0 mg IV 3–6 min prior to induction of anesthesia) and metoclopramide (10–20 mg IV 15–30 min prior to droperidol) was more effective in preventing nausea and vomiting than droperidol alone, and these patients spent a significantly shorter time in the PACU.[68]

Rao and colleagues found outpatient laparoscopy patients who received metoclopramide (10 mg alone or in combination with 300 mg cimetidine) had a significant decrease in nausea and vomiting compared to control or cimetidine-alone groups.[69] Patients were instructed to fast from midnight and take their tablets with a sip of water of the day of surgery just prior to starting from home to the ambulatory facility. Clinically, Rao and coworkers found that 10 mg metoclopramide IV relieves postoperative nausea and vomiting within 5 to 10 minutes and does not prolong PACU length of stay. Williams and colleagues feel that low-dose droperidol, metoclopramide, or a combination IV 15 to 30 minutes prior to induction of general anesthesia is ineffective as an antiemetic in outpatients given alfentanil for laparoscopic procedures.[70] Jorgensen and Coyle, on the other hand, found droperidol IV (0.02 mg/kg) immediately after induction reliably diminished the incidence of postoperative nausea and vomiting during alfentanil anesthesia.[71] A nasogastric tube was placed after induction to evaluate gastric contents. They noted no increase in duration of PACU stay.

For patients undergoing laparoscopic surgery insertion of an orogastric tube (with removal of gastric contents) after induction of anesthesia and tracheal intubation resulted in a significantly lower incidence of postprocedure vomiting compared to a control group.[72] Antiemetic efficacy of gastric suctioning has been noted.[73]

In comparing the effects of 20 mg domperidone, 2.5 mg droperidol, 10 mg metoclopramide, or placebo administered intravenously before induction of anesthesia in 199 women undergoing gynecologic ambulatory surgery, Madej and Simpson found that droperidol or metoclopramide significantly reduced the incidence of nausea and vomiting, whereas domperidone only decreased the incidence of postoperative nausea.[74] Droperidol has been found to be an effective antiemetic in doses as low as 0.25 mg IV in a group of ambulatory surgery D&C patients.[75] Wetchler and coworkers found droperidol (0.625–1.25 mg IV) immediately following intubation proved to be an effective antiemetic in outpatients undergoing laparoscopic tubal surgery.[76] The patients who received droperidol during anesthesia had a lower incidence of nausea and vomiting in the PACU, a significant decrease in the severity of emetic symptoms, and a shorter length of stay than the control group.

Valanne and Korttila administered droperidol (0.014 mg/kg) 5 minutes after induction of anesthesia.[77] Droperidol patients had less nausea (18%) or vomiting (7%) in comparison with patients given saline (27% and 11%, respectively).

Pandit and coworkers evaluated droperidol (5, 10, and 20 µg/kg) intravenously, metoclopramide (5 and 10 mg) orally, and a combination of the two drugs in adult women undergoing outpatient laparoscopy under general anesthesia[78] (Table 7-6). Oral metoclopramide alone had no effect on lessening the incidence of nausea and vomiting. Droperidol (10 and 20 µg/kg) and a combination of metoclopramide (10 mg) and droperidol (10 µg/kg) significantly decreased the incidence of nausea and vomiting in the PACU; however, only droperidol-treated (20 µg/kg) patients required no additional antiemetic therapy in the PACU. Pandit and col-

TABLE 7-6. Frequency of Nausea and Vomiting in the PACU
(percentage of 20 patients in each group)

Groups	No Nausea or Vomiting (%)	Nausea Only (%)	Nausea and Vomiting (%)	Any Nausea/ Vomiting (%)
Meto 5 mg plus placebo	45	30	25	55
Meto 10 mg plus placebo	55	25	20	45
Placebo plus Drop 5 µg/kg	60	20	20	40
Placebo plus Drop 10 µg/kg	75	20	5	25*
Placebo plus Drop 20 µg/kg	80	10	10	20*
Placebo plus placebo	35	25	40	65
Meto 10 mg plus Drop 10 µg/kg	75	20	5	25*

Chi-square tests were performed with raw numbers (percentage of total shown in the table)
*$P < 0.05$ Group 6 (placebo) significantly different from group 4 (droperidol 10 µg/kg), group 5 (droperidol 20 µg/kg), and group 7 (metoclopramide 10 mg plus droperidol 10 µg/kg).
SOURCE: Pandit SK et al.[78] Used with permission.

leagues conclude that 20 μg/kg droperidol IV is the optimum effective antiemetic dose. Droperidol did not significantly increase discharge time from the PACU compared to the patient group that received only placebo. Poler and White feel that droperidol (20 μg/kg IV) represents an acceptable compromise between decreased emetic sequelae and excessive postoperative sedation.[79] Dimenhydrinate (20 mg IV) prior to induction of anesthesia has proven to be effective in preventing postoperative nausea following outpatient surgical procedures.[80] Droperidol can potentiate drowsiness and, if administered during the final phases of recovery care, may increase the patient's length of stay. In an outpatient setting, the maximum antiemetic dose of droperidol should not exceed 2.5 mg; as the dose is increased above 1.25 mg, drowsiness becomes more noticeable.

Melnick noted two instances of extrapyramidal reactions (restlessness, anxiety, and acute dystonia) to low doses of droperidol (0.65 mg).[81] Although quite rare, these reactions can begin several hours after administration of droperidol. Caldwell and coworkers reported a case in which a healthy woman developed symptoms of severe dysphoria, agitation, and akathisia following preoperative metoclopramide (10 mg IV) administration.[82] Side-effects following metoclopramide administration have been reported (drowsiness and lassitude are the most frequent, feelings of anxiety and agitation are usually mild and transient), disappearing when the drug is discontinued. Benzotropine, a centrally acting anticholinergic (2 mg IM followed in 15 min by 2 mg IV) completely relieved the patients' symptoms. Although the benzodiazepines are used to treat akathisia, beta-blockers (i.e., propranolol) are considered a more effective treatment.

Alexander and coworkers noted a significant decrease in the incidence of postoperative nausea and vomiting in outpatients undergoing laparoscopic surgery when nitrous oxide was omitted from the anesthetic regimen.[83] Lonie and Harper evaluated a similar group of patients with comparable results.[84] Recent studies on women undergoing laparoscopic surgery do not consider nitrous oxide as a prime causative factor in the incidence of postprocedure nausea and vomiting[85,86] (Table 7-7). None of these studies looked at the relationship between nausea and vomiting occurrence after laparoscopy and day of menstrual cycle (Fig. 7-3).

The mechanism of vomiting (nitrous oxide) may be related to negative middle ear pressure during recovery, stimulating the vestibular system by placing trac-

TABLE 7-7. Nitrous Oxide: A Factor in Nausea and Vomiting?

Study		Percentage of Patients Having Nausea and Vomiting	
		Received N$_2$O	Did Not Receive N$_2$O
Alexander et al.[81]		61%	27.5%
Lonie and Harper[82]		29%	4%
Sengupta and Plantevin[83]	N	51%	39%
	V	18%	10%
Hovorka et al.[84]		34%	32%

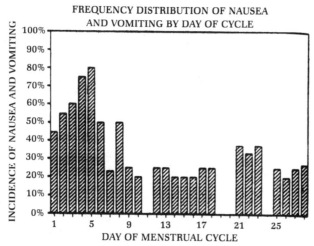

FIGURE 7-3. Frequency distribution of nausea and vomiting by day of cycle. (SOURCE: Lindblad T et al.[63] Used with permission.)

tion on the round window membrane.[87] Montgomery and coworkers studied this problem and found no association between postoperative negative middle ear pressure and postoperative vomiting in outpatient pediatric patients after nitrous oxide and halothane anesthesia.[88]

Our choice of induction agents does have an effect on nausea and vomiting. Ketamine-treated patients have a significant increase in the incidence of nausea (Table 7-8); there is at least a threefold increase when comparing etomidate-treated patients with thiopental- or methohexital-treated patients; propofol-treated patients have a significantly lower incidence of emetic symptoms compared to barbiturate-treated patients. As anesthesiologists, we do have choices over the agents and techniques that we use and should selectively look at those

TABLE 7-8. Comparison of Ketamine vs. Barbiturate Induction

| | Percent of Patients | |
Symptoms	Ketamine	Barbiturate
Nausea	42	22
Vomiting	30	10
Headache	39	25
Dizziness	73	38
Alert at Discharge	51	97
Frightening Dream	50	0
Request Again	55	90

SOURCE: Thompson GE et al: Experience with Outpatient Anesthesia. Anesth Analg 52: 881–887, 1973. Used with permission.

agents and techniques that create a lesser incidence of postanesthesia side-effects.

Local or regional anesthesia is an excellent choice for ambulatory surgery because of a low incidence of postoperative nausea and vomiting and earlier discharge of patients from the facility.[89] Epidural anesthesia is administered to 50% of laparoscopy cases at the Virginia Mason Hospital (Seattle, Washington). Following laparoscopy, nausea and vomiting were present in 38% of general anesthesia patients but in only 4% of those who had an epidural.[90]

The role of transdermal scopolamine (TS) in the prevention of nausea and vomiting has not been clearly defined. Pharmacokinetic studies have shown that the urinary excretion of scopolamine following the application of a single patch is similar to that seen during continuous low-dose intravenous infusion and that the drug continues to be absorbed for up to three days after initial application.[91] One would therefore expect that scopolamine, when administered in this fashion, would provide prolonged protection, as it does in motion sickness. Results, however, do not support this expectation.[92,93]

Tigerstedt and coworkers concluded that transdermal scopolamine does not reduce the overall incidence of postoperative emetic sequelae but noted that visual disturbances were more frequent in TS patients.[94] However, Bailey and colleagues found TS effective in reducing nausea, retching, and vomiting in women anesthetized for laparoscopy, although these problems still occurred in 37% of the TS-treated women.[95] The patch was applied behind an ear the night before surgery. Insignificant benefits from TS were noted in reducing postoperative emesis following pediatric eye surgery.[96] An unacceptable incidence of behavioral side-effects (hallucinations, extreme agitation) was noted. Routine use of scopolamine as a transdermal preparation for the prophylaxis of vomiting in the pediatric eye surgery patient is not recommended.

Dundee and coworkers noted that manual needling for five minutes at the P6 acupuncture point (Neiguan) resulted in a significant reduction in perioperative nausea and vomiting in 50 patients undergoing minor gynecologic procedures.[97] The application of low-frequency (10-Hz) electric current for five minutes to an acupuncture needle placed at the P6 point is as effective as manual needling in the reduction of postoperative emetic sequelae.[98] Transcutaneous electrical stimulation by means of a conducting stud or pressure over the P6 point provided a brief period (<1 hr) where nausea and vomiting were reduced; however, after one hour, the incidence of nausea and vomiting returned to the control-group level.[99]

There appears to be no effect on the incidence of nausea and vomiting in the immediate postoperative period in pediatric patients who receive intraoperative replacement of fluid intravenously compared with those who receive no intravenous supplements.[100] The level of activity on the first postoperative day was similar whether patients received fluid or not. This is in contrast to results reported in adult patients.[101]

A significant relationship was shown between postoperative emetic symptoms and the antagonism of neuromuscular blockade by neostigmine and atropine. The incidence of nausea and vomiting was significantly increased in patients whose neuromuscular blockade was reversed by neostigmine and atropine.[102] A significantly higher incidence of nausea and vomiting has been noted in pediatric patients who receive opioid premedication and those who have strabismus surgery, and a significantly lower incidence of vomiting was seen following anesthetics lasting less than 30 minutes and in children younger than three years.[103] Other studies have confirmed a significantly higher incidence of postoperative nausea and vomiting (up to 85%) in pediatric patients who undergo strabismus surgery.[104–107] Following orchiopexy, up to 5% of patients may have to be admitted because of drowsiness, nausea and vomiting, or more extensive surgery than planned.[108]

In separate studies, 75 μg/kg droperidol has been found to be more effective in reducing poststrabismus vomiting than 50 μg/kg.[104,105,107] When IV droperidol was given 30 minutes prior to the termination of surgery, 75 μg/kg reduced vomiting to 43% compared to 85% in the control group. When 75 μg/kg droperidol was administered during induction of anesthesia and before manipulation of the extraocular muscles, the incidence of vomiting was reduced from 47% in the control group to 10% in the droperidol group.[106] Droperidol (25 μg/kg) was effective in lessening the incidence of nausea and vomiting during the time the patient was in the facility; once the patient returned home, there appeared to be an increased incidence of nausea and vomiting in this group compared to the 50- and 75-μg/kg groups[109] (Fig. 7-4). Brown and colleagues recommend conservative management of children during and after strabismus surgery, involving gastric suctioning prior to extubation, complete replacement of preoperative fluid deficits, avoidance of narcotics, as well as a small dose of droperidol (20 μg/kg).[110] Antiemetic prophylaxis for pediatric patients undergoing strabismus procedures is more fully discussed in Chapter 4.

A recovery time of four to six hours after surgery would be considered prolonged in children following myringotomy or herniotomy, but because of nausea

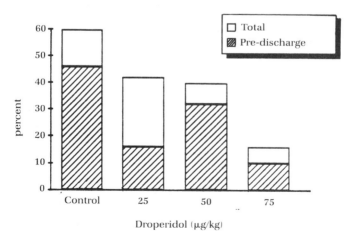

FIGURE 7-4. Incidence of vomiting after strabismus repair. (SOURCE: Eustis S et al.[109] Used with permission.)

TABLE 7-9. Nausea and Vomiting and Recovery Room Time

Procedure	DENTAL	KNEE ARTHRO	D&C	LAP	OVUM
N	32	73	90	175	59
Mean RR Time in Hours (SD)					
No N/V	2.23	1.87*	1.66*	2.21*	2.73*
	(.50)	(.53)	(.56)	(.90)	(.62)
N/V	2.32	2.23	2.46	2.81	3.45
	(.55)	(.63)	(.86)	(.63)	(.85)
All Patients**	2.24	1.94	1.77	2.41	3.10
	(.51)	(.57)	(.67)	(.80)	(0.83)
N/V%***	16	22	12	35	54
N/V% per Technique					
No Intra-op Narc.	12	17	11	30	52
Intra-op Narc.	33	37	17	42	60

*P<.05 for difference in RR time between patients with No N/V and N/V
**P<.03 for difference in RR time among all procedures
***P<.02 for difference in incidence of N/V among procedures
SOURCE: Pataky AO et al.[111] Used with permission.

and vomiting, it is not an unusual length of stay after strabismus or orchiopexy surgery. Intraoperative droperidol is recommended in these patients.

Pataky and coworkers evaluated the incidence of postoperative nausea and vomiting (general anesthesia) for the five most common procedures in the day-surgery unit at the University of Pennsylvania.[111] Depending on the procedure, 12% to 54% of patients experienced emetic symptoms (Table 7-9). Nausea and vomiting prolong PACU stay and increase per-patient labor costs.[112]

An important part of the preanesthesia interview is identifying the nausea-susceptible patient. A history of motion sickness or emesis following prior anesthetics elicited during the preanesthesia interview should alert the anesthesiologist to establish an anesthesia "game plan." When faced with this type of patient, one must carefully prioritize the use of antiemetics, gastric emptying (gastrokinetics or gastric suction), nitrous oxide, narcotic analgesics, anesthetic agents, local or regional block supplementation, and regional anesthesia. The nausea-susceptible patient should receive positive reassurance by all members of the staff to alleviate anxiety. The patient should be moved slowly at all times to avoid motion sickness. A warm blanket placed over such a patient may add to his or her sense of security. The patient should have limited pharyngeal suction at the conclusion of the procedure in order to avoid stimulation of the gag reflex and should be allowed to wake up slowly in the PACU.

In the PACU, droperidol (10 μg/kg) is the treatment of choice at MASC. For drowsy patients or those in whom droperidol treatment is ineffective, metoclopramide (0.15 mg/kg IV) is administered. We treat those patients who get nauseated when sitting up or when attempting to ambulate with ephedrine (10–25 mg IV). The use of ephedrine prophylactically to decrease postprocedure nausea and vomiting has both its advocates and detractors. Rothenberg and coworkers found ephedrine (0.5 mg/kg IM) prior to the conclusion of anesthesia was as effective as droperidol (0.04 mg/kg IM) and significantly more effective than placebo in reducing postoperative nausea and vomiting.[113] On the other hand, Poler and White found that ephedrine-treated patients (25 mg IM prior to the conclusion of the procedure) did not decrease emetic sequelae.[114]

When nothing seems to help, the situation should be explained to both the patient and the family member in attendance, and the option of spending a night in the hospital should be considered. Many patients will elect to recover at home. Patients should be instructed that if nausea and vomiting do not improve following rest at home, they should call the facility, their physician, or the emergency room if they feel it necessary to return to the hospital, and be admitted.

As we continue to evaluate prophylactic antiemetic therapies in the ambulatory setting, we must look at patient characteristics, anesthetic agents, and surgical procedures as well as other factors that appear to influence the incidence of postprocedure nausea and vomiting.

Postintubation Croup

Ambulatory surgery lends itself to managing the pediatric patient. The most serious immediate postintubation complication in the young child is laryngeal edema or tracheitis evidenced by hoarseness, croupy cough, and stridor. If not treated early and appropriately, the condition has the potential to progress to the point at which the child becomes restless, uses accessory muscles of respiration, and develops intercostal retraction. Tachypnea and fatigue set in, and the stage is set for a major problem. With improvements in technique and equipment, the incidence of postintubation croup appears to be decreasing from earlier reports of 6% to more recent reports of 1% of patients.[115-118] The overall incidence of croup (1%) in 7875 children intubated during a two-year period at the Children's Hospital Medical Center in Boston could be attributed to no single factor as a chief cause, but several—patient's age, intubation trauma, and length of surgery—were strongly related to the incidence of this complication.[117]

Mechanical trauma is related to a considerable extent to the anesthesiologist's experience with pediatric patients. The infantile larynx resembles a funnel, with the narrowest point situated at the lower border of the cricoid cartilage. The anesthesiologist may easily insert an endotracheal tube between the vocal cords only to find that the tube is too large to pass the cricoid constriction. A tube left in this position may produce subglottic swelling, whereas if the tube is forced through the cricoid narrowing, it may cause ischemia of the laryngeal mucosa followed by edema after extubation.[119] Despite all precautions and the use of flawless technique, subglottic edema may still occur.

By understanding the potential causes of postintubation croup, anesthesiologists may be able to lessen its incidence (Fig. 7-5). Contributing factors in the development of postintubation croup include[117]

1. Age of the patient. Children between one and four years of age are more likely to develop this complication.
2. Trauma related to intubation. Repeated attempts at intubation result in a higher incidence of postintubation croup.

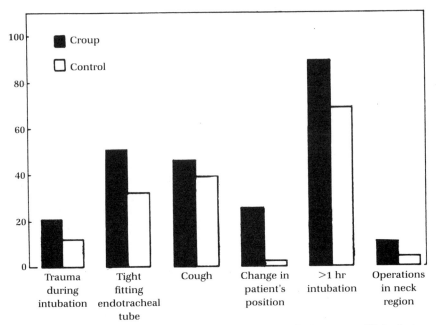

FIGURE 7-5. Contributing factors in the development of postintubation croup. All the factors shown increased trauma to the larynx. (SOURCE: Koka BV et al.[117] Used with permission.)

3. Size of the endotracheal tube. In patients in whom there was no leak around the endotracheal tube when positive pressure of approximately 25 cmH$_2$O was exerted on the breathing bag, postintubation croup was more prevalent.
4. Coughing with the endotracheal tube in place. There was a positive correlation between the development of croup and active coughing or straining by children at any time while the endotracheal tube was in place.
5. Changing the patient's position. A higher incidence of croup occurred in patients whose head changed position during surgery.
6. Duration of intubation. Longer periods of intubation were followed by more airway irritation.
7. Position of the patient. Operations performed in positions other than supine had a higher incidence of croup.
8. Site of the operation. Croup occurred more frequently following operations around the neck.

Symptom onset varies from immediately after extubation to a maximum of three hours. Epstein feels that in the pediatric outpatient population, symptoms that will require treatment will become evident within the first hour in the PACU.*

*Epstein BS: Personal communication, 1983.

There is no universal agreement as to the effectiveness of prophylactic regimens. Children treated prophylactically with 2% lidocaine (2 mg/kg) injected intravenously one minute prior to extubation had no laryngospasm, compared with a 20% occurrence in a nontreated group.[120] Subsequent intravenous injection of lidocaine (2 mg/kg) in the nontreated group controlled the spasm within 30 to 90 seconds. Moderate bradycardia was observed in one child, and transient respiratory depression occurred in two children. The study group (20 patients) was too small to evaluate the effectiveness of intravenous lidocaine in preventing hoarseness or croupy cough. Subjects given dexamethasone (0.3 mg/kg) and lidocaine (1 mg/kg) intravenously, separately and in combination, had a smaller incidence of postintubation croup than a control group.[121] Dexamethasone appeared to be more effective than lidocaine. When treatment of the early symptoms of laryngeal complications did not prove effective and signs of laryngeal obstruction became more evident, Deming and Oech combined intravenous diphenhydramine chloride (0.25–2.5 mg/kg) with dexamethasone (a single dose of 4 mg for infants under one year of age and 8 mg for older children).[124] Definite improvement was noted in 10 patients from 20 to 40 minutes after administration of this combination of drugs. When postintubation croup was treated with cool-mist inhalation alone and cool mist plus dexamethasone (4–8 mg) intravenously, fewer of the dexamethasone patients required additional treatment (intermittent positive-pressure breathing with epinephrine).[116] Most children with croup have a benign course. In mildly symptomatic patients, oxygen and cool mist are all that may be required.

By the very nature of the surgical procedures performed in an ambulatory setting, the severity of symptoms and percentage of patients experiencing postintubation croup are less than in an inpatient population. However, in view of the large number of ambulatory surgery pediatric patients, anesthesiologists should be aware of a simple, inexpensive, and effective means of handling postintubation croup. Racemic epinephrine will quickly and effectively manage this problem with minimal recurrence. Dilute 0.5 ml 2.25% racemic epinephrine with 3 ml sterile saline or water and deliver this through a face mask and nebulizer. This is easily accomplished with the patient seated in a parent's lap. By making a game of it, one usually encounters no resistance; we let the patient know that he or she can take the disposable face mask ("space mask") home. When patients receive racemic epinephrine, they should be observed in the PACU for a minimum of two hours in case of symptom recurrence. Additional factors to be considered are

1. The patient's age (a determinant of airway diameter)
2. Down's syndrome (frequently have subglottic stenosis)
3. The severity of the croup and how it responds to treatment
4. The reliability of the parents for home care
5. How far the family lives from the facility
6. Once home, how much time would elapse before the parents could access emergency care
7. Availability of support measures at home (for example, a humidifier)

The answers may influence the anesthesiologist's decision to discharge to home care or admit for observation.

Postanesthetic Delirium

Emergence from anesthesia may be accompanied by restlessness, disorientation, crying, moaning, or irrational speech. In its extreme form, excitement can be referred to as *emergence delirium*, in which the patient will scream, shout, and thrash wildly about.

Emergence delirium is prevalent among children and common in healthy adult patients, but as age increases, the incidence decreases. Among the more common factors contributing to delirium are pain, stress, anxiety, hypoxia, anticholinergic drugs, phenothiazines, barbiturates, ketamine, varying inhalation anesthetics, and distended urinary bladder. It is important to assess restlessness and delirium accurately in the postanesthetic patient and to treat the potential causes appropriately. Appropriate treatment may be simply medication for pain or reversing muscle relaxants or narcotic agents.

Longo first used the term *anticholinergic syndrome* in describing the central nervous system manifestations of toxicity from belladonna alkaloids and related compounds.[123] The symptom complex includes confusion, restlessness, agitation, dizziness, delirium, visual and auditory disturbances, stupor, and coma. In addition to belladonna alkaloids, phenothiazines and tricyclic antidepressants also may have a central anticholinergic action.

Physostigmine has been used successfully in treating the central anticholinergic syndrome. Sedation and delirium following diazepam and lorazepam, as well as sedation following the use of hydroxyzine and droperidol, have been reported to be completely relieved by the administration of physostigmine (1–2 mg) slowly intravenously.[23,124,125] Spaulding and coworkers noted an apparent increase in awareness following physostigmine administration but concluded that the accompanying ventilatory drive decrease may contraindicate its use in patients with diazepam-induced ventilatory depression.[126] The mechanism by which physostigmine reverses the effects of benzodiazepines is yet to be explained. Garber and colleagues were unable to speed the recovery process or improve psychomotor function in a group of outpatients undergoing dental extractions under intravenous diazepam sedation with a mixture of physostigmine and atropine.[127] The anticholinergic effects exerted by atropine may be the reason results differed from prior studies when physostigmine was used alone. Intravenous physostigmine (2.0 mg) administered intravenously 10 minutes after induction with 1.5 mg/kg ketamine resulted in significantly reduced PACU nystagmus, blurred vision, and length of stay but a higher incidence of nausea and vomiting.[128]

Although physostigmine's ability to reverse somnolence induced by anticholinergic drugs represents a specific antagonistic action, its reported ability to reverse postoperative somnolence induced by other depressant agents probably represents a nonspecific arousal response. Hannallah and coworkers administered physostigmine (60 µg/kg) intravenously over a period of 60 seconds in the PACU to pediatric outpatients who had received rectal methohexital induction for bilateral myringotomy.[129] There was no improvement in recovery score for the patients who received physostigmine compared with a control group. There was no slowing of the heart rate from physostigmine, and atropine was not used in any patient. Side-effects of physostigmine that occur infrequently are bradycardia, ventricular arrhythmias, abdominal cramping, nausea, and increased bronchial secretions. Atropine will counteract these muscarinic effects.

Flumazenil, a site-specific benzodiazepine antagonist (competitively displaces benzodiazepines at the specific central nervous system receptor site), has been developed recently. For patients undergoing termination of pregnancy under midazolam anesthesia, flumazenil (mean dose 0.4 mg IV in PACU) was an effective antagonist to the sedation induced by midazolam.[130] Amnesia was only abolished to a minor degree. Pharmacokinetic studies have shown an elimination half-life of 0.9 ± 0.2 hours for flumazenil. In view of this relatively short duration of action, there may be potential for benzodiazepine resedation. Flumazenil significantly reduced the degree of sedation following both midazolam and diazepam in patients who underwent gastroscopy.[131] No sign of resedation was found during the observation period of three hours; anterograde amnesia was effectively antagonized in both groups.

Postoperative Hypertension

Hypertension is one of the most common disease states encountered. It is present in up to 20% of patients, and it is very common in patients with coronary artery disease. Hypertension, if it occurs, is usually due to pain, anxiety, stressful emergence from anesthesia, hypoxia, hypercarbia, distention of the urinary bladder, or previous hypertension in which the patient was denied antihypertensive medications. All patients on hypertensive therapy should take their medication the morning of surgery.

It is important to determine the cause of postoperative hypertension. In the majority of patients, the condition results from pain and distress. In this setting, the best strategy is to treat the source of pain or distress. If hypertension is a result of a response to arousal, the patient should be allowed to wake up on his or her own and the hypertension should consequently resolve. The newer beta-blockers are very effective in managing an acute hypertensive episode. Esmolol may be preferred to labetalol because of a shorter elimination half-life (9 min). This results in less postoperative orthostatic hypotension. Esmolol is also more cardiac selective. To initiate esmolol therapy, a loading infusion of 0.5 mg/kg over one minute per bolus is followed by 1/10 of the loading infusion per minute for four minutes; then the drug is titrated to effect based on individual patient response.

Leslie and coworkers feel labetalol hydrochloride is an appropriate drug for the rapid treatment of hypertension following general anesthesia.[132] The initial dose of labetalol was 0.25 mg/kg administered over two minutes. If an adequate antihypertensive effect was not achieved within 10 minutes of the first labetalol dose, repeated doses were given at 10-minute intervals (0.5, 0.7, and 1.0 mg/kg). A total of 2.5 mg/kg labetalol could be administered over 40 minutes. No patients experienced any untoward side-effects such as hypotension, significant bradycardia, bronchospasm, or ECG changes. A single intravenous dose achieves full effect within 5 to 10 minutes.

Nifedipine, administered sublingually, has proven extremely effective in the treatment of severe hypertension and hypertensive crises. Adler and coworkers administered sublingual nifedipine (10 mg) to 19 elderly patients undergoing ophthalmologic surgery.[133] Blood pressure exceeded 200 mmHg systolic and/or 110 mmHg diastolic in all cases, and complicating cardiovascular problems and concomitant drug usage were common among these patients. An initial 10-mg sublingual dose of nifedipine was given followed by a second 10-mg dose if blood pressure was not reduced from baseline values within 20 minutes. A prompt antihypertensive response was achieved in all cases with no serious side-effects. To administer nifedipine sublingually, a 10-mg nifedipine capsule is placed into the barrel of a 3-ml syringe and the plunger is reinserted.[134] The diameter of the barrel is such that the capsule is self-oriented longitudinally. A 22-gauge needle (or larger) is used to pierce the capsule by means of the syringe orifice, keeping pressure against the capsule with the plunger. The syringe tip can then be placed sublingually and the contents of the capsule readily expelled with a somewhat firm push on the plunger. A single 10-mg dose of nifedipine given sublingually in the immediate preanesthetic or postanesthetic period is effective and safe for the management of hypertension.[135] Its onset of action is fast (2–15 min), its duration is long (3-5 hrs), and blood pressure level remains stable during its use.

Significant hypertension (mean 130 mmHg) not relieved by appropriate treatment of the cause will respond to a short-acting peripheral vasodilator. Hydralazine (2.5–5 mg) by slow intravenous bolus up to a total dose of 20 mg will usually control a transient hypertensive episode. Using a peripheral vasodilator to treat hypertension caused by hypoxia may cause a serious and profound drop in blood pressure as it counteracts compensatory vasoconstriction.[136] Hypertension, which may accompany emergence delirium, will respond to physostigmine.

Disseminated Intravascular Coagulation

White and coworkers described three patients who developed clinical and laboratory evidence of disseminated intravascular coagulation (DIC) after elective ambulatory midtrimester pregnancy terminations under general anesthesia.[137] Common to all three cases were fetal gestational age greater than 20 weeks, difficult fetal or placental extractions, and clinically significant hemorrhage (intraoperatively and 1–2 hr postoperatively). Patients at risk for developing DIC generally have gestations greater than 20 weeks with difficult extractions. White and coworkers recommend that all patients undergoing late midtrimester termination have blood sent to the hospital blood bank preoperatively for a type and screen and that these patients should remain in the PACU for a minimum of two to three hours with careful monitoring of blood loss. Where there is abnormal or increased bleeding, coagulation studies should be obtained to rule out DIC. The availability of blood and coagulation factors should be checked before anesthetizing this group of patients.

Coagulation function was prospectively studied in 25 patients undergoing intraamniotic instillation of hypertonic saline for the purpose of termination of pregnancy.[138] Consistent and statistically significant changes in platelet count, prothrombin time, plasma fibrinogen, and fibrin degradation products were found. Findings suggest that DIC is a sequelae of saline-induced abortion. Although anticoagulant therapy with heparin has been used with success in treating ongoing consumption coagulopathies, White and coworkers used procoagulants to replace factors that had been consumed.[137] Bick initiates anticoagulant therapy for acute DIC with 2500 to 5000 units of heparin subcutaneously every 8 to 12 hours, depending on the nature and severity of the bleeding.[139] He feels that mini-heparin therapy may be as efficacious as larger heparin doses.

Syncope

Symptoms of dizziness, drowsiness, weakness, and hypotension singly or in combination and of sufficient severity to prevent home readiness fall into my classification of *syncope*. Patients are not able to ambulate without support.

At the Phoenix Surgicenter, postoperative hypotension occurs in 16% of patients.[11] Usual causes are positional changes, pain, a full bladder, and analgesic or antiemetic drugs. Always rule out more serious possibilities, including hypoxia or myocardial problems. All our adult ambulatory surgery patients having services of the anesthesia department (general, spinal, epidural) receive 1000 ml intravenous fluids during operation and in the immediate recovery period. The intravenous line is maintained until patients retain oral fluids and ambulate. Keane and Murray assessed the value of infusing a total of 2 L intravenous fluids intraoperatively and postoperatively in 212 fasting patients undergoing minor surgical procedures.[101] The treated patients (108) recovered from the effect of surgery and anesthesia more quickly than patients without fluids. The results of improved quality of postoperative recovery—a shorter length of stay and a quicker return to work—especially in those patients who had some difficulty in recovering from anesthesia on previous occasions, encourages the more frequent use of intravenous fluids in ambulatory surgery patients. Although there was no statistically significant difference in symptoms of nausea, vomiting, headache, and drowsiness within the first six hours after minor gynecologic procedures for 50 patients who received 1 L intravenous fluids intraoperatively, compared with 50 patients who received no intravenous fluids, those patients who received intraoperative fluids exhibited a decreased incidence of dizziness within the first six hours and a decreased incidence of nausea when questioned at three days; the difference was statistically significant.[140] Depending on the severity of postoperative hypotension, one can treat the cause, administer oxygen, put the patient in a supine position, continue intravenous fluids, and if necessary, give a vasopresser drug (*i.e.*, ephedrine).

Orthostatic hypotension has not been a major problem in our facility. We attribute this to our two-phase recovery room and particularly to the use of reclining chairs in our second phase. By slowly being brought into an upright seated position, our patients are able to tolerate sitting and ambulating with minimal occurrence of hypotension. Patients who have had spinal or epidural anesthesia should be closely observed because their sympathetic block may outlast sensory and motor blocks. If you plan to use spinal or epidural anesthesia in your facility, be sure that an adequate explanation is provided for the postanesthesia care staff.

If narcotic drug administration is considered the cause of excessive drowsiness and an inability to ambulate, reversal can be accomplished with the use of naloxone. In clinical dosages, naloxone does not produce respiratory depression, even when used in the absence of narcosis. By titrating naloxone intravenously in repeated doses of 0.1 mg, one may be able to provide reversal of sedation and ventilatory depression without affecting pain control. In addition, depressed blood pressure may rise. There is potential for return to the narcotized state, particularly if long-acting narcotic drugs have been used.

Doxapram provides pure respiratory stimulation without a change in the patients' narcotized state. Minute volume is affected by first increasing the depth of ventilation and then the rate. Robertson and coworkers administered 80 mg doxapram intravenously to a group of ambulatory surgery patients who had received methohexital, nitrous oxide, and halothane.[8] This was associated with a significantly more rapid recovery from anesthesia. In a single dose of 1 to 1.5 mg/kg, doxapram effectively antagonized respiratory depression induced by morphine without affecting analgesic action.[141] Diazepam sedation during endoscopy, biopsy procedures, and minor surgery was effectively and safely reversed without any potentially serious side-effects.[142] Stephen and Talton administered single intravenous doses of 1.5 mg/kg or a sustained administration of 300 mg over a period of 30 minutes by intravenous drip and found the drug predictable, controllable, and therapeutically safe in patients who received inhalation anesthetics.[143] Although oxygen consumption increases moderately after doxapram administration, there is a concomitant increase in oxygen availability such that the extraction ratio does not change and there is no evidence of peripheral hypoxia.[144] Janis administered 1.0 to 1.5 mg/kg by slow intravenous push at the conclusion of the procedure, followed by a 0.1% infusion drip (5 mg/min) to hasten arousal in ambulatory surgery patients.[145] In healthy patients there were minimal effects on blood pressure and pulse rate and few complicating arrhythmias. Caution should be exercised in elderly patients with severe hypertension, irritable ventricular arrhythmias, or seizure disorders.

Reactive hypoglycemia has been reported as the cause of prolonged recovery.[146] Although exceedingly rare, this condition can be treated easily if suspected. Apparently, there is a wide variation in what constitutes a clinically significant level of hypoglycemia. Certain patients develop headache, weakness, vertigo, palpitations, and nausea, whereas others with similar blood glucose levels may be completely asymptomatic. In most instances, there is little physiologic rationale to support the diagnosis, but if a low blood glucose value is obtained, treatment of symptoms by administration of intravenous dextrose will be simple and effective.

Monitoring

Kataria and coworkers measured postoperative arterial oxygen saturation in pediatric outpatients during transportation (time of transport lasted 120–180 s) to the PACU.[147] At the conclusion of the procedure, after extubation, or at the conclusion of mask anesthesia, 100% oxygen was given for three minutes. Oxygen was then discontinued and patients were moved to the PACU in the left lateral position. SpO$_2$ was 100% in all patients before transport, and temperature was above 36°C. During transport, mean SpO_2 was 93.5% ± 0.55% (range 82%–100%). Desaturation was most notable in the 0- to 6-month age group, followed by the 7- to 12-month age group, and least in the 13-month to 14-year group. In a similar group of patients, Pullerits and coworkers noted that 28.1% of 71 healthy children had significant arterial desaturation as detected by pulse oximetry [only 9 of 20 (45%) were identified clinically].[148] Clinically significant desaturation ($SpO_2 \leq$ 90%, equivalent to $PaO_2 \leq 58$ mmHg) occurred in 27% of 110 pediatric ambulatory surgery patients.[149] Early detection of hypoxemia is more likely when the pulse oximeter is used as an adjunct to clinical assessment. Hypoxemia can be diagnosed with pulse oximetry before cyanosis or bradycardia is apparent. Other studies conclude that children recovering from anesthesia can become hypoxemic in the PACU.[150,151] The degree of wakefulness as measured by a PACU score cannot be used to establish an end point for oxygen supplementation.

After rectal methohexital administration, 10 of 24 patients developed an oxygen saturation less than 95% (four patients less than 90%).[152] It is recommended following rectal methohexital that patients not be left unattended and that they should be transported expeditiously with supplemental oxygen readily available. Brown and Kallar do not believe that a small degree of short-lived desaturation warrants the use of supplemental oxygen in healthy pediatric outpatients.[153] A preliminary study concluded that in the absence of preanesthetic medication, narcotics, nondepolarizing muscle relaxants, or airway obstruction, postoperative hypoxemia is not a clinically significant problem. Although there appear to be some differences of opinion, there is a definite consensus that the use of pulse oximetry is a valuable monitor in the pediatric PACU and should be used to determine the need for supplemental oxygen. Bissonnette and Scott demonstrated postoperative hypoxemia after minor procedures under general anesthesia.[154] The effect of duration of transport time while breathing room air was significant only for patients over 65 years of age. Although transient decreases in arterial oxygen saturation may be tolerated in young, health patients, this may not be true for patients with impaired coronary or cerebral perfusion. The authors encourage oxygen administration to patients over 65 years of age during transport to the PACU. Following elective diagnostic laparoscopy, in patients receiving 2 or 4 L O_2 in the PACU, oxygen saturation was well above normal values, whereas in patients receiving no oxygen, there was a decrease noted in SpO_2.[155] Increasing oxygen flow from 2 to 4 L/min appeared to have no major effect on oxygen saturation. Inpatients appear to be at significantly greater risk of becoming hypoxemic during recovery from anesthesia than ambulatory surgery patients.[156] Twenty-one of 149 inpatients (14.1%) had one or more hypoxemic measurements during their postoperative care compared to 1 of 92 outpatients (1.1%).

Length of Stay in the Postanesthesia Care Unit
According to Reed,[157]

> heavy, long-lasting premedication, an additional 100 to 200 mg of barbiturate, or extra depth with an inhalation agent may cause no deleterious effect in the healthy patient. The resulting increase in recovery time, however, will have an unfavorable impact on

the surgery outpatient who would otherwise safely ambulate; it could even create an 'anesthetic inpatient' out of what was meant to be an outpatient surgical procedure.

Many anesthesiologists feel that using inhalation anesthesia is superior to intravenous anesthesia for ambulatory surgery because the patient recovers more rapidly and is discharged from the facility more promptly. White feels that intravenous anesthetics would be more controllable and hence more like the volatile anesthetics if they were administered by continuous infusion rather than by intermittent injection.[158] By using a continuous infusion, the anesthesiologist minimized the "peaks and valleys" of drug concentrations, the amount of drug administered is less, and recovery time is shortened. In comparing fentanyl and ketamine given by continuous infusion to intermittent bolus as intravenous adjuvants to nitrous oxide for maintenance of general anesthesia following thiopental induction, the amount of drug decreased approximately 45% and time to awakening decreased approximately 60% with infusion techniques. Trieger scores were consistent with a more rapid recovery in the infusion groups; the incidence of common postoperative side-effects did not differ significantly between bolus and infusion groups.

Azar and coworkers assessed the neurologic state and psychomotor function of ambulatory surgery patients recovering from isoflurane, enflurane, and fentanyl balanced anesthesia.[159] Arousal scores at 20 minutes were highest in the fentanyl group, but at 40 minutes scores were similar in all three groups. Psychomotor function was depressed equally in all groups one hour after anesthesia but returned to normal at two hours. The return of psychomotor test scores to preanesthesia values suggested sufficient recovery of mentation and coordination for safe discharge two hours after anesthesia under the care of an accompanying responsible person.

Ideally, the ambulatory surgery patient should receive an agent capable of a rapid induction of surgical anesthesia and swift emergence followed by a rapid return to normal activity and appetite with no side-effects. In comparing the three major inhalational agents (halothane, enflurane, isoflurane) following a short anesthetic (<30 min), no single agent stands out as being superior to any of the others in the occurrence of postanesthesia side-effects or in getting the patient home in a timely manner.[160] Following fentanyl, halothane, or enflurane for ambulatory surgery laparoscopy, there were no significant differences in postanesthesia drowsiness, dizziness, headache, vomiting, muscle aches, and visual disturbances among the three anesthetic groups.[161]

Lecky and coworkers prospectively evaluated postoperative morbidity, duration of PACU stay, and cost for patients who received fentanyl or isoflurane for outpatient diagnostic laparoscopy.[162] There were no statistically significant differences between the groups in the proportion of patients with complaints of nausea, episodes of vomiting, or complaints of pain in the PACU. Duration of PACU stay was significantly longer for fentanyl patients. As administered in this study, isoflurane appeared to be a more reliable, less expensive anesthetic for outpatient diagnostic laparoscopy. Several other investigators have compared recovery from isoflurane with recovery from fentanyl, alfentanil, and sufentanil anesthetics in patients undergoing ambulatory surgery.[163–165] Although all studies found that each of these techniques provided satisfactory intraoperative conditions, all found a significant increase in the incidence of nausea and vomiting in the narcotic-based group. Gaskey and colleagues suggested that the incidence of nausea and vomiting after ambulatory surgery for gynecologic procedures rises directly in proportion to the amount of narcotic administered perioperatively.[166]

In 300 pediatric patients, there was very little difference in recovery at 15 and 30 minutes following a variety of ambulatory surgical procedures.[167] Incidence of recovery delirium in the isoflurane group (19%) was more than twice that in the halothane group (8%); nausea, vomiting, headache, and bad dreams were identical in all groups. There was a higher incidence of coughing and laryngospasm following extubation with the enflurane group. Steward compared recovery from enflurane and halothane in pediatric outpatients.[168] During the early recovery period, postanesthesia scores for the enflurane group were higher on admission to the PACU, but this was not statistically significant, and there was no difference in scores after 15 minutes and at the time of discharge. Examination of returned questionnaires showed that the majority of patients in both groups rapidly returned to a normal status and were considered by their parents to be bright and alert and to have a normal appetite. A higher incidence of bad dreams reported after enflurane in children was not demonstrated by Steward. Headache and muscle pains, however, seem to have occurred with somewhat greater frequency in the enflurane group. In comparing isoflurane with halothane and enflurane, the rate of postoperative recovery was comparable with any of the three agents; return to normal status at home occurred somewhat more rapidly with isoflurane than with either of the agents. Late complications (nausea, vomiting, lack of appetite) occurring at home were seen less frequently with isoflurane than with halothane or enflurane. Steward feels that halothane remains the potent inhalation agent of choice for pediatric patients in preference to enflurane. However, except for a slower induction time, isoflurane compares favorably with halothane. Although variations in PACU length of stay are present among the three major inhalational agents, initial studies have not established one agent as being superior for the ambulatory surgery patient.[169,170] Korttila and Valanne found that the longer the duration of enflurane anesthesia, the longer it took to recover.[171] This was not the case with isoflurane. Korttila and Valanne concluded from this and prior studies that of the three major inhaled anesthetics, isoflurane should be preferred in adult ambulatory anesthesia because of faster recovery following its usage.[172]

Dundee, in comparing ultrashort-acting barbiturates for ambulatory surgery, felt that only methohexital appeared to be an improvement over thiopental because of a more rapid return of consciousness.[173] In the real world of anesthesia, assuming a single intravenous bolus induction, there is very little difference in PACU length of stay between these two agents. Increasing the dose of rectal methohexital (15–30 mg/kg) improved the speed and efficacy of induction; it also prolonged postoperative recovery.[174] In addition, among the children monitored by pulse oximetry in the PACU, $SpO_2 < 95\%$ occurred in 45% of patients induced with 30 mg/kg compared to 0% for those induced with 15 mg/kg.

Fragen and Caldwell evaluated awakening times following thiopental or etomidate induction in 40 women scheduled for gynecologic ambulatory surgical procedures.[175] Awakening times were similar for both induction agents, but the incidence of nausea was higher after etomidate (55%) than after thiopental (15%). In studying only early recovery from anesthesia, Horrigan and coworkers found no difference in time or quality of recovery between etomidate-induced and thiopental-induced patients.[176] There was a threefold increase in nausea and vomiting in the etomidate group. Fentanyl supplementation of anesthesia significantly shortened the time before patients opened their eyes and were able to follow commands in both groups.

Millar and Jewkes compared anesthetic conditions, recovery and, side-effects through the first 48 hours postoperatively in patients who received propofol or thiopental-enflurane anesthesia with and without alfentanil.[177] Propofol patients had faster immediate recovery and were fit for discharge significantly sooner, and there was a significant reduction in postoperative morbidity in both the groups that received propofol up to 24 hours after discharge (Table 7-10). Visual analogue scores of postoperative well-being showed a significant improvement in both propofol groups; after thiopental and enflurane, scores were reduced and took 48 hours to return to preoperative values. The addition of alfentanil improved anesthetic conditions and reduced postoperative morbidity with both propofol and thiopental-enflurane. In 40 unpremedicated patients who underwent minor gynecologic surgery, mood state was less affected postoperatively in those pa-

TABLE 7-10. Recovery in Day Surgery Unit

	Propofol	Thiopentone, Enflurane	Alfentanil, Propofol	Alfentanil, Thiopentone, Enflurane
Time, minutes (SD) from end of operation to				
Eyes open	7.5 (3.4)*	10.7 (5.0)*	5.6 (2.9)*	9.2 (5.8)
Obey command	8.1 (3.5)*	12.1 (5.5)*	6.3 (3.0)*	9.9 (5.8)
Give date of birth	8.6 (3.7)*	12.9 (5.4)*	6.5 (3.1)*	10.6 (6.0)
Sit unaided	35 (11.2)*	59 (36.2)*	35 (16.4)*	40 (20.3)
Able to drink	39 (11.6)*	68 (42.6)*	40 (17.5)*	47 (29.5)
Able to eat	40 (11.8)*	72 (44.7)*	41 (17.4)*	51 (30.8)
Stand unaided	79 (37.6)*	119 (53.3)*	76 (26.7)*	93 (47.8)
Walk unaided	80 (37.5)*	119 (53.5)*	77 (26.7)*	93 (47.8)
Able to dress	90 (53.2)*	133 (60.6)*	82 (26.0)*	104 (49.4)
Fit for discharge	100 (52.6)*	146 (62.8)*	99 (34.0)*	119 (56.2)
Refused food	1§	6§	0§	4§
Analgesics	12 (41%)	11 (33%)	5 (16%)	9 (29%)
Antiemetics	0 (0%)	2 (6%)	0 (0%)	4 (13%)

*p < 0.001.
§p = 0.009.
SOURCE: Millar JM et al.[177] Used with permission.

tients induced with propofol than with thiopental.[178] Propofol patients had a definite sense of well-being after anesthesia. In a multicenter study (879 patients) following release of propofol in the United Kingdom, Sanderson and Blades examined its use outside a clinical trial program and within the context of a routine clinical setting.[179] Propofol was the main anesthetic agent for a range of ambulatory surgical procedures; supplementary agents were fentanyl, alfentanil, or nitrous oxide. The mean dose of propofol (intravenous infusion) was 10.6 mg/kg per hour. Recovery was rapid and with a low incidence of nausea (2.3%) and vomiting (1.5%). Elation and/or euphoria was frequently reported during recovery (12.2%). When propofol was used by continuous infusion, patient stays in the PACU were shorter.[180] Compared with a standard thiopental-enflurane technique, those patients who received propofol by continuous infusion had a significantly shorter PACU time and a lower incidence of nausea and vomiting.[181] Faster patient turnaround can result in less expense to the health care delivery system.

Conahan and coworkers examined the effect of heating and humidifying inspired gases on body temperature, recovery time, and apparent patient comfort.[182] Simple heating and humidification of inspired gas in patients undergoing laparoscopic ovum retrieval was associated with a 33% decrease in PACU stay. This time saving significantly reduced the per-case cost. The use of a relatively inexpensive heating system, eliminating almost an hour of PACU time, appeared to be a cost-effective approach to patient management in the ambulatory surgery population. Subsequent studies using a heated humidifier or a heat and moisture exchanger were unable to duplicate these findings.[183,184]

Hines and colleagues evaluated ambulatory surgical complications in the PACU.[185] For purposes of the study, reportable complications were listed as hypertension, hypotension, dysrhythmia, nausea and vomiting, drug reaction, respiratory difficulty (major and minor), cardiac events, and alterations in mental status. The overall PACU complication rate was 15.5%. Gynecologic and ophthalmologic procedures were associated with the highest overall rates (36% and 26%, respectively). Of patients who developed a PACU complication, those receiving a general anesthetic had a significantly higher incidence than those receiving regional anesthesia. Nausea and vomiting were the most frequently occurring PACU complications. Gynecologic surgery accounted for 39% of all nausea and vomiting reported, while ophthalmologic surgery had a nausea and vomiting rate of 33%. Patients who sustained a PACU complication had a 40% greater length of stay (145 vs. 107 min). Duration of anesthesia and ASA physical status did not have an impact on PACU complications. Patients over 42 years of age had the highest operating room complication rate (67%), while patients under 42 years of age experienced the greatest percentage of PACU complications (80%). Specific intraoperative factors, such as anesthetic technique and type of surgical procedure (gynecologic and/or ophthalmologic), and patient age are associated with an increased potential for the development of PACU complications.

Length of stay in the postanesthesia care unit not only depends on our choice of anesthetic agents, but also varies with the length of procedure, the criteria the facility uses to evaluate the patient for discharge, and other factors such as pain, nausea, vomiting, drowsiness, and dizziness. It is difficult to determine with great accuracy when patients can safely be allowed home, and the clinical judgment of the anesthesiologist must be the final determinant. Studies of postanesthesia care unit length of stay have produced differing results even with the same agents because dosage, length of surgery, and time spans between testings have all varied. Temporary arousal of patients to complete testing may allow them to score well even though certain areas of coordination are still impaired. If anesthetic agents that are appropriate for the ambulatory surgery patient are used, then anesthesia will not play a major role in increasing patients' length of stay in the PACU. The Phoenix Surgicenter reports that patients are usually ready for discharge within four hours. At George Washington University Hospital, the usual stay in the PACU is two to four hours, and at The Methodist Medical Center of Illinois, ambulatory surgery recovery stay averages two hours (25% are children with shorter lengths of stay).

"What's the hurry?" said the tortoise to the hare.* Ambulatory surgery facilities are not competing for record discharge times. Whether a patient is discharged in two or four hours following his or her procedure should not be the most important consideration. However, facilities cannot lose sight of the fact that time spent by patients and their families in the ambulatory facility can influence their level of satisfaction and can have a significant influence on health care costs. To meet the goal of discharging satisfied patients as soon as possible without compromising safety (and at the very least on the same day as their surgery), anesthesiologists and surgeons must be willing to modify techniques, facilities should regularly evaluate their discharge criteria, and physicians and staff should regularly discuss problem areas that affect length of stay.

WHEN TO FEED, WHAT TO FEED

Patients should be able to tolerate oral fluids with little or no nausea or vomiting prior to discharge. Berry feels that the patient's perception of hunger is one of the most helpful clinical signs in determining whether he or she is able to tolerate fluids.[186] When they are able, his pediatric patients are given oral fluids slowly (1 oz every 20 min for an hour) in the PACU, advancing their diet intake as tolerated. In our two-phase PACU, pediatric patients are transferred into phase 2 immediately upon reaching a postanesthesia recovery score of 10. Infants and small children who are alert and fussing are given water or a nippled bottle containing a solution of dextrose and water upon entry into phase 2 of recovery. We find that quickly giving clear oral fluids has a calming influence and makes for a smoother postoperative course. Infants who were not intubated during anesthesia and tolerate dextrose in water will quickly progress to milk, formula, or mother's milk. For those infants who had been intubated during anesthesia, even though we allow sips of water or dextrose and water, we do not allow milk products until one hour has elapsed from extubation. Our older pediatric patients are usually given water one half-hour after the conclusion of anesthesia. For our adult patients in phase 1 recovery who complain of a severe dry mouth, we have had no problem allowing them to rinse their mouth with water if they are alert,

*Tortoise T: Personal communication, 1990.

have progressed to the point that they can rest comfortably with the head of the stretcher elevated, and have no complaints of nausea. In phase 2 they receive water; if this is tolerated without nausea, they quickly progress to cola and 7-Up. Fluids given in our PACU are served at room temperature; we initially stay away from iced fluids and ice chips.

Patients are also given soda crackers to eat. If a patient insists on having tea or coffee, this is provided as long as nausea is minimal or absent. Patients are not given oral pain medications until they have tolerated liquids and soda crackers. Pain medications taken orally on an empty stomach are more likely to cause nausea and vomiting. At home, patients are instructed to take liquids and soda crackers prior to any oral pain medications.

MEASURING RECOVERY FROM ANESTHESIA

Assessment of recovery from anesthesia is increasingly significant as we see more extended operations requiring longer duration of anesthesia being performed on an ambulatory surgery basis. It is no longer sufficient to determine when a patient can leave the PACU; we must now know how to judge when a patient can be sent home safely after outpatient anesthesia. Steward divided recovery from general anesthesia into three stages:[187]

1. *Immediate recovery:* Return of consciousness, recovery of protective airway reflexes, and resumption of motor activity. This stage is short and can accurately be followed by the use of a postanesthesia scoring system.
2. *Intermediate recovery:* Return of coordination; disappearance of subjective feelings of dizziness. Following a short anesthetic, this stage lasts no more than one hour. At this time, the ambulatory surgery patient may be considered home ready in the company of a responsible person.
3. *Long-term recovery:* This stage may last hours or even days and is dependent on the length of anesthesia. Measurement requires use of precise psychomotor testing.

Korttila has looked at stages of recovery and some tests for their assessment (Table 7-11). Before patients can be considered fully recovered (e.g., able to drive), their psychomotor performance must return to the preanesthetic level. Carefully selected psychomotor tests or driving simulators can be used to assess patients' psychomotor recovery; however, these tests are complex and obviously cannot be used routinely in clinical practice.[188] Following intravenous sedation, psychomotor tests revealed considerable impairment of reactive and coordinative skills at 2½ hours, whereas neither the clinical nor the pencil-and-paper tests (used in Finland as sensitive indicators in assessing the performance of suspected drunken drivers) demonstrated significant impairment of performance a half hour after injection[189] (Table 7-12).

Cohen and MacKenzie gave patients a series of five tests of mental function just prior to anesthesia and during the second and third hour after entry into

TABLE 7-11. Stages of Recovery from Anesthesia and Tests Valid for Their Evaluation

Stage of Recovery	Tests of Recovery
Awakening	Opening eyes
	Answering
Immediate clinical recovery	Sitting steady
	Negative Romberg and other clinical tests
Fit to go home*	Maddox-Wing test
(hospital stay)	Paper and pencil tests
	Single reaction time tests
	Single coordination or attention tests
	Flicker fusion
"Street fitness"*	Flicker fusion
	Psychomotor test batteries
	EEG
Complete psychomotor recovery*	Carefully selected psychomotor test batteries
(fit to drive)	Driving simulators

*More than a single test is needed.
SOURCE: Korttila K.[206] Used with permission.

the PACU.[190] Although all patients appeared to have normal cognitive functioning at the time of discharge, there was a considerable degree of impairment of psychomotor ability. Doenicke and coworkers studied the effectiveness of psychological testings and feel that the tests do not adequately reflect the variations in cerebral function during the hours and days following anesthesia; fatigue plays a major role in the inaccuracies following repetitive testing.[191] To rule out the effect of fatigue on results, electroencephalography was used to assess depth and recovery from anesthesia following administration of different intravenous anesthetics.[192]

TABLE 7-12. Combination of Tests Used by Korttila

Clinical:
  Walking on a straight line
  Romberg test with open eyes
  Picking up matches
  Numerical countdown test
  Horizontal nystagmus
  Postrotary nystagmus
Pencil-and-paper:
  Bender motor gestalt
  Burdon-Wiersma
Psychomotor:
  Reactive skills
  Coordinative skills
  Attention
  Critical flicker fusion

SOURCE: Korttila K.[186] Used with permission.

TABLE 7-13. Stages of Recovery and Some Tests for Their Assessment

Stage of Recovery	Test of Recovery
Awakening and recovery of vital reflexes	Patient can open eyes and answer questions. Patient can maintain and guard his or her own airway.
Immediate clinical recovery	Patient can stand unaided.
Home readiness*	Patient can walk on a straight line. Paper and pencil tests. Maddox wing test. Simple coordination and reaction time tests.
Street fitness	Flicker fusion test. Psychomotor test batteries.
Full recovery (complete psychomotor recovery)	Carefully selected psychomotor test batteries. Real driving tests.
Psychologic recovery	Psychologic tests.

*For overall minimal criteria for discharge, see Table 7-14
SOURCE: Korttila K.[194] Used with permission.

The success of any ambulatory surgical program depends on appropriate and timely discharge of patients. Postanesthesia scoring systems can provide the necessary information to guide transfer from one phase of recovery to another. However, they do not provide absolute information to assess home readiness after ambulatory surgery (Tables 7-13 and 7-14). Unfortunately, we do not have cognitive or psychomotor tests that can be recommended as standard criteria for discharging ambulatory surgery patients after anesthesia. A variety of clinical, pencil-and-paper, and psychomotor tests have been used, singly or in combina-

TABLE 7-14. Guidelines for Safe Discharge after Day Surgery

1. Patients must have a responsible "vested" adult to escort them home and stay with them at home.
2. Patient's vital signs must have been stable for at least one hour.
3. Patient must have no evidence of respiratory depression.
4. Patient must be:
    Oriented to person, place, time
    Able to dress himself or herself
    Able to walk out without assistance
    Able to maintain orally administered fluids*
    Able to void*
5. Patient must not have:
    More than minimal nausea or vomiting
    Excessive pain
    Bleeding
6. Patient should stay at least one to two hours after extubation.
7. Patient must be discharged by the person who gave anesthesia or his or her designee. Written instructions for the postoperative period at home including a contact place and person need to be reinforced.

*The role of these variables as criteria for discharge remains to be established.
SOURCE: Korttila K.[194] Used with permission.

tion, as a means of measuring patient recovery from anesthesia. The majority are too involved and impractical for a busy clinical setting. Although psychomotor tests provide useful objective data on residual drug effects, their validity in assessing a patient's suitability for discharge after ambulatory surgery needs further evaluation. Korttila and coworkers feel that we need outcome studies to evaluate the usefulness of cognitive and psychomotor tests in evaluation of home readiness after ambulatory surgery.[193] The main problems associated with the clinical use of these tests are improvement of test results when the tests are repeated (training effect) and large individual variations in drug effects on the test results.[194]

Before considering the range of tests that have been applied to the assessment of recovery, one must consider extraneous factors that may affect test performance. Almost any test requires an indication of how well the patient can perform it before operation. The same conditions should pertain for preoperative baseline performance as in the postoperative test. Environmental factors (excessive noise, undue heat, flickering lights) that may have a distractive effect on the patient must be minimized.[195]

The postoperative test must then be carried out under as similar conditions as possible. The following factors are relevant: environmental factors; wearing similar clothes (loose-fitting slippers may impede tests involving walking); wearing of glasses, contact lenses, or hearing aides; and the investigator (the way in which test instructions are given). Most tests need to be practiced to achieve a reasonable baseline performance. There is a steep learning curve that is followed by a peak in performance, and subsequently, as the patient becomes bored with the test, performance declines.

Tests of recovery may be categorized into one of the following three types:*

> Clinical tests
> Paper-and-pencil tests
> Psychomotor tests

Before choosing or using any test of recovery, there are several questions to be considered:

> Is it practical to perform the test after an operation?
> Is the length of the test appropriate?
> Is the interest factor right?
> Is the test sensitive enough to pick up small differences in performance?
> Is it possible to get a reasonable baseline?
> Is the test appropriate to the deficiency under study?

---

*For those readers wishing a complete description of tests of recovery, the editor recommends obtaining copies of the following monographs published in the United Kingdom: Cooper G: Recovery from anaesthesia. Anaesth Rounds. 19: 1-23, 1986 (monograph presented by the Pharmaceuticals Division of Imperial Chemical Industries PLC); and Hindmarch I: Psychological testing after anaesthesia. Anaesthetists Information Services Monograph Series No 4 (Monograph presented by Janssen Pharmaceutical Limited).

A variety of tests have been used in studies evaluating recovery from anesthesia: Trieger dot, choice reaction time, *p*-deletion, Maddox-Wing, digit symbol substitution, critical flicker fusion, and quantitative Romberg. Clyburn and colleagues utilized the Trieger test to evaluate quality of recovery in 60 ambulatory surgery patients who received either midazolam or diazepam with fentanyl and etomidate for induction and maintenance of anesthesia.[196] No significant difference was noted in quality of recovery. White and coworkers used Trieger tests to help evaluate comparison of alfentanil with fentanyl for ambulatory surgical anesthesia. Compared with fentanyl, recovery of psychomotor function was more rapid and postoperative drowsiness and sedation were less with alfentanil.[197] Hargreaves used both Maddox-Wing and digit-symbol substitution tests to determine recovery in patients who received a premedication of midazolam (15 mg), temazepam (20 mg), or placebo.[198] Although both midazolam and temazepam produced anxiolysis compared with placebo (midazolam being superior), slower recovery was noted in the midazolam patients.

In comparing propofol with methohexital and thiopental for induction of anesthesia in ambulatory patients, Mackenzie and Grant used the Leeds psychomotor tester (single apparatus capable of measuring critical flicker fusion threshold and choice reaction time scores).[199] Postanesthetic recovery was superior with propofol, with virtual absence of side-effects and rapid recovery with little impairment of psychomotor function 30 minutes after anesthesia. Using a computerized force platform (body sway) and the digit-symbol substitution test, Korttila and coworkers noted a significant difference in patient recovery for propofol-treated patients compared with the thiopental group.[200] Milligan and colleagues compared recovery in outpatients who received incremental propofol (continuous infusion or propofol followed by isoflurane).[201] Recovery was assessed using both clinical and psychomotor criteria (choice reaction time and *p*-deletion tests). Initial recovery was more rapid in the incremental propofol group. Vielle and associates measured psychomotor performance using the serial four-choice reaction time for patients receiving propofol or thiopental-isoflurane.[202] Psychomotor performance tests showed an increased reaction time in the thiopental-isoflurane group, but the difference was not statistically significant. However, quality of recovery was significantly better for the propofol-treated patients. Similar results were noted when comparing recovery in patients receiving propofol versus enflurane.[203] When comparing a sedative infusion of midazolam or propofol during local and regional anesthesia, Negus and White utilized visual analogue scores (VAS) and the digit-symbol substitution test (DSST).[204] The sedation VAS and DSST scores during the perioperative period demonstrated a more rapid return to baseline following propofol. Overall, propofol by continuous infusion appears to be an excellent alternative to midazolam for sedation during local and regional anesthesia. Millar and Jewkes consider propofol to be the present anesthetic agent of choice for ambulatory surgery because of improved quality of recovery and reduced postoperative morbidity.

The tendency of a patient to sway in a standing position after administration of a drug may be an index of patient safety. Jansen and coworkers determined postural stability of patients before and 90 minutes after oral administration of diazepam (0.2 mg/kg).[205] A quantitative Romberg test, the indication of body sway, was used in the study. There was a statistically significant increase in mean postural sway after premedication with diazepam, especially with the eyes open; the tendency of swaying was not aggravated when the patients closed their eyes. The study demonstrated that a patient's visual perception of surroundings adds no safety in the standing position after premeditation. Jansen and coworkers believe that patients should not be allowed to ambulate after premedication.

The complexity of brain function is such that there is no single test that delineates when a patient is sufficiently recovered to go home. Reliance has to be placed on clinical assessment and modifying the activities of patients for at least the ensuing 24 hours. Once discharge criteria have been met, clinical judgment becomes the single most important factor in determining the patient's home readiness. Psychological tests whose results do not coincide with clinical judgment in no way indicate that the patient should not be sent home. The patient should be allowed home once clinical discharge criteria have been met, but he or she should be transported home and watched over by a responsible person.

Perhaps in no other area must anesthesiologists be more acutely aware of the variations that occur in the PACU following anesthetic intervention than when dealing with the ambulatory surgery patient. The literature can be helpful in decision making; however, only by personal evaluation of the effects that the varying agents have on individual patients, such as nausea, vomiting, headache, dizziness, drowsiness, and length of stay in the PACU, can anesthesiologists decide which agents are more desirable than others for their ambulatory surgery patients.

WHEN CAN A PATIENT DRIVE?

Clinically, we consider the patient recovered from anesthesia when he or she is capable of responding to commands in the PACU and performing other simple tasks, whereas from the patient's standpoint, recovery often signifies the return to normal function in a familiar environment. As anesthesiologists, we are interested in patients meeting specific criteria for discharge home; patients are more interested in when can they drive a car or go back to work.

Korttila assigned certain tests as specific indicators of return of particular functions in patient recovery from anesthesia[206] (Table 7-11). The less complex the test, the less sensitive it is in evaluating complete psychomotor recovery. Driving simulators, reaction timers, and complex psychodiagnostic testing are of value, providing reasonably reliable and objective information about the duration of effects of anesthetic agents, and can serve as points of reference for a facility when establishing discharge criteria.[172,207,208]

A member of the legal profession in the United Kingdom writing about anesthetics and driving stated, "After most general anaesthetics it is safer to advise against driving for 48 hours."[209] Members of the Anaesthetic Subcommittee of the Association of Anaesthetists immediately challenged the statement. The 48-hour rule was refuted with the conclusion that a patient who has had a good night's sleep after an anesthetic should be able to drive the following day.[210] Herbert and coworkers monitored ambulatory surgery patients for two days following hernia surgery with a choice reaction time test.[211] Reaction times gradually returned to baseline values during the first 24 hours, but there was a slowing during the second postoperative day. This occurred in patients who had been breathing spontaneously during surgery but not in those whose breathing was assisted. The authors feel that it is wise to extend the warning not to drive to at least 48 hours postoperatively. If the duration of anesthesia is less than 30 minutes, Korttila recommends that patients not drive for 24 hours; if the duration is two hours or more, it may be safer to advise them not to drive for 48 hours.[194]

There is an obvious difficulty in establishing firm conclusions from data provided by heterogeneous groups administered varying doses of different anesthetic agents and tested in different ways. Until such time as results conform and definite conclusions can be drawn, a period of 24 hours before resuming driving is a reasonable time to recommend following most of the commonly used ambulatory surgical anesthetic agents.[212]

EEG readings following barbiturate induction returned to normal within 30 minutes, but 2½ and 3½ hours later, drowsiness appeared. At 4½ hours, a transitory sleep stage ensued, and this persisted for up to 12 hours.[213] These results provide substance to recommendations that following anesthesia, patients should be accompanied by a responsible person, refrain from activities in which a decrease in alertness might be a hazard (driving a car, making crucial business decisions), and abstain from alcohol for 12 to 24 hours.

DISCHARGE CRITERIA

Ambulatory surgery facilities go to great length to develop criteria for patient selection; it is of equal importance to have criteria for patient discharge. Although the varying psychomotor tests can provide us with information that is usable in developing criteria, the majority of tests are too complex, time-consuming, and cumbersome to be used in a clinical setting. Practical discharge criteria must be tailored to the particular facility, size of the PACU, and number of postanesthesia care nurses and must not compromise patient safety.

Patients should be informed before being discharged home that they may experience pain, headache, nausea, vomiting, dizziness, and muscle aches and pains not related to the incision for at least 24 hours following surgery and anesthesia. Fahy and Marshall found that women are more likely to be affected than men, that the incidence of postanesthesia morbidity among patients undergoing anesthesia for the first time (49.1%) was higher than that of patients who had a previous anesthetic experience (29.4%), and that increasing the length of surgery over 20 minutes was associated with both the occurrence and severity of symptoms.[16] When halothane is a part of the anesthetic technique, a higher incidence of headache within the first 24 hours has been reported.[213]

In 100 consecutive outpatients who were provided no written instructions at discharge, Ogg found that 31% of patients went home unaccompanied by a responsible adult; 73% of car owners drove within 24 hours of surgery, with 30% driving within 12 hours; 9% of patients drove themselves home; and a bus driver returned to work on the same day, driving a busload of passengers a distance of

95 miles.[214] Patients in this study reported postoperative symptoms of headache (27%), drowsiness (26%), nausea (22%), and dizziness (11%). Fifty percent of medical outpatients do not follow physicians' instructions, but the addition of written and verbal education techniques at discharge has a marked impact on improving compliance.[215]

Malins studied compliance following ambulatory surgery.[216] Generalized written instructions on admission to the outpatient area were given to a group of patients without any discussion or explanation. A second group was given instructions on admission specific to the patient's postanesthetic activities, and these instructions were read to the patient, who was asked to retain the form and take it home on discharge. Between 77% and 95% of patients in the first group did not remember getting any instructions as to postanesthetic activities, and they consequently drove cars, operated machinery, and drank alcoholic beverages in less than 24 hours. The group who kept the written instructions that had been read to them were in compliance 88% to 96% of the time. Only 1 of 30 patients failed to remember being told not to drive for 24 hours, whereas 22 of 30 patients in the first group claimed they did not remember this instruction. Another problem area that surfaced during this study was the number of patients undergoing general anesthesia who did not understand or speak any English. In areas with high immigrant populations, consent forms, procedural explanations, and discharge information may have to be written in appropriate languages, and the services of an interpreter should be provided. Case 12 in Chapter 8 provides an excellent example of how an unrecognized language barrier created a problem.

Simple general anesthetic techniques affect patient memory retention in the immediate postoperative period.[217] Inhalation and narcotic techniques cause impairment of recall of new material at one hour postanesthesia even though patients appear clinically fit for discharge. At three hours postanesthesia, recall of new material in all patients returns to normal.

Hippocrates said, "Keep an eye on the faults of your patients; they often lie about what medicines they are taking." Two thousand years later, we can still say that patient compliance is less than perfect. In the medicolegal climate of today, providing patients with written discharge instructions should be part of every facility's discharge policy.

Following discharge, patients should continue their recovery at home in bed. The discharge examination does not determine the patient's readiness to return to normal activities but establishes whether he or she can safely be released for a trip home. The Phoenix Surgicenter prefers the term *home readiness* to *street fitness*.[218] To be ready for the ride home, Surgicenter patients, in addition to a responsible person in attendance, must have[157]

1. Stable vital signs for at least one half hour
2. No new signs or symptoms postoperatively that may threaten a safe recovery (*e.g.*, the patient with mild shoulder pain following laparoscopy will be released home, but a patient with more than mild ab-

dominal pain following a diagnostic D&C will be detained for further observation)

3. Cessation of oozing or bleeding when bleeding was a feature of the operation
4. No nausea or emesis for a half hour or evidence that it is waning
5. Good circulation in and return of sensation to the operated extremity when a tourniquet has been used
6. No evidence of swelling or impaired circulation in an extremity when a cast has been applied.
7. Voided clear urine following cystoscopy
8. The ability to recognize time and place
9. Little or no dizziness after changing clothes and sitting for 10 minutes
10. No pain not subject to control by oral analgesics

After a state of home readiness has been established, the responsible nurse notifies the anesthesiologist, and together they make sure that the applicable requirements of the Surgicenter's postoperative checklist are satisfied. This is known as *informed discharge*.[157]

1. Dietary instructions are given: Clear liquids until the stomach is settled, then progress to regular feedings. No alcohol should be taken (unless by physician's order) for at least 12 hours.
2. Pain is provided for: Medication appropriate to the need.
3. Prescriptions are checked: The patient or responsible person has prescriptions for all medications ordered by the surgeon.
4. Surgeon's instructions are reviewed: Limitation of activity, elevation of operated extremity, when to return to office, anticipated complications, whom to call in event of unanticipated complications.
5. Anesthesiologist's instructions are given:
   a. "You may feel sleepy and somewhat sluggish for several hours." "Don't drive until tomorrow." "Postpone important decisions until tomorrow."
   b. "You may have a sore throat for a few hours" (if patient was intubated). Instruct patient in use of saltwater gargles, humidifying devices, aspirin, or acetaminophen, and advise to call if soreness persists more than a day.
   c. "You may have some muscular soreness for a day or two" (soreness, which follows the use of succinylcholine, may be more pronounced than any other discomfort). It is often, but not always, relieved by the medication prescribed for relief of pain at the operative site. Aspirin is recommended for the relief of this soreness, and a warm bath is suggested if not contraindicated by the surgical procedure.
6. Return dentures, valuables, and clothes.

7. The patient is reassured that he or she has behaved properly. The patient should be informed that dreaming often occurs, and an opportunity should be afforded for the patient to discuss any dream that may be remembered.
8. The patient is informed that a follow-up call is routine and is to be expected.

Patients often expect to drive, travel, return to work, and participate in a variety of activities following what they assume to be a short procedure carrying with it very little morbidity. It is important that they be made aware of how they may feel within the first 24 to 48 hours following their procedure. At the Virginia Mason Hospital, guidelines include the following points.[146]

1. The first night after surgery must be within one-hour traveling time from hospital.
2. A responsible adult should accompany the patient home.
3. A staff anesthesiologist should discuss at least the following five Ds prior to discharge.
   a. Do not drive.
   b. Do not drink.
   c. Beware of dizziness.
   d. Don't make critical decisions.
   e. Discuss any questions or problems with us (call or come in).

Hospital staff evaluate the patient's ability to walk prior to discharge, and this, plus the anesthesiologist's interview, forms the basis for their discharge criteria.

Fragen and Shanks use additional discharge criteria for ambulatory surgery patients who have received nondepolarizing muscle relaxants[219] (Table 7-15). The degree of recovery following muscle relaxant use can be assessed clinically, but this requires cooperation by the patient (i.e., head lift, negative inspiratory force, grip strength, and evidence of diplopia). Use of a peripheral nerve stimulator with a T4/T1 greater than 70% usually correlates with a clinical impression of adequate reversal. Patients should be watched closely and treated immediately if residual curarization is suspected.

TABLE 7-15. Discharge Criteria for Patients Who Have Received
Nondepolarizing Muscle Relaxants

---

1. A minimum of 1 half-hour must elapse past full recovery of grip strength.
2. A minimum of 2½ hours must elapse after the end of surgery and anesthesia.
3. Vital signs must be stable.
4. If unusual muscle weakness or adverse effects unrelated to muscle relaxant administration occurs, patients will be kept in the hospital until the adverse reaction is controlled or reversed.
5. The patient must be able to tolerate all fluids, void, and walk without assistance.
6. No other complications must be present.

SOURCE: From Fragen and Shanks.[219] Used with permission.

In addition to achieving a postanesthesia recovery score of 10, our patients must meet other discharge criteria that are incorporated into our phase 2 PACU record (see section on Forms and Policies):

1. Vital signs stable: This includes temperature, pulse, respiration, and blood pressure when appropriate. Vital signs should remain stable (*i.e.*, blood pressure ±20 mmHg) for a period of not less than a half hour and be consistent with patient's age and preanesthesia levels.
2. Ability to swallow and cough: The patient must demonstrate ability to swallow fluids and be able to cough.
3. Ability to walk: The patient demonstrates ability to perform movement consistent with age and development level (sit, stand, walk).
4. Minimal nausea, vomiting, dizziness:
   a. Minimal nausea: Absence of nausea, or if nausea is present, patient can still swallow and retain some fluids.
   b. Minimal vomiting: Vomiting is either absent or, if present, does not require treatment. Following vomiting that requires treatment, patient should be able to swallow and retain fluids.
   c. Minimal dizziness: Dizziness is either absent or present only upon sitting and patient is still able to perform movement consistent with age.
5. Absence of respiratory distress: The patient exhibits no signs of snoring, obstructed respiration, stridor, retractions, or croupy cough.
6. Alert and oriented: The patient is aware of surroundings and what has taken place and is interested in returning home.

Patients have their dressings checked and are walked to the bathroom to void. Patients receiving spinal or epidural anesthesia must void before leaving the facility. Nursing staff reviews the authorization form (see section on Forms and Policies) completed prior to the procedure and the surgeon's postoperative orders (preprinted for specific procedures by our facility on a copy of their office letterhead) with the patient and responsible person. These orders are reviewed annually by the surgeon according to recommendations of the Joint Commission on Accreditation of Healthcare Organizations (JCAHO). Specific discharge instructions are given to patients who have had services of the anesthesia department (see section on Forms and Policies), and additional instructions are included for patients who have had spinal or epidural anesthesia.

Our postspinal patients are instructed to rest in bed for 24 hours. They may be propped up on pillows, sit up to eat, and have bathroom privileges, but we prefer that they wait until the next day before resuming appropriate normal activities. They are instructed to call if they develop a headache not relieved by acetaminophen, a stiff neck, or elevated temperature. Similar instructions are given to epidural patients, but we are more liberal in allowing them to be up and out of bed.

Complete bed rest (flat in bed) for 24 hours to prevent postdural puncture headache (PDPH) was first recommended in 1902 by Sicard and is a ritual still followed without question by many physicians.[220] Jones, in studying the effects of recumbency for 4 to 12 hours following spinal anesthesia with 20- to 25-gauge needles in 1134 hospitalized patients, found that there was not a predictable pattern relating the time spent recumbent to the occurrence of PDPH.[221] As soon as motor function permits, he sees no reason to delay ambulation and feels that this approach would also result in better patient acceptance of spinal anesthesia. Carbaat and van Crevel performed diagnostic lumbar punctures with 18-gauge needles in 50 patients who were kept ambulant and 50 patients who were kept on 24-hour bed rest following the procedure.[222] The average incidence of PDPH (37%) was the same on 7-day follow-up in both groups. Does recumbency have some rationale? Coombs and Porter performed 17 spinal taps—single punctures with 25-gauge needles—at L3–4 on 10 female and 7 male volunteers ages 24 to 35, all members of an anesthesia health care team, for radioimmunoassay studies.[223] All taps were done between 6:30 A.M. and 7:45 A.M., and all volunteers then worked a full day. Classic spinal headaches occurred in 9 of the 17, including the two authors. An epidural blood patch was required in two cases. A point is made for recumbency.

A prospective evaluation of 302 outpatients who received spinal anesthesia reported that the overall incidence of headache (11%) was significantly increased in female compared to male patients.[224] There was no correlation between headache and the number of attempts, needle gauge, experience of anesthesia personnel, or surgical procedure. No headache was reported in any patient over 55 years of age. Six female patients required epidural blood patches. The overall incidence of backache (32%) was not related to position, number of attempts, site of lumbar puncture, or patient age. Although backache was a frequent complaint, only five patients rated theirs as severe. Mulroy and coworkers found no difference in PDPH incidence based on age, sex, or use of Greene or Quincke point needles.[225] Incidence of headache was 5.2% for the outpatient group compared with 1.2% for inpatients. In patients over 50 years of age, the incidence of headache was 3.6% for the outpatients (threefold higher incidence than inpatients). Of the patients over the age of 50, only 1.8% were required to return to the hospital for an epidural blood patch (EBP). The 1.8% incidence of EBP in older patients is equivalent to the 2% rate of unplanned hospitalizations from many facilities following outpatient anesthesia.

Spinal or epidural anesthesia should not be denied the ambulatory surgery patient based only on his or her intention to go home on the day of the procedure. Burke considers spinal anesthesia with a 26-gauge needle for laparoscopy to be safe and satisfactory and to provide excellent relaxation with significant freedom from morbidity and mortality.[226] In his study, pain during the procedure was minimal and limited to transient mild neck or shoulder discomfort. Of 1063 patients, 240 were discharged on the day of surgery. There was an overall headache incidence of 1.3%. When laparoscopy anesthesia is either spinal or epidural, approximately 40% of patients complain during the procedure of mild shoulder or neck discomfort that is readily relieved by intravenous administration of a short-acting narcotic (fentanyl or alfentanil). Explaining this to the patient prior to the procedure will dispel fears that the anesthesia is wearing off, and this mild discomfort will be well tolerated when appropriately treated.

When is it safe to permit patients to ambulate following spinal or epidural anesthesia? The sequence of return of function generally accepted is motor, then sensory, and finally sympathetic. Several studies examining the sequence of return of function have found recovery of sympathetic activity occurring prior to complete regression of the subarachnoid block.[227–229] Pflug and coworkers consider the ability to urinate a final indication of reversal of sympathetic paralysis, since an intact, functioning sympathetic nerve supply to the bladder and urethra is necessary for this function.[228]

In our facility, patients who have received spinal or epidural anesthesia are transferred from our phase 1 recovery (patient on stretcher) to our phase 2 recovery (patient on recliner) after return of sensation and motor strength. As with our other patients, they are gradually brought into an upright seated position prior to ambulation. Suitable criteria for ambulation after spinal anesthesia include normal perianal (S4–5) pinprick sensation, plantar flexion of the foot, and proprioception of the big toe. At the Day Surgery Unit of the Brigham and Women's Hospital, discharge criteria after spinal anesthesia include return of normal sensation, ability to ambulate (return of strength and proprioception), and ability to urinate (return of sympathetic nervous function).* Their patients are encouraged to "take it easy" for the remainder of the operative day, as are their other patients, and to maintain good fluid intake. They are told not to lift heavy objects or strain, but ambulation, activity, and position are not otherwise limited. Patients are encouraged to call the unit if any postoperative problem occurs, such as headache. Discharge after epidural anesthesia is evaluated by the same three criteria. Postspinal ambulatory surgery patients at the Virginia Mason Hospital are instructed to resume normal but quiet activity (no dancing, no weightlifting), and there are no bed rest restrictions.†

Following a major peripheral nerve block, discharge criteria should include return of normal sensation and motion. Variations are acceptable, and each ambulatory surgery facility should establish criteria they consider practical and medically appropriate. Is there a difference if residual, sensory, or motor block involves the upper or lower extremity? What if there is only a patch of numbness after a minor peripheral block? These are the questions that should be asked and answered before patients are discharged. Philip does not think it prudent to discharge a patient with residual sensory or motor block of the lower extremity.* There is the possibility of injury after a fall, which may be due to a patient's overestimation of return of function or to a lack of experience with crutches. However, patients are discharged with residual sensorimotor impairment after an upper extremity major nerve block. Even when appropriate agents are used, the duration of action is sometimes exceptionally long. Patients are discharged

---

*Philip BK: Personal communication, 1984.
†Thompson G: Personal communication, 1984.

with the extremity in a sling. They are reminded that the normal sensation that would protect the extremity against injury is absent and are cautioned particularly not to smoke cigarettes or cook. Patients are given the name and telephone number of an anesthesiologist or the Day Surgery Unit written on their discharge instruction sheet and told to call the next day. Instructions and precautions are documented in the chart. Patients are reassured that nothing has "gone wrong"; a block *does* sometimes persist for a long time, and sensation and motion are expected to return shortly. A patch of numbness after a minor peripheral nerve block often does not warrant a sling but requires similar precautionary instructions against injury and use of fire. At George Washington University In and Out Surgery, patients who have received regional anesthesia must have complete return of sensory and motor function in the affected extremity.* However, criteria for discharge may be modified at the discretion of the anesthesiologist. As each facility attempts to establish its own policies, the question must be asked, "Is the use of crutches to go home considered more acceptable following arthroscopic surgery than following prolonged sensorimotor anesthesia (major block)?" Specific discharge criteria will depend on how this question is answered by the physicians in the individual ambulatory facility.

The ambulatory surgery facility should have a plan that addresses patient discharge to home care:

1. Are patient support systems conducive to home management of postoperative care?
2. Has adequate information been provided for home care of postoperative and postanesthetic sequelae?
3. Has physiological stability been achieved?
4. Is the recovery of cognitive and psychomotor function sufficient to manage postoperative care?

In many settings, assessment of the postoperative home care environment and initiation of discharge instructions begin several days in advance of surgery. A preadmission program allows for identification and resolution of physiological and home care problems.[230] In addition, preoperative and postoperative teaching can be conducted without the immediate stress of impending surgery.

Criteria used for discharging inpatients from the PACU cannot be applied to ambulatory surgery patients. Kitz and coworkers designed a study to identify the factors nurses consider in evaluating ambulatory surgery patients for discharge from the PACU to home care.[231] Significant agreement was found among the ambulatory surgery unit nurses surveyed with regard to the particular factors and their relative importance in evaluating ambulatory surgery patients for discharge to home (Table 7-16). While the first three items parallel factors evaluated in the APARS, the remaining items, including ability to ambulate, clarity of vision, and level of rehydration, are unique to an ambulatory surgery patient.

*Levy M-L: Personal communication, 1984.

TABLE 7-16. Rank-Ordered List of Factors Considered for Discharge

Rank	Item
1	Adequacy of respiratory function
2	Stability of vital signs
3	Level of orientation
4	Swelling/drainage of operative site
5	Degree of pain
6	Temperature
7	Degree of vomiting
8	Level of alertness
9	Level of rehydration
10	Skin color
11	Ability to ambulate
12	Clarity of vision
13	Ability to void
14	Degree of nausea

SOURCE: Kitz DS et al.[231] Used with permission.

Because more extensive procedures requiring longer duration of anesthesia are currently being performed and will continue to be performed as ambulatory surgery, assessment of recovery from anesthesia takes on increasing significance. Not only must we know how to anesthetize patients to provide rapid recovery with as little postanesthetic cognitive and psychomotor impairment as possible, we also must be able to judge clinically when these patients can be sent home. Our goal is to assess home readiness rather than street fitness.

Nursing staff should assess the adult who will take the patient home to determine whether the individual is in fact a responsible person. We have had "responsible" persons who appeared intoxicated. We did not question the ability of these persons to take care of the patient at home, but we made certain that another adult was present to drive the patient home and stay with him or her during the early recovery period. The term *responsible* is defined in Chapter 2 of this book as someone physically and intellectually capable of taking care of the patient at home. There is an additional precaution ambulatory surgery facilities might consider: Have both the patient and responsible person sign the medical record signifying that they have both understood and received verbal and written discharge instructions.

At our facility, additional considerations are as follows:

1. Patients whose anesthetic management has included endotracheal intubation remain for a minimum of 1½ hours following extubation.
2. Patients receiving depressant medication for relief of pain, nausea, or vomiting must be observed for a minimum of 1 hour.

Patients are told that they will receive a telephone call the next day from one of our postanesthesia care nurses to find out how they are recovering from their surgery and anesthesia. Some facilities give patients a follow-up postcard with instructions to fill in comments on recovery and return it within one or two weeks. Patients appreciate the facility that cares enough to follow up.

Patients should never leave with the impression that they are being rushed out of the facility. This is avoided by having postanesthesia room personnel who are sympathetic, understanding, and compassionate, as well as *upbeat* in caring for the patient. In the words of Francis Weld Peabody, "The secret of the care of the patient is in caring for the patient."[232]

The anesthesiologist plays a major role in the compacted perioperative care provided to the ambulatory surgery patient. Managing common postanesthesia care unit problems quickly and effectively is equal in importance to appropriate patient selection and choice of anesthesia technique if patients are to return home on the same day that surgery is performed.

REFERENCES

1. Levy ML, Coakley CS: Organization and experience with outpatient anesthesia in a large university hospital. Int Anesthesiol Clin 14(2): 131, 1976
2. Brody DC: Criteria for patient care. Curr Rev Recov Room Nurses 19: 155, 1983
3. Apgar V: A proposal for a new method of evaluation of the newborn infant. Anesth Analg 32: 260, 1953
4. Carignan G, Kerri-Szanto M, Lavelle JP: Post-anesthetic scoring system. Anesthesiology 25: 396, 1964
5. Aldrete JA, Kroulik D: A postanesthetic recovery score. Anesth Analg 49(6): 924, 1970
6. Figueroa M: The post-anesthesia recovery score: A second look. South Med J 65: 791, 1972
7. Steward DJ: A simplified scoring system for the post operative recovery room. Can Anaesth Soc J 22(1): 111, 1975
8. Robertson GS, MacGregor DM, Jones CJ: Evaluation of doxapram for arousal from general anaesthesia in outpatients. Br J Anaesth 49: 133, 1977
9. Staertow C: Recliners are advantageous in the recovery. Same Day Surg 7(11): 141, 1983
10. Patterson JF, Bechtoldt AA, Levin KJ: Ambulatory surgery in a university setting. JAMA 235(3): 266, 1976
11. Dawson B, Reed WA: Anaesthesia for day-care surgery: A symposium: III. Anaesthesia for adult surgical outpatients. Can Anaesth Soc J 27(4): 409, 1980.
12. Meridy HW: Criteria for selection of ambulatory surgical patients and guidelines for anesthetic management: A retrospective study of 1553 cases. Anesth Analg 61(1): 921, 1982
13. Dhamee MS, Gandhi SK, Kalbfleisch JH, et al: Morbidity after outpatient anesthesia: A comparison of different endotracheal anesthetic techniques for laparoscopy. Anesthesiology 57(3): A375, 1982
14. Doctor NH, Hussain Z: Bilateral pneumothorax associated with laparoscopy. Anaesthesia 28: 75, 1973
15. Soderstrom RM, Butler JC: A critical evaluation of complications in laparoscopy. J Reprod Med 10: 245, 1973
16. Fahy A, Marshall M: Post-anaesthetic morbidity in outpatients. Br J Anaesth 41: 433, 1969
17. Anderson S, McGuire R, McKeown D: Comparison of the cognitive effects of premedication with hyoscine and atropine. Br J Anaesth 57: 169, 1985
18. Clark AJM, Hurtig JB: Premedication with meperidine and atropine does not prolong recovery to street fitness after outpatient surgery. Can Anaesth Soc J 28: 390, 1982

19. Coakley CS, Levy ML: Anesthesia for ambulatory surgery. J Ark Med Soc 68: 101, 1971
20. Levy ML, Coakley CS: Survey of in and out surgery, first year. South Med J 61: 995, 1968
21. Ahlgren EW, Bennett EJ, Stephen CR: Outpatient pediatric anesthesiology: A case series. Anesth Analg 50(3): 402, 1971
22. Nagel EL, Forster RK, Jones D, et al: Outpatient anesthesia for pediatric ophthalmology. Anesth Analg 52: 558, 1973
23. Larson GF, Hurlbert BJ, Wingard D: Physostigmine reversal of diazepam-induced depression. Anesth Analg 56(3): 348, 1977
24. Mackenzie JW, Bird J: Timolol: A non-sedative anxiolytic premedicant for day cases. Br Med J 298: 363, 1989
25. Aldrete JA: Are intramuscular injections obsolete in the recovery room? Curr Rev Recov Room Nurses 5(18): 147, 1983
26. White PF: Pain management after day-case surgery. Curr Opin Anaesthesiol 1: 70, 1988
27. Feeley TW: The recovery room. In Miller RD (ed): Anesthesia, 2d ed, pp 1921–1945. New York, Churchill-Livingstone, 1986
28. Epstein BS, Levy ML, Thein MH, et al: Evaluation of fentanyl as an adjunct to thiopental–nitrous oxide–oxygen anesthesia for short surgical procedures. Anesthesiol Rev 2(3): 24, 1975
29. Hunt TM, Plantevin OM, Gilbert JR: Morbidity in gynaecological day-case surgery: A comparison of two anaesthetic techniques. Br J Anaesth 51: 785, 1979
30. Soni V, Burney R: Anesthetic techniques for laparoscopic tubal ligation. Anesthesiology 55(3): A145, 1981
31. Sanders RS, Sinclair ME, Sear JW: Alfentanil in short procedures. Anaesthesia 39: 1202, 1984
32. Jellico EJA: A comparison of alfentanil, halothane and enflurane for day-case gynaecological surgery. Anaesthesia 40: 810, 1985
33. Short SM, Ruthefoord CF, Cebel PS: A comparison between isoflurane and alfentanil supplemented anaesthesia for short procedures. Anaesthesia 40: 1160, 1985
34. White PF, Chang T: Effect of narcotic premedication on the intravenous anesthetic requirement. Anesthesiology 61: A389, 1984
35. Shandling B, Steward D: Regional analgesia for postoperative pain in pediatric outpatient surgery. J Pediatr Surg 15(4): 477, 1980
36. Steward DJ: Experiences with an outpatient anesthesia service for children. Anesth Analg 52: 877, 1973
37. Steward DJ: Postoperative pain relief in children. Curr Rev Clin Anesth 5: 179, 1985
38. Hinkle AJ: Percutaneous inguinal block for the outpatient management of post-herniorrhaphy pain in children. Anesthesiology 67: 411, 1987
39. Cross GD, Barrett RF: Comparison of two regional techniques for postoperative analgesia in children following herniotomy and orchidopexy. Anaesthesia 42: 845, 1987
40. Epstein RH, Larijani GE, Wolfson PJ, et al: Plasma bupivacaine concentrations following ilioinguinal-iliohypogastric nerve blockade in children. Anesthesiology 69: 773, 1988
41. Khiroya RC, Davenport HT, Jones JG: Cryoanalgesia for pain after herniorrhaphy. Anaesthesia 41: 73, 1986
42. Sinclair R, Cassuto J, Hogstrom S, et al: Topical anesthesia with lidocaine aerosol in the control of postoperative pain. Anesthesiology 68: 895, 1988
43. Casey W, Rice L, Hannallah RS, et al: A comparison between bupivacaine instillation versus ilioinguinal/iliohypogastric nerve block for postoperative analgesia following inguinal herniorrhaphy in children. Anesthesiology 72: 637, 1990
44. Baggish MS, Lee WK, Miro SJ, et al: Complications of laparoscopic sterilization: Comparison of two methods. Obstet Gynecol 54: 54, 1979
45. Dobbs FF, Kuman V, Alexander JI, et al: Pain after laparoscopy related to posture and ring versus clip sterilization. Br J Obstet Gynaecol 94: 262, 1987
46. Chi IC, Cole LP: Incidence of pain among women undergoing laparoscopic sterilization by electrocoagulation, the spring-loaded clip, and the tubal ring. Am J Obstet Gynecol 133: 397, 1979
47. Thompson RE, Wetchler BV, Alexander CD: Infiltration of the mesosalpinx for pain relief after laparoscopic tubal sterilization with Yoon rings. J Reprod Med 32: 537, 1987

48. Alexander CD, Wetchler BV, Thompson RE: Bupicavaine infiltration of the mesosalpinx in ambulatory surgical laparoscopic tubal sterilization. Can Anaesth J 34: 362, 1987

49. Cook PT, Lambert TF: An investigation of the effectiveness of bupivacaine applied to the abdominal wall and fallopian tubes in reducing pain after laparoscopic tubal ligation. Anaesth Intensive Care 14: 148, 1986

50. McGlinchey J, McLean P, Walsh A: Day case penile surgery with penile block for postoperative pain relief. Ir Med J 76(7): 319, 1983

51. Tree-trakarn T, Pirayavaraporn S: Postoperative pain relief for circumcision in children: Comparison among morphine, nerve block, and topical analgesia. Anesthesiology 62: 519, 1985

52. Tree-trakarn T, Pirayavaraporn S, Lertakyamanee J: Topical analgesia for relief of post-circumcision pain. Anesthesiology 67: 395, 1987

53. Elder PT, Belman AB, Hannallah RS, et al: Postcircumcision pain: A prospective evaluation of subcutaneous ring block of the penis. Reg Anesth 9: 48, 1984

54. Hannallah RS, Broadman LM, Belman AB, et al: Control of post-orchidopexy pain in pediatric outpatients: Comparison of two regional techniques. Anesthesiology 61: A429, 1984

55. Takasaki M, Dohi S, Kawahata Y, et al: Dosage of lidocaine for caudal anesthesia in infants and children. Anesthesiology 47: 527, 1977

56. Broadman LM, Hannallah RS, Norrie WC, et al: Caudal analgesia in pediatric outpatient surgery: A comparison of three different bupivacaine concentrations. Anesth Analg 66: S19, 1987

57. Wolf AR, Valley RD, Fear DW, et al: Bupivacaine for caudal analgesia in infants and children: The optimum concentration. Anesthesiology 69: 102, 1988

58. Knos GB, Sung YF, Powell RW: Effect of local marcaine infiltration on postoperative pain and morbidity in ambulatory surgery. Anesth Analg 68: S149, 1989

59. Broadman LM, Patel RI, Feldman BA: Peritonsillar infiltration with bupivacaine hydrochloride 0.25% and epinephrine 1:200,000 prior to tonsillectomy in children. Anesthesiology 63: A347, 1985

60. Milligan KA, Mowbray MJ, Mulrooney L, et al: Intraarticular bupivacaine for pain relief after arthroscopic surgery of the knee joint in daycase patients. Anaesthesia 43: 563, 1988

61. Katz JA, Kaeding CS, Hill JR, et al: The pharmacokinetics of bupivacaine when injected intraarticularly after knee arthroscopy. Anesth Analg 67: 872, 1988

62. Wetchler BV, Alexander CD, Davis A, et al: Transnasal butorphanol for pain control following ambulatory surgical procedures: A pilot study (abstr). In proceedings of the Annual Meeting of the Society for Ambulatory Anesthesia, Scottsdale, Arizona, 1988

63. Lindblad T, Beattie WS, Buckley DN, et al: Increased incidence of postoperative nausea and vomiting in menstruating women. Can J Anaesth 36: S78, 1989

64. Jensen S, Wetchler BV: The obese patient: An acceptable candidate for outpatient anesthesia. J Am Assoc Nurse Anesthetists 50: 369, 1982

65. Anderson R, Crohg K: Pain as a major cause of postoperative nausea. Can Anaesth Soc J 23(4): 366, 1976

66. Craig J, Cooper GM, Sear JW: Recovery from day-case anaesthesia: Comparison between methohexitone, althesin and etomidate. Br J Anaesth 54: 447, 1982

67. Cohen SE, Woods WA, Wyner J: Antiemetic efficacy of droperidol and metoclopramide. Anesthesiology 60: 67, 1984

68. Doze VA, Shafer A, White PF: Nausea and vomiting after outpatient anesthesia: Effectiveness of droperidol alone and in combination with metoclopramide. Anesth Analg 66: S41, 1987

69. Rao TLK, Madhavareddy S, Chinthagada M, et al: Metoclopramide and cimetidine to reduce gastric fluid pH and volume. Anesth Analg 63: 1014, 1984

70. Williams JJ, Goldberg ME, Boerner TF, et al: A comparison of three methods to reduce nausea and vomiting after alfentanil anesthesia in outpatients. Anesth Analg 68: S311, 1989

71. Jorgensen NH, Coyle JP: Effect of intravenous droperidol upon nausea and vomiting using alfentanil anesthesia. Anesth Analg 68: S139, 1989

72. McCarroll SM, Mori S, Bras PJ, et al: The effect of gastric intubation and removal of gastric contents on the incidence of postoperative nausea and vomiting. Anesth Analg 70: S262, 1990

73. Kraynack BJ, Bates MF, Gintautas J: Antiemetic efficacy of ranitidine, metoclopramide and gastric suctioning in outpatient laparoscopy. Anesth Analg 70: S218, 1990

74. Madej TH, Simpson KH: Comparison of the use of domperidone, droperidol and metoclopramide in the prevention of nausea and vomiting following gynaecological surgery in day cases. Br J Anaesth 58: 879, 1986

75. Shelley ES, Brown HA: Antiemetic effect of ultralow-dose droperidol. Presented at the Annual Meeting of the American Society of Anesthesiologists, Chicago, 1978

76. Wetchler BV, Collins IS, Jacob L: Antiemetic effects of droperidol on the ambulatory surgery patient. Anesthsiol Rev 9: 23, 1982

77. Valanne J, Korttila K: Effect of a small dose of droperidol on nausea, vomiting and recovery after outpatient enflurane anaesthesia. Acta Anaesthesiol Scand 29: 359, 1985

78. Pandit SK, Kothary SP, Pandit UA, et al: Dose-response study of droperidol and metoclopramide as antiemetics for outpatient anesthesia. Anesth Analg 68: 798, 1989

79. Poler SM, White PF, Margrabe D, et al: Nausea and vomiting in outpatients: Use of droperidol prophylaxis. Anesthesiology 71: A134, 1989

80. Bidwai AV, Meuleman T, Thatte WP: Prevention of postoperative nausea with dimenhydrinate (Dramamine) and droperidol (Inapsine). Anesth Analg 68: S25, 1989

81. Melnick BM: Extrapyramidal reactions to low-dose droperidol. Anesthesiology 69: 424, 1988

82. Caldwell C, Rains G, McKiterick K: An unusual reaction to preoperative metoclopramide. Anesthesiology 67: 854, 1987

83. Alexander GD, Skupski JN, Brown EM: The role of nitrous oxide in postoperative nausea and vomiting. Anesth Analg 63: A175, 1984

84. Lonie DS, Harper NJN: Nitrous oxide anaesthesia and vomiting. Anaesthesia 41: 703, 1986

85. Sengupta P, Plantevin OM: Nitrous oxide and day-case laparoscopy: Effects on nausea, vomiting and return to normal activity. Br J Anaesth 60: 570, 1988

86. Hovorka J, Korttila K, Erkola O: Nitrous oxide does not increase nausea and vomiting following gynaecological laparoscopy. Can J Anaesth 36: 145, 1989

87. Perreault L, Normandin N, Planadon L, et al: Middle ear pressure variations during nitrous oxide and oxygen anaesthesia. Can Anaesth Soc J 29: 428, 1982

88. Montgomery CJ, Vaghadia H, Blackstock D: Negative middle ear pressure and postoperative vomiting in pediatric outpatients. Anesthesiology 68: 288, 1988

89. Mulroy MF: Regional anesthesia: When, why, why not? In Wetchler BV (ed): Outpatient Anesthesia, Vol 2, pp 82–92. Philadelphia, JB Lippincott, 1989

90. Bridenbaugh LD, Soderstrom RM: Lumbar epidural block anesthesia for outpatient laparoscopy. J Reprod Med 23: 85, 1979

91. Shaw JE: Transdermal drug delivery: Potentials and limitations. In Lemberger L, Reidenberg MM (eds): Proceedings of the Second World Conference on Clinical Pharmacology and Therapeutics. Bethesda, Md, 1983

92. Aronson JK, Sear JW: Transdermal hyoscine (scopolamine) and postoperative vomiting (editorial). Anaesthesia 41: 1, 1986

93. Uppington J, Dunnet J, Blogg CE: Transdermal hyoscine and postoperative nausea and vomiting. Anaesthesia 41: 16, 1986

94. Tigerstedt I, Salmela L, Aromaa U: Double-blind comparison of transdermal scopolamine, droperidol and placebo against postoperative nausea and vomiting. Acta Anaesthesiol Scand 32: 454, 1988

95. Bailey PL, Bubbers SJM, East KA, et al: Transdermal scopolamine reduces postoperative nausea and vomiting. Anesthesiology 69: A641, 1988

96. Gibbons PA, Nicholson SC, Betts EK, et al: Scopolamine does not prevent post-operative emesis after pediatric eye surgery. Anesthesiology 61: A435, 1984

97. Dundee JW, Chestnutt WN, Ghaly RG, et al: Traditional Chinese acupuncture: A potentially useful antiemetic? Br Med J 293: 583, 1986

98. Ghaly RG, Fitzpatrick KTJ, Dundee JW: Antiemetic studies with traditional Chinese acupuncture. Anaesthesia 42: 1108, 1987

99. Dundee JW, Ghaly RG, McKinney MS: P6 acupuncture antiemesis comparison of invasive and noninvasive techniques. Anesthesiology 71: A130, 1989

100. Blackstock D, DaSilva CA, Demars PD, et al: Intravenous fluid administration does not reduce nausea and vomiting in children. Can J Anaesth 36: S126, 1989

101. Keane PW, Murray PF: Intravenous fluids in minor surgery: Their effect on recovery from anaesthesia. Anaesthesia 41: 635, 1986
102. King MJ, Milazkiewicz R, Carli F, et al: Influence of neostigmine on postoperative vomiting. Br J Anaesth 61: 403, 1988
103. Rowley MP, Brown TCK: Postoperative vomiting in children. Anaesth Intensive Care 10: 309, 1982
104. Abramowitz MD, Oh TH, Epstein BS, et al: The antiemetic effect of droperidol following outpatient strabismus surgery in children. Anesthesiology 59: 579, 1983
105. Abramowitz MD, Epstein BS, Friendly DS, et al: The effect of droperidol in reducing vomiting in pediatric strabismus outpatient surgery. Anesthesiology 55: A329, 1981
106. Lerman J, Eustis S, Smith DR: Effect of droperidol pretreatment on postanesthetic vomiting in children undergoing strabismus surgery. Anesthesiology 65: 322, 1986
107. Hardy JF, Charest J, Girouard G, et al: Nausea and vomiting after strabismus surgery in preschool children. Can Anaesth Soc J 33: 57, 1986
108. Caldamone AA, Rabinowitz R: Outpatient orchiopexy. J Urol 127: 286, 1982
109. Eustis S, Lerman J, Smith D: Droperidol pretreatment in children undergoing strabismus repair: The minimal effective dose. Can Anaesth Soc J 33: S115, 1986
110. Brown RE, James DJ, Weaver RG, et al: Low-dose droperidol vs. standard-dose droperidol for prevention of vomiting after pediatric strabismus surgery. Anesth Analg 70: S37, 1990
111. Pataky AO, Kitz DS, Andrews RS, et al: Nausea and vomiting following ambulatory surgery: Are all procedures created equal? Anesth Analg 67: S163, 1988
112. Metter SE, Kitz DS, Young ML, et al: Nausea and vomiting after outpatient laparoscopy: Incidence, impact on recovery room stay and cost. Anesth Analg 66: S116, 1987
113. Rothenberg D, Parnass S, Newman L, et al: Ephedrine minimizes postoperative nausea and vomiting in outpatinets. Anesthesiology 71: A322, 1989
114. Poler SM, White PF: Does ephedrine decreased nausea and vomiting after outpatient anesthesia? Anesthesiology 71: A995, 1989
115. Goddard JE, Phillips OC, Marcy JH: Betamethasone for proplylaxis of postintubation inflammation: A double blind study. Anesth Analg 16: 348, 1967
116. Jordan WS, Graves CL, Elwin RA: New therapy for postintubation laryngeal edema and tracheitis in children. JAMA 212: 585, 1970
117. Koka BV, Jeon IS, Andre JM, et al: Postintubation croup in children. Anesth Analg 56(4): 501, 1977
118. Pender JW: Endotracheal anesthesia in children: Advantages and disadvantages. Anesthesiology 15: 495, 1954
119. Eckenhoff JE: Some anatomic considerations of infant larynx influencing endotracheal anesthesia. Anesthesiology 12: 405, 1951
120. Baraka A: Intravenous lidocaine controls extubation laryngospasm in children. Anesth Analg 57: 506, 1978
121. Phillalamarri ED, Tadoori PR, Abadir AR: Prophylactic effect of dexamethasone and/or lidocaine on post extubation croup in children. Anesthesiology 57(3): A429, 1982
122. Deming MC, Oech SR: Steroid and antihistamine therapy for post-intubation subglottic edema in infants and children. Anesthesiology 22: 933, 1961
123. Longo VG: Behavioral and electroencephalographic effects of atropine and related compounds. Pharmacol Rev 18: 965, 1966
124. Blitt CD, Petty WC: Reversal of lorazepam delirium by physostigmine. Anesth Analg 54(5): 607, 1975
125. Rosenberg H: Physostigmine reversal of sedative drugs (letter). JAMA 229: 1168, 1974
126. Spaulding BC, Choi SD, Gross JB, et al: The effect of physostigmine on diazepam-induced ventilatory depression: A double-blind study. Anesthesiology 61: 551, 1984
127. Garber JG, Ominsky AJ, Orkin FK, et al: Physostigmine-atropine solution fails to reverse diazepam sedation. Anesth Analg 59: 58, 1980
128. Toro-Matos A, Rendon-Platas AM, Avil-Valez E, et al: Physostigmine antagonizes ketamine. Anesth Analg 59: 7644, 1980
129. Hannallah RS, Abramowitz MD, McGill WA, et al: Physostigmine does not speed recovery

following rectal methohexital induction in pediatric outpatients. Anesthesiology 57(3): A412, 1982

130. Wolff J, Carl P, Clausen TG, et al: RO15-1788 for postoperative recovery: A randomized clinical trial in patients undergoing minor surgical procedures under midazolam anaesthesia. Anaesthesia 41: 1001, 1986

131. Jensen S, Knudsen L, Kirkegaard L, et al: Flumazenil used for antagonizing the central effects of midazolam and diazepam in outpatients. Acta Anaesthesiol Scand 33: 26, 1989

132. Leslie JB, Kalayjian RW, Sirgo MA, et al: Intravenous labetalol for treatment of postoperative hypertension. Anesthesiology 67: 413, 1987

133. Adler AG, Leahy JJ, Cressman MD: Management of perioperative hypertension using sublingual nifedipine: Experience in elderly patients undergoing eye surgery. Arch Intern Med 146: 1927, 1986

134. Schiller EC: An easy way to administer sublingual nifedipine. Anesthesiology 65: 239, 1986

135. Sodeyama O, Ikeda K, Matsuda I, et al: Nifedipine for control of postoperative hypertension. Anesthesiology 59(3): A18, 1983

136. Estafanous FG: Postoperative hypertension: Incidence and management. Curr Rev Recov Room Nurses 5: 11, 1983

137. White PF, Coe V, Dworsky WA, et al: Disseminated intravascular coagulation following midtrimester abortions. Anesthesiology 58: 99, 1983

138. Laros RK, Collins J, Penner JA, et al: Coagulation changes in saline-induced abortion. Am J Obstet Gynecol 116: 277, 1973

139. Bick RL: Disseminated intravascular coagulation. Hosp Physician 24: 34, 1986

140. Spencer EM: Intravenous fluids in minor gynaecological surgery: Their effect on postoperative morbidity. Anaesthesia 43: 1050, 1988

141. Gupta PK, Dundee JW: Post-operative pain relief with morphine combined with doxapram and naloxone. Anaesthesia 29: 33, 1974

142. Allen CJ, Gough KR: Effect of doxapram on heavy sedation produced by intravenous diazepam. Br Med J 286: 1181, 1983

143. Stephen CR, Talton I: Investigation of doxapram as a post-anesthetic respiratory stimulant. Anesth Analg 43: 628, 1964

144. Kim SI, Winnie AP, Carey JS, et al: Use of doxapram in the critically ill patient: Does increased oxygen consumption reflect an oxygen dividend or an oxygen debt? Crit Care Med 1: 252, 1973

145. Janis KM: Outpatient anesthesia in geriatric setting. Int Anesthesiol Clin 20: 87, 1982

146. Thompson CE, Remington JM, Millman BS, et al: Experiences with outpatient anesthesia. Anesth Analg 52(6): 881, 1973

147. Kataria BK, Harnik EV, Mitchard R, et al: Postoperative arterial oxygen saturation in the pediatric population during transportation. Anesth Analg 67: 280, 1988

148. Pullerits J, Burrows FA, Roy WL: Arterial desaturation in healthy children during transfer to the recovery room. Can J Anaesth 34: 470, 1987

149. Chripko D, Bevan JC, Archer DP, et al: Decreases in arterial oxygen saturation in paediatric outpatients during transfer to the postanaesthetic recovery room. Can J Anaesth 36: 128, 1989

150. Soliman IE, Patel RI, Ehrenpreis MB, et al: Recovery scores do not correlate with postoperative hypoxemia in children. Anesth Analg 67: 53, 1988

151. Smith DC, Canning JJ, Crul JF: Pulse oximetry in the recovery room. Anaesthesia 44: 345, 1989

152. Voss S, Rockoff M, Brustowicz, et al: Oxygen saturation in children following administration of rectal methohexital. Anesth Analg 67: S247, 1988

153. Brown MD, Kallar SK: Hypoxemia in children following general anesthesia in the ambulatory surgery center. Anesthesiology 63: A460, 1985

154. Bissonnette B, Scott AA: Arterial oxygen saturation in adults during transport from the operating room to the recovery room. Can J Anaesth 34: S86, 1987

155. Vegfors M, Cederholm I, Lennmarken C, et al: Should oxygen be administered after laparoscopy in healthy patients? Acta Anaesthesiol Scand 32: 350, 1988

156. Buschman A, Morris R, Warren D, et al: Pulse oximetry and the incidence of hypoxemia during recovery from anesthesia. Anesthesiology 67: A481, 1987

157. Reed WA: Recovery from anesthesia and discharge. In Shultz R (ed): Outpatient Surgery, p 45. Philadelphia, Lea & Febiger, 1979

158. While PF: Use of continuous infusion versus intermittent bolus administration of fentanyl or ketamine during outpatient anesthesia. Anesthesiology 59: 294, 1983

159. Azar I, Karambelkar DJ, Lear E: Neurological state and psychomotor function following anesthesia for ambulatory surgery. Anesthesiology 60(4): 347, 1984

160. Carter JA, Dye AM, Cooper GM: Recovery after day-case anaesthesia: The effect of different inhalational anaesthetic agents. Anaesthesia 40: 545, 1985

161. Dhamee MS, Gandhi SK, Munshi CA, et al: Anesthetic techniques for laparoscopy: Morbidity after outpatient anesthesia. Anesthesiol Rev 13: 15, 1986

162. Lecky JH, Kitz DS, Andrews RW, et al: Fentanyl vs. isoflurane in outpatient diagnostic laparoscopy: An evaluation of perioperative morbidity and cost. Anesthesiology 67: A433, 1987

163. Rising S, Dodgson MS, Steen PA: Isoflurane vs. fentanyl for outpatient laparoscopy. Acta Anaesthesiol Scand 29: 251, 1985

164. Melnick BM, Chalasani J, Hy NTL: Comparison of enflurane, isoflurane and continuous fentanyl infusion for outpatient anesthesia. Anesthesiol Rev 11: 36, 1984

165. Zuurmond WWA, van Leeuwen L: Recovery from sufentanil anaesthesia for outpatient arthroscopy: A comparison with isoflurane. Acta Anaesthesiol Scand 31: 154, 1987

166. Gaskey NJ, Ferriero L, Pournaras L, et al: Use of fentanyl markedly increases nausea and vomiting in gynecological short stay patients. AANAJ 54: 309, 1986

167. Horne JA, Ahlgren EW: Halothane and isoflurane for outpatient surgery: A pediatric case series. In Abstracts of the American Society of Anesthesiologists Meeting, p 269. 1973

168. Steward DJ: A trial of enflurane for paediatric outpatient anaesthesia. Can Anaesth Soc J 24(5): 603, 1977

169. Hoyal RHA, Prys-Roberts C, Simpson PJ: Enflurane in outpatient paediatric dental anaesthesia. Br J Anaesth 52: 219, 1980

170. Padfield A, Mullins SRC: Recovery comparison between enflurane and halothane techniques: A study of outpatients undergoing cystocopy. Anaesthesia 35: 508, 1980

171. Korttila K, Valanne J: Recovery after outpatient isoflurane and enflurane anaesthesia. Anesth Analg 64: 185, 1985

172. Korttila K, Tammisto T, Ertama P, et al: Recovery, psychomotor skills and simulated driving after brief inhalational anesthesia with halothane or enflurane combined with nitrous oxide and oxygen. Anesthesiology 46: 20, 1977

173. Dundee JW: Ultrashort-acting barbiturates for outpatients. Acta Anaesthiol Scand [Suppl] 17: 17, 1965

174. Forbes RB, Murray DJ, Dillman JB, et al: Postoperative recovery following induction of anaesthesia with rectal methohexitone. Can J Anaesth 36: S109, 1989

175. Fragen RJ, Caldwell N: Comparison of a new formulation of etomidate with thiopental: Side effects and awakening times. Anesthesiology 50: 242, 1979

176. Horrigan RW, Moyers JR, Johnson BH, et al: Etomidate vs. thiopental with and without fentanyl: A comparative study of awakening in man. Anesthesiology 52: 362, 1980

177. Millar JM, Jewkes CF: Recovery and morbidity after daycase anaesthesia: A comparison of propofol with thiopentone-enflurane with and without alfentanil. Anaesthesia 43: 738, 1988

178. McDonald NJ, Mannion D, Lee P, et al: Mood evaluation and outpatient anaesthesia: A comparison between propofol and thiopentone. Anaesthesia 43: 73, 1988

179. Sanderson JH, Blades JF: Multicentre study of propofol in day case surgery. Anaesthesia 43: 70, 1988

180. Cork RC, Scipione P, Vonesh MJ, et al: Propofol infusion vs. thiopental/isoflurane for outpatient anesthesia. Anesthesiology 69: A563, 1988

181. Pandit SK, Kothary SP, Randel GI, et al: Recovery after outpatient anesthesia: Propofol versus enflurane. Anesthesiology 69: A565, 1988

182. Conahan TJ, Williams GD, Apfelbaum JL, et al: Airway heating reduces recovery time (cost) in outpatients. Anesthesiology 63: A166, 1985

183. Conahan TJ, Kitz DS, Andrews RW, et al: Airway heating does not affect recovery time or postoperative complaints in outpatients. Anesthesiology 69: A278, 1988

184. Goldberg ME, Jan R, Gregg CE, et al: The heat and moisture exchanger does not preserve body temperature or reduce recovery time in outpatients undergoing surgery and anesthesia. Anesthesiology 68: 122, 1988

185. Hines RL, Barash PG, Dubow H, et al: Ambulatory surgical complication in the postoperative period: We can't just walk away. Anesth Analg 68: S122, 1989

186. Berry FA: Pediatric outpatient anesthesia. In ASA Ed: S. G. Hershey Refresher Courses in Anesthesiology, Vol 10, p 17. Philadelphia, JB Lippincott, 1982

187. Steward DJ, Volgyesi G: Stabilometry: A new tool for the measurement of recovery following general anaesthesia for outpatients. Can Anaesth Soc J 25(1): 4, 1978

188. Korttila K: Recovery and driving after brief anaesthesia. Anaesthetists 30: 377, 1989

189. Korttila K: Recovery after intravenous sedation: A comparison of clinical and paper and pencil tests used in assessing later effects of diazepam. Anaesthesia 31: 724, 1976

190. Cohen RL, MacKenzie AI: Anaesthesia and cognitive functioning. Anaesthesia 37: 47, 1982

191. Doenicke A, Gurtner T, Kugler J, et al: Experimentelle untersuchungen uber das ultrakurz-narkotikum propanidid mit serumcholinesterase-bestimmungen, EEG, psychodiagnostischen tests und kreislaufanalysen. In Horatzk K, Frey R, Kindler M (eds): Anaesthesiology and Resuscitation, 4th ed. Berlin, Springer-Verlag, 1965

192. Doenicke A, Kugler J, Schellenberger A, et al: The use of electroencephalography to measure recovery time after intravenous anaesthesia. Br J Anaesth 38: 580, 1966

193. Korttila K, Ghoneim MM, Jacobs L, et al: Time course of mental and psychomotor effects of 30 percent nitrous oxide during inhalation and recovery. Anesthesiology 54: 220, 1981

194. Korttila K: How to assess recovery from outpatient anesthesia. In Barash PG (ed): ASA Refresher Courses in Anesthesiology, Vol 16, pp 133–144. Philadelphia, JB Lippincott, 1988

195. Cooper G: Recovery from anaesthesia. Anaesth Rounds. 19: 1, 1986

196. Clyburn P, Kay NH, McKenzie PJ: Effects of diazepam and midazolam on recovery from anaesthesia in outpatients. Br J Anaesth 58: 872, 1986

197. White PF, Coe V, Shafer A, et al: Comparison of alfentanil with fentanyl for outpatient anesthesia. Anesthesiology 64: 99, 1986

198. Hargreaves J: Benzodiazepine premedication in minor day-case surgery: Comparison of oral midazolam and temazepam with placebo. Br J Anaesth 61: 611, 1988

199. Mackenzie N, Grant IS: Comparison of the new emulation formulation of propofol with methohexitone and thiopentone for induction of anaesthesia in day cases. Br J Anaesth 57: 725, 1985

200. Korttila K, Nuotto E, Lichtor L: Recovery and psychomotor effects after brief anesthesia with propofol and thiopental. Anesth Analg 68: S151, 1989

201. Milligan KR, O'Toole DP, Howe JP, et al: Recovery from outpatient anaesthesia: A comparison of incremental propofol and propofol-isoflurane. Br J Anaesth 59: 1111, 1987

202. Vielle G, Gardaz JP, Jermond M, et al: Outpatient anesthesia with propofol: A comparative evaluation on recovery and psychomotor performance. Anesthesiology 69: A566, 1988

203. Pandit SK, Kothary SP, Randel GI: Recovery after outpatient anesthesia: Propofol versus enflurane. Anesthesiology 69: A565, 1988

204. Negus JB, White PF: Use of sedative infusions during local and regional anesthesia: A comparison of midazolam and propofol. Anesthesiology 69: A711, 1988

205. Jansen EC, Wachowiak-Andersen G, Munster-Swendsen J, et al: Postural stability after oral premedication with diazepam. Anesthesiology 63: 557, 1985

206. Korttila K: Minor outpatient anaesthesia and driving. Mod Probl Pharmacopsychiatry 11: 91, 1976

207. Green R, Long HA, Elliot CJR, et al: A method of studying recovery after anaesthesia. Anaesthesia 8: 189, 1963

208. Korttila K, Linnoila M, Ertama P, et al: Recovery and simulated driving after intravenous anesthesia with thiopental, methohexital, propanidid or alphadione. Anesthesiology 43: 291, 1975

209. Harvard JA: Medical Aspects of Fitness to Drive. London, Medical Commission on Accident Prevention, 1976

210. Baskett P, Vickers M: Driving after anaesthetics. Br Med J 1: 686, 1979

211. Herbert M, Healy EGJ, Bourke JB, et al: Profile of recovery after general anaesthesia. Br Med J 286: 1539, 1983
212. Cundy JM: Medical aspects of fitness to drive. Anaesthesia 34: 1056, 1979
213. Doenicke A, Kugler J, Laub M: Evaluation of recovery and "street fitness" by EEG and psychodiagnostic tests after anaesthesia. Can Anaesth Soc J 14(6): 567, 1967
214. Ogg TW: An assessment of post-operative outpatient cases. Br Med J 4: 573, 1972
215. Blackwell B: Treatment adherence. Br J Psychiatry 129: 510, 1976
216. Malins AF: Do they do as they are instructed? A review of outpatient anaesthesia. Anaesthesia 33: 832, 1978
217. Ogg TW, Fischer HBJ, Bethune DW, et al: Day case anaesthesia and memory. Anaesthesia 34: 784, 1979
218. Reed WA, Ford JL: The surgicenter: An ambulatory surgical facility. Clin Obstet Gynecol 17(3): 17, 1974
219. Fragen RJ, Shanks CA: Neuromuscular recovery after laparoscopy. Anesth Analg 63: 51, 1984
220. Sicard JA: Leliquide Cephaalo-rachidien, p 55. Paris, Mason and Gauthier-Villars, 1902
221. Jones RJ: The role of recumbency in the prevention and treatment of postspinal headache. Anesth Analg 53: 788, 1974
222. Carbaat PAT, van Crevel H: Lumbar puncture headache: Controlled study on the preventative effect of 24 hours' bed rest. Lancet 2: 113, 1981
223. Coombs DW, Porter JG: Lumbar puncture headache. Lancet 2: 87, 1981
224. Perz RR, Johnson DI, Shinozaki T: Spinal anesthesia for outpatient surgery. Anesth Analg 67: S168, 1988
225. Mulroy MF, Neal JM, Bridenbaugh LD, et al: Is postspinal headache more frequent in outpatients? Presented at the American Society of Regional Anesthesia Annual Meeting, Boston, 1989
226. Burke RK: Spinal anesthesia for laparoscopy: A review of 1063 cases. J Reprod Med 21: 59, 1978
227. Daos FG, Virtue RW: Sympathetic block persistence after spinal or epidural analgesia. JAMA 183: 285, 1963
228. Pflug AE, Aasheim GM, Foster C: Sequence of return of neurological function and criteria for safe ambulation following subarachoid block (spinal anaesthesic). Can Anaesth Soc J 25: 133, 1978
229. Roe CF, Cohn FL: Sympathetic blockade during spinal anesthesia. Surg Gynecol Obstet 136: 265, 1973
230. Cramer C: Ambulatory surgery: Nursing considerations. Curr Rev Post Anesth Care Nurs 9: 174, 1988
231. Kitz DS, Robinson DM, Schiavone PA, et al: Discharging outpatients: Factors nurses consider to determine readiness. AORN J 48: 87, 1988
232. Peabody FW: The care of the patient. JAMA 88: 877, 1927

Appendix 7A

■ ■

STANDARDS FOR POSTANESTHESIA CARE
(Approved by House of Delegates on October 12, 1988)

These Standards apply to postanesthesia care in all locations. These Standards may be exceeded based on the judgment of the responsible anesthesiologist. They are intended to encourage high quality patient care, but cannot guarantee any specific patient outcome. They are subject to revision from time to time as warranted by the evolution of technology and practice.

Standard I

All patients who have received general anesthesia, regional anesthesia, or monitored anesthesia care shall receive appropriate postanesthesia management.

1. A Postanesthesia Care Unit (PACU) or an area which provides equivalent postanesthesia care shall be available to receive patients after surgery and anesthesia. All patients who receive anesthesia shall be admitted to the PACU except by specific order of the anesthesiologist responsible for the patient's care.
2. The medical aspects of care in the PACU shall be governed by policies and procedures which have been reviewed and approved by the Department of Anesthesiology.
3. The design, equipment and staffing of the PACU shall meet requirements of the facility's accrediting and licensing bodies.
4. The nursing standards of practice shall be consistent with those approved in 1986 by the American Society of Post Anesthesia Nurses (ASPAN).

Standard II

A patient transported to the PACU shall be accompanied by a member of the anesthesia care team who is knowledgeable about the patient's condition. The patient shall be continually evaluated and treated during transport with monitoring and support appropriate to the patient's condition.

Standard III

Upon arrival in the PACU, the patient shall be re-evaluated and a verbal report provided to the responsible PACU nurse by the member of the anesthesia care team who accompanies the patient.

1. The patient's status on arrival in the PACU shall be documented.
2. Information concerning the preoperative condition and the surgical/anesthetic course shall be transmitted to the PACU nurse.
3. The member of the Anesthesia Care Team shall remain in the PACU until the PACU nurse accepts responsibility for the nursing care of the patient.

Standard IV

The patient's condition shall be evaluated continually in the PACU.

1. The patient shall be observed and monitored by methods appropriate to the patient's medical condition. Particular attention should be given to monitoring oxygenation, ven-

tilation and circulation. While qualitative clinical signs may be adequate, quantitative methods are encouraged.

2. An accurate written report of the PACU period shall be maintained. Use of an appropriate PACU scoring system is encouraged for each patient on admission, at appropriate intervals prior to discharge, and at the time of discharge.

3. General medical supervision and coordination of patient care in the PACU should be the responsibility of an anesthesiologist.

4. There shall be a policy to assure the availability in the facility of a physician capable of managing complications and providing cardiopulmonary resuscitation for patients in the PACU.

Standard V

A physician is responsible for the discharge of the patient from the postanesthesia care unit.

1. When discharge criteria are used, they must be approved by the Department of Anesthesiology and the medical staff. They may vary depending upon whether the patient is discharged to a hospital room, to the ICU, to a short stay unit, or home.

2. In the absence of the physician responsible for the discharge, the PACU nurse shall determine that the patient meets the discharge criteria. The name of the physician accepting responsibility for discharge shall be noted on the record.

Addendum: The Board of Directors of the American Society of Anesthesiologists at its March 1990 meeting accepted a proposed modification of STANDARD IV.

The patient's condition shall be evaluated continually in the PACU.

1. The patient shall be observed and monitored by methods appropriate to the patient's medical condition. Particular attention should be given to monitoring oxygenation, ventilation and circulation. While quantitative clinical signs may be adequate, quantitative methods are encouraged. During recovery from all anesthetics, a quantitative method of assessing oxygenation such as pulse oximetry shall be employed.*

   Under extenuating circumstances the responsible anesthesiologist may waive the requirements marked with an asterisk (*); it is recommended that when this is done, it should be so stated (including the reasons) in a note in the patient's medical record.

The above modification will not become part of the Standards for Postanesthesia Care until final action by the House of Delegates in October 1990. If approved, date of implementation will be determined by the House of Delegates.

Complications

8

■ ■

HERBERT E. NATOF, BARBARA GOLD, DEBORAH S. KITZ

Complications: There is probably no subject in medicine in which the search for pure truth is as evasive. Complications highlight our failures, betray our ignorance, and reaffirm that the mastery of our skills has limitations. And yet, as practitioners of medicine we must have a realistic understanding of the potential dangers of ambulatory surgery if we are to establish preventive measures and be prepared for prompt and effective treatment.

This chapter focuses not only on anesthesia complications but on the full range of complications associated with the ambulatory surgery setting. The role of the anesthesiologist in both the hospital-affiliated and freestanding centers frequently assumes many of the characteristics of a primary care physician. The anesthesiologist serves a central and crucial role in the preoperative screening process and plays a significant and broad role in the postoperative phase of care. Emphasizing this point, Brown states, "Never has the role of anesthesiologist been more challenged than in outpatient evaluation."[1]

It is essential from the onset to formulate a simple and uniform definition of the term *complication.* One of the pervasive pitfalls of any discussion of complications is the lack of a uniform definition, and the practicing physician finds himself or herself trying to evaluate information based on different ideas and concepts. In 1981, the Federated Ambulatory Surgery Association (FASA) established the following definition of a complication for the purposes of collecting data: an untoward response or abnormal condition resulting from treatment and care associated with ambulatory surgery.

A *major complication* is defined as an untoward response or abnormal condition *having the potential for serious harm.* Major complications include hemorrhage, infection, serious anesthetic complications, any medical problem requiring hospitalization, and other potentially harmful occurrences. A *minor complication* is an untoward response with minimal or no potential for serious harm and includes transient episodes of nausea and vomiting, weakness, headache, muscle aching, sore throat, and dizziness.

It is evident that any simple definition of a concept as complex as complications will have many gray areas in spite of our best efforts to seek uniformity. The reader may consider these examples:

1. The patient who complains of unusual pain postoperatively but heals normally
2. The patient who manifests premature ventricular contractions during the course of anesthesia but requires no specific therapy and has no sequelae
3. The patient who has an apparent sterilizing procedure but becomes pregnant one year later
4. The patient who develops a benign episode of laryngospasm that relents without specific therapy
5. The patient whose bunionectomy heals in an overcorrected position

Should any or all of these patients be classified as a complication case? There is no clear and authoritative answer, and the decision ultimately must be based on the individual evaluation of each case and a consensus of established criteria. In general, we would not classify as a complication an anesthetic or surgical event that was a relatively common deviation from the norm and required no special treatment or action on the part of the surgeon or anesthesiologist and presented no substantive danger to the patient. In addition, we would not classify as a complication a less-than-satisfactory surgical result unless it posed an increased risk to the general health of the patient. The vast majority of complications, however, are clearly identified by this definition and need not be subjected to arbitrary interpretation.

After collecting and studying ambulatory surgery complication data for the past 10 years, there are certain general concepts that emerge from our search for truth in this area.

▓ GENERAL CONCEPT NO. 1

The incidence of many major complications is related to specific surgical procedures such as tonsillectomy or adenoidectomy, laparoscopy, arthroscopy of the knee, augmentation mammaplasty, and other plastic and reconstructive operations. This does not mean that the same complications would be less likely to occur in the inpatient setting, nor does it mean that major complications cannot occur in association with other surgical procedures. It does mean that one can predict with reasonable confidence that certain major complications are more likely to occur in patients scheduled for certain specific operative procedures.

A corollary to this concept is that the types and incidence of major complications are generally related to the incidence of the specific surgical procedures being performed in an ambulatory surgery center. Each center has its own profile that will influence the occurrence of complications.

GENERAL CONCEPT NO. 2

Given any specific surgical procedure or anesthetic experience, there is the potential for the same complications whether the patients are inpatients in a hospital or outpatients in an ambulatory surgery facility.

There are several identifiable exceptions to this concept. First, there is considerable evidence that the incidence of infection is substantially less among ambulatory surgery patients. This is an important and unique advantage to patients whose surgery is performed in the ambulatory surgery setting. Second, there is circumstantial evidence, based on many case reports, that complications resulting from errors in patient identification such as "wrong surgery performed," medication errors, and incorrect entry of laboratory results occur with less frequency in the ambulatory surgery setting.

The diminished infection rate is probably due to the separation of ambulatory patients from the reservoir of nosocomial infections prevalent within the general hospital population. The paucity of identification errors is most likely due to the overall simplicity of the routine admission and preparation process of the ambulatory surgery setting. In addition, most ambulatory surgery patients do not receive preoperative sedative medications and are quite aware of what is happening until the anesthetic is begun.

Furthermore, there is some evidence that certain surgical procedures have fewer complications when performed in the ambulatory surgery setting. Williamson has performed over 3000 outpatient cataract procedures and has stated that the ambulatory patient has less chance of experiencing pneumonia, cross-infection, and pulmonary embolism.[2] Nabatoff and Aufses have reported on 2000 patients who had varicose vein surgery using general anesthesia in the ambulatory setting.[3] These authors reported wound healing that seemed better than usual, no significant hematomas, and no wound infections. Importantly, there were no instances of phlebitis or embolism.

GENERAL CONCEPT NO. 3

If something can go wrong—given a sufficient number of patients over a sufficient period of time—it will. This adaptation of Murphy's famous law is all too familiar to experienced physicians who have seen unfortunate and tragic events occur in spite of prudent precautions and care.

A recently opened ambulatory surgery center experienced the deaths of two apparently healthy patients within a five-week period in 1983. Examination of one of the two anesthesia machines used to administer inhalation anesthesia revealed a malfunctioning vaporizer valve. Information released by the center's administrator implied that a similar malfunction in the other anesthesia machine may have been implicated in the other death.

LOOKING AT COMPLICATIONS FROM DIFFERENT PERSPECTIVES

Complications in the ambulatory surgery setting may be viewed in an instructive fashion from many perspectives. We will consider three: the minor complication compared to the major complication, the relationship of complications to the phase of patient care, and the general etiology of complications.

Magnitude of Complication

Minor Complications

There appears to be little difference in the incidence of minor complications within the inpatient and the ambulatory settings when similar surgical procedures are compared. Minor complications may cause discomfort and anxiety but do not pose a threat to the life or limb of the patient. However, the ambulatory patient and his or her family should be well informed about potential minor complications prior to discharge.

The hospitalized patient who experiences an episode of nausea, muscle aching, or sore throat at 2 o'clock in the morning may be reassured by a concerned nurse. The uninformed ambulatory surgery patient may suffer unnecessary anxiety and sleeplessness at home. Ambulatory surgery patients should be told about the potential for minor complications such as muscle aching after the use of succinylcholine, the shoulder discomfort associated with laparoscopy, the sore throat following intubation, the frequent occurrence of nausea and vomiting after eye muscle surgery, and the feeling of generalized weakness after a particularly long anesthetic. The basic key to dealing with minor complications in ambulatory surgery patients is predischarge reassurance and information. These brief case reports illustrate.

■ CASE REPORT NO. 1

A 30-year-old woman called her surgeon early on the first postoperative day after an ambulatory diagnostic laparoscopy. With "tears in her voice," she reported that she had not slept because of a "gnawing" sore throat that became more painful and more frightening during the course of the night. She was sure that something "dreadful" had happened. The surgeon explained that the sore throat was due to a tube that was inserted by the anesthesiologist and necessary for safe anesthesia. Clearly, a few words of explanation by either the anesthesiologist or one of the postanesthesia care unit (PACU) nurses would have prevented the patient's anxiety.

■ CASE REPORT NO. 2

In contrast to the case described above, a seven-year-old child was scheduled for a myringotomy and adenoidectomy. The patient vomited once in the PACU but manifested no other problems. The PACU nurses informed the parents prior to discharge that their daughter might have some additional nausea and vomiting. The parents were instructed to call their surgeon if there was persistent vomiting or bleeding. They were reassured that an occasional bout of vomiting after surgery and anesthesia was not unusual or cause for concern. The following day, one of the PACU nurses called the mother to check on the patient's condition (an excellent routine practiced in many ambulatory surgery centers). The mother reported that the child vomited once after the car ride home and once several hours later, but was now drinking fluids without any problem. The mother commented that "the excellent instructions and reassurance made them very comfortable, and they had not been overly concerned about the two bouts of vomiting."

Major Complications

Major complications associated with ambulatory surgery have several unique aspects. First, the adjective *major*, as it has been defined for the ambulatory setting, has certain quantitative implications that need emphasis. Within the framework of hospital inpatient surgery, we tend to think of major complications as catastrophic or imminently life-threatening occurrences such as massive hemorrhage, septicemia, pulmonary emboli, or myocardial infarction. Although these critical complications may rarely occur among ambulatory surgery patients, a major complication in the ambulatory setting is much more likely to be a postoperative hematoma, localized wound infection, or persistent nausea and vomiting. Hence the term *major complication* must be viewed within the context of its definition—an untoward response with the potential for serious harm.

Second, the majority of major ambulatory complications occur after the patient has been discharged from the ambulatory surgery center. This fact emphasizes once again the importance of precise, clear postoperative instructions and the availability and cooperation of the surgeon.

▎ CASE REPORT NO. 3

A two-month-old infant was scheduled for a bilateral inguinal herniorrhaphy under general anesthesia. The operating room and PACU phases of care went well. The infant was hospitalized at 1:30 A.M. on the first postoperative day because of a fever of 104°F rectally and purulent drainage from the left incisional area. The patient was treated with intravenous antibiotics and fluids. In view of the rapidity and virulence of the infection, it was assumed that the organism was beta-hemolytic *Streptococcus*. All personnel who participated in the surgery had nose and throat cultures performed. No pathogens were discovered. Culture of the wound drainage of the patient grew *Staphylococcus aureus*. In spite of antibiotic therapy, the patient developed drainage from the right inguinal incision several days later. After one week of treatment in the hospital, the patient made a complete recovery, and there was no disruption of the hernia repair.

▎ CASE REPORT NO. 4

A 34-year-old woman was scheduled for a laparoscopic tubal sterilization. The surgeon observed at the time of surgery that there were multiple adhesions in the right lower quadrant of the abdomen, and the right tube was freed and grasped with difficulty. The remainder of the surgery was uneventful, and the patient did well in the PACU. She manifested abdominal distention and discomfort on the first postoperative day and was subsequently hospitalized by her surgeon. She was observed in the hospital for several days, and on the fourth postoperative day, the abdomen was explored, revealing a segment of inflamed small bowel that had become entrapped in the right lower quadrant adhesions. The bowel was released, and some of the adhesions excised. The patient made a prompt and uneventful recovery.

Postoperative instructions given by an ambulatory surgery center should include a warning that the patient should contact his or her attending surgeon promptly in the event of unusual pain, bleeding, or other unexpected symptoms. Many ambulatory surgery centers have qualified personnel call each patient on the first postoperative day and provide valuable patient follow-up. The patient described above wisely called her doctor when she experienced increasing distention of her abdomen, and her problem was prudently managed.

Phase of Patient Care
We also can view complications from the perspective of the phase of patient care: Complications may occur in the operating room, in the PACU, and after discharge.
Many of the most serious and life-threatening complications happen while the patient is in the operating room. Therefore, the anesthesiologist, surgeon, and nursing staff should be prepared to respond promptly and offer effective treatment.

Complications in the Operating Room
■ CASE REPORT NO. 5
An 11-month-old girl who appeared poorly developed and who manifested poor muscle tone was scheduled for bilateral myringotomy. The anesthesiologist noted that the infant also had a history of poor weight gain and had been followed by the neurology department of a large university hospital. The infant was scheduled for bilateral myringotomy and had been cleared by her neurologist. Approximately one minute into a nitrous oxide, oxygen, halothane inhalation induction (the halothane concentration was set at 1.5%), the infant manifested marked bradycardia and suddenly stopped breathing. The anesthesiologist was unable to properly ventilate the infant even after insertion of an oropharyngeal airway. The infant was immediately intubated and respiration was supported by the administration of only oxygen. The pulse returned to a normal rhythm in approximately 30 seconds, but spontaneous respiration did not return for approximately 10 minutes. The myringotomy was performed, and the patient recovered in the PACU without further difficulty. Since the initial experience, this patient has returned for three additional myringotomies without any further problems.

CASE REPORT NO. 6

A 32-year-old woman was scheduled for a laparoscopic tubal coagulation on an ambulatory basis. Upon insertion of the primary trocar, massive bleeding emerged through the trocar cannula. An emergency laparotomy was immediately performed. The hemorrhage, which originated at the hypogastric artery, was partially controlled using direct pressure while proximal and distal control of the artery was secured using clamps. A vascular surgeon was called and arrived approximately 45 minutes later and performed a primary closure of the laceration. The blood volume was maintained using plasma expanders and the subsequent administration of 5 units of whole blood. The patient made a complete recovery after a 2½-week period of hospitalization.

CASE REPORT NO. 7

A 39-year-old woman was scheduled for a laparoscopic tubal cautery using general anesthesia. The procedure was performed without difficulty, but fresh bleeding was observed within the abdominal cavity. The site of bleeding could not be identified through the laparoscope, and an emergency laparotomy was performed. A large retroperitoneal hematoma was discovered, the abdomen was closed, and the patient was transferred to a hospital immediately. In spite of the prompt transfer and a second laparotomy performed at the hospital, the patient died seven hours later. Postmortem examination revealed massive retroperitoneal hemorrhage and a diffuse bleeding diathesis.

CASE REPORT NO. 8

A seven-year-old girl was scheduled for a bilateral myringotomy and adenoidectomy using nitrous oxide, oxygen, halothane anesthesia. There was copious bleeding from the adenoid bed following the use of the adenotome and subsequent curettement. The bleeding was partially controlled with direct pressure. A preoperative partial prothrombin time (PPT) was normal, and the screening medical history revealed no family history of bleeding or clotting problems. Several conservative measures were used to control the bleeding, including electrofulguration and persistent pressure. The adenoid bed continued to ooze, and after 75 minutes, the surgeon inserted a posterior pack. There was no further evidence of bleeding, and the patient had a smooth and stable course in the PACU. She was transferred directly to a hospital for skilled observation. The posterior pack was removed the next day, and she was discharged from the hospital. There were no further problems, and the child had a normal recovery at home.

Complications in the PACU

Of all the phases of patient care in the ambulatory setting, the PACU phase requires a nursing staff that is alert, knowledgeable about potential complications, and endowed with superior communication skills and an abundant capacity for reassuring both patient and family.

CASE REPORT NO. 9

A five-and-a-half-year-old boy was scheduled for a rectal biopsy under general anesthesia. There was no unusual bleeding during the course of surgery, and the patient emerged satisfactorily in the PACU. Although the patient's vital signs remained stable, the PACU nurses expressed concern about his malaise and pallor. There was no evidence of external bleeding. The surgeon was requested to return to the center and examine the patient. Gentle but thorough examination by the surgeon revealed a large quantity of blood concealed in the bowel above the level of the surgery. The patient was transferred to a hospital for observation and blood replacement. He was discharged three days later in excellent condition.

CASE REPORT NO. 10

A 41-year-old woman was scheduled for a right capsulotomy under general anesthesia. The surgery and the initial postoperative period in the PACU were normal. Approximately 1 hour after surgery, the patient complained of increasing pain in the right breast. The PACU nurses followed the patient carefully and observed an increase in breast size. The surgeon was notified and returned to the center. Removal of the dressings revealed a very large hematoma. The patient consented to a second anesthetic and surgery for evacuation of the hematoma and control of the bleeding. The second procedure went well, and the patient's vital signs remained remarkably stable in spite of a blood loss of approximately 1200 ml. The patient requested that she be allowed to go home rather than to a hospital for observation. The surgeon allowed the patient to be discharged home, but she and her husband were given detailed and specific instructions and warning information. She was followed very carefully by her surgeon. She made an excellent recovery without any further problems.

CASE REPORT NO. 11

A 12-year-old girl underwent a tonsillectomy and adenoidectomy under general anesthesia. The anesthetic and operative phases of care were uneventful. The tonsil and adenoid beds were dry when the procedure was completed, and the pharynx was cleared of mucus and blood before and after removal of the endotracheal tube. Upon arrival in the PACU, the patient was not awake. She had a clear airway, good ventilation, and stable vital signs. Approximately 10 minutes after her arrival in the PACU, the patient coughed once or twice, manifested severe laryngospasm, and became cyanotic. The PACU nurses who were at her cart side (since she had not emerged from the anesthetic) immediately called for the anesthesiologist and administered oxygen using a portable ventilator and intermittent positive pressure. The PACU emergency cart, which was equipped with a full range of intubation equipment, was brought to the area. The girl's color was deeply cyanotic, and her pulse slowed to approximately 40 beats per minute. The anesthesiologist was just about to administer succinylcholine when the spasm relented and the patient's color and pulse rapidly returned to normal. After the patient awoke, the pharynx was cleansed with gentle suction, revealing a small amount of bloody mucus. The laryngospasm was probably triggered by the mucus in an emerging patient still in a state of "light" anesthesia. Although laryngospasm is usually a benign problem when managed properly, failure to observe and care for this patient properly could possibly have resulted in serious damage.

Postdischarge Complications

Every ambulatory patient should clearly understand who to call in the event of a complication or problem. The patient also should be aware of the common complications associated with the surgery performed. It is the experience of most ambulatory surgery centers that the three most common major complications in the postdischarge period are bleeding, infection, and persistent nausea and vomiting.

The risk of bleeding can, in general, be predicted based on the surgical procedure. Tonsillectomy and adenoidectomy patients usually do not bleed after discharge for the first 24 hours. The incidence of bleeding in these patients increases during the first week, peaking between the 7th and 10th days. These patients rarely bleed after the 12th day. In contrast, patients who undergo circumcision, submucous resection, rhinoplasty, face lift, and blepharoplasty, if they are going to bleed, usually do so during the first 48 hours. Cervical conization patients are most likely to have bleeding problems between the 7th and 12th postoperative days. Patients who have an augmentation mammaplasty or capsulotomy will usually bleed with hematoma formation during the first four postoperative days. Patients scheduled for arthroscopy of the knee (particularly with lateral release surgery) will usually bleed during the first 48 hours, resulting in hemarthrosis.

■ CASE REPORT NO. 12

A six-year-old Chinese boy was scheduled for a tonsillectomy and adenoidectomy. The parents seemed to understand the admission questions, the preoperative interview with the anesthesiologist, and conversations with the nurses in the PACU. The child did well while in the center, and the parents were given the usual explicit postoperative instructions. Everyone was sure the parents comprehended the instructions. The nurses at the ambulatory surgery center subsequently found out that the child bled seriously on the sixth postoperative day, but the parents ignored the problem. The child was finally brought to an emergency room of a hospital when he become extremely pale and poorly responsive. It was then discovered that the parents understood very little English, did not comprehend the discharge information, and had "faked out" the surgeon, anesthesiologist, and nursing staff by shaking their heads appropriately and using several English words.

This case illustrates the vital importance of communication in the ambulatory setting. The patient or a responsible relative, friend, or companion must fully understand the postoperative instructions and be able to assist during the preoperative interview. A lapse in communication due to language, diminished mental function, or physical disability may cause serious problems. We strongly encourage the patient's relative or friend to be present when the postoperative instructions are reviewed prior to discharge. The residual effects of the anesthesia may alter the ability of the patient to fully understand what is said, and sometimes patients have amnesia for this phase of their care.

CASE REPORT NO. 13

A five-year-old boy was scheduled for eye muscle surgery. The patient's surgical procedure went smoothly under nitrous oxide, oxygen, halothane anesthesia. The patient received only atropine as a premedicant. He did well in the PACU except for one episode of vomiting. The follow-up telephone call on the first postoperative day revealed that the patient had vomited three or four times during the night and was not drinking fluids. The mother was instructed to call the surgeon later in the day if the vomiting did not subside. By 4:00 P.M., the child was febrile, with a rectal temperature of 104°F, lethargic, and had continued to vomit. He was hospitalized by his surgeon and treated with intravenous fluids. The child was discharged after two days in the hospital, and there were no further problems.

CASE REPORT NO. 14

A 19-year-old woman was scheduled for a diagnostic dilatation and curettage (D&C) because of irregular menses. The patient was anesthetized using thiopental and nitrous oxide, oxygen, and halothane. She had a normal operative and anesthetic course. After awakening in the PACU, the patient wept continuously and complained of severe abdominal cramping. She received only modest relief from oral acetaminophen. The following day, the patient's mother called the surgeon and reported that her daughter had profound generalized weakness, bordering on paralysis, and could not walk. The patient was hospitalized, and a neurologist was called as a consultant. No organic disease was discerned, and the patient was seen by a psychiatrist. She was discharged in good condition after one week in the hospital with the diagnosis of anxiety reaction.

General Etiology

Complications also may be viewed from the perspective of general etiology: the complication may be due to anesthetic drugs or the conduct of anesthesia, the conduct of the surgery, preexisting disease, fortuitous occurrences, or a combination of several factors.

Etiology Related to Anesthesia

There was a time when we did not equate death with an outpatient procedure. However, at the 1986 meeting of the Federated Ambulatory Surgery Association

(FASA), a report of mortality statistics revealed 17 deaths in approximately 1.1 million procedures.* Deaths have occurred in freestanding, hospital-affiliated, and office-based ambulatory facilities, reinforcing the old cliché that there are no "minor anesthetics."

The most common anesthetic problem resulting in serious morbidity and mortality appears to be violation of the fundamental principles of proper ventilation and clear airway. The two clinical situations that pose recurrent problems in the ambulatory setting are laparoscopy performed with general anesthesia and use of the conscious sedation technique, particularly for nasal and facial surgery.

Although we personally believe that routine endotracheal intubation is not essential for the conduct of safe anesthesia for laparoscopy, the anesthesiologist must exercise constant attention to ventilation and be prepared to intubate the patient at the first indication of inadequate ventilation. We recommend routine intubation if the surgeon requires excessive degrees of Trendelenburg position (usually more than 5–10 degrees) or uses larger than normal volumes of gas (resulting in intraabdominal pressures exceeding 15–20 mmHg) and for patients with special problems such as obesity, cardiac or pulmonary disease, or other serious preexisting problems.

The conscious sedation technique has many advantages for ambulatory surgery patients, such as prompt emergence, a low incidence of nausea and vomiting, and usually a rapid return to clear mental function and general vitality. However, this technique, which is used in association with local anesthesia administered by the surgeon, involves potent respiratory depressants such as narcotics, barbiturates, and tranquilizers. The safety of this technique depends on the constant observation of ventilation and the respiratory airway. These guidelines are especially crucial when the technique is used for nasal and facial surgery: The anesthesiologist must ensure that the oropharyngeal airway is clear of blood and that there is no glossopharyngeal obstruction. The anesthesiologist must exercise constant vigilance with this valuable but potentially hazardous technique. Pulse oximetry is extremely valuable when conscious sedation is used.

One would suspect that a serious and recurring problem among ambulatory surgery patients would be aspiration of gastric contents, including partially digested food, due to the limitations of control in the preoperative period. However, the incidence of vomiting and aspiration is relatively low. This favorable result may well be due to the special emphasis of preoperative instructions and the thorough questioning of patients about ingestion of food and liquids upon arrival at the ambulatory surgery center. This potentially serious complication, however, is an ever-present danger in the ambulatory setting.

The potential for a malignant hyperthermic crisis is equally present in both outpatient and inpatient surgical settings. In the ambulatory surgery facility geographically separate from a hospital, a full complement of dantrolene sufficient to properly treat an adult patient should be immediately available. Treatment

---

*Reed WA: Personal communication, 1986.

objective should be reversal of metabolic crisis, stabilization, and transfer to a hospital bed for further observation and treatment.

The final topic of complications directly related to anesthesia is reactions to local anesthetic drugs. Based on information voluntarily submitted to FASA in 1982, over 15,000 patients had surgery performed using local anesthesia in 31 ambulatory surgery centers. This figure does not include the use of local anesthetic drugs in other patients who were classified under conscious sedation. If these data are extrapolated to encompass the experiences of ambulatory surgery centers throughout the United States, it is evident that an enormous number of patients are administered local anesthetic drugs.

In most cases, the volume, concentration, and rapidity of injection of the drugs are well within safe criteria, and the surgical procedure is limited to excision of small, superficial lesions. However, there is a large number of patients scheduled for surgery such as augmentation mammaplasty, rhinoplasty, submucous resection, rhytidectomy, and multiple podiatric procedures who are receiving marginally safe or unsafe amounts of local anesthetic drugs usually injected over a brief period of time and often injected into potentially vascular areas where rapid absorption or inadvertent intravascular entry may occur.

The monitoring of patients having surgery with local anesthesia varies considerably among ambulatory surgery centers. The extremes of patient care range from a policy requiring trained anesthesia personnel to attend every patient to only casual observation of the patient undergoing extensive surgery. A common-sense approach based on the pharmacology of the local anesthetic drugs and the data gathered over the years about complications would suggest that patients receiving large volumes and concentrations of local anesthetic drugs, particularly if they are injected over a relatively short period of time or into potentially vascular areas, should be carefully observed and their vital signs monitored by trained personnel during and after surgery.

■ CASE REPORT NO. 15

A 29-year-old woman was scheduled for multiple corrective procedures of both feet. The surgeon injected a total of 83 ml of a mixture of equal parts of 2% lidocaine and 0.5% bupivacaine into the operative sites of both feet. The patient was sedated by an anesthesiologist. The surgery was performed by two surgeons, each working independently on one of the patient's feet and each using a tourniquet above the ankle. The operating room phase of care went well without any hint of a problem. Upon arrival in the PACU, however, the patient manifested grossly jerky movements of the upper extremities, difficulty in swallowing, and inability to talk clearly. The anesthesiologist remained with the patient, administered oxygen and assisted ventilation, and carefully monitored her vital signs. During the next 45 minutes, the symptoms gradually abated, and the patient returned to a normal state. This patient received amounts of local anesthetic drugs in excess of recommended safe doses. It is very likely that very high levels of lidocaine reached the systemic circulation when the ankle tourniquets were released.

■ CASE REPORT NO. 16

A 19-year-old man was scheduled for a rhinoplasty on an ambulatory basis. The surgery was performed with local anesthesia administered by the surgeon and intravenous sedation administered by an anesthesiologist. The amounts of the narcotic and barbiturate are unknown. Approximately 30 minutes after the onset of surgery, the surgeon commented that the blood looked very dark. The anesthesiologist checked the patient and discovered that he was both apneic and pulseless. In spite of all attempts to resuscitate the patient, he was pronounced dead some 40 minutes later. This case is typical of several similar cases involving a planned conscious (in this instance unconscious) sedation technique. It is very likely that death resulted from one or a combination of these factors: central depression of respiration, glossopharyngeal obstruction, or blood in the pharynx or trachea and a diminished or absent cough reflex. This patient was not properly monitored, and the case illustrates the crucial importance of constant observation of ventilation and airway when this technique is used.

■ CASE REPORT NO. 17

A 28-year-old woman was scheduled for a laparoscopic tubal sterilization under general anesthesia. The patient was anesthetized with sodium thiopental followed by a nitrous oxide, oxygen, halothane routine. No endotracheal tube was used. The anesthetist thought she had a good airway, but admitted later that she could not clearly see "any chest movement." The surgeon noted that the patient appeared pale and dusky as the drapes were removed at the end of the procedure. Examination of the patient revealed no palpable pulse or other vital signs. Attempts to resuscitate the patient were futile. This case illustrates what can happen when the anesthetist is either unaware or unsure of proper ventilation during laparoscopic surgery. The anesthetist should not hesitate for one second to intubate the laparoscopy patient if there is any question about adequate ventilation. If the anesthetist is not skilled in managing these patients without an endotracheal tube, then each of these patients should be routinely intubated.

■ CASE REPORT NO. 18

A 21-year-old man was scheduled for a submucous resection under only local anesthesia (the type and concentration were not reported). Packs soaked in a 10% cocaine solution were inserted into both nostrils prior to the injection of local anesthesia. Approximately five minutes after the local had been injected and the cocaine packs removed, the patient became unresponsive and pulseless. The surgeon called for help and attempts were made to restore a normal heartbeat. The patient was finally pronounced dead some 45 minutes after the discovery of the arrest. The medical record failed to document if the patient was monitored or even observed at any time during the use of local and topical anesthesia.

▉ CASE REPORT NO. 19

A 69-year-old woman in good general health but with a history of hiatal hernia was scheduled for dental extractions. The anesthetic was a barbiturate, narcotic, muscle relaxant technique. When the anesthesiologist performed laryngoscopy prior to intubation, it was noted that a large amount of clear gastric contents was in the posterior pharynx. This was suctioned and an endotracheal tube inserted. The surgery was completed in 20 minutes, but the anesthesiologist had ventilation problems because of bronchospasm. Immediately upon the patient's entry into the PACU, a chest film was obtained and a preliminary diagnosis made of aspiration pneumonitis. The patient was admitted into the hospital and placed in the care of a pulmonary specialist. She received aggressive treatment for the problem. She did not require any further intubation or ventilatory support and was discharged in satisfactory condition one week following her procedure. Patients with hiatal hernia are considered "at risk" for aspiration and should be treated appropriately.

▉ CASE REPORT NO. 20

An 11-year-old boy (46-kg) was scheduled for an adenoidectomy and bilateral myringotomy. The patient was in good general health, and there was no family history of problems associated with anesthesia. The patient was anesthetized using 200 mg thiopental IV and 40 mg succinylcholine IV. The patient was intubated and received nitrous oxide, oxygen, halothane anesthesia. The surgery and anesthesia were uneventful. However, the anesthesiologist noted that there was no return of spontaneous respiration after approximately one-half hour. Examination of the IV site revealed no evidence of infiltration. A tentative diagnosis of succinylcholine apnea secondary to cholinesterase deficiency was made by the anesthesiologist. The surgery was completed about 35 minutes after the administration of the muscle relaxant. The patient was ventilated manually and kept in the operating room. The parents were informed of the problem and reassured. Two hours after the start of anesthesia, the patient began to breathe spontaneously and subsequently responded to the endotracheal tube. The patient was extubated about 20 minutes later. He was kept in the operating room and observed for an additional half hour. The patient had good ventilation and demonstrated good muscle activity and was able to lift his head without difficulty. The patient was moved to PACU. The anesthesiologist instructed the nurses to continue ECG monitoring and to move the resuscitation cart close to the patient's cart. (Pulse oximetry was not in general use at the time.) In addition, the anesthesiologist requested that a PACU nurse remain with the patient. The boy's mother was invited to stay with her son. He appeared normal and conversed with his mother. Approximately one-half hour after the patient had arrived in the PACU, the ECG displayed increasing premature ventricular contractions and the boy suddenly stopped breathing. Since the necessary equipment was at the cart-side, he was immediately ventilated and intubated again by the original anesthe-siologist. The mother was badly shaken but was calmed by the nursing staff. The anesthesiologist supported respiration using a portable manual ventilator and supplemental oxygen. The arrythmia subsided promptly, but spontaneous res-piration did not return for almost one hour. Following extubation there were no further problems. Subsequent blood testing of the patient, mother, father, and two siblings revealed low cholinesterase levels in the patient and a younger sib-ling who had never had a anesthetic experience.

The pathophysiology of this case is unclear. However, the case illustrates that good patient care depends on vigilance and skilled physicians and nurses re-gardless of whether the setting is inpatient or outpatient. Although most cata-strophic ambulatory surgery complications resulting in death appear to be re-lated to anesthetic drugs and the conduct of anesthesia, the overall majority of major complications are related to the surgery.

Etiology Related to Surgery

The single most prevalent surgical complication is hemorrhage. For the purposes of definition, *hemorrhage* in ambulatory surgical patients is defined as bleeding of sufficient quantity to require special attention and treatment. The volume of blood loss is not the primary criterion, since it can rarely be accurately measured. The definition of hemorrhage should include adenoidectomy patients requiring a posterior pack; patients who must return to an operating room, emergency room, or physician's office for additional suturing, cautery, packing, or pressure dressings; patients with postoperative hematoma requiring evacuation; and pa-tients requiring laparotomy for intraabdominal bleeding.

Approximately 1% to 4% of all tonsillectomy and adenoidectomy (T&A) pa-tients bleed sufficiently to require special treatment during either the operating room, PACU, or postdischarge phase of care. Most of the bleeding episodes will occur after discharge from the ambulatory surgery center.

The most urgent and serious episodes of hemorrhage are associated with lap-aroscopy. The laceration of a major intraabdominal blood vessel upon insertion of the primary trocar creates one of the most critical situations in the ambulatory surgery facility, as well as in the hospital inpatient setting. Every ambulatory sur-gery center must have a plan for immediate response to this potentially fatal complication. A sterile laparotomy tray, as well as plasma expander fluids, should be immediately available. The abdomen should be entered without delay and the hemorrhage controlled by any and all means until a primary repair of the lacer-ation can be performed. The center's plan for obtaining blood should be initiated as soon as a blood sample can be drawn for type and crossmatch. In some cases, the use of noncrossmatched O negative blood may be life saving. Probably the single most important aspect of treatment is having the center's professional nursing staff well informed about their duties in the event of this complication.

Less serious episodes of bleeding associated with laparoscopy may occur within the abdominal wall owing to the introduction of the secondary trocar or may occur intraabdominally as a result of the freeing of preexisting adhesions.

The laparoscopy procedure is associated with other serious major complications such as bowel burn, laceration of the bowel or other hollow viscus, bowel obstruction secondary to perforation or adhesions, and peritonitis secondary to unrecognized bowel perforation. Since the introduction of the bipolar coagulation technique, bowel burns have been virtually eliminated. Two cases of intraabdominal explosion following the use of nitrous oxide as the filling gas have been reported in the literature.[4]

Although the incidence of wound infection is low among ambulatory surgery patients, several cases of fulminating streptococcal septicemia have occurred in women who had undergone augmentation mammaplasty. It is not clear why such infections may take such a rampant course in these patients; however, the virulence of these rare infections has prompted some plastic surgeons to use prophylactic antibiotics in their breast augmentation patients.

▓ CASE REPORT NO. 21

A 64-year-old man was scheduled for excision of multiple bilateral nasal polyps under general endotracheal anesthesia. There was generous bleeding during the performance of the procedure, which lasted almost 105 minutes. Upon arrival in the PACU, the patient bled through the nasal packs and blood clots were suctioned from his oropharyngeal area. The patient was restless but cooperative. In view of his persistent bleeding, the patient was transferred directly to a hospital for observation. Upon arrival at the hospital, the patient removed his packs and was subsequently scheduled for emergency surgery under general anesthesia to reinsert them. When the patient arrived in the hospital PACU following the second operation, blood continued to soak the newly inserted nasal packing. He was again returned to the operating room for further packing. The patient never awakened from the second anesthetic and died four days later. Postmortem examination revealed an iatrogenic defect in the cribriform plate with a laceration of the brain.

▓ CASE REPORT NO. 22

A 39-year-old woman was scheduled for a laparoscopic tubal sterilization and D&C. The surgeon accidentally perforated the dome of the bladder during the insertion of the primary trocar. The perforation was observed upon insertion of the laparoscope. A urologist was called and performed a cystoscopy in order to assess the damage. A laparotomy was subsequently performed and the perforation repaired. An open tubal ligation was performed at the same time. The patient was transferred to a hospital for postoperative care after stable emergence in the ambulatory surgery center PACU.

▓ CASE REPORT NO. 23

A 39-year-old woman underwent a bilateral augmentation mammaplasty under local anesthesia. The surgery went smoothly and the patient was discharged in good condition. The following day the patient called her surgeon and complained of fever, chills, and generalized weakness. The patient was hospitalized later on the same day. The patient was treated with intravenous antibiotics, and drainage material from the right breast was cultured. Despite intensive antibiotic therapy, the patient died on the third postoperative day. Culture of the breast drainage material grew beta-hemolytic streptococci.

■ CASE REPORT NO. 24

A nine-year-old boy was scheduled for excision of a papillary lesion of the left upper cheek area. The patient was anesthetized and intubated without difficulty. The operative site was prepped with Betadine paint and draped with a combination paper and plastic drape with adhesive on the perimeter of one side. After the lesion was excised, the area was cauterized using an Accu-Temp hand-held, battery-operated cautery unit. The red hot heating element of the unit accidentally made contact with the combination paper and plastic drape. The site of contact burst into flames, which were promptly smothered by the surgeon. However, several areas of the drape distant from the original point of contact began to smolder. The drape was then removed immediately from the patient's face. Subsequent examination of the facial area revealed several areas of second- and third-degree burns.

Etiology Related to Preexisting Conditions

The variations of complications that may arise as a result of preexisting disease are limitless and may include such diverse complications and disease entities (which have actually occurred) as subglottic edema in a child with congenital tracheal stenosis, a fulminating episode of bronchospasm in a patient with extrinsic asthma, an arrhythmia in a patient with prolapse of the mitral valve resulting in cardiac arrest, uncontrolled bleeding in a patient with a familial coagulation disturbance, and severe postoperative psychoneurotic behavior in a patient with a history of serious emotional problems.

This discussion focuses on three significant problem areas associated with preexisting conditions that may be present in ambulatory patients: intraoperative or postoperative myocardial infarction, disruption of metabolic control in insulin-dependent patients with diabetes mellitus, and certain complications occurring in pregnant patients (pregnancy is not a preexisting disease, but it is a preexisting condition that presents some unique complications in the ambulatory setting).

MYOCARDIAL INFARCTION. Tinker studied the relationship of myocardial infarction to surgical and anesthetic experiences.[5] His review and cogent observations were presented at the refresher course lectures at the annual meeting of the American Society of Anesthesiologists in 1982, and his comments are generously referred to in this discussion. Many of the important aspects of his review are as appropriate for ambulatory patients as for hospital inpatients.

Tarhan and coworkers reported that the overall risk of perioperative infarction was 6% in patients who had a history of a previous myocardial infarction.[6] However, if the myocardial infarction had occurred within 3 months prior to the surgical and anesthetic experience, the risk for a recurrent myocardial infarction increased to 37%. The risk diminished to 16% if the interlude between the first myocardial infarction and the surgical experience was between three and six months. The mortality rate as a result of repeat myocardial infarction in Tarhan's study was 50%!

Tinker also reported on Mahar's review of surgical patients who had survived previous coronary bypass surgery. Mahar and coworkers studied 99 postbypass patients who underwent a total of 168 subsequent noncardiac operations without a single perioperative myocardial infarction[7] Tinker also presented data gathered by Backer and colleagues and Lang and coworkers.[5,8] Backer and his group studied over 10,000 patients who underwent ophthalmic surgery using local or retrobulbar block anesthesia. Of the patients in this group, 195 had a documented previous myocardial infarction; almost one-half of these patients had more than one surgical procedure. Not a single perioperative reinfarction occurred. Lang and coworkers reported very similar results in patients who had eye surgery under general anesthesia. Tinker commented, "This implies that the magnitude of the surgery, not the type of anesthesia is responsible for these good results." He further observed, "The other relevant point for anesthesiologists is that these seemingly very fragile patients, many of whom are quite elderly with many other medical problems, scheduled for ophthalmic surgery, are in fact not at great risk of perioperative myocardial infarction."

Tinker's comments are important and have been substantially corroborated as changes in Medicare policy have shifted many elderly patients scheduled for cataract and other surgery to the ambulatory setting.

DIABETES MELLITUS. Our experience at Northwest Surgicare suggests that the ambulatory setting is ideal for many diabetic patients scheduled for certain types of surgical procedures. Diabetes mellitus is a common disease, and there is a large population of insulin-dependent patients. The method we use works remarkably well, and we have experienced no complications related to insulin management.

The primary objective is to restore the diabetic patient's insulin balance as smoothly as possible to the preoperative state. We have observed that the sooner these patients return to their own environment, accustomed diet, and activity, the less severe will be the disturbance to their insulin balance and associated changes in their metabolism.

There is substantial variation among the individual responses of diabetic patients receiving insulin ranging from relative stability on a day-to-day basis to marked "brittleness," manifested by episodes of hypoglycemia (insulin reactions) and periods of high blood glucose. In general, diabetic children and young adults are more likely to fall into the latter group. If the patient has a history of poor or complicated insulin control, the case should be thoroughly discussed with the patient's physician. The patient may not be a candidate for ambulatory surgery.

The traditional methods of managing the insulin-dependent diabetic patient for surgery within the hospital setting are predicated on the administration of fractional doses of the patient's normal insulin requirements (usually one-third to one-half) and the continuous administration of an intravenous glucose infusion. The patient's balance is fine-tuned by obtaining frequent blood sugar determinations and using supplemental regular insulin as needed. If everyone involved in the patient's care (laboratory personnel, nurses, and physicians) works together diligently, the method works reasonably well.

When the traditional method is applied to the ambulatory setting, there are obvious problems. The question of how much insulin to administer and when to administer it is difficult to coordinate with the patient's physician. One frequently used management routine is to administer one-half the patient's normal insulin requirement on the morning of surgery. This dose may be too much or too little depending on the specific metabolic characteristics of the patient, the type and quantity of intravenous fluids, the length and stress of the surgery, and other factors. In the hospital setting, medical personnel can provide proper attention, making the necessary adjustments with supplemental insulin and regulating the intravenous fluids. Not only is this method difficult in the ambulatory surgery setting, but it also creates many problems for the patient after discharge from the center. The diabetic ambulatory surgery patient will usually resume almost normal meals after returning home, frequently resulting in high blood sugars for the remainder of the day of surgery. The presence of hyperglycemia during this period may increase the incidence of infection.

We often use a different management approach for the insulin-dependent patient that has worked very well in the ambulatory setting. The basic principles also can be adapted for diabetic patients managed by diet and one of the blood sugar lowering drugs. The method is relatively simple and effective, and we call it *moving the sun in the sky.* Each of these patients has a baseline fasting blood sugar determination preoperatively and may have one or more repeat blood sugar tests performed in the PACU using one of the "home-type" colorimetric techniques. The ultimate success of the process depends on the absence of persistent vomiting. We have been very fortunate and have not had a single patient who experienced recurrent vomiting in the postoperative period. It is axiomatic that vomiting mandates hospitalization and intravenous support until the patient can return to a normal diet and insulin balance. If the patient is scheduled for local anesthesia only, he or she is instructed to take a usual insulin dose and have meals at the accustomed intervals.

If the patient is scheduled for surgery using general or intravenous sedation, every attempt should be made to start as early as possible. This is one of the more compelling situations for maximum cooperation related to scheduling. These patients are instructed to omit their normal morning injection and bring their insulin with them. They are instructed to arrive at the center early in order to manage a possible hypoglycemic episode due to the absence of a normal breakfast. We allow these patients to remain in the reception area; however, they are told to notify our personnel immediately if they perceive an impending insulin reaction. If this happens preoperatively, the patient is moved promptly to the PACU, and the hypoglycemia is reversed by means of an intravenous glucose infusion. The patient's status can be monitored with blood sugar tests if necessary.

After completion of surgery, the intravenous infusion is maintained until the patient is almost ready to go home. The blood sugar test is repeated at least once in the postoperative period. Barring nausea and vomiting, the patient is instructed to pretend that he or she has just awakened and to take the usual and normal dose of insulin and have normal meals with the usual time intervals between meals—hence the name *moving the sun in the sky*. The insulin dose may be increased or decreased if the last blood sugar test results were substantially high or low, and the dose may be moderately increased if the patient's activity is to be markedly restricted at home.

For example, if the patient is moved into the PACU at 9:30 A.M. and is ready to be discharged at 11:00 A.M., the patient may take insulin prior to leaving the facility (if he or she lives close to the center) or immediately upon arrival at home. The patient is instructed to have a normal breakfast 20 minutes after the insulin injection, lunch four hours later, and dinner approximately five hours after lunch (which in this example would be between 8:30 and 9:00 P.M.). The following day the patient takes a normal dose of insulin and has normal meals spaced at a normal interval. All we have done is artificially "move the sun in the sky." The later the insulin is administered on the day of surgery, the greater will be the risk of an insulin reaction the next morning after the normal dose of insulin is taken at the customary time. Therefore, these patients should be cautioned that they may be more vulnerable to an insulin reaction on the first postoperative morning and may require additional carbohydrate at breakfast time.

PREGNANCY. The pregnant patient poses at least two potentially serious complications. The first problem may have both a medical and legal component.[9] The anesthesiologist may or may not be aware that the patient is pregnant at the time of the ambulatory surgery (not all ambulatory surgery facilities perform pregnancy testing prior to administering anesthesia). At some point in the future, the patient may allege or blame a miscarriage or a retarded or deformed child on the anesthetic experience at the ambulatory surgery facility. It is prudent to ask every female patient of childbearing age if she is pregnant before administering anesthesia or performing surgery. Northwest Surgicare has incorporated this specific question into its preoperative medical screening process. If the patient is pregnant or suspects that she is pregnant, have a forthright and informative discussion with the patient about the potential hazards to the fetus. Do not hesitate to cancel the procedure if there is any reluctance on the part of the patient to go ahead, particularly if the surgery could be postponed without any difficulty. Obviously, if the patient elects to proceed, avoid suspected teratogenic drugs such as certain antiemetics and tranquilizers and carefully document all this information on the chart.

The second complication associated with the pregnant patient may have even more serious consequences. A very large number of pregnant women come to ambulatory facilities for termination of the pregnancy. It is one of the most common ambulatory surgical procedures performed in the United States. It is essential that the tissue removed be examined by a trained pathologist and the results of the examination reported to the surgeon as soon as possible. There have been several catastrophic cases of ruptured ectopic pregnancy following an abortion procedure. This complication may be due to failure of the surgeon to request examination of the tissue, failure to promptly inform the surgeon of the results of the examination, or failure of the surgeon to respond properly to the pathology results. The absence of chorionic villi or other conception tissue in the specimen material should immediately alert the surgeon to the potential of an undiagnosed ectopic pregnancy.

CASE REPORT NO. 25

A 53-year-old man was scheduled for a minor podiatric procedure using local anesthesia plus intravenous sedation administered by an anesthesiologist. The patient was moderately obese and had a 20-year history of cigarette smoking. The operating room and PACU phases of care went well without any problems. Approximately 48 hours after discharge, the patient was hospitalized because of chest pain. He spent several days in the coronary care unit of a hospital with a diagnosis of myocardial infarction. The patient had a benign hospital course. No bypass surgery was recommended after a cardiac workup that included a coronary angiogram. During his hospitalization, the patient told his internist that he had experienced occasional chest pain for several weeks prior to his surgery but had told no one.

CASE REPORT NO. 26

A 27-year-old woman visited an abortion clinic and consented to the termination of an apparent first trimester pregnancy. The procedure was performed without any unusual problems. The patient returned to her apartment after the surgery. She was found dead several days later by a neighbor. Postmortem examination revealed a ruptured ectopic tubal pregnancy with exsanguination within the abdominal cavity. Material removed from the patient at the time of the abortion had never been examined by a pathologist.

CASE REPORT NO. 27

A 36-year-old woman was scheduled for a diagnostic laparoscopy. She had a 15-year history of asthma related to allergic and emotional factors. The patient was administered a nitrous oxide, oxygen, halothane anesthetic following thiopental induction. There were no problems during the operating room phase of care. Approximately one half-hour after the patient awakened in the PACU, she began to wheeze and manifested labored respiration. Auscultation of the chest revealed bilateral, diffuse wheezing breath sounds. The asthmatic episode was promptly treated with intravenous aminophylline administered by drip infusion. The wheezing and dyspnea gradually abated over the next hour. The patient had normal breath sounds prior to discharge, and follow-up revealed that she had no further problems.

Etiology Related to Fortuitous Occurrences
Rarely, there are complications that occur without any rhyme or reason. These complications reflect no deficiency in medical care and seem only to corroborate that there is a capricious nature to life that defies our best efforts to practice safe and knowledgeable medicine.

■ CASE REPORT NO. 28
A 25-year-old man had a vasectomy performed on an ambulatory surgery basis under local anesthesia. Following the procedure, he rested in the reception area before starting on his way home. Approximately 15 minutes later the police pulled his body from his wrecked automobile. He had apparently lost control of the car and crashed into a building. Postmortem examination of the patient revealed a ruptured intracranial aneurysm with massive bleeding. There had been no history of any previous problems in this young man.

■ CASE REPORT NO. 29
A healthy 39-year-old woman elected to have a diagnostic D&C performed under local anesthesia. Her temperature and vital signs were normal on the day of surgery. She had no other complaints or symptoms at the time. On the first postoperative day, she became acutely ill with a cough, fever, and chills. She was seen by her family doctor, and chest radiography revealed viral pneumonia.

■ CASE REPORT NO. 30
A 25-year-old man was scheduled for an arthroscopy and arthrotomy of the right ankle under local anesthesia and intravenous sedation administered by an anesthesiologist. There were no problems during the operative or the PACU phases of care. On the second postoperative day, the patient complained of severe abdominal pain and was hospitalized by his family doctor. The patient was admitted to the hospital with a diagnosis of an "acute abdomen." He spent one week in the hospital and was discharged with a diagnosis of acute gastritis.

Etiology Related to Multiple Factors
There are complications in which the general etiology may be attributed to more than one factor. It may be difficult or impossible to apportion the significance of each individual factor properly, but one cannot rule out that each factor bears a relationship and contributes to the etiology of the complication.

■ CASE REPORT NO. 31
A 58-year-old man with a history of hypertension was scheduled for a hair transplant under local anesthesia and intravenous sedation administered by an anes-

thesiologist. The surgeon had intended to implant 100 plugs, but the surgery was abandoned after the placement of 25 plugs because of uncontrolled bleeding. The patient required two 500-ml units of plasma expander and was transferred to a general hospital for observation. A hematologic workup established the diagnosis of von Willebrand's disease. This case report implicates multiple factors, including the history of hypertension, the decision to perform the cosmetic surgery in the first place, and the undiagnosed coagulation disease.

■ CASE REPORT NO. 32

A thin, frail 72-year-old woman was scheduled for cataract surgery using retrobulbar block anesthesia. According to her family, she had lost a significant amount of weight during the past year without any plausible explanation. In addition, she had a history of angina pectoris and coronary artery disease. The ophthalmologic surgeon instructed the circulating nurse to administer 5 mg diazepam in a single dose intravenously. Approximately 5 to 10 minutes later, the circulating nurse noted that the patient's hands and nail beds appeared blue. The drapes were removed, and no respiration or heartbeat could be discerned. Despite closed-chest cardiac massage, the patient's heart action was never restored. This case implicates many factors, including failure to investigate the patient's weight loss and prepare the patient properly for surgery, inadequate monitoring of the vital signs during the procedure in view of her fragile general condition, and the rapid administration of a respiratory depressant drug without proper observation.

■ CASE REPORT NO. 33

A 39-year-old woman was scheduled for multiple podiatric procedures under general anesthesia. In spite of a past history of six episodes of thrombophlebitis, the surgeon elected to use a pneumatic thigh cuff inflated to 450 mmHg for a period of 100 minutes. The patient had no problems during either the operating room or PACU phases of her care. She was discharged in good condition but developed signs and symptoms of thrombophlebitis on the fourth postoperative day. She was hospitalized for 11 days while receiving anticoagulant therapy. She made a satisfactory recovery without any further problems. However, a potentially serious complication might have been prevented if some other method for the management of bleeding had been used. It is also possible that this patient was not a candidate for ambulatory surgery and should have had preoperative and postoperative anticoagulant treatment.

■ CASE REPORT NO. 34

A 59-year-old man was scheduled for excision of redundant gingival tissue. The patient had a long history of alcoholism, recent onset of mild hypertension, and a morbid fear of doctors. He had refused to have the surgery performed under local anesthesia in the oral surgeon's office. Shortly after the onset of surgery using general, endotracheal anesthesia (nitrous oxide, oxygen, halothane), he manifested an irregular pulse followed by ventricular fibrillation. Closed-chest cardiac compression was started promptly, and the patient's color improved almost immediately. The patient was electrically defibrillated without difficulty, and a normal sinus rhythm ensued. Spontaneous respiration returned shortly thereafter, and there were no blood pressure problems. The anesthesiologist felt certain that satisfactory circulation had been restored within a safe period of time. However, the patient did not regain consciousness for several days and was left with diminished cerebral function.

COMPLICATION STATISTICS AND DATA: TRYING TO FIND THE TRUTH

What is a Complication?

One thing becomes clear when considering complications associated with ambulatory surgery: There is no generally accepted, specific definition of *complications*. Rather, authors have defined broad categories of untoward events or focused on specific postoperative events. For example, Shah and coworkers, in their early comparison of inpatient and ambulatory care for children, categorized complications as mild, moderate, and severe.[10] Mild complications did not require active intervention (e.g., cough); moderate complications required intervention by a nurse or parent (e.g., medication change or change of dressing); and severe complications necessitated intervention by a physician.

In a survey of patients cared for at a single surgical facility, one of us (Natof) defined a complication as "an untoward response or abnormal condition with the potential for serious harm resulting from the treatment and care associated with ambulatory surgery."[11] Transient nausea and vomiting, dizziness, sore throat, weakness, and headache were explicitly excluded from the survey. This definition and explicit exclusions also were used in the multifacility study of complications that Natof conducted on behalf of the Federated Ambulatory Surgery Association.[12]

Earlier in this chapter, complications were categorized as minor complications (those which cause discomfort or anxiety but pose no or minimal potential for serious harm) and major complications (untoward responses or abnormal conditions with the potential for serious harm). Minor complications include myalgias and transient nausea and vomiting. Major complications include wound infection and postoperative hematoma.[13,14] Despite the lack of specificity with regard to a definition of complications, investigators have found that even minor problems, such as nausea or myalgias, may delay discharge or time to resumption of normal activities for ambulatory surgery patients.[15] This suggests that any untoward event may be important to consider in examining the clinical and administrative aspects of ambulatory surgery.

Have Complications Occurred?

A multipronged approach is necessary to determine the incidence of complications among ambulatory surgery patients. Orkin outlined three approaches to identifying complications from an organizational perspective: (1) structure assessment (*i.e.*, examining qualifications and adequacy of personnel and physical resources), (2) process assessment (*i.e.*, determining adherence to criteria or standards of care), and (3) outcome assessment (*i.e.*, evaluating morbidity, mortality, duration of PACU stay, and patient satisfaction).[16] Accreditation and regulatory organizations frequently use one or more of these approaches to examine complications.

The American Society of Anesthesiologists (ASA) developed a document that outlines methods for evaluating complications. The ASA includes the basic qualifications and responsibilities of anesthesia personnel (including department directors), standards for preoperative evaluation and intraoperative monitoring, information to be recorded on anesthesia records, and factors to be considered in examinations of PACU incidents.[17]

As part of a comprehensive "quality and appropriateness" effort, the Joint Commission on Accreditation of Healthcare Organizations (JCAHO) has developed documents to assist in the examination of anesthesia care. *Monitoring and Evaluation*, for example, provides a step-by-step guide for the establishment, implementation, and review of a program to evaluate anesthesia care.[18] The document also provides examples of indicators of untoward events, criteria for determining acceptable quality of care, and steps to address potential problems. Although the events listed as indicators of potential problems may be most common among inpatients, they certainly are important to consider for ambulatory surgery patients (*e.g.*, heart rate less than 40 or greater than 140 beats per minute during anesthesia, intraoperative cardiac arrest). Other events, such as protracted somnolence or protracted vomiting requiring hospital admission, may be added for the ambulatory setting, particularly as outpatient surgery becomes more prevalent.

The JCAHO's *Ambulatory Health Care Standards Manual* may serve as another guide for the development of a general quality assessment and/or complications review program.[19] In fact, one chapter is devoted to surgical and anesthesia services. The specific items listed in the manual are now used as part of JCAHO's accreditation process.

Intraoperative Complications

Intraoperative complications, such as aspiration, ECG changes, and reactions to anesthetic agents, usually may be assessed by examining nursing, surgical, and anesthesia records. These sources provide information on the patient's clinical status prior to, during, and immediately following the event.

Postoperative Complications

As with intraoperative events, complications that occur in the immediate postoperative period are most readily assessed from PACU records. Determining the incidence of complications that occur in the period following acute recovery poses a greater challenge for ambulatory surgery patients than for surgery inpatients. Whereas inpatients are monitored and observed by trained personnel in this period, ambulatory surgery patients are discharged to home, where monitoring and observation are not available.

Perioperative Records

Review of perioperative records, including anesthesia, surgical, and PACU records, is another approach to determining the incidence of postoperative complications. In fact, this method is usually the most feasible, particularly if the records require clear and consistent delineation of untoward events. For retrospective analyses, perioperative records are the most common source of complication data.

Metter and coworkers[15] and Pataky and colleagues,[20] for example, reviewed perioperative records to determine the incidence of postoperative nausea and vomiting among specific groups of ambulatory surgery patients. They also used the records as sources of information regarding patients' demographic characteristics, anesthesia technique, and surgical procedure. Meridy,[21] Patel and Hannallah,[22] and Hines and coworkers[23] also used this approach in their studies of complications among general populations of ambulatory surgery patients. One approach to assessing the relatively more serious perioperative complications is to identify ambulatory surgery patients who required hospital admission.

Types of Complications

Major complications in the ambulatory surgery setting are rare, undoubtedly contributing to the rapid growth of outpatient surgery practices. Factors that are usually associated with increased inpatient anesthetic morbidity and mortality such as advanced age, ASA physical status, major surgery, and emergency surgery have not been prevalent in the ambulatory setting.[24,25] However, a substantial number of minor, yet distressing, complications such as nausea, vomiting, and myalgias often occur following ambulatory surgery, and these events may present major impediments to patient discharge and disrupt the smooth operation of an ambulatory surgery unit.

Many studies have documented the types of complications that occur within individual practices and are briefly summarized here. As early as 1975, Brindle and Soliman surveyed 500 ASA physical status 1 outpatients who underwent bilateral tubal ligation and found that the incidence of minor complications was substantial: 43% of patients complained of muscular pain, 28% of sore throat, 17% of headache, 23% of nausea and vomiting, and 16% of cough.[26] Additionally, 41% of patients claimed to feel "dizzy" and 30% complained of an inability to concentrate, which usually resolved within five days after surgery. Despite this seemingly high incidence of relatively minor complaints, there were no major complications. The Federated Ambulatory Surgery Association surveyed a total of 87,492 patients treated in 43 freestanding ambulatory surgery centers where most patients (80%) were adult and 98% were ASA physical status 1 or 2.[12] Only a fraction of complications occurred in the operating room or PACU (14% and 17%, respectively), whereas the majority (69%) occurred after discharge. The most common complications that occurred in the operating room were airway obstruction ($n = 12$), arrhythmias ($n = 11$), and hemorrhage ($n = 9$). In the PACU, the most common complications were hemorrhage ($n = 22$), hypotension ($n = 28$), and persistent nausea ($n = 13$). Following discharge, hemorrhage and wound infection accounted for the majority of complications. Additionally, of 87,492 patients, 3 suffered a perioperative cardiac arrest, from which they survived, and 82 patients (0.09%) required hospital admission.

In a prospective survey of 13,433 patients treated at a single freestanding ambulatory center between 1974 and 1978, Natof found only 106 (0.8%) complications.[11] The most common complications were hemorrhage, infection, and nausea and vomiting. Other complications that were less frequent but potentially more serious included laryngospasm ($n = 2$), respiratory arrest ($n = 1$), and bronchospasm ($n = 1$). There were no cardiac arrests. The hospital admission rate was 0.12% (16 of 13,433).

In the postoperative period, a prospective study of 3477 ambulatory surgery patients reported complications ranging from hypotension, hypertension, arrhythmias, nausea and vomiting, drug reactions, respiratory distress, cardiac events, and alterations in mental status.[23] The overall complication rate in the PACU was 15.5%, with the majority of complications occurring in gynecologic and ophthalmologic patients. Nausea and vomiting were the most frequent complications, especially among these same patient subgroups. There were no cases of cardiac arrest or myocardial infarction. Although major complications such as cardiac arrest, myocardial infarction, aspiration, and death are rare in the ambulatory setting, relatively minor complications such as nausea and vomiting, myalgias, and dizziness are quite common. While the clinical ramifications of complications are of utmost concern, it is also important to consider the administrative implications of such untoward events (e.g., extended PACU stay, increased nursing costs, revised scheduling practices, and unanticipated hospital admission).

Types of complications that occur in ambulatory surgery patients have been documented; several outpatient studies have focused on specific complications that are either common (e.g., nausea and vomiting) or potentially devastating (e.g., hypoxemia).

Nausea and Vomiting
The incidence of postoperative nausea and/or vomiting in the ambulatory setting is considerable (20%–80%) and depends on the patient population.[11,27–29] Postoperative vomiting also delays patient discharge and is a leading cause of unanticipated admission.[15,21,30–32] As a result, several studies have examined the role of different antiemetic regimens in the ambulatory setting. However, postoperative emesis has been difficult to study because of confounding variables, including the type of surgical procedure, anesthetic agents, and patient population. Although various drugs, including droperidol, metoclopramide, hydroxyzine, and prochlorperazine, have been evaluated, one has not emerged as a singularly effective prophylactic antiemetic.

Droperidol has been found to be useful in some circumstances, such as strabismus repair, where it has reduced postoperative vomiting by almost 50%.[33] However, other studies are less convincing. For example, in a study of 150 outpatients scheduled for dilatation and evacuation under general anesthesia, 56% of controls vomited postoperatively as compared with 44% of patients who received intramuscular (IM) droperidol. In contrast, only 10% of patients who received IM hydroxyzine experienced postoperative nausea and vomiting.[27] Young and coworkers found no significant difference in the incidence of postoperative nausea and vomiting among patients receiving droperidol, metoclopramide, and prochlorperazine or placebo in a randomized double-blind prospective trial of 100 healthy women who underwent outpatient bilateral tubal ligation.[29] In patients undergoing dental surgery with general anesthesia, intravenous (IV) droperidol was effective in decreasing nausea and vomiting within the first hour postoperatively.[34] However, patients who received droperidol had greater difficulty with postoperative psychomotor testing. Droperidol also has been associated with prolonged recovery, and there have been two case reports of extrapyramidal reactions, including dystonia and motor restlessness, occurring approximately three hours after outpatients received prophylactic low-dose (0.625 mg IV) droperidol.[27,28,35]

In summary, while several agents have been shown to be useful in controlling postoperative nausea and vomiting for specific groups of ambulatory surgery patients, no antiemetic appears to be universally effective. Although various anesthetics and surgical procedures may contribute to nausea and vomiting in the PACU, other causes for persistent nausea, such as hypotension and pain, should be excluded before therapeutic antiemetics are given.

Hypoxemia

With the advent of pulse oximetry, hypoxia has been found to occur with surprising frequency in the ambulatory setting. Raemer and coworkers studied 108 outpatients having gynecologic surgery and found that moderate intraoperative desaturation (O_2 saturation 85%–90%) occurred in 10% of patients and that severe desaturation (<85%) occurred in 5%.[36] Risk factors for moderate desaturation were nonlaparoscopic gynecologic surgery, obesity, age greater than 35 years, and the lithotomy position. Risk factors for severe intraoperative hypoxemia were obesity and age greater than 35. In the recovery period, postoperative hypoxemia (O_2 saturation < 90%) was more prevalent in inpatients versus outpatients (14% vs. 1%).[37] Risk factors for developing postoperative hypoxemia were advanced ASA physical status, age greater than 40, obesity, lengthy surgical procedure, surgical procedures on body cavities, large intraoperative fluid administration, and breathing room air postoperatively. In another study of hypoxemia in the postoperative period, 4% of 164 female outpatients with normal body habitus who breathed room air upon arrival in the PACU developed O_2 saturations ≤ 90% without clinical signs of hypoxemia.[38] Desaturation occurred between 3 and 32 minutes after arrival in the PACU and was not predictable. Additional data from the ASA closed claims study support the view that the vast majority of preventable mishaps could have been detected earlier with the use of pulse oximetry.[39]

It is clear from the preceding studies that even though outpatients undergo relatively minor surgical procedures, they can and do experience hypoxemia both intraoperatively and postoperatively, often without warning. Consequently, routine use of intraoperative pulse oximetry and postoperative oxygen supplementation are recommended.

Pulmonary Aspiration

Although pulmonary aspiration is a relatively rare occurrence, it represents one of the more serious potential complications in the outpatient setting. Ong and coworkers compared inpatients with outpatients who were having minor surgical procedures and found that outpatients had both a larger gastric volume and a lower pH than inpatients.[40] Furthermore, outpatients who were at highest risk for aspiration (*i.e.*, gastric volume > 25 ml and pH < 2.5) were indistinguishable by age, weight, or duration of fast.

With the suggestion that outpatients may be at higher risk for aspiration than inpatients, different agents that increase gastric pH and lower gastric volume have been investigated. Sodium citrate has been found to be very effective for increasing gastric pH.[41] When given approximately 30 to 90 minutes prior to induction, only 16% of patients had gastric pH lower than 2.5 as compared with 88% of controls. However, sodium citrate also substantially increased the gastric volume; this effect was attenuated with metoclopramide (10 mg IV).

Both cimetidine and ranitidine, when given as a single oral dose approximately five hours preoperatively, have been shown to raise gastric pH among outpatients.[42,43] Because of the prevalence of low gastric pH among outpatients, routine use of H_2 blockers (*e.g.*, cimetidine) has been recommended.[42] However, aspiration of gastric contents is a very infrequent complication, and it has yet to be shown that any of these regimens result in a lower incidence of aspiration.[11,12,26,41,42,44] Furthermore, H_2 antagonists add cost and are associated with a myriad of side-effects such as headache, rash, dizziness, and hepatitis.[45]

Thus it appears that while select groups of ambulatory surgery patients may have a theoretically higher risk of aspiration as demonstrated by lower gastric pH and higher gastric volume, judicious use of sodium citrate and metoclopramide or an H_2 antagonist may be effective in attenuating this risk.

Unanticipated Admission Following Ambulatory Surgery

Although we cannot disregard the incidence of sore throat, pain, bleeding, syncope, arrhythmias, or nausea and vomiting, the singular yardstick in ambulatory surgery by which we can measure the perceived severity of a problem of complication is whether it resulted in the unanticipated admission of the patient into the hospital. Unexpected hospital admission following ambulatory surgery has been used as an index of outpatient morbidity and complications. Depending on statistics reviewed, unanticipated admission rates vary between 0.1% and 5%.[21,46–49] In 1980, the Phoenix Surgicenter reported their overall hospital transfer rate of 0.2% increased to 0.59% for patients over the age of 64 and increased to 1.41% for ASA physical status 3 patients.[50] The most common causes for transfer included bleeding, inadequate pain control, and the need for further elective operation. Most well-organized ambulatory surgery facilities will have a hospitalization rate of less than 1%.[50] However, the rate may be higher in ambulatory centers with a large proportion of geriatric and ASA physical status 3 patients.[51]

Although admission following ambulatory surgery is uncommon, occurring in approximately 1% of patients, nevertheless, it is instructive to examine the risk factors and reasons for admission. Meridy retrospectively studied 1533 ambulatory surgery patients treated between 1979 and 1980.[21] Except for dental procedures, he found no relationship between duration of anesthesia or PACU stay and the need for admission. The admission rate was 2.4%, and all admitted patients received general anesthesia. The most common reasons for admission were nausea and vomiting, postoperative pain, and "errors in [surgical] diagnosis." Patel and Hannallah found that 90 of 10,000 pediatric ambulatory surgery patients required admission.[22] The most common reasons for admission were protracted vomiting, complicated surgery, and croup.

A case-control study by Gold and coworkers examined unanticipated admission following outpatient surgery among 9616 patients at a university hospital and identified several factors that were associated with unanticipated admission.[32] The admission rate was 1%, and factors independently associated with an increased likelihood of admission were general anesthesia, type of procedure (specifically, lower abdominal procedures), lengthy procedures (i.e., lasting longer than one hour), postoperative vomiting, and age (Table 8-1). Physical status was not independently associated with a greater likelihood of admission. The most common reasons for admission were postoperative nausea and vomiting, pain, and bleeding. Among outpatients having eye surgery at another university facility, Freeman and coworkers found that the most common reasons for admission were nausea and vomiting, pain, drowsiness, hypertension, and intraoperative ophthalmic complications.[31] The admission rate was 1.3%. Variables that were independently associated with admission were time of completion of surgery (i.e., late afternoon), higher intraoperative fentanyl dose, and preoperative leukocytosis (WBC > 11,000/mm^3). Factors not associated with admission were age, ASA physical status, screening systolic or diastolic blood pressures, type of ophthalmologic procedure, and type of anesthesia (local vs. monitored anesthesia care vs. general anesthesia).

TABLE 8-1. Multivariate Logistic Regression Analysis of Factors Associated With Admission

Factor	Odds Ratio	95% Confidence Interval
General anesthesia	5.18*	2.60–10.30
Emesis	3.03*	1.35–6.81
Abdominal surgery	2.89*	1.07–7.79
Operating room time >1 h	2.72*	1.46–5.08
Age (30-y intervals)	2.56*	1.32–4.94
Laparoscopy	1.71	0.69–4.22
Drive >1 h	1.49	0.79–2.80

*$p < 0.05$

The preceding data indicate that unanticipated admission is an uncommon event associated with several different factors. However, hospital admission appears to be largely a function of the surgical procedure (i.e., type of surgery, type of anesthesia, length of procedure) rather than underlying patient characteristics (i.e., ASA physical status).

Complications and the Elderly

As more procedures such as cataract extraction are mandated "outpatient procedures," the utilization patterns of ambulatory surgery facilities have increasingly become a function of the type of procedure rather than a function of age.[52] Consequently, many ambulatory facilities are caring for elderly patients, many of whom have clinically important underlying medical problems.

The physiologic and functional vulnerability of elderly patients, especially during the perioperative period, is well-documented.[53,54] However, relatively little is known about the attendant complications experienced by elderly patients who undergo ambulatory surgery. One profile of 100 consecutive cataract patients revealed that their average age was about 75 and 84% had at least one coexisting important medical problem.[55] Hypertension was the most common disorder, occurring in 47% of patients, and atherosclerotic cardiovascular disease occurred in 38% of patients. Perioperative complications among these cataract patients included hypertension, either intraoperatively or postoperatively, postoperative confusion, and cerebrovascular accident.

Although elderly patients would appear at greater risk for perioperative complications compared to younger patients, studies examining discrete complications, such as unanticipated admission, have not found this to be universally true.[53,54] For example, as discussed earlier, a case-control study that included elderly patients who underwent ophthalmologic surgery found that age was not independently associated with unanticipated admission.[31] However, survey data of geriatric patients suggest that age may be a contributor toward unanticipated admission. Octogenarians with coronary disease and arrythmias undergoing cataract surgery with monitored anesthesia care experienced an admission rate of 18%; the ages of admitted patients were significantly greater than those of patients not requiring admission.[55] Wetchler reports an admission rate of 4.6% for patients older than 60 receiving general anesthesia versus 1.4% for their overall patient population at the Methodist Medical Center of Illinois Ambulatory SurgiCare.* While the influence of advanced age on hospital admission is debatable, more investigation is needed to resolve this issue. In addition, the impact of ambulatory anesthesia and surgery on the physiologic and functional status of the elderly remains to be determined.

Pediatric Complications

Ambulatory surgery is well suited for minor procedures in children due to minimal separation from family and home. The pediatric outpatient population pre-

*Wetchler BV. Personal communication, 1989.

sents its own unique set of challenges, but fortunately, major complications have been rare and the majority of events have been relatively minor in nature. Patel and Hannallah examined postanesthesia complications in 10,000 pediatric ambulatory surgery patients between 1983 and 1986.[22] These patients underwent a variety of procedures, including hernia repair, strabismus surgery, myringotomy, adenoidectomy, and dental restorations. The rate of unanticipated hospital admission was 0.9%, and the most common reason for admission was postoperative vomiting, which accounted for 33% of all admissions (Table 8-2). Other common reasons for admission were complicated surgery (17% of admissions), croup (9%), and parental request (7%). Approximately 50% of families were contacted postdischarge, and about a third of those patients complained of various complications that included vomiting, cough, sleepiness, sore throat, fever, and hoarseness.

Children who have upper respiratory tract infections (URI) at the time of surgery have a greater risk of developing perioperative complications. Liu and coworkers prospectively studied 388 patients less than 11 years of age who underwent elective ambulatory surgery during winter months.[57] Of patients with URI symptoms, 31% experienced critical incidents, including laryngospasm, cyanosis, and bradycardia, compared with only 14% of patients without URI symptoms. In addition, one study of younger children (age 1–4 years) who underwent simple otolaryngologic procedures revealed that a greater proportion of children with URI symptoms developed transient hypoxemia postoperatively.[58] In contrast, Tait and coworkers prospectively studied 489 patients with and without URI symptoms who underwent myringotomy.[59] No difference in perioperative complications, which included laryngospasm, arrhythmias, and apnea, was found. However, none of these patients underwent tracheal intubation. Thus, while a consensus is lacking, there is compelling evidence to suggest that children with URI symptoms who undergo even minor outpatient procedures are at greater risk for developing perioperative airway complications.

TABLE 8-2. Reasons for Admission to the Hospital from PACU*

Reason	No. of Patients (%)
Protracted vomiting	30 (33%)
Complicated surgery	15 (17%)
Croup	8 (9%)
Parental request	6 (7%)
Fever	6 (7%)
Bleeding	3 (3%)
Sleepiness	2 (2%)
Others	20 (22%)
TOTAL	90 (100%)

*Overnight hospital admission rate—90 of 10,000 patients (0.9%).
SOURCE: Patel and Hannallah.[22] Used with permission.

Another potential complication, with devastating consequences and of special relevance to pediatric outpatients, is postoperative apnea. Although this particular problem area is discussed in Chapters 4 and 9 (Case 7), its consequences make it worthy of additional review and summary in this section. Preterm infants (*i.e.*, those less than 37 weeks) undergoing minor procedures are known to be particularly vulnerable to this complication.[60] However, what is the optimum age for safely anesthetizing an ex-preterm infant on an outpatient basis? Liu and coworkers prospectively examined 214 infants (173 full-term, 41 preterm) and found that all infants who developed postoperative apnea had a post-conceptual age of less than 41 weeks.[61] In a subsequent study of 47 preterm infants who underwent surgery at less than 60 weeks post-conceptual age, 51% of infants had apneic episodes.[62] These apneic episodes began as early as two hours but as late as 12 hours postoperatively. The risk of postoperative apnea was greater in younger patients, with the greatest risk being among infants less than 42 weeks post-conceptual ages. Of note, there were three ambulatory surgery patients in this study who developed apnea. They were 43, 52, and 54 weeks post-conceptual age, who were otherwise healthy and presented for elective hernia repair. In two patients, apnea occurred in the PACU; however, in one patient, apnea occurred 12 hours postoperatively. In light of these findings, the authors recommend monitoring preterm infants who are less than 60 weeks post-conceptual age for 12 hours postoperatively, which effectively precludes ambulatory surgery. Other studies also have documented postoperative apnea in ex-preterm infants of up to 51 weeks post-conceptual age.[63] Because of the limited number of patients evaluated and differences in study design, the exact "window of vulnerability" is unknown.

Anticipating Complications

Although patient safety is a high priority for every anesthesiologist, complications are bound to occur. Fortunately, several modalities exist for avoiding or at least anticipating complications. These include thorough preoperative evaluation and appropriate patient selection. In the ambulatory setting, the preoperative evaluation process raises unique questions that must be addressed if complications are to be avoided. What is the patient's physiologic *and* functional status? Will patients be able to return home just a few hours after surgery or would they benefit from prolonged postoperative care? What medical benefit would they derive from inpatient care as opposed to outpatient care?

Ambulatory surgery facilities have developed their own styles for preoperative evaluation, and they usually fall into one of three categories. Patients may be evaluated on the day of surgery, which may be convenient. While this may be perfectly suitable for young and healthy patients, evaluating older and chronically ill patients on their way to the operating room can be fraught with problems and delays. A second approach is to have patients complete a screening questionnaire several days to weeks preoperatively, which is then reviewed by the nursing and anesthesia staff. This is then followed up with a telephone interview to verify the questionnaire, give preoperative instructions, and have the patient talk with the anesthesiologist if necessary. With this approach, potential problems can be resolved before the date of surgery. Patel reported an increase in surgery cancellations when comparing patients who were not screened prior to surgery with those who were screened (Table 8-3). At the time of the preanesthesia interview (on day of surgery) there was also a significant increase in the number of unscreened patients whose status was changed to "admit after procedure" (P.M. admission) compared to the prescreened population. The third approach is to have the patient actually visit the ambulatory surgery facility for a preanesthetic evaluation. While this approach is more time-consuming and labor-intensive for both staff and the patient, potential problems can be resolved early and the patient is able to develop a rapport with both the nursing and anesthesia staff. Despite these various styles, there are few data to suggest that any one of these approaches is best or prevents complications. They all have advantages and disadvantages, depending on the patient population and available resources. However, all ambulatory surgery practices, but especially those with complicated, elderly, or high-risk patients, require a consistent and thorough preoperative screening process.

Postdischarge Follow-up

Postdischarge follow-up is necessary to identify untoward events or conditions that occur among ambulatory surgery patients after the acute phase of recovery. Telephone calls and mailed surveys seem to be the most common approaches to postdischarge follow-up. In Patel and Hannallah's study of pediatric patients, nursing staff made telephone calls to parents on the first postoperative day.[22] Parents were asked about specific complications, including vomiting, drowsiness, and fever, as well as other complaints.

Postoperative telephone surveys are commonly used to determine complications among patients enrolled in clinical studies of anesthetic agents and adjuncts. In some studies, 80% to 95% of patients are contacted, particularly when work telephone numbers are requested from patients.[29,64] Mailed questionnaires or personal interviews also may be used to assess postdischarge complications. Shah and coworkers included visits by nurses and personal interviews of parents, administered by a study nurse, in their comparison of inpatient and ambulatory care for children.[10] The nurses assessed postoperative complications, and par-

TABLE 8-3. Outcome of Patients Who Were Screened vs. Those Not Screened by Telephone Interview

	Screened	Unscreened
Surgery completed as scheduled	79%	71%
Surgery postponed	5.4%	6.5%
Surgery canceled*	4.3%	8.2%
Not on final schedule	5.9%	5.3%
Changed to P.M. admission*	0.3%	1.3%

*$p < 0.05$.
SOURCE: Patel RI: Personal communication, 1989.

ents were queried about their attitudes toward inpatient and ambulatory surgical care.

Considering the Approaches

Several factors should be taken into account when assessing biases in approaches to collecting data regarding complications. First, no single approach will capture all the complications occurring among a population of ambulatory surgery patients. Review of records of patients admitted to the hospital following ambulatory surgery will reveal the more serious and acute complications. Review of perioperative records will not include information about postdischarge complications. Similarly, postdischarge surveys will not reveal information about intraoperative complications and are subject to patient availability.

Other factors to consider are the methodologic drawbacks of these approaches to data collection. Patient questionnaires and telephones surveys, for example, have inherent methodologic flaws, including recall and nonresponse biases.[65] *Recall bias* may be described as "selective memory," whereby respondents only recall the events or conditions that stand out in their minds rather than all events. In this context, recall bias may result in gathering information about the most "troublesome" complications (as perceived by the patients) rather than the complete array of complications.

Nonresponse bias occurs when less than 100% of the persons surveyed respond. The impact of nonresponse bias on conclusions drawn from survey data varies depending on the time at which the survey was conducted and the size of the respondent and nonrespondent groups (among other things). Patel and Hannallah, for example, collected postdischarge information from 50% of patients' parents.[22] Results indicate that the postdischarge complication rate was 34.5%. However, a viable hypothesis may be that the overall complication rate actually was much lower; the nonrespondents may have been able to leave home, since all their children were asymptomatic. On the other hand, the total and respondent sample sizes were relatively large (10,000 and 5000, respectively), potentially minimizing any effect of incomplete follow-up.

As long as surgeons perform surgery and anesthesiologists administer anesthesia, complications are a foregone conclusion. Accurate documentation may vary depending on the definition of a complication and the willingness to report complications.

REFERENCES

1. Brown BR Jr: Outpatient Anesthesia. Philadelphia, FA Davis, 1978
2. Williamson DE: The cataract patient: The postoperative regimen. In Brockhurst RJ, Boruchoff SA, Hutchinson BT, et al (eds): Controversy in Ophthalmology. Philadelphia, WB Saunders, 1977
3. Nabatoff RA, Aufses AH: Ambulatory surgery: Experience with 2000 patients. Mt Sinai J Med 46: 354, 1979
4. Robinson JS, Thompson JM, Wood AW: Fire and explosion hazards in operating theatres: A reply and new evidence. Br J Anaesth 51: 908, 1979

5. Tinker JH: Assessment of perioperative risk in patients with myocardial ischemia. 1982 American Society of Anesthesiologists Annual Refresher Course Lectures. Las Vegas, Nev., October 22–26, 1982

6. Tarhan S, Moffitt EA, Taylor WF, et al: Myocardial infarction after general anesthesia. JAMA 239: 2566, 1978

7. Mahar LJ, Steen PA, Tinker JH, et al: Perioperative myocardial infarction in patients with coronary artery disease with and without aorta-coronary artery bypass grafts. J Thorac Cardiovasc Surg 26: 533, 1978

8. Backer CL, Tinker JH, Robertson DM, et al: Myocardial reinfarction following local anesthesia for ophthalmic surgery. Anesth Analg 59: 257, 1980

9. Olson MD: Legal issues. Same Day Surg 8: 26, 1984

10. Shah CP, Robinson GC, Kinnis C, Davenport HT: Day care surgery for children: A controlled study of medical complications and parental attitudes. Med Care 10: 437, 1972

11. Natof HE: Complications associated with ambulatory surgery. JAMA 244: 1116, 1980

12. Federated Ambulatory Surgery Association: FASA Special Study I. Alexandria, Va., FASA, 1986

13. Natof HE: Complications. In Wetchler BV (ed): Anesthesia for Ambulatory Surgery. Philadelphia, JB Lippincott, 1985

14. Levy M-L: Complications: Prevention and quality assurance. Anesthesiology Clin North Am 5: 137, 1987

15. Metter SE, Kitz DS, Young ML, et al: Nausea and vomiting after outpatient laparoscopy: Incidence, impact on recovery room stay cost (abstr). Anesth Analg (66: S116, 1987

16. Orkin FK: Risk management and quality assurance in outpatient anesthesia care. Risk Management Quality Assurance 2: 152, 1988

17. American Society of Anesthesiologists: Peer Review in Anesthesiology. Park Ridge, Ill., American Society of Anesthesiologists, 1988

18. Joint Commission on Accreditation of Healthcare Organizations: Monitoring and evaluation: Anesthetic services. Chicago, Ill., JCAHO, 1987

19. Joint Commission on Accreditation of Healthcare Organizations: Ambulatory Health Care Standards Manual. Chicago, Ill., JCAHO, 1988

20. Pataky AO, Kitz DS, Andrews RW, Lecky JH: Nausea and vomiting following ambulatory surgery: Are all procedures created equal? Anesth Analg 67: S163, 1988

21. Meridy HW: Criteria for selection of ambulatory surgical patients and guidelines for anesthetic management: A retrospective study of 1553 cases. Anesth Analg 61: 921, 1982

22. Patel RI, Hannallah RS: Anesthetic complications following pediatric ambulatory surgery. A 3-year study. Anesthesiology 69: 1009, 1988

23. Hines RL, Barash PG, Dubow H, et al: Ambulatory surgical complication in the postoperative period: We can't just walk away (abstr). Anesth Analg 68: S122, 1989

24. Cohen MM, Duncan PG, Tate RB: Does anesthesia contribute to operative mortality? JAMA 260: 2859, 1988

25. Cohen MM, Duncan PG: Physical status score and trends in anesthetic complications. J Clin Epidemiol 41: 83, 1988

26. Brindle GF, Soliman MG: Anaesthetic complications in surgical outpatients. Can Anaesth Soc J 22: 613, 1975

27. McKenzie R, Wadhwa RK, Uy NTL, et al: Antiemetic effectiveness of intramuscular hydroxyzine compared with intramuscular droperidol. Anesth Analg 60: 783, 1981

28. Cohen SE, Woods WA, Wyner J: Antiemetic efficacy of droperidol and metoclopramide. Anesthesiology 60: 67, 1984

29. Young ML, Kitz DS, Andrews R, et al: Efficacy of antiemetic prophylaxis in patients receiving general anesthesia for outpatient surgery. Anesthesiology 69: A449, 1988

30. Pandit SK, Kothary SP, Pandit U, et al: Antiemetic effect of oral metoclopromide vs. intravenous droperidol for outpatient laparoscopic procedures. Anesthesiology 67: A425, 1987

31. Freeman LN, Schachat AP, Manolio TA, et al: Multivariate analysis of factors associated with unplanned admission in "outpatient" ophthalmic surgery. Ophthal Surg 19: 719, 1988

32. Gold B, Kitz DS, Lecky JH, et al: Unanticipated admission to the hospital following ambulatory surgery. JAMA Vol. 262 p. 3008–3010, 1989

33. Abramowitz MD, Oh TH, Epstein BS, et al: The antiemetic effect of droperidol following outpatient strabismus surgery in children. Anesthesiology 59: 579, 1983

34. Valanne J, Korttila K: Effect of a small dose of droperidol on nausea, vomiting and recovery after outpatient enflurane anaesthesia. Acta Anaesthesiol Scand 29: 359, 1985

35. Melnick BM: Extrapyramidal reactions to low dose droperidol. Anesthesiology 69: 424, 1988

36. Raemer DB, Warren DL, Morris R, et al: Hypoxemia during ambulatory gynecologic surgery as evaluated by the pulse oximeter. J Clin Monit 3: 244, 1987

37. Morris RW, Buschman A, Warren DL, et al: The prevalence of hypoxemia detected by pulse oximetry during recovery from anesthesia. J Clin Monit 4: 16, 1988

38. Murray RS, Raemer DB, Morris RW: Supplemental oxygen after ambulatory surgical procedures. Anesth Analg 67: 967, 1988

39. Dull DL, Tinker JH, Caplan RA, et al: ASA closed claims study: Can pulse oximetry and capnometry prevent anesthetic mishaps? Anesth Analg 68: S74, 1989

40. Ong BY, Palahniuk RJ, Cumming M: Gastric volume and pH in outpatients. Canad Anaesth Soc J 25: 36, 1978

41. Manchikanti L, Grow JB, Colliver JA, et al: Bicitra (sodium citrate) and metoclopramide in outpatient and anesthesia for prophylaxis against aspiration pneumonitis. Anesthesiology 63: 378, 1985

42. Manchikanti L, Roush RJ: Effect of preanesthetic glycopyrrolate and cimetidine on gastric fluid pH and volume in outpatients. Anesth Analg 63: 40, 1984

43. Gonzalez ER, Butler SA, Jones MK, et al: Cimetidine versus ranitidine: Single-dose, oral regimen for reducing gastric acidity and volume in ambulatory surgery patients. Drug Intell Clin Pharm 21: 192, 1987

44. Miller CD, Anderson WG: Silent regurgitation in day case gynaecological patients. Anaesthesia 43: 321, 1988

45. Physicians Desk Reference, 42d ed, pp 1026, 1380, 2031. Oradell, N.J., Medical Economics Co., Inc, 1988

46. Ahlgren EW: Pediatric outpatient anesthesia. Am J Dis Child 126: 36, 1973

47. Coakley CS, Levy ML: Anesthesia for ambulatory surgery. J Ark Med Soc 68: 101, 1971

48. Caldamone AA, Rabinowitz R: Outpatient orchiopexy. J Urol 127: 286, 1982

49. Patterson JF, Bechtoldt AA, Levin KJ: Ambulatory surgery in a university setting. JAMA 235: 266, 1976

50. Dawson B, Reed WA: Anaesthesia for adult surgical outpatients. Can Anaesth Soc J 27: 409, 1980

51. White PF: Outpatient anesthesia. In Miller RD (ed): Anesthesia, pp 1895–1919. New York, Churchill-Livingstone, 1986

52. Lagoe RJ, Bice SE, Abulencia PB: Ambulatory surgery utilization by age level. Am J Public Health 77: 33, 1987

53. Galazka SS: Preoperative evaluation of the elderly surgical patient. J Fam Pract 27: 622, 1988

54. Johnson JC: Surgery in the elderly. In Goldmann DR (ed): Medical Care of the Surgical Patient, pp 578–590. Philadelphia, JB Lippincott, 1982

55. Fisher SJ, Cunningham RD: The medical profile of cataract patients. Geriatr Clin North Am 1: 339, 1985

56. Kareti RKP, Callahan H, Draper GA: Factors leading to hospital admission of elderly patients following outpatient eye surgery: A medicare dilemma. Anesth Analg 68: S144, 1989

57. Liu LMP, Ryan JF, Coté CJ, et al: Influence of upper respiratory infection on critical incidents in children during anesthesia. Presented at the 9th World Congress of Anaesthesiologists, Abstract No. AO786, 1988

58. DeSoto H, Patel RI, Soliman IE, et al: Changes in oxygen saturation following general anesthesia in children with upper respiratory infection signs and symptoms undergoing otolaryngological procedures. Anesthesiology 68: 276, 1988

59. Tait AR, Knight PR: The effects of general anesthesia on upper respiratory tract infections in children. Anesthesiology 67: 930, 1987

60. Steward DJ: Preterm infants are more prone to complications following minor surgery than are term infants. Anesthesiology 56: 304, 1982

61. Liu LMP, Coté CJ, Goudsouzian NG, et al: Life-threatening apnea in infants recovering from anesthesia. Anesthesiology 59: 506, 1983

62. Kurth CD, Spitzer AR, Broennle AM, et al: Postoperative apnea in preterm infants. Anesthesiology 66: 483, 1987

63. Malviya S, Swartz J, Lerman J: Are all preterm infants less than 60 weeks post-conceptual age at risk for postoperative apnea? Anesth Analg 68: S177, 1989

64. Lecky JH, Kitz DS, Andrews RW, et al: Alfentanyl vs. isoflurane in outpatient laparoscopy: An evaluation of morbidity and cost (abstr). Anesth Analg 68: S158, 1989

65. Abramson JH: Survey Methods in Community Medicine: An Introduction to Epidomiological and Evaluative Studies, 3rd ed. New York, Churchill-Livingstone, 1984

In the Real World

9

HARRY C. WONG, CYNTHIA ALEXANDER NKANA

The patients discussed in this chapter are actual cases that have been seen in ambulatory surgery facilities in the United States. The discussion and responses are not meant to establish standards of care, but rather to present individual methods of management. In certain case presentations, the opinions of the discussant and the respondent differ. These differences may involve anesthetic management or the question of whether the patient is an acceptable candidate for an ambulatory surgical procedure. We are not attempting to establish a correct approach; we are hoping our readers will consider these cases in the light of how they might apply to their own local setting. In addition, this chapter highlights some of the different approaches required by ambulatory surgery patients that may necessitate changes in our practice patterns.

▪ CASE REPORT NO. 1
A 2-year-old girl is scheduled for a hernia repair. The mother states that approximately 20 years ago the child's grandfather died while under anesthesia for a minor surgical procedure. At that time, his temperature increased to 104°F. There is also a history of the mother's brother having a "near death" under anesthesia with a temperature rise during the anesthetic procedure. Neither parent has been exposed to an anesthetic agent. The child has no history of orthopedic problems, and laboratory studies, including creatinine phosphokinase (CPK) levels, are in the normal range.

475

Discussion
Frederic A. Berry, M.D.
Professor of Anesthesiology and Pediatrics, University of Virginia Health Science Center, Charlottesville, Virginia

The most important question in this case is where should patients who are malignant hyperthermia–susceptible be managed? If the answer is in a routine hospital setting rather than an ambulatory surgical center, then this discussion is finished. However, there are those who hold the opinion that as long as trigger-free anesthetics are administered, the surgery can be performed safely in an ambulatory surgery setting. A *trigger-free anesthetic* is an anesthetic that avoids the use of volatile anesthetics or succinylcholine. The next issue to be addressed would be if a patient with malignant hyperthermia (MH) susceptibility is anesthetized in an ambulatory care facility, then (1) should ABGs and/or end-tidal CO_2 determinations be available for immediate diagnosis and (2) should dantrolene be immediately available on the premises? The answers to these questions are not easy, since in many ambulatory centers there is no blood gas machine. Sending samples to another facility may delay the results. This raises the question of whether or not end-tidal CO_2 sampling is sufficient to make a diagnosis of MH. When the minute ventilation is controlled and remains essentially the same, a rising end-tidal CO_2 would indicate a hypermetabolic state and the diagnosis would be MH.

The other concern is the immediate availability of dantrolene. Apparently, there are a great number of ambulatory surgery centers in the United States that do not have dantrolene immediately available. If dantrolene were not available, then I would not give an anesthetic to any patient, much less this patient who has MH susceptibility.

If the decision were made to proceed with surgery—and there are those clinicians who would hold such an opinion—then the induction technique would be either with rectal methohexital, intravenous barbiturate, or intramuscular ketamine. The maintenance of anesthesia would be with some form of a nitrous oxide, narcotic technique with a nondepolarizing muscle relaxant. This patient would be a good candidate for either supplemental ilioinguinal/iliohypogastric nerve block or a caudal anesthetic. Either of these techniques would reduce the anesthetic requirement as well as the muscle-relaxant requirement and provide the patient with a smooth postoperative period of analgesia. In addition, I would avoid the use of the nondepolarizing muscle relaxant pancuronium because the vagolytic and sympathomimetic properties of this drug will cause a tachycardia that may add to the diagnostic confusion, since tachycardia is an early sign of MH.

There is no apparent benefit to the prophylactic administration of dantrolene. The issue has been well studied, and there is no indication for the preoperative administration of dantrolene. Another issue is whether or not at the time of hernia repair a muscle biopsy should be performed for MH. However, the consensus at the present time is that muscle biopsies for MH should not be performed on children under the age of 5.

The final issue is postoperative observation. In the study reported earlier, in which there were no instances of an episode of MH in a large group of MH-susceptible patients who were anesthetized with a trigger-free anesthetic, four of the 965 patients had an MH episode in the PACU, one of which was treated with dantrolene. It is hard to tell exactly from this study the significance of the episode and whether or not it would have cleared with the same conservative management that was used to treat the others. In summary, it would appear that although the majority of clinicians would operate on this patient in a routine hospital setting, there are some that would do the procedure in an ambulatory surgery center but with certain backups, such as (1) blood gas and end-tidal CO_2 monitoring and (2) dantrolene. The occurrence of postoperative MH episodes in patients in whom a trigger-free anesthetic was used is somewhat bothersome. As we gain more experience with this disease and are able to diagnose it more accurately, then perhaps some of these clinical conundrums can be answered.

SUGGESTED READINGS

1. Ryan CA, Al-Ghamdi AS, Gayle M, Finer NN: Osteogenesis imperfecta and hyperthermia. Anesth Analg 68: 811, 1989
2. Berry FA, Lynch C III: Succinylcholine and trismus. Anesthesiology 70: 161, 1989
3. Rosenberg H. Management of patient in whom trismus occurs following succinylcholine (reply to letter). Anesthesiology 68: 654, 1988
4. Gronert GA: Management of patient in whom trismus occurs following succinylcholine (letter). Anesthesiology 68: 653, 1988
5. Van Der Spek AFL, Fang WB, Ashton-Miller JA, Stohler CS, Carlson DS, Schork MA: Increased masticatory muscle stiffness during limb muscle flaccidity associated with succinylcholine administration. Anesthesiology 69: 11, 1988
6. Van Der Spek AFL, Fang WB, Ashton-Miller JA, Stohler CS, Carlson DS, Schork MA: The effects of succinylcholine on mouth opening. Anesthesiology 67: 459, 1987
7. Hein HAT, Roeur N, Jantzen J-P: Malignant hyperthermia: Are we really prepared? (letter). Anesthesiology 66: 448, 1987

Response
Eugene H. Flewellen, M.D.
Trinity Anesthesiology Associates, Carrollton, Texas

Contrasted with the early 1960s when malignant hyperthermia (MH) was first described, most present-day clinicians possess sufficient knowledge of the syndrome to feel comfortable in the management of these patients. I concur with Dr. Berry that the ambulatory surgery center is an appropriate setting for anesthetizing the MH-suspect patient, provided that capnography and access to dantrolene are ensured.

Capnography allows a continuous evaluation of the metabolic state when alveolar ventilation remains constant and provides an early diagnostic tool. Arterial blood gas analysis provides diagnostic support but should not be considered mandatory before reaching the MH diagnosis or instituting therapy.

Dantrolene sodium has been firmly established as a therapeutic agent for MH. Therapy should begin immediately after diagnosis, since promptness is the key to successful outcome. I begin treatment with a dose of 2.5 mg/kg IV and have sufficient drug available to administer 10 mg/kg.

The role of dantrolene MH prophylaxis is less well established. I prefer the intravenous route just prior to induction rather than oral dosing to avoid the potential gastrointestinal side-effects and to better ensure sufficient drug blood level. Dantrolene prophylactic dosing varies between 1 and 2.5 mg/kg depending on the degree of suspicion of MH propensity and the magnitude of the proposed surgical procedure. The study cited by Dr. Berry was not designed to assess efficacy of prophylactic dantrolene. I would be more likely to employ prophylaxis in the ambulatory rather than the hospital setting. I do not administer prophylaxis before brief (<30 min) or minor noncavitary procedures.

The value of halothane-caffeine muscle contracture testing remains controversial. Proponents of testing are now addressing diagnostic accuracy issues, which in the past have made most clinicians skeptical of the negative test result. Hopefully, proponents will be persuasive in gaining credibility for the negatively diagnosed patient, allowing for better counseling of families and routine anesthetic management.

The safe duration of postanesthetic observation has not been examined scientifically. I cautiously discharge the suspect patient after 4 to 6 hours provided that no evidence of MH has arisen. The responsible party should be informed of the early signs of MH, have the ability to communicate with a physician, and have the means to expeditiously transport the patient back to a medical facility.

CASE REPORT NO. 2

A 24-year-old woman, ASA physical status 1, is having a McDonald's cerclage under epidural anesthesia. The epidural block was performed with an 18-gauge Tuohy needle, and a "wet tap" occurred. The needle was withdrawn, and a satisfactory epidural was performed one interspace higher. Prior to discharge to home care, what measures could the anesthesiologist undertake to decrease the possibility of postdural puncture headache?

Discussion
Cynthia Alexander Nkana, M.D.
Clinical Instructor of Anesthesia, University of Illinois College of Medicine at Peoria; Associate Medical Director, Ambulatory SurgiCare, The Methodist Medical Center of Illinois, Peoria, Illinois

Headache is the most common problem following dural puncture and provides much frustration for the patient and anesthesiologist. Its incidence has been reported to be between 2% and 36% after spinal anesthesia using 25- to 22-gauge needles,[1] up to 76% after myelography, and between 24% and 80% after accidental dural puncture using an 18- to 16-gauge needle.[2]

Pregnant patients have a slightly higher overall incidence of postdural puncture headache (PDPH) than nonpregnant patients. The onset of PDPH usually occurs 24 to 48 hours following the dural puncture; in some cases, it may appear sooner, particularly when a large-gauge needle was used, as is commonly the case for epidural procedures.

The etiology of PDPH is thought to be secondary to leakage of cerebrospinal fluid through the dural puncture site into the epidural space with descent of the medulla and pons in the cranial cavity in the upright position resulting in postural headache. A second theory proposes that the decline in quantity and pressure of cerebrospinal fluid causes compensatory dilatation of the cerebral vasculature. These dilated cerebral vessels actually produce the characteristic "upright" headache.

In response to these two theories, treatment to prevent PDPH has centered around maintaining cerebrospinal fluid pressure. Crawford advocated the infusion of normal saline into the epidural space following dural puncture.[3] Injection or infusion of fluid into the epidural space to reduce the pressure differential across the site of the dural puncture and lessen the rate of fluid loss was associated with a pressure increase only lasting a few minutes. Rice and Dabbs[4] repeated the use of epidural injections of saline for the treatment of postdural puncture headaches but obtained only temporary relief. Saline injection (60 ml + 60 ml over a 24-hr period) or continuous infusion (1.5 L over 24 hrs) prophylactically by means of an epidural catheter reduced the incidence of PDPH. The number of patients was small in these two studies.

In response to the second theory, caffeine benzoate infusion has gained acceptance to treat PDPH.[5] Caffeine benzoate causes constriction of cerebral vessels. Jarvis and coworkers have shown that 80% of patients infused with 1 L D_5 lactated Ringer's solution containing caffeine benzoate (500 mg) followed by an additional infusion of 1 L D_5 lactated Ringer's solution resulted in significant improvement of symptoms.[5]

Technique appears to decrease the incidence of PDPH. Orienting the bevel of a 22- or 25-gauge needle parallel to the longitudinal dural fibers significantly diminishes the incidence of headache following subarachnoid anesthesia.[6] Norris and coworkers addressed the relationship between headache and needle bevel orientation following dural puncture with 17- and 18-gauge needles.[7] Of 1558 women who received epidural anesthesia for labor, the overall incidence of dural puncture was 2.6%. Seventy-three percent of the parturients in whom dural puncture occurred with a needle bevel perpendicular to dural fibers developed moderate to severe headaches, whereas only 31% did so with a parallel needle orientation. A potential drawback of the parallel insertion technique is the need to rotate the needle bevel 90 degrees after identifying the epidural space. Experts differ as to the advisability of this maneuver, since it may actually increase the risk of a dural puncture.[8]

Of all the modalities used to treat postdural puncture headache, none is as effective as the epidural blood patch. Once attempts have been made to hydrate the patient, encourage bed rest, and "wait and see" if a headache develops, the epidural blood patch is the next modality of treatment. Crawford[9] and Loeser[10] advise against using the epidural blood patch as a prophylactic measure. In many patients it is unnecessary, and there is evidence of a high failure rate when it is done soon after the dural puncture. This is presently being reassessed by Dr. Pietro Colonna-Romano. In evaluating 33 patients who had a dural puncture with a 17-gauge Touhy needle, Dr. Colonna-Romano found that those patients who prophylactically received an epidural blood patch (15 ml autologous blood) through the epidural catheter had a PDPH incidence of 18%. This was in contrast to a 77% incidence of PDPH in parturients who received only conservative therapy (i.e., hydration, bed rest, minor analgesics). "The potential for morbidity is small, and if a small percent of patients can be spared the onset of a postdural headache, it is worth proceeding at the time of the epidural procedure."* With an epidural blood patch, it is necessary to emphasize to patients the importance of avoiding Valsalva maneuvers (bending, lifting, or straining) in order to prevent patch "blowout." Mulroy and associates have demonstrated that postlumbar puncture headaches occur three to four times more frequently in outpatients than in inpatients who receive spinal anesthesia under similar conditions.[11] Is this related to early ambulation?

Presented with this patient, my approach would be conservative—hydration, bed rest, and diligent follow-up. The epidural catheter would not be removed, however, until the patient was ready for discharge. If symptoms of a PDPH appeared prior to discharge, I would perform an epidural blood patch through the catheter using 15 ml autologous blood and then proceed with conservative therapy. If symptoms appeared later (after 24 hrs), an epidural blood patch should be performed quickly on an outpatient basis. More than 90% of patients respond to one epidural blood patch.

REFERENCES

1. Harrison LM, Harmel MH: The comparative incidence of postlumbar puncture headache following spinal anesthesia administered through a 20 and 24 gauge needle. Anesthesiology 14: 390, 1953
2. Brownridge P: The management of headache following accidental dural puncture in obstetric patients. Anaesth Intensive Care 11: 4, 1983
3. Crawford JS: Prevention of headache consequent upon dural puncture. Br J Anaesth 44: 598, 1972
4. Rice GG, Dabbs HC: The use of peridural and subarachnoid injection of saline solution in the treatment of severe postspinal headache. Anesthesiology 11: 17, 1950
5. Jarvis AP, Greenawalt JW, Fagraeush: Intravenous caffeine for postdural puncture headache. Reg Anesth 11: 42, 1986
6. Mihic DN: Postspinal headache in relationship of needle bevel to a longitudinal dural fibers. Reg Anesth 10: 76, 1985
7. Norris M, Leighton B, DeSimone C: Needle bevel direction in headache after inadvertent dural puncture. Anesthesiology 70: 729, 1989
8. Meiklejohn BH: The effect of rotation of an epidural needle. Anaesthesia 42: 1180, 1987
9. Crawford JS: Experience with epidural blood patch. Anaesthesia 35: 513, 1980
10. Loeser, EA, Hill GE: Time vs. success rate for epidural blood patch. Anesthesiology 2: 147, 1978
11. Anesthesiol News 15(7): 1989

*Colonna-Romano P: Personal communication, 1989.

Response*

The occurrence of a "wet tap" when attempting an epidural is a problem everyone will face if they do many epidural anesthesias. Dr. Alexander Nkana has presented a good discussion of the etiology and the debate of the methods to reduce the incidence of postspinal headaches. However, in this specific case (*i.e.*, a dural puncture, an 18-gauge Tuohy needle, a young woman), the patient would have a 50% or greater chance of developing a PDPH.[1,2] I would explain these facts and the potential incidence of problems related to PDPH that may occur at home and explain the treatment option of epidural blood patch to the patient. While there is controversy on the use of prophylactic epidural blood patches, considering the high potential for headache occurring in this patient, I would recommend a prophylactic blood patch before discharge and provide written discharge instructions warning against straining, bending, and lifting to prevent possible patch "blowout."

REFERENCES

1. Mulroy MF: Spinal headaches: Management and avoidance. In Brown DL (ed): Problems in Anesthesia. Philadelphia, JB Lippincott, 1987
2. Mulroy MF: Regional anesthesia: When, why, why not? In Wetchler BV (ed): Problems in Anesthesia. Philadelphia, JB Lippincott, 1988

▧ CASE REPORT NO. 3

A 5-ft, 3-in, 148.6-kg woman is scheduled for a D&C for postmenopausal bleeding. The procedure was attempted in the gynecologist's office, but the cervix could not be visualized and the patient was unable to lie in the supine position. The patient is a hypertensive who is well controlled with medications. What preoperative investigations would you require for this patient, and how would the perioperative anesthesia management be handled. Is this an acceptable candidate for an ambulatory facility?

Discussion

Susan L. Polk, M.D., M.S.Ed.
Assistant Professor, Chief, Section on Education, University of Chicago, Department of Anesthesia and Critical Care, Chicago, Illinois

Is This Patient Morbidly Obese?

Morbid obesity is defined as being twice the ideal body weight (height in centimeters minus 100 = ideal body weight in kilograms) or having a body mass index (weight in kilograms divided by height in meters squared) greater than 30.[1] This patient more than qualifies using both formulas. The definition is important from a risk-assessment standpoint because morbidly obese patients have a perioperative mortality rate twice to three times that of the normal population. There is

*Uncredited responses are by Dr. Wong and/or Dr. Alexander Nkana.

a long list of conditions commonly associated with morbid obesity that should guide the preoperative evaluation and help to plan the ensuing anesthetic.[2]

Medical Conditions Associated with Morbid Obesity

PULMONARY. Morbidly obese patients have an increased oxygen requirement and increased carbon dioxide production because of the large mass of tissue that must be served, and because their reduced compliance results in an increased work of breathing. At the same time, their ventilation is inefficient because of the decreased functional residual capacity leading to a ventilation-perfusion mismatch. They are usually hypoxemic, and as the disease progresses, they become polycythemic and hypercarbic and eventually develop pulmonary hypertension and right-sided heart failure. Many obese patients suffer from periodic alveolar hypoventilation (obstructive and central sleep apnea), which leads to exquisite sensitivity to respiratory depressant drugs. Pickwickian syndrome is seen in 5% to 10% of morbidly obese patients late in the course of the disease and is characterized by hypoxemia and hypercarbia at rest, persistent acidosis, episodic somnolence, biventricular failure, and an inability to ventilate when lying down.

CARDIAC. Morbidly obese patients have an increased circulating blood volume and hence increased cardiac output. Systemic hypertension (systolic > 150 mmHg or diastolic > 90 mmHg) occurs in about 60% of otherwise healthy morbidly obese patients. Combined with the pulmonary hypertension due to chronic hypoxemia, these factors lead to biventricular enlargement and eventually failure. Ischemic heart disease is common, as is vascular disease.

OTHER ASSOCIATED DISEASES. Morbidly obese patients are at a high risk for hiatal hernia, insulin-resistant diabetes, and liver dysfunction, which may not be evident in routine screening tests but which alters the metabolism and excretion of drugs. Hypercoagulability has been shown to be prevalent in this population.[3] Finally, there is a high incidence of psychological problems that may contribute to prolonged recovery period with inactivity after surgery.

Assessing the Risks of Anesthesia and Surgery in This Patient

This patient is hypertensive and could not lie down when the D&C was attempted under local anesthesia. We already suspect there is an element of cardiac disease because of the presence of hypertension, and now we must determine if the inability to tolerate the supine position indicates upper airway obstruction, circulatory failure, or simply a further reduced pulmonary compliance. The preoperative assessment must begin with a thorough medical history, which includes a search for signs and symptoms of both obstructive and central sleep apnea, of congestive heart failure, and of ischemic heart disease. It is prudent to assume that there is a significant deficit in hepatic function, which would result in altered metabolism and clearance of many anesthetics and adjuncts.[4] Patients with sleep apnea of moderate duration develop a central component that results in depression of the central respiratory drive, especially while unconscious and most especially in the presence of even very small amounts of sedatives, narcotics, or anesthetic agents.[5]

I would obtain a hemoglobin and hematocrit in order to assess polycythemia or anemia; an ECG and chest x-ray to assess cardiac status, the pulmonary circulation, and the degree of restrictive disease; an arterial blood gas to determine the baseline; and a fasting glucose to rule out diabetes. If there is evidence of chronic hypoxemia and hypercarbia on blood gasses, pulmonary function tests should probably be evaluated as well. The presence of arrhythmias, congestive failure, or myocardial ischemia would require a more intensive cardiac workup under the direction of a cardiologist in order to stabilize and treat the condition as much as possible prior to anesthesia, as well as to aid the anesthesiologist in planning anesthetic technique and monitoring. Coagulation studies should be obtained, since liver disease may cause a reversible coagulopathy that could contribute to the morbidity of the procedure. Hypercoagulability requires that prophylaxis for venous thrombosis be instituted prior to surgery and continued until full ambulation is achieved, since thromboembolic phenomena are the leading cause of postoperative mortality in the morbidly obese patient.

Can This Procedure Be Done in an Outpatient Unit?

A D&C is a minor procedure, but there are no minor anesthetics in morbidly obese patients. This patient needs general anesthesia, an endotracheal tube, controlled ventilation, and, arguably, invasive monitoring. A regional anesthetic would most likely not be possible for her, because she would not tolerate the lithotomy position with spontaneous ventilation. Paul and coworkers documented that in otherwise normal morbidly obese patients who were awake and unsedated, change from the sitting to the supine position resulted in the following physiologic changes: 17.9% increase in A-V oxygen difference, 11% increase in oxygen consumption, 17.7% increase in venous admixture, 35.5% increase in cardiac output, 35.8% increase in cardiac index, 31% increase in mean pulmonary artery pressure, 44% increase in pulmonary artery occlusion pressure, 21.5% decrease in peripheral resistance, 6% decrease in heart rate, and no change in (A-a) D_{O_2}, respiratory rate, or mean arterial blood pressure.[6] Not only is this patient at risk for ventilatory insufficiency, but if her heart proves to be at all compromised, she is likely to go into acute pulmonary edema, ventricular fibrillation, and die, simply because of her positioning.

Under what conditions could this procedure be done in an ambulatory unit? If her heart were found to be normal, her blood pressure well controlled, her blood gases normal for her age, she were either not diabetic or in good control, and her coagulation status normal, this patient could be discharged after awakening and becoming fully ambulatory. However, I would have to be satisfied that she was motivated enough to remain ambulatory at home and that an informed observer would pay close attention to her so that she would maintain a semirecumbent position and not go to sleep and stop breathing.

Findings that would lead me to suggest hospitalization would include any element of congestive failure, chronic hypercarbia, or hypoxemia; signs of liver dysfunction; and evidence of hypercoagulability. I believe that the presence of any degree of hypoxemia beyond that expected for her age would preclude her being anesthetized as an outpatient. Vaughan and coworkers reported that in otherwise normal morbidly obese patients after abdominal surgery, Pa_{O_2} fell continuously through the second postoperative day to a low of about 20 mmHg below baseline and did not return to normal for a week.[7] Even though a D&C does not result in the pulmonary dysfunction that abdominal surgery does, I would still not be comfortable sending this patient home until I documented that she was not becoming more hypoxic, at least through the first night.

Could the patient breathe adequately in the postoperative period? The need for postoperative mechanical ventilation has been associated with (among other things) age greater than 50 years, cardiac disease, CO_2 retention, and uncooperativeness.[8] While most anesthesiologists avoid postoperative mechanical ventilation whenever possible, it is commonly required in the presence of prolonged sedation and obesity, whether or not central sleep apnea is present. Prolonged sedation can be expected in morbidly obese patients because of their increased fat content as well as their hepatic dysfunction. Maintaining the sitting position contributes to adequate ventilation, and administration of supplemental oxygen is an absolute requirement until proven otherwise.

Risk factors for thromboembolic phenomena include increased pulmonary blood volume, polycythemia, hypercoagulability, and prolonged immobilization. Prophylaxis requires activity, even passive in the critically ill, as well as intravenous dextran and subcutaneous heparin, which should be continued until the patient is fully ambulatory.

In conclusion, this patient is at great risk for postoperative morbidity involving cardiac function, ventilation, oxygenation, and thromboembolism. A few hours of monitoring might not be adequate, especially in view of her age and her previous experience with the attempt under local anesthesia. Only under the most favorable circumstances could she be expected to recuperate at home without constant observation and support.

REFERENCES

1. Vaughan RW: Definitions and risks of Obesity. In Brown BR (ed): Anesthesia and the Obese Patient, pp 1–7. Philadelphia, FA Davis, 1982
2. Vaughan RW: Anesthetic management of the morbidly obese patient. IARS 1987 Refresher Course Lectures, 11–18
3. Kakkar VV, Howe CT, Nicholaides AN, et al: Deep vein thrombosis: Is there a "high risk" group? Ann Surg 120: 527, 1970
4. Weinstein JA, Matteo RS, Ornstein E, et al: Pharmacodynamics of vecuronium and atracurium in the obese patient. Anesth Analg 67: 1149, 1988
5. Sullivan CE, Issa FG, Berthon-Jones M, Saunders NA: Pathophysiology of sleep apnea. In Saunders NA, Sullivan CE (eds): Sleep and Breathing, p 325. New York, Marcel Dekker, 1984
6. Paul DR, Hoyt JL, Boutros AR: Cardiovascular and respiratory changes in response to change of posture in the very obese. Anesthesiology 45: 73, 1976
7. Vaughan RW, Engelhardt RC, Wise L: Postoperative hypoxemia in obese patients. Ann Surg 180: 877, 1976
8. Vaughan RW, Wise L: Choice of abdominal incision in the obese patient. Ann Surg 120: 527, 1975

Response

The morbidly obese patient is always a challenging problem for the anesthesiologist. Despite the pressures from the payors of health care, we must continue to exercise our best medical judgment for the safety of each individual patient. The patient with significant concurrent health problems may require hospitalization even for minor surgical procedures.[1] Dr. Polk has outlined an excellent approach in the preanesthesia evaluation of this patient. The decision whether to perform this patient's operation in an ambulatory surgery unit may depend on the facility's support and location. This patient should probably be cared for only in a unit that has immediate access to blood gas analysis if her baseline blood gases and pulmonary functions are abnormal. It also would be recommended that the patient and family be informed that because of her obesity and potential pulmonary problems, she would be scheduled as a possible admission following surgery, but should she do extremely well and is motivated to go home, she might be able to be discharged on the day of surgery. This is a better psychological approach than to schedule this patient as an outpatient and then require admission if the patient's postanesthesia parameters are not adequate for discharge.

In reference to anesthesia technique, I would consider a regional technique only if the patient were agreeable and bony landmarks were palpable. If general anesthesia is to be used for such a short operative procedure, it would be difficult to justify the cost-benefit ratio of invasive lines, which could add risk and prolong the procedure. It would be my recommendation that the duration of general anesthesia be kept as short as possible (position and prep prior to IV induction) using primarily inhalation anesthesia and avoiding paralysis (increased changes in ventilation-perfusion mismatch that occur with paralysis) unless absolutely necessary.[2]

REFERENCES

1. Jensen S, Wetchler BV: The obese patient: An acceptable candidate for outpatient anesthesia. J Am Assoc Nurse Anesth 50: 369, 1982
2. Froese AB, Bryon AC: Effect of anesthesia and paralysis on diaphragmatic mechanics in man. Anesthesiology 41: 3, 1974

CASE REPORT NO. 4

A 2-year-old black child is scheduled for inguinal hernia repair; hemoglobin is 10 g. The mother states that the child had no problems surrounding birth and there is no history of sickle cell anemia in the family. The mother is unsure if the child has been tested. What additional preoperative studies do you feel are necessary prior to administering an anesthetic to this child.

Discussion

Eric T. Kunichika, M.D.

Instructor and Special Fellow in Anesthesiology and Pediatrics, University of Florida-College of Medicine, Department of Anesthesiology, Gainesville, Florida

Shirley A. Graves, M.D.
Professor of Anesthesiology and Pediatrics, University of Florida-College of Medicine, Department of Anesthesiology, Gainesville, Florida

Between 7% and 9% of all black Americans are carriers of the sickle cell gene—and they have sickle cell trait. Under normal circumstances, sickle cell trait is not associated with anemia and does not impair survival. However, hypoxia, acidosis, and vascular stasis, all of which may occur during anesthesia, can promote sickling in patients with sickle cell trait.[1]

Patients with sickle cell disease (Hgb SS) and combination hemoglobinopathies such as Hgb SC and Hgb S–β-thalessemia do have increased morbidity and mortality. The patient's history and physical examination can provide clues to the presence of sickle cell disease. Sickled red blood cells have a survival time of only approximately 12 days and may result in anemia, hyperbilirubinemia, and hepatosplenomegaly. Compensatory erythroid hyperplasia is evident on a peripheral blood smear as reticulocytosis. Sequestration, hemolytic, aplastic, and vaso-occlusive crises are associated with sickle cell disease. Before 6 months of age, the presence of fetal hemoglobin (Hgb F) shifts the oxyhemoglobin curve to the left and increases oxygen affinity for hemoglobin. This will partially ameliorate the propensity of Hgb S to become deoxygenated and sickle. Newborns with sickle cell disease typically have less than 20% Hgb S and are protected against vaso-occlusive events until at least 3 to 4 months of age.

In vitro studies of Hgb SS have demonstrated that intracellular deformation occurs when oxygen saturation is less than 85% (Pa_{O_2} 40–50 mmHg).[2] Normal mixed venous saturation approximates 75%. Therefore, patients with sickle cell disease are constantly sickling. Sickle-trait cells do not sickle until oxygen saturation decreases below 40% (Pa_{O_2} 25–30 mmHg). In normal circumstances, oxygen saturation remains well above this level in both the arterial and the venous circuits and sickling does not occur. However, induction of anesthesia may be associated with conditions that can cause even sickle-trait cells to sickle. Laryngospasm, hypoventilation, hypoxia, acidosis, hypothermia, anemia, and surgery- or tourniquet-induced venous stasis can all create conditions conducive to red cell sickling. Pediatric patients are particularly prone to episodes of arterial desaturation. As many as 28% to 35% of patients monitored with pulse oximetry were found to have arterial saturation of 90% or less during emergence or transport to the PACU.[3,4] Venous saturation would expectedly be correspondingly lower. Special care should be taken when administering anesthetics to patients with sickle cell trait. Therefore, a previously untested black child scheduled for anesthesia and surgery should be examined and screened for the sickle cell gene. An associated anemia lends additional credence to further hematologic testing. However, the degree of anemia is not always associated with the severity of sickle cell disease. This is particularly true of SC hemoglobinopathy.

Initial laboratory evaluation of a patient with the potential for the sickle cell gene should include a complete blood count, reticulocyte count, peripheral blood smear, and a sickle cell preparation. Should testing or history indicate that the sickle cell gene is present, further laboratory analysis with hemoglobin electrophoresis is indicated. The peripheral blood smear is not normal in sickle cell disease. The presence of cells with sickle morphology, even in small numbers, confirms the diagnosis of sickle cell disease. In contrast, red cells of sickle-trait patients have essentially normal morphology.

After 6 months of age, the sodium metabisulfite test may be the sickle cell preparation selected. It involves placing a drop of 2% sodium metabisulfite on a drop of fresh blood on a coverslip sealed with petrolatum. Under high power and low light, the preparation is examined for the presence of sickled cells. Severe iron deficiency, the presence of certain poikilocytes, and the presence of a low percentage of Hgb S can lead to misinterpretation of this test result.

The Sickledex reaction is a newer sickle cell preparation in which the Sickledex reagent is added to a blood sample with the Sickledex test solution. The relative insolubility of Hgb S will cause precipitation of the suspension and a positive test. Hypergammaglobulinemia and hyperproteinemia will cause false-positive results; low concentrations of Hgb S will cause false-negative results. Both sickle preparation tests are quick and easy to perform, but neither can distinguish sickle cell trait from sickle cell disease; this is accomplished through the use of one of two types of hemoglobin electrophoreses. Cellulose acetate electrophoresis utilizes the relative negative charge of Hgb A to separate hemoglobin variants into distinct bands. Citrate agar electrophoresis is used to confirm the results of cellulose acetate testing. This test uses solubility differences, as well as relative charge, to differentiate the hemoglobinopathies.

Children younger than 6 months have enough Hgb F to make the use of the sickle preparation tests difficult. If a diagnosis is needed, hemoglobin electrophoresis is the ideal test. Many states now use electrophoresis for mandatory neonatal screening.

In summary, the patient in this case and all untested black or mulatto patients should receive sickle cell screening prior to surgery. Special precautions must be taken in patients possessing the sickle cell gene. Although a sickle preparation test is used as a screening tool prior to surgery, the only definitive test is hemoglobin electrophoresis. Hemoglobin electrophoresis should be performed to confirm the presence, type, and percentage of abnormal hemoglobin in anyone at risk of having the hemoglobin S gene. If hemoglobin electrophoresis cannot be obtained, sickle cell trait is the most likely diagnosis with a positive sickle preparation, a normal hemoglobin, a normal reticulocyte count, and a normal blood smear. The blood smear should be examined by, or under the direction of, a knowledgeable hematologist or pathologist. However, this does not replace hemoglobin electrophoresis.

Anesthesia and surgery in patients with sickle cell disease require inpatient care. Sickle-trait patients can be cared for in the ambulatory care setting provided precautions are taken to avoid dehydration, hypoxia, cardiovascular compromise, and extremes of temperature and pH.

REFERENCES

1. Esseltine DW, Baxter MR, Bevan J: Sickle cell states and the anaesthetist. Can J Anaesth 35: 385, 1988

2. Bromberg PA, Jensen WN: Blood oxygen dissociation curves in sickle cell disease. J Lab Clin Med 70: 480, 1967
3. Pullerits J, Burrows FA, Roy WL: Arterial desaturation in healthy children during transfer to the recovery room. Can J Anaesth 34: 470, 1987
4. Tyler IL, Tantisira B, Winter PM, et al: Continuous monitoring of arterial oxygen saturation with pulse oximetry during transfer to the recovery room. Anesth Analg 64: 1108, 1985

Response

L. Reuven Pasternak, M.D., M.P.H.

Assistant Professor, Anesthesiology and Critical Care Medicine, Director, Ambulatory Surgery Programs, The Johns Hopkins Hospital Baltimore, Maryland

The preoperative evaluation of patients for surgery occasionally requires that the anesthesiologist assume the role of primary care provider in identifying potential health problems that have not been screened or managed. When a history and a physical examination are noncontributory, their inclusion in an at-risk population may require additional testing to ensure that this condition is not present. Such an approach is designed both to guarantee a safe anesthetic and to assist in overall health care management. Sickle cell disease and trait are examples of such a condition. Screening for these disorders in all black children is indicated, regardless of family history or presence of anemia. It is our policy that lacking a negative screening at some time after 6 months of age, all black children should be tested for these conditions before undergoing surgery.

It is well known that the factors precipitating sickle crises in susceptible patients include hypoxia, dehydration, and acidosis. Where patients have a history of frequent intervention for such events, major residual morbidity, or any episode requiring admission within the preceding 12 months, we have admitted them preoperatively to ensure full hydration at the time of surgery. However, during the past 4 years, we have come to observe that lacking this extreme history, these patients can be managed on an outpatient basis without significant distress.

As is often the case, we were called on to evaluate the possibility of performing these cases on an outpatient basis by patients and their families, who preferred not to be hospitalized if at all possible. In addressing this issue, we determined what was to be accomplished with preoperative and postoperative admission that could not be achieved at home. Specifically, we addressed the extent to which the risk factors of dehydration, hypoxia, and acidosis could be prevented in the ambulatory surgery setting.

Clearly, these patients generally do well at home, sleeping through the night without intravenous fluids and repleting themselves with normal oral intake during the following morning and throughout the day. Unless they have experienced significant respiratory compromise, hypoxia is also not present while breathing room air. Finally, as long as dehydration, hypotension, and hypoxia are absent, acidosis is also an extremely unlikely event. Thus, if hydration is the only preoperative concern, we have found it quite satisfactory to have these patients arrive at the ambulatory surgery preparation site at 7 A.M. on the morning of surgery where an IV infusion is immediately started to ensure adequate hydration.

The procedure is scheduled to start no earlier than 10 A.M. and no later than noon to ensure adequate time for administration of fluids before surgery and for postoperative observation. Those patients who require transfusion to reduce their Hgb S concentrations below 40% do so the day before surgery under the direction of the pediatric hematology service and then return the following day for their procedure. The 1-day delay does not significantly affect the Hgb S concentration, and its performance during "daylight" operations allows for better observation and determination of adequate care than transfusing overnight, when nurses are limited and busy with other patients more in need of inpatient care.

The issues relating to hypoxia, hypotension, dehydration, and acidosis associated with respiratory compromise, blood loss, and postoperative problems such as nausea and vomiting are clearly of major concern in patients with sickle cell disease. However, judicious anesthetic practice involves avoidance of these conditions in all pediatric patients. Appropriate attention to fluid and airway management is always maintained. The well-documented oxygen desaturation observed postoperatively in the PACU is managed by administration of supplemental oxygen to all patients until they are considered for discharge to the step-down unit before going home.

A procedure such as inguinal hernia repair usually entails minimal blood loss and is generally short in duration. Given an uneventful perioperative course where the preceding risk factors are avoided through the recovery period, the issue is then whether discharge home places these patients at risk. Again, the issues of concern to the patient with sickle cell disease are also important in the management of any patient. Discharge for all patients is conditional on their being alert, without any respiratory distress, fully hydrated and voiding, and taking oral fluids without evidence of nausea or emesis.

The ability of the patient with sickle cell disease to meet these stringent criteria has allowed us to manage these individuals as outpatients for the past several years. We have done so while meeting the other critical requirement—this being timely follow-up to determine the postoperative status within 24 hours of discharge. To date, none of these patients has required admission or emergency evaluation after discharge. Furthermore, both patients and families are grateful that hospital stays have been avoided.

▓ CASE REPORT NO. 5

A 25-year-old man on renal dialysis needs a new A-V access shunt; hemoglobin is 8.0 g and hematocrit is 25%.

Discussion
Surinder K. Kallar, M.D.
Professor of Anesthesiology, Director of Ambulatory Anesthesia, Virginia Commonwealth University, Medical College of Virginia Hospitals, Richmond, Virginia

Patients with chronic renal failure undergoing an A-V access shunt procedure can be handled safely on an ambulatory basis, but they present several problems to the anesthesiologist, including hypertension, anemia, electrolyte imbalance, and acidosis. They are often on antihypertensive medication and have previously been treated with steroids and immunosuppressants. Various psychological symptoms related to their disease and hemodialysis, especially depression, may also occur. As a result of impaired erythropoietin production, it is not uncommon for these patients to have a hemoglobin concentration of 5 to 8 g. This degree of anemia is well tolerated if the cardiovascular and respiratory systems are normal. Preoperative transfusion is usually not indicated. The decreased oxygen-carrying capacity of blood is normally compensated by an increased cardiac output, often to levels twice normal. Therefore, it is important to minimize or prevent cardiac depression during anesthesia. Coagulopathies are common and must be remembered in considering regional anesthetic technique. Electrolyte abnormalities include hyperkalemia, hypermagnesemia, and high blood urea nitrogen (BUN) levels. Hyperkalemia, the most serious electrolyte abnormality, can cause cardiac conduction abnormalities and dysrhythmias. Serum potassium concentration should not be more than 5.5 mEq/L and can be controlled with preoperative dialysis. Hypermagnesemia can potentiate depolarizing and nondepolarizing muscle relaxants. A high BUN level is accompanied by decreased tolerance to barbiturates. The blood-brain barrier may not be intact in the presence of uremia, and this can increase the incidence of excessive drug effects. General anesthetic agents must be administered in small doses compared to those administered to patients with normal BUN levels. Regardless of the blood volume status, these patients tend to respond to induction of anesthesia as if they were hypovolemic, and this is accentuated if they are on antihypertensive drugs. The patients are often on multiple therapies, and possible drug interactions include digitalis and potassium concentration, antibiotics interfering with muscle relaxants, and corticosteroids causing suprarenal exhaustion and hypotension. Patients receiving corticosteroids should be pretreated with the appropriate increased dose before operation. A deficiency of plasma proteins may cause a prolonged or exaggerated effect of those drugs which are highly protein bound (i.e., thiopental, bupivacaine). Deficiency of gammaglobulin renders these patients more liable to infection and necessitates meticulous aseptic technique and frequent antibiotic administration.

Ideally, the anesthetic for creation of an A-V shunt also should provide satisfactory vasodilation of the vessel for the anastomosis and help in the prevention of thrombosis. Both general anesthesia and regional anesthesia have been used successfully. Ideally, the patient should be dialyzed 1 day prior to surgery. Laboratory work should include a hematocrit and serum electrolytes. If the patient is debilitated, smaller doses of all anesthetics should be administered. General anesthesia should be induced slowly with a barbiturate to minimize hypotension. Maintenance of anesthesia should consist of nitrous oxide in oxygen and a short-acting narcotic such as fentanyl or alfentanil and low concentration of isoflurane or enflurane. Narcotics are used to maintain cardiovascular stability, and volatile agents are used to control intraoperative hypertension. However, the high incidence of associated liver disease in patients with chronic renal disease should be considered when selecting these agents.

Chronic renal disease alters the response to nondepolarizing muscle relaxants. Prolonged responses are predictable if the usual muscle relaxant dose is given to the patient with severely limited or no renal function. The choice of nondepolarizing drugs is between *d*-tubocurarine, pancuronium, vecuronium, and atracurium. Gallamine and metocurine are dependent on renal excretion and should be avoided. Initial doses of the drugs should be reduced at least 50%, and subsequent doses should be determined by the response observed. In the past, the use of succinylcholine in patients with chronic renal disease was complicated by diminished cholinesterase activity caused by absorption onto hemodyalysis membranes, which lead to an exaggerated potassium release; however, this does not occur with currently used hemodyalysis membranes and the response to succinylcholine is not altered in these patients.

Local infiltration and brachial plexus block anesthesia are frequently employed for shunt creation. Brachial plexus block (BPB) provides the highest A-V fistula blood flow with the least hemodynamic changes, abolishes vasospasm, and provides optimal surgical conditions by producing maximal vascular dilation as a result of a regional sympathetic blockade.[1] The increase in brachial artery blood flow in BPB patients is due to an increase in diameter and mean blood velocity. BPB appears to be the anesthetic technique of choice.[1]

The duration of the block produced by local anesthesia is shortened by about 40% in these patients.[2] It is thought that elevated tissue blood flow secondary to the increased cardiac output results in a more rapid clearance of the agents from the active site. Lidocaine, mepivacaine, or bupivacaine can be used. Potential toxicity of bupivacaine in patients with end-stage renal failure should be kept in mind.[3] If hyperkalemia and acidosis are present, the patient may have increased myocardial irritability; therefore, local anesthetic solutions containing epinephrine should not be used. Adequacy of coagulation should be confirmed and the presence of uremic neuropathies excluded before regional anesthesia is performed.

REFERENCES

1. Mouquet C, Bitker MO, Bailliart O, et al: Anesthesia for creation of a forearm fistula in patients with endstage renal failure. Anesthesiology 70: 909, 1989
2. Bromage PR, Gertel M: Brachial plexus anesthesia in chronic renal failure. Anesthesiology 36: 488, 1972
3. Gould DB, Aldrete JA: Bupivacaine cardiotaxicity in a patient with renal failure. Acta Anaesthesiol Scand 27: 18, 1983

Response

This presentation covers the major physiologic derangements one would encounter with a patient in chronic renal failure. Both general and regional anesthesia can provide adequate analgesia and anesthesia for this group of patients. The anesthesiologist must remember that the patient with chronic renal failure has less physiologic reserve and will respond more quickly and more seriously to hypoxia, hypotension, infection, and myocardial depressant drugs. At our facility, the anesthetic of choice would be a brachial plexus block, allowing the patient to maintain his baseline physical status while providing adequate anesthesia for the surgical procedure. In addition, because many ESRD patients are very familiar with hospitals and procedures, many will tolerate A-V shunt placement under local anesthesia with monitored anesthesia care. Should intravenous supplement to local anesthesia be necessary, small doses of midazolam (0.5 to 1 mg increments) or infusion of alfantenil (0.25 to 0.5 µg/kg/min) will provide satisfactory sedation.

CASE REPORT NO. 6

A three-year-old, 17-kg uncooperative child diagnosed as having a brain tumor is scheduled for a six-week course of radiation therapy as an outpatient. A ventriculoperitoneal shunt was placed during prior surgery. Therapy will be performed daily, taking 15 to 30 minutes with the child in the prone position. The anesthesiologist must be out of the room during actual therapy but will be able to visualize the child and have intercom contact.

Discussion
William K. Hamilton, M.D.
Vice Dean, UCSF School of Medicine, Professor of Anesthesia, University of California, San Francisco, California

Claire Brett, M.D.
Associate Professor of Anesthesia and Pediatrics in Residence, UCSF School of Medicine, Professor of Anesthesia, University of California, San Francisco, California

The anesthetic management of small children requiring daily anesthetic administration in physical situations prohibiting immediate attendance presents many conditions that must be considered. These include the following:

1. The anesthesia required needs to be very light because there will be a minimum of what we usually consider surgical stimulation. Anesthesia must prevent movement and be deep enough to avoid vomiting, laryngospasm, and other complications of light anesthesia *per se.*

2. Daily anesthesia for a period of 6 weeks must be accomplished using drugs that will allow dietary and food intake sufficient to satisfy metabolic needs for a growing child. Weight gain may not be maintained in a 3-year-old child, but weight loss should be avoided. Our early experiences with lytic cocktails and various forms of parenteral sedation were most unsatisfactory.

3. Daily anesthesia also provides us with a challenge to make the experience pleasant or at least not unpleasant. Such discomforts as needlesticks and postoperative nausea should not be part of the experience. We have had parents complain to us of nocturnal excitement and apparent hallucinations associated with the use of ketamine. Following this, we abandoned the use of that drug.

4. Closely associated with the preceding is the need to keep recovery time at an absolute minimum. Since the patient is ambulatory, it is almost an intolerable encumbrance on parents to have to wait long periods of time for recovery. In summary, it is worth every effort to have a comfortable, happy child with minimal stress and discomfort to the parents already faced with catastrophic realization.

5. Our own view is that spontaneous respiration has a great deal of inbuilt safety. Fortunately, requirements for this procedure do not include need for muscle relaxation and postoperative analgesia, and therefore, drugs that compromise respiration can be minimized or avoided.

6. Although frequent tracheal intubation seems to be well tolerated, there are complications from endotracheal tubes and the act of intubation and increased anesthetic complexity (pharmacologic and mechanical) associated therewith. These considerations direct us to avoid tracheal intubation. The prone position required for this patient should actually be optimal for airway maintenance in an unconscious patient. Our satisfaction with using insufflation techniques for brief periods of radiotherapy has been supplemented by experience with longer time periods that include the prone position.[1]

We do not have the experience that allows us to accurately compare the outcome of various anesthetic approaches to this specific problem. It is our belief that we can best meet these requirements with nitrous oxide and isoflurane and oxygen induced by means of mask and maintained with insufflation through a nasopharyngeal catheter or oropharyngeal airway. We believe that this can best be accomplished with no premedication and no intravenous drugs. Isoflurane is chosen over halothane because of the unknown chances of hepatic toxicity with repeated administration of the latter. This is apparently an extremely small risk in small children, but to the extent that it exists at all, there is no reason to accept it. Our unproven clinical impression is that recovery from isoflurane provides patients with less hangover than does halothane. We have not had sufficient experience with enflurane. There are many who profess that isoflurane induction in children is difficult. We do not find it so. We elect to use nitrous oxide because we believe it facilitates induction, and if it adds something to the maintenance of anesthesia, we are happy to accept this benefit.

Others may be able to manipulate and administer nonvolatile drugs to provide the preceding conditions, repeated attempts have taught us that we cannot.

We are aware of the alleged dangers of specific increases in intracranial pressure as a result of inhalation anesthetic agents. On the other hand, inhalation anesthesia was the anesthetic of choice for many, many years in neurosurgery without known complications from these agents *per se*. This child had a functioning shunt, but even in its absence, this potential disadvantage would be less than those imposed by other approaches.

The airway must be *meticulously* guarded by positioning and perhaps the use of nasal or oral airways. These may actually facilitate the delivery of agents and oxygen by insufflation. The possibility of insufflation gas flows inflating the stomach must be recognized. Careful positioning of insufflation catheters and a guaranteed route of egress of insufflated gases will minimize this potential hazard.

The precise choice of drugs and techniques is of less importance than careful attention to the listed principles. These cases are not easy. That's why experts are needed.

REFERENCE

1. Brett CM, Wara WM, Hamilton WK: Anesthesia for infants during radiotherapy: An insufflation technique. Anesthesiology 64: 402, 1986

Response
The problems related to daily anesthesias for a child receiving radiation therapy are well covered by Drs. Hamilton and Brett. I would concur that the method they advise—mask inhalation induction, anesthesia maintained by insufflation by means of nasopharyngeal catheter or through an oral pharyngeal airway with spontaneous ventilation, and no intravenous supplement—would be the technique I also would choose. There are, however, two issues to which I would like to speak. First, insufflation anesthesia is a technique commonly used years ago, but I would question whether it is being taught in many training programs currently. I agree that the need for repeated short anesthesias in a prone position makes insufflation anesthesia almost the ideal technique, yet it would be my impression that most young anesthesiologists would not feel comfortable without an endotracheal tube and an IV in this patient. While this would certainly require significantly more instrumentation, the anesthesiologist administering the anesthesia must reach his or her own comfort level and confidence in the anesthesia technique. Other concerns that could be raised about insufflation anesthesia are (1) unknown inhaled anesthetic concentration, (2) inability to assist ventilation, (3) exposure to waste gases, and (4) drying of mucous membranes.

Second, I believe inhalation inductions with halothane are much smoother and more pleasant than those with enflurane or isoflurane. Since this procedure must be repeated so often, it would be best to use the most pleasant inhalation technique, and I would accept what possible hepatotoxic risk there is with the use of halothane to make it the most pleasant experience for this patient. Recovery time from the different inhalation agents for this patient without supplemental parenteral medication would be insignificant.

REFERENCE

1. Roth AG: The pediatric problem patient. In Wetchler BV (ed): Problems in Anesthesia. Philadelphia, JB Lippincott Co. 1988.

■ CASE REPORT NO. 7

A 4-month-old, 4.9-kg infant is scheduled for an inguinal hernia repair. History from the mother reveals that the child was 4 weeks premature and was in the newborn intensive care unit for 3 weeks. The child suffers from periodic apnea and is monitored at home.

Discussion
Charles J. Coté, M.D.
Associate Professor of Anaesthesia, Associate Anesthetist, Massachusetts General Hospital, Harvard Medical School, Boston, Massachusetts

Gregory[1] and Steward[2] first noted the high incidence of postoperative apnea in ex-premature infants (*i.e.*, infants < 37 weeks gestational age). Since then, a great deal of attention has been devoted to defining the population at risk. Gregory reported that 25% of preterm infants suffered from postoperative apnea, while Steward reported 6 of 33 ex-premature infants. Both these studies were flawed because they were retrospective. However, both increased our awareness of this problem. Our anesthesia group prospectively examined a large series of full-term and premature infants undergoing a variety of surgical procedures.[3] A total of 173 full-term and 41 ex-premature infants were studied. Of the 41 ex-premature infants, 15 had a history of neonatal apnea: six developed postoperative apnea, two were ventilated because of the nature of their surgery, and 7 recovered uneventfully. The post-conceptual age of all patients who developed apnea was less than 41 weeks; none of the older children developed apnea. Although all types of surgical procedures were included, 3 of the 6 infants who developed apnea had had inguinal herniorrhaphies. There was no association of apnea with ASA physical status classification.

Welborn and coworkers prospectively studied 86 infants undergoing inguinal herniorrhaphy repair; 38 were ex-premature infants.[4] Of 16 ex-premature infants, 12 were more than 44 weeks post-conceptual age and none developed postoperative apnea. Of 22 ex-premature infants, 18 were less than 44 weeks post-conceptual age and none developed postoperative apnea, but 14 of these 18 developed periodic breathing. The authors concluded that outpatient inguinal herniorrhaphy could be safely performed in ex-premature infants of more than 44 weeks post-conceptual age who were free of major cardiac, neurologic, endocrine, and metabolic diseases. The ASA physical status classification of these patients was not reported.

Kurth and coworkers examined preoperative and postoperative pneumograms in 47 ex-premature infants of less than 60 weeks post-conceptual age.[5] These infants underwent a variety of surgical procedures including seven laparotomies, seven ventriculoperitoneal shunts, four central line placements, and 26 inguinal herniorrhaphies. Episodes of apnea were observed after 25 of 49 operations. Three infants for inguinal hernia repair experienced apnea; one (43 weeks post-conceptual age) had prolonged apnea with episodes up to 12 hours postoperatively, two were more than 44 weeks post-conceptual age (52 and 54 weeks) and developed prolonged apnea only in the recovery room. Apnea events were inversely related to post-conceptual age and positively related to a history of necrotizing enterocolitis. Only one infant required mechanical ventilation. The preoperative pneumogram was not felt to be a reliable test in predicting post-operative apnea. The authors concluded that preterm infants younger than 60 weeks post-conceptual age should be monitored postoperatively for at least 12 apnea-free hours in order to prevent apnea-related complications. The major defect of this study was that the length of the preoperative pneumogram was relatively brief and may in fact have missed infants having subclinical apnea spells. It is interesting that 14 of 18 patients who had abnormal preoperative pneumograms had abnormal postoperative pneumograms. This suggests that the pneumogram, if abnormal, is highly but not 100% predictive of postoperative apnea.

Mestad and associates studied 100 ex-premature infants scheduled for in-guinal herniorrhaphy or lacrimal duct probing.[6] They found that infants of less than 40 weeks post-conceptual age or infants with a history of apnea or lung disease were the infants at risk for developing postoperative apnea. The absence of apnea in recovery did not guarantee that apnea would not occur later. Vanik and coworkers prospectively examined 102 ex-premature infants of less than 60 weeks post-conceptual age who underwent inguinal herniorrhaphy repair.[7] Ten infants experienced 11 episodes of apnea; six were preextubation, one in the recovery room, and four after release from the recovery room. All infants who experienced apnea after release from the recovery room were less than 47 weeks post-conceptual age.

The case of the infant presented for discussion has several interesting areas of concern. First, although described as 4 months old, the child is actually only 52 weeks post-conceptual age; it is very important for the anesthesiologist to deter-mine the post-conceptual age rather than the chronological age, since the inci-dence of apnea is inversely related to post-conceptual age.[5] Second, this child is somewhat unusual because he continues to experience periodic apnea and is monitored for apnea at home. It appears that this child still has a respiratory pattern consistent with immaturity of the respiratory center. This history should alert the anesthesiologist to inquire as to actual episodes of apnea and when they last occurred, whether the child is taking any medication for the apnea (amino-phylline or caffeine), and whether there are any siblings who have had sudden infant death syndrome (SIDS). If the child is on medication, then the child should continue this medication up to and including the morning of surgery. Any child who is currently having apnea, no matter what the post-conceptual age, should be admitted to an intensive care unit and monitored for apnea, since several studies have demonstrated postanesthetic apnea in such patients.[3,5,6] The anes-thesiologist also should question the necessity for a surgical procedure when a child is still in danger of postoperative apnea; obviously, the risk of delayed sur-gery must be balanced against the risk of postoperative apnea. For the patient at hand, the answer is easy: If surgery is necessary, then the child should not be an outpatient and should be admitted to an apnea-monitored bed.

More difficult questions are: When is it "safe" to anesthetize an infant who is no longer experiencing apnea? When is it safe to anesthetize even a full-term "normal" infant as outpatient? Each of the published studies has limitations and problems with methodology. None has a very large series of ASA physical status

1 and 2 patients undergoing the same operative procedure with the same anesthetic technique by the same anesthesiologist, the same surgeon, or the same operating room conditions; the two largest series are still in abstract form.[6,7]

Many factors contribute to the development of apnea, including hypothermia, anemia, abnormalities of glucose and calcium homeostasis, anesthetic agents, and perhaps anesthetic technique.[8,9] The bottom line is that a history of prematurity is a red flag that means these infants must be observed very carefully for episodes of postoperative apnea. When can these infants be safely operated upon (i.e., for herniorrhaphy)? The sum total of cases reported in the literature is approximately 325; therefore, it is difficult to make definitive statements that are all-inclusive. It has been our experience and that of others, with a limited number of infants, that the majority of healthy ex-premature infants, even those with a neonatal but not a current history of apnea, who are of more than 46 weeks post-conceptual age may be safely anesthetized as outpatients.[3,4,6,7] It must be emphasized, however, that it is safer to err on the conservative side than to discharge a patient who later gets into trouble.[5] Until more extensive, meticulous prospective studies are carried out, it is reasonable to admit all ex-premature infants of less than 50 weeks post-conceptual age and monitor them for possible apnea; the infants at greatest risk are those of less than 46 weeks post-conceptual age with a history of apnea. Obviously, there must be a middle ground between the conservative 60 weeks recommended by Kurth and associates and our early recommendations of 46 weeks. It appears that as the child matures, the tendency toward apnea greatly diminishes, but no one yet knows at which post-conceptual age all babies are "safe." Recent reports of full-term infants developing postoperative apnea suggest that perhaps any newborn has the potential to develop postoperative apnea.[10,11] This risk is significantly increased with a history of prematurity, further increased with a history of neonatal apnea, and still further increased by a history of current apnea spells.[3-7] Perhaps infants should be the first case of the day and be observed for a prolonged period of time, and if there is the slightest suggestion of a problem, even the full-term infant should be admitted and monitored. Finally, there is a suggestion, as yet unsubstantiated, that regional anesthesia may result in a lower incidence of postanesthetic respiratory problems.[12]

REFERENCES

1. Gregory GA: Outpatient anesthesia. In Miller RD (ed): Anesthesia, p 1329. New York, Churchill-Livingstone, 1981
2. Steward DJ: Preterm infants are more prone to complications following minor surgery than are term infants. Anesthesiology 56: 304, 1982
3. Liu LMP, Coté CJ, Goudsouzian NG, et al: Life-threatening apnea in infants recovering from anesthesia. Anesthesiology 59: 506, 1983
4. Welborn LG, Ramirez N, Oh TH, et al: Postanesthetic apnea and periodic breathing in infants. Anesthesiology 65: 658, 1986
5. Kurth CD, Spitzer AR, Broennle AM, Downes JJ. Postoperative apnea in preterm infants. Anesthesiology 66: 483, 1987
6. Mestad PH, Glenski JA, Binda RE Jr: When is outpatient surgery safe in preterm infants? (abstr). Anesthesiology 69: 744, 1988

7. Vanik PE, Warner LO, Teitelbaum DH, et al: Inguinal herniorrhaphy in young infants: Perioperative problems. Presented at the Section on Anesthesiology, American Academy of Pediatrics, May 1988
8. Gregory GA, Steward DJ: Life-threatening perioperative apnea in the ex-"premie." Anesthesiology 59: 495, 1983
9. Schute FJ: Apnea. Clin Perinatol 4: 65, 1977
10. Tetzlaff JE, Annand DW, Pudimat MA, Nicodemus HF: Postoperative apnea in a full-term infant.
    Anesthesiology 69: 426, 1988
11. Noseworthy J, Duran C, Khine HH: Postoperative apnea in a full-term infant. Anesthesiology
    70: 879, 1989
12. Harnik EV, Hoy GR, Potolicchio S, et al: Spinal anesthesia in premature infants recovering from
    respiratory distress syndrome. Anesthesiology 64: 95, 1986

Response

Dr. Coté has done an excellent job in discussing the problems facing the anesthesiologist asked to anesthetize young infants and post-premature children for
ambulatory surgical procedures. It is impossible to try to establish a specific age
at which it would be considered "safe" to administer anesthesia for ambulatory
surgery. Each patient must be individually evaluated by the anesthesiologist. The
guidelines are fairly clear, however, that age should be uniformly counted from
date of conception and not, therefore, to be confused by postbirth age. The evidence is also clear that ex-premature's who have had problems with apnea are
also the infants who have problems with apnea following anesthesia and surgery.
Therefore, these are the infants who must be monitored carefully in the postanesthesia period. We are not provided with this child's birth weight. Since this
child only weighs 10 lbs 4 months after birth, it also may be a clinical indicator
of failure to thrive that would also influence the decision to provide this patient's
anesthesia and surgery as an inpatient for adequate postanesthesia monitoring.

CASE REPORT NO. 8

A 16-year-old girl with documented mitral valve prolapse who is prone to par-
oxysmal supraventricular tachycardia is scheduled as an outpatient to have extraction of four severely impacted third molars. Her cardiologist recommends she
receive antibiotic prophylaxis intravenously. The patient is allergic to penicillin.

Discussion
Solomon Aronson, M.D.
*Assistant Professor, Anesthesia and Critical Care, University of Chicago, Director
of Cardiovascular Anesthesia, L.A. Weiss Memorial Hospital, Chicago, Illinois*

This case presents the anesthesiologist in the ambulatory surgery center with
two important issues. The first is the perioperative risks to patients with mitral
valve prolapse, and the second is the antibiotic prophylaxis for this lesion.
   Since Barlow's description in 1963, mitral valve prolapse (MVP) has been increasingly recognized and diagnosed and has now been described as the most
common valvular cardiac abnormality in this country. In men, the incidence is

approximately 2% to 4% in all age groups; in women, the incidence varies with age. Between ages 20 and 29, the incidence is approximately 17%, declining with each subsequent decade to 1.4% over 80 years of age. Mitral valve prolapse has been reported to be present in 6.3% of otherwise healthy young women (ages 17–54).

Since mitral valve prolapse is such a prevalent disease, it is important to identify subgroups of patients with this lesion who may be at high risk, and conversely, it is also important to identify those patients with MVP who are at little or no risk. This approach would enable one to provide reassurance to the patient who is considered at low risk and permit the development of an efficient risk-benefit strategy for providing optimal care.

The principal anatomic and histologic abnormalities found in the syndrome of MVP are redundancy and degeneration of the leaflets, dilatation of the mitral valve annulus, and variable chordal pathology. During ventricular systole, the redundant leaflets prolapse into the left atrium. Because of this pathology, MVP is a lesion with highly variable clinical features. These features include a nonejection systolic click and/or the echocardiographic finding of prolapsing movement of one or both mitral valve leaflets with or without a late or holosystolic murmur.

The information about the true risk of patients with mitral valve prolapse is rather sketchy and is focused primarily on clinical studies that suggest MVP is associated with progressive mitral insufficiency, dysrhythmias, and bacterial endocarditis. Furthermore, most studies seem to indicate that the propensity for any of the preceding risks is more likely in highly symptomatic patients, especially those patients with late or holosystolic murmurs.

The vast majority of patients with MVP are asymptomatic. Palpatations appear to be one of the most common symptoms, reported in nearly 50% of patients with MVP; however, when compared to matched control groups, patients with MVP do not have a significantly greater incidence of dysrhythmias than patients without MVP.

Therefore, for an anesthesiologist with the task of taking care of a patient with MVP, the first question to be answered is whether a murmur of mitral insufficiency is present? Then the patient should be classified as having either a high or low risk, and treatment strategies to provide safe and efficient care should be considered.

The issue concerning antibiotic prophylaxis is an especially interesting one in the context of this case because the American Heart Association (AHA) recently issued an update on their recommendations for infective endocarditis in general and MVP in particular. Clinical studies have suggested that we challenge the overall risk(cost)-benefit ratio of antibiotic prophylaxis for infective endocarditis. Calculations indicate that, overall, fewer than 10% of cases of endocarditis are theoretically preventable. The general focus of the AHA recommendations was on less emphasis for parenteral administration of agents and a decrease in the duration of antibiotic administration. The recommendations for MVP, in particular, state that the risk of developing endocarditic is low and that the risk-benefit ratio is uncertain. The AHA recommends prophylaxis specifically for MVP with murmur of mitral insufficiency.

At this point, clinical judgment is necessary for deciding whether antibiotic prophylaxis is required for MVP or not. The potential problem with the AHA recommendation is that the degree of insufficiency may be variable in patients with MVP, depending on hemodynamic and volume-loading conditions. In addition, several reports have challenged the cost(risk)-benefit ratio for MVP prophylaxis, especially with penicillin, and have suggested that erythromycin is preferable. One report clearly recommended prophylaxis for patients with MVP and isolated mitral valve murmurs.

Finally, the issue of the type of procedure should be considered. While procedures on the oral cavity and respiratory tract (except fiberoptic bronchoscopy) have been shown to cause bacteremia, most diagnostic procedures on the gastrointestinal tract are associated with a low percentage of bacteremia. Considering the strong recommendation of the AHA that patients be separated into high- and low-risk lesion groups who undergo high- or low-risk procedures and the controversy that surrounds a low-risk lesion such as MVP, in particular, I recommend that this patient be given antibiotic prophylaxis only if there is a holosystolic murmur associated with her MVP. If this patient, scheduled to undergo a high-risk procedure, the extraction of four impacted third molars, has MVP with a holosystolic murmur (high-risk lesion), then a reasonable indication for antibiotic prophylaxis exists.

Once this decision is made, the proper timing and method of antibiotic administration are important. The AHA recommendations for prophylaxis mention that oral antibiotic regimens may be used for routine dental procedures. One approach to this problem is to administer a single 3-g dose of oral amoxicillin 1 hour before the procedure. Amoxicillin has been shown to be much more effective than equivalent doses of penicillin V in reducing bacteremia after tooth extraction. Ten hours after a patient receives 3 g amoxicillin, blood levels are bactericidal for most oral streptococci. According to Durak and Petersdorph, in order to prevent endocarditis, it is necessary to have bactericidal activity in plasma 9 hours after a bacterial challenge; therefore, the 10 hours of activity provided by the amoxicillin regimen give an adequate margin of safety. If a further margin of safety is desired (which is probably not necessary), the amoxicillin dose could be repeated 6 hours after the procedure or probenecid could be given with the initial dose. Considering the potentially low rate of compliance of patients for ambulatory surgical procedures, the single oral dose seems preferable.

In this case, in which a penicillin allergy is present, substitution with 1 g erythromycin orally 1 hour before the procedure would be indicated. Again, if a further margin of safety were desired, a second dose (500 mg) could be repeated 6 hours later.

REFERENCES

1. Savage, Garrison, Devereaux, et al: Mitral valve prolapse in the general population: I. Epidemiologic features: The Framingham study. Am Heart J 106: 571, 1983
2. Savage, Garrison, Devereaux, et al: Mitral valve prolapse in the general population: II. Clinical features: The Framingham study. Am Heart Journal 106: 577, 1983

probably diminished by his not being exposed to the hospital environment. While there are no hard data that say the risk of infection or of cross-contamination from other patients is less in the ambulatory setting than in the inpatient setting, logic would dictate it be so. Second, the sooner a patient regulates his or her own fluids and electrolytes—that is, the sooner the physicians let the patient's body control its own functions—the less likely it is that iatrogenesis imperfecta will cause problems. Third, from the current history, I see no contraindication to the patient undergoing ambulatory surgery, but a lot depends on the adequacy of the history. Was chest pain asked about? Was exercise tolerance asked about? Does the patient have any other complicating factors, such as a familial history of malignant hyperthermia? Has the patient had reasonable anesthesia experiences in the past without complications? Is the patient able to take in food prior to leaving the postanesthesia care unit? Is a spinal planned? What is the patient's home situation, and is there someone who can get him back to the ambulatory, emergency room, or hospital setting should he not be able to hold down food?

My own management for this patient, were I to see him in our outpatient anesthesia clinic a week or so prior to surgery, would be to go through a careful history with him, which we now do with an automated device. That automated device would undoubtedly suggest tests indicated, including an ECG, and suggest salient points of history that I would then discuss with the patient. The automated device does not change the amount of time I spend with the patient; I still spend 15 to 20 minutes with each patient, more with complex patients, less with straight-forward patients, but the device highlights areas that I must discuss. Were I to find the patient to be a suitable candidate, meaning that he had an individual vested in his care to go home with and he understood the basic ground rules of care and of seeking help when it is needed, I would schedule him to be the first case in the morning. I would have him bring his insulin and insulin syringes with him, and as soon as I started an IV with 100 ml D_5 half-normal saline per hour per 70 kg, I would then give him half of each type of his insulin. I would have told him to bring a carton of orange juice with him should he get hypoglycemic on the way and to let us know if that should happen. Were he to have signs of autonomic dysfunction, such as early satiety, impotence, abnormal sweating, and so on, I would treat him with metoclopramide 10 mg IM 1½ hours prior to the start of surgery. That dose is what is necessary to cause appropriate gastric emptying and ridding of solids from the stomach. I would then use the anesthetic technique I thought most appropriate for removing a Baker's cyst. This would depend on the patient, but it might well involve an epidural or a spinal anesthetic if the patient did not have autonomic dysfunction or might involve a general anesthetic. If the patient had autonomic dysfunction, I would certainly take care to intubate him after treatment with metoclopramide to facilitate gastric emptying of solids. I would plan on having the patient awake and able to take in liquids easily prior to sending him home.

Thus the qualifications for acceptance for ambulatory surgery would be the same as acceptance for inpatient surgery, with the thought that the reduced risk of nosocomial infections, iatrogenesis imperfecta, and early self-regulation of fluids and electrolytes would be beneficial. The risk of ambulatory surgery for this patient might be the advent of painless ischemia or lack of appropriate treatment of pain, but assuming that the latter can be dealt with and that the former is excluded prior to his leaving the ambulatory facility, I would consider this patient a suitable candidate for anesthesia in the ambulatory setting.

Response
Nearly a third of insulin-dependent diabetes (IDDM) are diagnosed after age 30. The patients with maturity-onset IDDM have progressive loss of beta-cell function, and within 5 years of diagnosis, 85% become insulin dependent.[1]

Once the patient begins insulin therapy, it is important to monitor and maintain control of glucose levels. There should be communication with the internist and the patient prior to surgery. The anesthesiologist must have a clear understanding of the patient's medical history, including episodes of ketoacidosis, any signs of neuropathy or autonomic dysfunction, and general compliance of the patient to his insulin regimen.[2] If there is a history of poor compliance to glucose monitoring and insulin therapy, then I would not recommend that this patient have the procedure as an outpatient. A patient must demonstrate that he or she is capable and willing to handle the chronic medical problem in the postoperative period. If by history it is apparent that the patient has been noncompliant, certainly this will not improve after the patient has received an anesthetic.

Prior to the scheduled day of surgery, the patient should receive a telephone call and specific instructions regarding NPO, arrival time, medication management (insulin should be brought to the facility), and identification of the responsible adult who will be present. Upon arrival at the ambulatory center, a method of assessing the patient's fasting blood (*i.e.*, Accucheck) should be performed. An IV solution containing dextrose should be started at 100 ml per hour, the Accucheck result should be obtained, and the patient's insulin dose should be determined. It may range from no insulin required to one-third to one-half the usual morning dose.

Returning the insulin-dependent diabetic to normal activity should be a major factor when deciding on a choice of anesthesia. Whenever possible, a local anesthetic should be used. The patient must be carefully evaluated prior to a regional or general anesthetic. Once the patient has recovered from the anesthetic, he should resume his normal oral intake of calories. Since several hours would have elapsed since the patient's arrival at the facility, and prior to discharge, a second Accucheck could be obtained. It is also advisable that the patient do a home glucose check and receive an afternoon telephone call (about 4 P.M.) to follow up on his status and to determine if additional insulin is needed. Orange juice should be kept at the patient's bedside to counteract any signs of hypoglycemia. Within 24 hours, the patient should resume his normal insulin and food schedule.

Insulin-dependent diabetics can have surgical procedures performed very safely in an ambulatory surgery facility. These patients should be well controlled and capable of and willing to follow instructions to maintain control of their diabetes.

REFERENCES

1. Irvine WJ, Sawers JSA, Feek CM: The value of islet cell antibody in predicting secondary failure of oral hypoglycemic agent therapy in diabetes mellitus. J Clin Lab Immunol 2: 23, 1979
2. Tattersall RB, Scott AR: When to use insulin in the maturity-onset diabetic. Postgrad Med J 63: 859, 1987

CASE REPORT NO. 10

A 42-year-old woman is scheduled for an incisional ventral hernia repair. The patient states that she takes 40 mg furosemide every day for fluid retention. The patient has noted occasional lightheadedness, fatigue, and palpitations. A potassium level drawn on the morning of surgery is 2.7 mEq/L.

Discussion
K. C. Wong, M.D., Ph.D.

Professor of Anesthesiology and Pharmacology, Chairman, Department of Anesthesiology, University of Utah School of Medicine, Salt Lake City, Utah

The magnitude of hypokalemia presenting in this patient is not unusual for someone who has been taking furosemide regularly without oral potassium supplementation. Since this is a chronic loss of body potassium, it can be assumed that the intracellular loss of potassium is proportional to the extracellular loss. The ratio of intracellular-to-extracellular potassium concentration (about 40:1) is important for maintaining cardiac resting membrane potential. The patient is not having persistent cardiac arrhythmias. Nevertheless, the ability of her myocardium to resist the development of arrhythmias could be reduced.

Although it has been traditionally taught that elective surgery should not be performed in patients whose serum potassium is below 3 mEq/L or in digitalized patients whose serum potassium is below 3.5 mEq/L, there are no hard data to substantiate these recommendations. There are only anecdotal case reports to suggest that these recommendations are intuitively "reasonable." Having been interested in this clinical problem for many years, I have not been able to substantiate in animal models that hypokalemia increases the incidence of arrhythmias during anesthesia.[1] Likewise, two recent prospective studies in 597 surgical patients did not demonstrate a correlation between intraoperative ventricular arrhythmias and preoperative hypokalemia,[2,3] even among the high-risk cardiac surgery patients.[3] However, asphyxia[4] or epinephrine overdose[1] has produced significant cardiovascular compromise in the hypokalemic dog. I am convinced that hypokalemia can add to cardiovascular difficulties in patients who are subjected to severe physiologic trespasses, for example, hypoxia, hypotension, or surgical manipulation that can compromise cardiopulmonary function.

The rate of potassium loss appears to be more important; hypokalemia occurring over hours or days may be more ominous than hypokalemia occurring over weeks or months; presumably the latter has had time for physiologic compensatory mechanisms to take place. Although no hard data are available, it is also reasonable to conclude that hypokalemia also can contribute to cardiovascular instability in the presence of cardiovascular disease and cardiovascular depressant drugs. Optimal preparation of a hypokalemic patient is *not* based on hypokalemia alone, but on all of the preceding factors.

Finally, should the hypokalemic patient receive intravenous potassium to replace lost body potassium? Replacement of cellular potassium loss cannot be accomplished overnight. Potassium administration is not innocuous. As many as 1 in 200 patients receiving potassium may suffer a morbid or fatal episode of hyperkalemia.[5]

With this discussion in mind, I would use a routine general anesthesia that will allow quick recovery and would pay special attention to maintaining normal acid-base balance intraoperatively. When the environment is conducive to a regional anesthesia, a spinal or epidural could be done with equal safety. At the time of discharge, I would encourage the patient to eat more bananas.

REFERENCES

1. Wong KC, Tseng KC, Puerto BA, et al: Chronic hypokalemia on epihephrine-induced dysrhythmias during halothane, enflurane, or methoxyflurane with nitrous oxide anesthesia in dogs. Anaesth Sinica 21: 139, 1983
2. Vitez TS, Soper LE, Wong KC, et al: Chronic hypokalemia and intraoperative dysrhythmias. Anesthesiology 63: 130, 1985
3. Hirsch IA, Tomlinson DL, Slogoff S, et al: The overstated risk of preoperative hypokalemia. Anesth Analg 67: 131, 1988
4. Wong KC, Port JD, Steffins J: Cardiovascular responses to asphyxial challenge in chronically hypokalemic dogs. Anesth Analg 62: 991, 1983
5. Burke GR, Gulyassy PF: Surgery in patients with renal disease and related electrolyte disorders. Med Clin North Am 63: 1191, 1979

Response

The problem of hypokalemia in a patient scheduled for elective surgery is faced by anesthesiologists on a daily basis. Decreased body potassium levels can generally be traced to either a decreased intake or an excessive loss of potassium in the urine or sweat. The plasma potassium concentration is 98% intracellular. Many factors—changes in pH, neuronal and hormonal changes, nutritional status—can affect the distribution of intracellular and extracellular potassium. Furosemide, a potent loop of Henle diuretic, inhibits salt resorption.[1]

Hypokalemia may produce muscle weakness that may affect the cardiac, smooth and skeletal muscles. Symptoms may range from weakness and paralysis to respiratory insufficiency. Cardiac effects include arrhythmias such as premature atrial and ventricular beats, atrial ventricular block, possibly ventricular tachycardia, and fibrillation. ECG changes, including depressed ST segments, a flattened T wave, increased prominence of the U wave, and prolongation of the QT interval, all indicate abnormalities in ventricular repolarization.

Hypokalemia has the potential for increased morbidity and mortality. It must be remembered that this is an elective procedure. Potassium repletion is best accomplished orally. Orange juice and bananas are a good source of potassium, but they provide little chloride. Each facility must establish its own guidelines for safe patient care and follow those guidelines in all circumstances. *Question:* Is this patient in the best possible condition for her medical problem? If the answer is no, then we would not proceed.

REFERENCES

1. Forbes GB, Lewis AM: Total Na, K and Cl in adult man. J Clin Invest 35: 596, 1956
2. Linshaw MA: Potassium homeostasis and hypokalemia. Pediatr Clin North Am 34(3): 649, 1987

■ CASE REPORT NO. 11

A 22-month-old infant presents to the ambulatory surgery unit for bilateral myringotomy and tube insertion. He has an axillary temperature of 37.9°C (100.2°F), and the mother states that he has had a runny nose and cough over the last 2 days, there has been no history of fever or chills at home, his cough has not awakened him at night, and his cough has improved over the last 24 hours. After auscultation of the child's chest, which reveals no rhonchi or wheezes, and examination of the mouth, which demonstrates minimal pharyngeal erythema, the anesthesiologist must decide whether to proceed or postpone the procedure.

Discussion

Eugene K. Betts, M.D.

Senior Anesthesiologist and Director, Division of Anesthesiology, Bruce E. Miller Fellow in Pediatric Anesthesia and Critical Care Medicine, Department of Anesthesiology and Critical Care Medicine, The Children's Hospital of Philadelphia, Philadelphia, Pennsylvania

Administering general anesthesia to a patient who manifests signs and symptoms of upper respiratory tract pathology remains an area of controversy among health care providers. Upper respiratory infections (URIs) are the most common infectious diseases of childhood. Children average 5 to 8 URIs per year, especially during the first 2 years of life.[1] Making an accurate diagnosis of URI, differentiating infectious from noninfectious etiologies, and being aware of the currently available evidence concerning administration of a general anesthetic to patients with a URI will help the anesthesiologist choose the appropriate management for this patient.

Tait and Knight use the presence of any two of the following criteria to define the presence of a URI:[2] (1) sore or scratchy throat, (2) sneezing, (3) rhinorrhea, (4) congestion, (5) malaise, (6) nonproductive cough, (7) fever < 101°F, or (8) laryngitis. Combinations of 1 and 5, 2 and 3, 3 and 6, or 4 and 6 require the presence of one additional symptom to differentiate a URI from noninfectious causes, such as allergic or vasomotor rhinitis. The patient's parents frequently judge well in making this distinction in their child. Complications associated with the administration of general anesthesia during a noninfectious rhinitis are infrequent, whereas the frequency of complications during or immediately after the course of an infectious URI remains controversial.

Tait and Knight retrospectively reviewed the cases of 3585 children who underwent various surgical procedures at the University of Michigan's C. S. Mott Children's Hospital and found a complication rate of 1.61% in healthy patients, 1.64% in patients with URI symptoms, and 5.31% in asymptomatic patients with a recent URI (previous 2 weeks).[3] Complications included laryngospasm (1.26%), bronchospasm (0.17%), stridor (0.08%), and breath holding (0.14%). The total incidence of respiratory complications was statistically different ($p < 0.05$) only between control patients and asymptomatic patients with recent URIs. Most of these patients were intubated, a factor that did not increase the incidence of complications. A subsequent prospective study by the same authors of 489 pediatric patients undergoing myringotomies under halothane, N_2O, O_2 anesthesia delivered by face mask revealed no statistically significant differences in perioperative complications among asymptomatic children (1.23%), children with URIs (1.28%), and symptomatic children who did not fulfill the URI criteria or asymptomatic children with a URI in the previous 2 weeks (2.38%).[2] These two studies indicate the acceptability of proceeding with general anesthesia in uncomplicated patients presenting for superficial surgery with URI symptoms.

Other reports, however, present a different view. McGill and coworkers reported intraoperative pulmonary dysfunction in 11 asymptomatic patients, 10 of whom had had a URI in the 4 weeks preceding the administration of the general anesthetic.[4] DeSoto and associates demonstrated an increased incidence of oxygen desaturation in the recovery room in children with an active URI or a URI in the previous week.[5] This desaturation responded to short-term administration of supplemental oxygen. Other studies have shown an increase in bronchial reactivity for up to 7 weeks after a URI,[6] a decrease in FVC and flow rates during URIs,[7] and impaired clearance of mucus from the trachea for at least a week after the disappearance of URI symptoms.[8] These data suggest postponement of general anesthesia for 4 to 7 weeks after the onset of a URI.

We are prospectively comparing the incidences of perioperative oxygen desaturation, laryngospasm, and bronchospasm among ASA physical status 1 or 2 children with an active URI, a recent URI, or no history or current evidence of a URI. These children are undergoing a variety of largely superficial procedures. Approximately 75% undergo tracheal intubation. Our work thus far indicates no significant differences in these variables among the three groups totaling 209 patients. Our findings, like those of Koka and coworkers,[9] have also shown no correlation between the presence of a URI and the occurrence of postintubation croup.

In the case presented here, the child fulfills the diagnosis of an active URI based on Tait and Knight's criteria (criteria 3, 6, and 7). Assuming this child is otherwise healthy and based on the available data, we would proceed with anesthetizing this patient for bilateral myringotomy and tube placement. We would administer supplemental oxygen in the recovery room, as is our standard for all patients. However, the presence of signs of lower respiratory tract pathology (rhonchi, wheezes, rales, fever $> 101°F$) or the presence of preexisting pulmonary or cardiac disease would make us recommend postponement of anesthesia and surgery for 4 to 6 weeks.

The frequency of URIs in this child is not mentioned, but it is conceivable that these could recur every 4 to 6 weeks in a child less than 2 years old, especially from the fall through the spring months. Therefore, for those anesthesiologists who feel compelled to delay anesthesia and surgery for 4 to 6 weeks after a URI, the ideal time for performing the procedure might never arrive. We feel the available studies provide convincing information to assure us of the safety of proceeding with this surgical procedure under the presented circumstances.

REFERENCES

1. Behrman RE, Vaughan VC: Nelson's Textbook of Pediatrics, p 870. Philadelphia, WB Saunders, 1987
2. Tait AR, Knight PR: The effects of general anesthesia on upper respiratory tract infections in children. Anesthesiology 67: 930, 1987
3. Tait AR, Knight PR: Intraoperative respiratory complications in patients with upper respiratory tract infections. Can J Anaesth 34(3): 300, 1987
4. McGill WA, Coveler LA, Epstein BS: Subacute upper respiratory infection in small children. Anesth Analg 58: 331, 1979
5. DeSoto H, Patel RI, Soliman IE, Hannallah RS: Changes in oxygen saturation following general anesthesia in children with upper respiratory infection signs and symptoms undergoing otolaryngologic procedures. Anesthesiology 68: 276, 1988
6. Empey DW, Laitinen LA, Jacobs L, Gold WM, Nadel JA: Mechanisms of bronchial hyperreactivity in normal subjects after upper respiratory tract infection. Am Rev Respir Dis 113: 131, 1976
7. Collier AM, Pimmel RL, Hasselblad V, Clyde WA, Knelson JH, Brooks JG: Spirometric changes in normal children with upper respiratory infections. Am Rev Respir Dis 117: 47, 1978
8. Wong JW, Keens TG, Wannamaker EM, Crozier DN, Levison H, Aspin N: Effects of gravity on tracheal mucus transport rates in normal subjects and in patients with cystic fibrosis. Pediatrics 60(2): 146, 1977
9. Koka BV, Jeon IS, Andre JM, MacKay I, Smith RM: Postintubation croup in children. Anesth Analg 56(40): 501, 1977

Response

It is not uncommon for anesthesiologists to see the picture provided by this case. Young children scheduled for bilateral myringotomy and ear tube placement may present with low-grade fever, rhinorrhea, and cough. In this case, additional information is provided that the chest is clear to ausculation, the pharynx does not reveal evidence of an infectious process, and the cough has not awakened this child from sleep. It also would be reassuring to have the history from the mother state that the child's activity, dietary intake, and sleep patterns also had been normal and on physical examination to find a subacute otitis media to explain the low-grade fever.

We would concur with Dr. Betts and proceed with anesthesia for this patient, but we would monitor this patient carefully with pulse oximetry in the PACU.

While each patient must be handled individually, Dr. Betts has described Tait and Knight's criteria for the diagnosis of URI. Certainly evidence of lower airway involvement (laryngitis, bronchitis, wheezes, or rales) and a history of changes in normal activities, dietary intake, and sleep patterns are strong clinical indicators to defer anesthesia and surgery in patients who present with these symptoms.

▧ CASE REPORT NO. 12

A seven-month-old infant (healthy, normal gestation) is scheduled for removal of a cyst from the mandible. During the preanesthesia interview, the mother states that the infant's sister died of "crib death" two years ago at six months of age. Would you proceed on an outpatient basis?

Discussion

Mark A. Rockoff, M.D.
Vice Chairman and Clinical Director, Department of Anesthesia, Children's Hospital Medical Center, Associate Professor of Anaesthesia (Pediatrics), Harvard Medical School, Boston, Massachusetts

Mary Ellen McCann, M.D.
Instructor in Anaesthesia (Pediatrics), Harvard Medical School, Assistant in Anesthesia at Children's Hospital Medical Center, Boston, Massachusetts

Sudden infant death syndrome (SIDS) is defined as the sudden and unexpected death of an apparently well infant whose death remains unexplained after the performance of an adequate autopsy.[1] It is the leading cause of mortality in the United States for infants after the neonatal period, occurring in approximately 1 in 500 live births. The peak incidence occurs between two and three months of age, with 90% of cases occurring within the first six months of life. It is extremely rare to occur after one year of age. Deaths from SIDS tend to recur within families; the rate among siblings of victims is about five times that for the population at large, and twins of SIDS victims appear to be at particular risk.[2]

The cause of SIDS is unclear, and the etiology appears to be multifactorial.[3] Studies done in infants with near-miss SIDS episodes have shown that some infants have an abnormal respiratory pattern with periods of apnea and periodic breathing detectable by pneumography.[4] Whether this is related to the well-recognized apnea of prematurity is unknown, although premature infants are at much greater risk of SIDS than full-term babies. In addition, it has been shown that near-miss SIDS infants have an impairment in their ventilatory response to carbon dioxide breathing during sleep, a finding also seen in preterm infants.[5] Interestingly, one study also documented a similar finding in parents of SIDS victims, and siblings of SIDS victims have been shown to have an increase in periodic breathing.[6,7] Furthermore, some episodes of apnea may be obstructive (rather than central), and obstructive sleep apnea in older patients appears to have a familial basis.[8] These findings lend additional support to the concept that there is an inheritable factor in this disorder. Other studies have shown that some infants have an abnormal ECG (with either a short or prolonged QT segment) or that there is more liability and poorer stabilization of heart rate after stimulation.[9] Gastroesophageal reflux can cause laryngospasm and hypoxia leading to sudden death, and rarely seizure activity or brainstem abnormalities have been implicated as causes of apnea and bradycardia.[10]

Whether there are any unusual effects of anesthesia and/or surgery in infants "destined" to become SIDS victims is unknown. There is little published in this regard, although one retrospective review of a small number of patients suggested that anesthesia is not a trigger for SIDS.[11] Much literature does exist, however, that clearly documents apnea and bradycardia following general anesthesia in very young infants, particularly those who are less than 44 weeks postconceptual age and for an even longer period in those born prematurely. Because of all these concerns, anesthesia for patients at increased risk of SIDS cannot be taken lightly.

The preoperative medical evaluation of an infant considered at risk for SIDS is not likely to be revealing, since most infants are well by definition. Many infants whose siblings have died of SIDS have already had pneumograms, but these are not reliable predictors of future episodes. Some of these infants have already been placed on a home apnea monitor and their caretakers taught basic life support.

Based on this information, this seven-month-old infant is most safely managed following surgery and anesthesia as an inpatient. While this may be considered very conservative therapy and be unnecessary for most patients, the available studies to date indicate (at least to us) that the benefits outweigh the risks. Since the reason for admission is to monitor the patient closely postoperatively, a cardiac and respiratory monitor (and/or pulse oximeter) should be employed overnight. This duration of monitoring should be sufficient if no problems develop, since extrapolation of data from studies of premature infants developing apnea following anesthesia suggests that infants who do have problems manifest them initially within the first 12 hours after surgery.[12] Alarm parameters should be clearly defined, such as apnea greater than 20 seconds, heart rate less than 90 beats per minute, or oxygen saturation less than 95%. Considering the anxiety experienced by families who have lost a previous child to SIDS, this period of overnight observation is usually well understood, accepted, and frequently desired.

In conclusion, it is prudent to admit this infant for monitoring following anesthesia. While there is little scientific evidence linking anesthesia to an increased risk of death from SIDS in full-term infants, this is a cautious approach to the infant who is a sibling of a SIDS victim. Healthy babies with risk factors for SIDS who are older than one year of age should have outgrown this problem and can have anesthesia and surgery done on an outpatient basis.

REFERENCES

1. Valdes-Dapena M: Sudden infant death in infancy. In Nelson, Vaughn, McKay, Behrman (eds): Nelson's Textbook of Pediatrics, p 1980. Philadelphia, WB Saunders, 1979
2. Smialek JE: Simultaneous sudden infant death syndrome in twins. Pediatrics 77: 816, 1986
3. Valdes-Dapena M: Sudden infant death syndrome: A review of the medical literature 1974–1979. Pediatrics 66: 597, 1980
4. Haidmayer R, Kurz R, Kenner T, Wurm H, Pfeiffer KP: Physiologic and clinical aspects of respiratory control in infants with relation to the sudden infant death syndrome. *Klin. Wochenschr* 60: 9, 1982
5. Shannon DC, Kelly DH, O'Connor K: Abnormal regulation in infants at risk for sudden infant death syndrome. N Engl J Med 297: 747, 1977
6. Schiffman PL, Westlake RE, Santiago TV, Edelman NH: Ventilatory control in parents of victims of sudden infant death syndrome. N Engl J Med 302: 486, 1980

7. Kelly DH, Walker A, Cahen L, Shannon DC: Periodic breathing in siblings of sudden infant death syndrome victims. Pediatrics 66: 515, 1980
8. Strohl KP, Saunders NA, Feldman NT, Hallet M: Obstructive sleep apnea in family members. N Engl J Med 299: 969, 1978
9. Salk L, Grellong BA, Dietrich J: Sudden infant death: Normal cardiac habituation and poor autonomic control. N Engl J Med 291: 219, 1974
10. Kenigsburg K, Griswold P, Buckley B, Gootman N, Gootman P: Cardiac effects of esophageal reflux (GER) and sudden infant death syndrome (SIDS). J Pediatr Surg 18: 542, 1983
11. Steward D: Is there a risk of general anesthesia triggering SIDS? Possibly not! Anesthesiology 63: 326, 1985
12. Kurth CD, Spitzer AR, Broenne AM, Downs JJ: Postoperative apnea in preterm infants. Anesthesiology 66: 483, 1987

Response

When approaching a family in which a child has already died from SIDS, it is important to be sympathetic to the family and available to answer any questions that they may have (somewhat difficult in that the etiology of SIDS is poorly understood). It has been postulated that there is an inherited factor to the disorder. However, a study by Peterson and coworkers suggests that the risk of SIDS in siblings of SIDS victims is inflated.[1] There is no current evidence to suggest that general anesthesia may trigger SIDS or the infant apnea syndrome.[2] There are some infants, however, who do seem to be at greater risk for the development of SIDS, such as premature infants, infants with the infant apnea syndrome, and infants who have had bronchopulmonary dysplasia. When faced with a child who does not fall into any of these groups, there is no clearcut evidence that the child is at greater risk for developing SIDS. If there is any history of this child having periods of apnea at home, the prudent approach would be to observe the child (must be monitored) within the hospital setting postanesthesia.

If the surgical removal of this cyst can be delayed, this would be the best approach. SIDS is extremely rare after 1 year of age. After that time, even if there is a familial tendency for SIDS, the incidence drops precipitously. Let's plan on delaying this child's procedure until after one year of age, if possible. Parent comfort level must enter into any decision making.

REFERENCES

1. Peterson DR, Sabotta EE, Daling JR: Infant mortality among subsequent siblings of infants who died of sudden infant death syndrome. Pediatrics 108: 911, 1986
2. Steward DJ: Is there a risk of general anesthesia triggering SIDS? Possibly not! Anesthesiology 63: 326, 1985

▊ CASE REPORT NO. 13

A 38-year-old woman arrives in the ambulatory surgery unit scheduled for excision of a large lipoma on her anterior thigh. She has a history of asthma and takes theophylline SR (250 mg) twice a day and utilizes an albuterol (Alupent) inhaler four times a day. Her most recent asthmatic attack was four months ago, and she required hospitalization and intravenous theophylline therapy. She takes 2.5 mg

Brethine on a PRN basis but has not used it since discharge from the hospital. She has been followed by an internist, and theophylline levels have been in a therapeutic range.

Discussion
Marina D. Bizzarri-Schmid, M.D.
Instructor in Anaesthesia, Harvard Medical School, Anesthesiology, Brigham and Women's Hospital, Boston, Massachusetts

Beverly K. Philip, M.D.
Assistant Professor of Anaesthesia, Harvard Medical School, Anesthesiology/Director, Day Surgery Unit, Brigham and Women's Hospital, Boston, Massachusetts

Asthma is defined as a disorder "characterized by increased responsiveness of the trachea and bronchi to various stimuli, resulting in widespread narrowing of the airways. These changes are reversible either spontaneously or as a result of therapy."[1] The two major types of asthma are extrinsic (childhood onset, seasonal variation, specific allergens) and intrinsic (adult onset, perennial, no specific allergen), which is more severe. Nonallergic stimuli for the attack include respiratory infection, cold, exercise, and psychogenic factors. The stimulus causes release of trigger agents such as leukotrienes, histamine, prostaglandins, and chemotactic factors, which produce smooth-muscle contraction, vasodilatation, edema, mucus secretion, and eosinophilia. The typical asthma attack begins with coughing and wheezing followed by chest tightness and dyspnea.[1]

Treatment of asthma consists of acute and chronic management. The acute attack must be treated promptly with oxygen and sympathomimetic drugs. Maintenance therapy may include sympathomimetic agents, methylxanthines, and cromones. Severe cases may warrant the use of corticosteroids. The potential side-effects of these drugs must be carefully considered.

The evaluation of the patient with a history of asthma should include a history of the patient's general health, activity level, medications, recent upper or lower respiratory tract infections, and compromising factors such as obesity and smoking. The anesthesiologist should also ascertain if there have been any problems with anesthesia in the past, such as difficult airway or intubation and bronchospasm or laryngospasm. A physical examination should be performed with special attention to the upper airway, lungs, and body habitus. If sneezing and rhinorrhea are present, one should determine if there is an allergic or infectious etiology. If an infection is suspected, laboratory data should include a WBC with a differential. A theophylline level may be indicated in the presence of symptoms of inadequate therapy or toxicity. Stress-dose steroids may be indicated during surgery.[2]

This particular patient requires chronic oral and inhalational therapy and recently was hospitalized and treated with intravenous medication. Therefore, her asthma is severe, and she must be considered at increased risk for intraoperative and postoperative complications. It is important to determine compliance with her medical regimen, precipitating factors, frequency and severity of attacks, and speed of resolution. Inspection of the airway and auscultation of the lungs are essential. Any indication of an infection or wheezing must be taken seriously, and postponement of surgery should be considered. According to Cecil, "One of the most important nonspecific irritants is respiratory tract infection, particularly by viral agents. Both lower and upper respiratory infections may initiate or aggravate bronchospasm."[1] The patient should be instructed to take her usual medications with a sip of water on the morning of surgery and to use the albuterol inhaler before surgery.

The scheduled surgery involves the lower extremity. We believe that a regional technique is definitely the anesthesia of choice. The specific technique (spinal vs. epidural) and local anesthetic agent will be determined by the expected duration of surgery. The agent chosen should allow sufficient time for the surgery and still permit discharge the same day. Spinal anesthesia using 5% hyperbaric lidocaine would be ideal for a procedure of less than two hours. However, one must always be prepared to induce general anesthesia at any point. Thus it would be unwise to proceed with surgery if the patient were not in the best possible condition. Supplementation with intravenous medication also may be given if required. Anxiety, which itself can cause attacks in some patients, should be treated with the judicious use of benzodiazepines and non-histamine-releasing narcotics. Barbiturate sedation should be avoided because it can precipitate bronchospasm. Sedation should be carefully controlled to avoid the need for airway manipulation. Essential monitoring includes ECG, blood pressure, pulse oximeter, and precordial stethoscope. Arterial blood gas analysis may be required.

If general anesthesia must be given, the risks and benefits of different techniques should be considered. Although inhalational agents are often recommended, intravenous drugs carefully administered may be well tolerated. Minimal instrumentation of the airway is preferable. The case under discussion could be performed with mask anesthesia. Histamine-releasing agents should be avoided.[2-4]

This patient can undergo the planned procedure, ideally under regional anesthesia, in an ambulatory unit. The unit should have facilities available for immediate treatment of an acute attack and access to a hospital. If the patient suffers an asthma attack, hospitalization may be necessary. Consider the following statement from the most recent edition of *Cecil's Textbook of Medicine:* "In more than one half of asthmatic patients, inhalation of specific allergens causes an immediate bronchoconstriction that resolves within minutes to hours and then recurs six to ten hours later. An appreciation of late-onset reactions is reshaping our thinking about asthma: It is not solely a syndrome of brief and reversible airways obstruction but also a disease involving a progressive, multistage inflammatory response." After ambulatory anesthesia, this patient may be discharged to home with a companion, provided she has been free of asthma symptoms.

Patients with asthma can be safely managed in an ambulatory surgery unit provided their disease is well controlled, the medical personnel are aware of the possibility of acute and delayed reactions, the unit is prepared to handle such emergencies, and hospital facilities are available.

REFERENCES

1. Wyngaarden JB, Smith LH (eds): Cecil's Textbook of Medicine, 18th ed. pp 403–410. Philadelphia, WB Saunders, 1988
2. Yao F, Artusio JF, Jr (eds): Anesthesiology: Problem-Oriented Patient Management, pp 3–18. Philadelphia, JB Lippincott, 1983
3. Hirshman CA, et al: Mechanism of action of inhalational anesthesia on airways. Anesthesiology 56: 107, 1982
4. Downes H, Hirshman CA, Leon DA: Comparison of local anesthetics as bronchodilator aerosols. Anesthesiology 58: 216, 1983

Response

There is little to add to the fine discussion of this obese asthmatic patient. Motivated patients with obesity and asthma that is well controlled are reasonable candidates for extremity surgery on an ambulatory basis. I would agree with Drs. Bizzarri-Schmid and Philip that regional anesthesia would be the first choice of anesthesia technique for this patient. However, other regional techniques besides spinal or epidural anesthesia also should be considered. First, local anesthesia depending on the size of the lesion and patient acceptance could well be the anesthesia of choice. Second, the history states that the lipoma is on the anterior thigh, and a femoral nerve block, supplemented, if necessary, by a lateral femoral cutaneous and/or obturator nerve block, may also be a better alternative than epidural or spinal anesthesia. Depending on the patient's weight distribution, peripheral nerve blocks may be technically easier to perform than an epidural or spinal anesthesia. Epidural anesthesia would be the preferred technique over spinal anesthesia, especially in a young woman, because of the potential for postspinal headache. Even though regional anesthesia is the technique of choice, all patients should be optimally prepared, because general anesthesia may be necessary. Should general anesthesia be required, drugs that may trigger bronchospasm or histamine release should be avoided, and if tracheal intubation is necessary, lidocaine spray of the vocal cords and trachea should be performed prior to intubation to reduce the chances of reactive bronchospasm from placement of the endotracheal tube.

REFERENCE

1. Hirshman CA: Perioperative management of the patient with asthma. Presented at ASA Annual Meeting, Refresher Course, San Francisco, CA, 1988

◼ CASE REPORT NO. 14

An apprehensive 80-year-old man requests general anesthesia for cataract surgery. Upon arrival his blood pressure is 190/110 mmHg. He takes one Dyazide every morning. The patient states that his blood pressure has never been this high. Preoperative ECG reveals minor ST changes and rare PVCs. There are no acute changes.

Discussion
Edward D. Miller, Jr., M.D.
E. M. Papper Professor of Anesthesiology and Chairman, Department of Anesthesiology, College of Physicians and Surgeons of Columbia University, New York, New York

This patient presents to the ambulatory surgery center with hypertension. Whether the patient's hypertension is secondary to underlying renal disease or more commonly to essential hypertension is not readily apparent. However, if the patient had been followed by his local medical doctor, it is unlikely that an elevation in BUN and creatinine would not have been detected prior to this visit. Other stigmata of renal failure also would be present and would alert the anesthesiologist to the fact that hypertension was due to renal dysfunction and the surgery would then be postponed. If it can be assumed that the patient has essential hypertension, then the question arises should this procedure be postponed or should the case be done at the time the patient presents himself.

The important information that should be sought is whether this degree of hypertension is abnormal for the patient. The patient states that the blood pressure has never been this high, but if old records were available, they might either confirm or suggest that the hypertension had been more severe in the past. In this particular case, it would seem appropriate to sedate the patient with intravenous midazolam, allow him to lie quietly in the holding area, and then have the blood pressure taken several times to see what the trend would be. If the blood pressure tends to decrease with sedation, then further therapy is not appropriate. If, however, the blood pressure remains elevated or actually increases, then it would be appropriate to treat this patient with either 10 mg sublingual nifedipine PO or intravenous labetalol. Since this patient has some rare PVCs, the use of labetalol may have a specific advantage.

The patient has requested general anesthesia. While general anesthesia can be safely administered to this patient, the chances of his developing significant hypertension intraoperatively are great. It would be in the best interest of the patient to convince him that a retrobulbar or peribulbar block would be more appropriate. Specifically, I would recommend small amounts of local anesthetic containing epinephrine. The use of epinephrine in this patient would not be detrimental for two reasons. First, the total amount of local anesthetic given for such a block is very low, and therefore, the amount of epinephrine administered would be relatively small. Second, the amount of epinephrine given could potentially stimulate peripheral beta receptors and cause vasodilatation in the vascular bed, with a resultant decrease in diastolic blood pressure. The fact that the patient has ventricular arrhythmias would not dissuade me from using epinephrine-containing solutions, because if the arrhythmias got worse, they could be treated either with intravenous lidocaine or an intravenous beta blocker.

If the patient cannot be convinced that local anesthesia would be the best approach for this procedure, then general anesthesia should be administered. The main concern in the hypertensive patient is that the patient responds in an exaggerated manner to various procedures. Specifically, at the time of intubation and at the time of wakeup, the patient may respond with increases in blood pressure and heart rate that would not be seen in a normotensive patient. This is due to the fact that the patient with long-standing hypertension has increased vascular reactivity, and this particular patient also evidences stiffening of the arterioles. This stiffening means that there is less compliance of the vascular tree and that when the heart is stimulated, the full force of contraction of the left ventricle is transmitted to the vessels. In a normally compliant individual, systolic blood pressure rises only a small degree. However, in patients with long-standing hypertension, the ejection of blood from the left ventricle into a noncompliant vascular tree results in excessive increases in systolic blood pressure. Second, there is an alteration in the vascular smooth muscles so that there is an increase in resistance, and diastolic blood pressure remains elevated. This increase in resistance is the result of increased vascular smooth-muscle tone and hypertrophy of these vascular smooth muscles. Therefore, diastolic blood pressure is high and sympathetic stimulation results in increases in vascular resistance, which is exaggerated compared to normotensive patients. These two factors result in increases both in systolic and diastolic pressure.

What can one do to minimize the increases in blood pressure at the time of stress—specifically, at the time of induction and intubation and at the time of extubation and emergence from anesthesia? Several approaches have been used, and all may be successful but none is foolproof. The use of narcotics prior to intubation has been shown to decrease the incidence of hypertension. In an elderly patient such as this, 25 to 50 μg fentanyl may be appropriate. If at the time of laryngoscopy there is a sudden increase in blood pressure or heart rate, it might be better to stop the laryngoscopy, ventilate the patient, and titrate more narcotic. It should be pointed out that emphasis has often been placed on the absolute blood pressure, but heart rate is a much more important determinant of damage to the myocardium. The main area of concern for the anesthesiologist in such a patient is to prevent myocardial ischemia secondary to increased demands. The fact that the patient has hypertension increases the oxygen demand by his myocardium, but on top of this, the increases are much greater if tachycardia also occurs. Other methods to decrease myocardial oxygen demand would be the use of intravenous lidocaine prior to intubation, the use of intravenous labetalol, or the use of short-acting beta blockers such as esmolol. In general, though, small doses of narcotics and generous amounts of barbiturates at the time of induction will minimize the increases that are seen.

Postoperatively, the patient should be observed for increases in blood pressure and heart rate, and the patient also should be appropriately monitored to see if ST-segment changes have occurred as well as any increase in the number of ventricular arrhythmias. Blood pressure control in the postoperative setting can be achieved through the use of either intravenous labetalol or calcium-channel blockers. The patient should be instructed to start his medications the next day following the procedure. Patients are often instructed to take their medicines on the day of surgery, but in this particular case, the use of a diuretic rarely would have much significance in terms of blood pressure control. However, if the patient were on calcium-channel blockers, an alpha blocker, or a drug such as clonidine, then the PO medication on the day of surgery is much more important than in this particular circumstance.

The patient who comes to the ambulatory surgery center with an elevation in his blood pressure probably has underlying essential hypertension. With diastolic blood pressures less than 120 mmHg, the anesthesiologist has a variety of drugs that will allow him or her to proceed with the surgical procedure. However, a patient whose diastolic blood pressure is greater than 120 mmHg or who shows signs of myocardial ischemia or ventricular arrhythmias should be postponed until an appropriate workup can define the degree of myocardial dysfunction. In elective surgical procedures, antihypertensive therapy should be begun prior to the surgical procedure and blood pressure should be well controlled. The arbitrary use of a blood pressure of 120 mmHg must be put into the context of the whole patient and what other underlying diseases are present.

Response
In this scenario, the patient must be aware of the potential for increased morbidity associated with hypertension and general anesthesia. Careful explanation should be given relating to the safety of a regional (*i.e.*, peribulbar, retrobulbar block) anesthetic and its postoperative course with less side-effects. There is nothing wrong with letting the patient know that a regional would be your choice (if in fact that is true). If the patient then chooses to proceed with the general anesthetic, every effort should be made to prevent further increases in blood pressure during induction and emergence from anesthesia. In addition to the antihypertensive medications mentioned by Dr. Miller, 0.5 to 1 mg/kg lidocaine IV prior to intubation may be helpful in blunting the hypertensive response associated with laryngoscopy. This also may affect the patient's PVCs. Hypertensive patients also merit close observation in the postoperative period. One must always be on guard that these patients have an increased risk of myocardial infarction and other systemic disturbances.[1]

REFERENCE
1. Estafanous FG: Postoperative hypertension: Incidence and management. Curr Rev Recov Room Nurses 5: 11, 1983

CASE REPORT NO. 15
A 3-year-old child with a history of chronic hypertrophic tonsillitis is scheduled for a T&A. The child has cerebral palsy and is quite combative. What approach can be used to smooth his anesthetic course?

Discussion
Ramesh I. Patel, M.D.
Associate Professor, George Washington University Medical Center, Department of Anesthesiology, Children's National Medical Center, Washington, D.C.

Cerebral palsy is a term used to describe a group of diverse nonprogressive syndromes that affect the brain and impair motor function.[1] The clinical manifestations may include mental retardation, learning difficulties, seizures, and motor deficit with hypertonia and contractures. A child with mild cerebral palsy with minimal hypertonia and no respiratory obstruction may be scheduled to undergo tonsillectomy on an ambulatory basis. On the other hand, a patient with severe hypertonia, muscle contractures, or severe upper airway obstruction should be admitted overnight to the hospital following tonsillectomy. The extent of this 3-year-old child's impairment is not clear from the preceding history; therefore, precise recommendations for or against ambulatory surgery cannot be made. Segal and coworkers have studied 892 patients and have concluded that it is safe to perform T&A on an ambulatory basis in a healthy child.[2] Chiang and associates have reported a series of 40,000 tonsillectomies performed on an outpatient basis without a death.[3] They emphasize careful preoperative medical evaluation and selection of patients.

If the history of combativeness is known prior to the day of surgery, we will try to schedule this patient as a second or third case of the day. Our ambulatory admission area is full of patients and parents early in the morning because the first case in every room starts at 7:30 A.M. Later on in the day, there is staggering of cases. A combative child in a room full of other children and parents may present logistic problems. Isolating the child and the family in a private location is another alternative.

Generally, I do not prefer to premedicate such patients with sedatives or hypnotics, but some patients may benefit from premedication. If premedication is administered, patients should be closely watched for signs of respiratory obstruction and respiratory depression. Induction of anesthesia is smoother through intravenous or intramuscular route. The presence of parents during induction reduces anxiety and leads to reduced agitation and resistance by the patient. At CNMC, parents will accompany the child to the induction room. One of the parents will then give a firm hug to the child, and the outstretched arm will be held by the anesthesiologist. Care should be taken so as not to show the needle to the child. Anesthesia can then be induced with thiopental 4 to 6 mg/kg through a 25-gauge butterfly needle if the child has visible veins. In the absence of visible veins, an intramuscular injection of 3 to 4 mg/kg ketamine mixed with 0.2 mg atropine should be administered through a 23-gauge needle. Rectal methohexital (30 mg/kg) is used at other institutions. Dose of any induction agent should be tailored according to the weight of the patient, combativeness, and degree of airway obstruction. Monitors are applied after the child is induced. We use pulse oximeter and a precordial stethoscope in the induction room. Intravenous muscle relaxants are administered following mask ventilation. Succinylcholine is not contraindicated in a child with cerebral palsy and can be safely used to facilitate tracheal intubation.

Use of intraoperative narcotics will depend on the degree of airway obstruction and the degree of motor impairment. A child who has obstructive apnea or has a severe handicap should not receive intraoperative narcotics, but narcotics could be judiciously titrated in the recovery room. Peritonsillar infiltration with local anesthetics containing epinephrine 1:200,000 reduces operative blood loss but may not reduce perioperative pain.[4] It is recommended that all children receive supplemental oxygen during transport and in the recovery room if Sp_{O_2} is not measured. The decision to discharge a patient with cerebral palsy who has undergone tonsillectomy should be based on the degree of physical impairment, presence or absence of obstructive apnea and bleeding, status of hydration, degree of pain, and social environment. My own preference would be to admit this patient overnight to the hospital for observation and to ensure adequate hydration and treatment of pain.

REFERENCES

1. Low NL, Carter S: Static encephalopathies. In Rudolph AM, Hoffman JIE (eds): Pediatrics, pp 1594–1597. New York, Appleton and Lange, 1987
2. Segal C, Berger G, Barker M, Marshak G: Adenotonsillectomies on a surgical day-clinic base. Laryngoscope 93: 1205, 1983
3. Chiang TM, Sukis AE, Ross DE: Tonsillectomy performed on an outpatient basis: Report of a series of 40,000 cases performed without a death. Arch Otolaryngol 88: 307, 1968
4. Broadman LM, Patel RI, Feldman BA, Sellman GL, Milmoe G, Camilon F: The effects of peritonsillar infiltration on the reduction of intraoperative blood loss and post-tonsillectomy pain in children. Laryngoscope 99: 578, 1989

Response

Dr. Patel has presented a thorough and intelligent management plan for any child who is uncooperative or combative. From our experience at Methodist Ambulatory SurgiCare, intramuscular ketamine (2–3 mg/kg), methohexital (5–8 mg/kg), or midazolam (0.08–0.1 mg/kg) provide satisfactory sedation. The future is promising for other less invasive ways of providing sedation—sufentanil administered nasally[1] or transmucousal fentanyl lollipops.[2]

The key to this discussion is careful observation and monitoring of any child receiving intramuscular (or rectal) sedation. If no induction room is available, a parent should be encouraged to accompany this child to the operating room, where appropriate monitoring and availability of items to provide respiratory support are immediately available. An appropriately placed precordial stethoscope and pulse oximeter are minimal requirements for patient monitoring during this induction.

This child might benefit from prolonged postoperative observation (6–8 hrs) with a parent present to provide comfort. However, if there were no surgical contraindication to sending the patient home, this child's postoperative emotional course might be much smoother in its own home environment rather than the strange environs of the hospital. If parents are both capable of and comfortable with managing this child at home following surgery, I would encourage this approach.

In review, I would schedule this child for a procedure in the ambulatory unit at 8:00 A.M. The child, parents, and a member of the nursing staff should proceed to a quiet area prior to this child's surgery. In the quiet area or the operating room (with a parent present), preinduction sedation should be provided.

REFERENCES

1. Henderson J, Bradsky D, Fisher D, et al: Fentanyl given transmucousally from lollipops. Anesthesiology 68: 671, 1988
2. Streisand JB, Hague B, van Vreeswijk HAL: Oral transmucousal fentanyl premedication in children. Anesth Analg 66: 5170, 1987

CASE REPORT NO. 16

This patient is a 46-year-old man who is scheduled for extraction of all remaining teeth. The patient has severe rheumatoid arthritis and has been on prednisone (20 mg daily) for the last 5 years. On physical examination, the patient is of normal size and weight, opens his mouth well, and has good mobility in his neck. Should there be concern over the patient's long use of prednisone?

Discussion

Albert T. Cheung, M.D.
Clinical and Research Fellow in Anaesthesia, Harvard Medical School, Massachusetts General Hospital, Boston, Massachusetts

Bart Chernow, M.D., F.A.C.P.
Physician-in-Chief, Sinai Hospital of Baltimore, Professor of Medicine, Anesthesiology and Critical Care, Johns Hopkins University School of Medicine, Baltimore, Maryland

Patients on long-term glucocorticoid therapy subjected to surgery can have an abnormal physiologic response to surgical stress. Exogenous glucocorticoids, through negative feedback, suppress the normal production and release of corticotrophin-releasing factor (CRF) and adrenocorticotrophic hormone (ACTH), which leads to adrenal gland atrophy. The normal augmentation of glucocorticoid production during surgical stress is therefore impaired in these patients and they are at risk of developing acute adrenocortical insufficiency precipitated by anesthesia or surgery. The anesthesiologist caring for these patients is therefore confronted with several problems. The first problem is to determine which patients are at risk for underlying glucocorticoid-induced secondary adrenal insufficiency. The second problem is to determine the appropriate supplemental dose of corticosteroid that will be required to "cover" the stress of the procedure. Finally, the underlying problem for which glucocorticoid therapy was instituted and other long-term side-effects of chronic glucocorticoid therapy should be recognized as independent risk factors.

Attention was brought to the problem of "secondary" adrenal insufficiency caused by discontinuation of glucocorticoid therapy in a case report that appeared in 1952.[1] In this report, cortisone therapy was discontinued several days prior to elective surgery in a patient who had been on chronic cortisone therapy for rheumatoid arthritis. Postoperatively, the patient died of shock, and the postmortem examination showed bilateral adrenal gland atrophy. In the accompanying editorial, supplemental glucocorticoid therapy was recommended for all glucocorticoid-treated patients when subjected to the stress of surgical operations, trauma, or acute infections. As a result of this devastating consequence, the use of perioperative glucocorticoid prophylaxis has persisted as the standard of care for patients on chronic glucocorticoid therapy.

Not all patients on chronic glucocorticoid therapy have underlying adrenal insufficiency. Among a variety of preoperative laboratory tests available to detect underlying adrenal insufficiency, the rapid ACTH stimulation test is the most useful, because it is easy to perform and provides a quick result. This test is performed by comparing plasma cortisol concentrations before and 30 minutes following the IV administration of 250 μg synthetic ACTH (Cosyntropin, Cortrosyn). An increase in plasma cortisol concentration by more than 7 μg/dl and to a concentration greater than 18 to 20 μg/dl 30 minutes after the ACTH injection is associated with a normal endogenous cortisol response to surgery.[2] However, the test is seldom necessary, since the routine provision of perioperative prophylactic glucocorticoids to all patients with the potential for underlying adrenal insufficiency carries little risk in itself. A general rule is to provide glucocorticoid "coverage" for patients taking exogenous corticosteroids for a period exceeding one week during the previous 6 months. When uncertainty exists, the rapid ACTH stimulation test is useful to confirm the adequacy of adrenocortical function. Preoperative serum sodium and potassium concentrations should be measured in all patients on chronic high-dose glucocorticoid therapy, since a recent case report[3] suggests that severe mineralocorticoid deficiency may occur in rare patients. The presence of hyponatremia, hyperkalemia, and metabolic acidosis should alert the clinician to this problem.

The appropriate dose and timing of perioperative glucocorticoid therapy is the subject of considerable controversy. Initially, overcompensation was the general rule, but a greater understanding of the adrenocortical response to graded degrees of surgical stress have allowed the individualization of dosage regimens to mimic the normal pattern of cortisol production in the perioperative period. In patients undergoing uncomplicated oral surgery, cortisol production peaks several hours after surgery and normalizes by 24 hours postoperatively.[4] This pattern of cortisol production can be reproduced by the intravenous administration of 25 mg hydrocortisone preoperatively and 50 mg postoperatively and the resumption of the usual maintenance therapy on postoperative day 1. Furthermore, the endogenous cortisol response to stress can be attenuated by the use of analgesics and nerve blocks to control postoperative pain. The duration of glucocorticoid use and the requirements for maintenance therapy also must be considered when deciding on the appropriate dose of prophylactic therapy.[5]

In addition to adrenal suppression, chronic glucocorticoid therapy has other effects that can complicate perioperative management. Glucocorticoid therapy can cause immunosuppression and increase susceptibility to infections. Poor wound healing, skin and bone fragility, and glucose intolerance are also characteristic problems of chronic glucocorticoid use. The underlying disease for which glucocorticoid therapy was instituted is also of importance. For example, in this case, rheumatoid arthritis may present difficulties in airway management.

In summary, with proper attention to managing the problems present in patients on chronic glucocorticoid therapy, there is no evidence that they are at an increased risk of perioperative mortality or morbidity when treated in an ambulatory care setting.

REFERENCES

1. Fraser CG, Preuss FS, Bigford WD: Adrenal atrophy and irreversible shock associated with cortisone therapy. JAMA 149: 1542, 1952
2. Kehlet H, Binder C: Value of an ACTH test in assessing hypothalamic-pituitary-adrenocortical function in glucocorticoid-treated patients. Br Med J 2: 147, 1973
3. Jacobs TP, Whitelock RT, Edsall J, Holub DA: Addisonian crisis while taking high-dose glucocorticoids. JAMA 260: 2082, 1988
4. Banks P: The adreno-cortical response to oral surgery. Br J Oral Surg 8: 32, 1970
5. Napolitano LM, Chernow B: Guidelines for corticosteroid use in anesthetic and surgical stress. Int Anesthesiol Clin 26: 226, 1988

Response

Better insight to changes in cortisol levels associated with the stress of surgery have lead to a more rational approach to glucocorticoid replacement. The dosages of hydrocortisone that I use to prophylax patients who have been on chronic prednisone therapy also have decreased markedly. Historically, it was quite common for a patient to receive 300 mg hydrocortisone to blunt the surgical response to stress. A popular regimen calls for the administration of 200 to 300 mg hydrocortisone per 70-kg body weight in divided doses on the day of surgery. Symreng and coworkers advocate the infusion of 25 mg cortisol IV before the induction of anesthesia, followed by continuous infusion of 100 mg cortisol during the following 24 hours.[1]

This patient should take his morning dose of prednisone followed by 25 mg hydrocortisone IV preinduction and 50 mg IV postoperatively. Many anesthesiologists administer 100 mg hydrocortisone IV prior to surgery. It should be stressed to the patient that within 24 hours he should resume his normal maintenance dose of prednisone. The occurrence of acute adrenal crisis is life-threatening, and the goal is to provide supplemental steroids in the minimum drug dosage necessary to protect the patient.

REFERENCE

1. Symreng T, Karlberg BE, Kagedal B, et al: Physiological cortisol substitution of long-term steroid-treated patients undergoing major surgery. Br J Anaesth 53: 949, 1981

▨ CASE REPORT NO. 17

A 37-year-old man who is on the surgical schedule at 9:00 A.M. for a right inguinal hernia repair admits to the anesthesiologist that he uses cocaine on a daily basis. After further questioning, the patient states that he took his "regular fix" of cocaine at approximately 2 A.M. and that this lasts him approximately 12 hours. Can a substance abuser, either acute or chronic, be managed safely in an ambulatory surgery setting?

Discussion
Kenneth Zahl, M.D.
Director of Outpatient Anesthesiology, Assistant Professor of Anesthesiology, The Mt. Sinai Medical Center, New York, New York

The initial answer to this question is a resounding no! Although the data and literature on the anesthetic management of the substance abuser are limited, I believe that the studies and arguments (although occasionally anecdotal) that I will present are compelling enough to support my response.

In order to answer this question, I will assume that this is an elective procedure; if not (e.g., incarcerated hernia), then one could, and should, manage this more safely as an inpatient emergency. In my opinion, one of the primary considerations in patient selection for ambulatory surgery is patient reliability and appropriateness of the home environment. This patient appears to be a chronic cocaine abuser, not a recreational user. There is a high correlation of polysubstance abuse and alcoholism among all substance abusers. Although cocaine is considered to be the recreational drug of the 1980s, purchase and possession of cocaine are illegal in the United States. Over time, many people will develop criminal habits to obtain money for cocaine. To actually obtain the drug usually requires clandestine activity. These patients are notoriously unreliable historians. For example, if the patient admits to taking cocaine at 2:00 A.M., might he not also have violated the instructions to be NPO? What type of reliable escort will this patient have? What home environment will this patient come from? I would be hard pressed to believe that this patient would not continue to abuse drugs postoperatively, in violation of our postoperative orders.

It is also conceivable that the timing of the ingestion could have been later (i.e., closer to 9:00 A.M.), since most addicts would realize that they would be denied care if they admitted to recent drug ingestion. Recent cocaine use may have anesthetic implications related to its lethal cardiovascular effects. Publicity related to deaths of young athletes has dramatized the lethality of cocaine or its newer formulation, known as "crack." It has been accepted that cocaine use can be temporally related to myocardial ischemia[1] or infarction.[2] Patients exhibiting ischemia or an infarction may have normal coronary arteries,[3] but apparently most patients have preexisting coronary artery disease.[2]

Recently, in many New York City emergency rooms, cocaine users have presented with fatal intoxications related to a syndrome of hyperpyrexia, rhabdomyolysis, and renal failure.[4,5] According to Dr. Lewis Goldfrank, director of emergency medicine at Bellevue Hospital, up to one patient per month may present with this syndrome (personal communication). Treatment consists of sedation with diazepam, intubation and paralysis with pancuronium if needed, intravenous hydration, treatment of hypertension and tachycardia, and vigorous cooling with ice and fans. This syndrome has been reproduced in dogs,[6] and pancuronium, chlorpromazine, and induced hypothermia were found to be protective of the hyperthermic, but not the cardiovascular effects of cocaine. Since this syndrome could mimic malignant hyperthermia, I believe it would be unwise to electively give anesthesia to someone with a history of acute cocaine ingestion.

To answer the other question, let us assume that the patient admits to occasional cocaine abuse, but no recent intake. This patient, as in the case of other complicated patients, should not be evaluated for the first time on the day of surgery by the anesthesiologist. Adequate time and thought are required to decide on what is the best course of management. In this case, I would have surgery scheduled for later in the morning, in order to obtain a stat toxic screen of the urine and blood for cocaine or benzoylecgonine (its major metabolite). In addition, I would check for other illicit drugs and alcohol on the morning of surgery. I have been surprised in several cases by the results of the toxic screen in patients who claimed to have had no recent drug use. I would carefully question and examine the patient for evidence of intravenous drug use. IV drug users have a high incidence of HIV infection and hepatitis and also may have SBE or renal failure. Alcoholics have a high incidence of liver disease (with attendant coagulopathy, thrombocytopenia, and hypoglycemia), organic brain syndrome, delerium tremens, withdrawal seizures, and anemia. I also would examine the patient for the classic findings of chronic alcoholism and liver disease (i.e., spider angiomata, hypersplenism, jaundice, ascites, neurologic impairment, and so on). Owing to the increased possibility of multiple organ disease, I would order a CBC, platelet count, coagulation profile, SMA 20, and ECG where I normally would not do so in a patient of this age.

If the physical examination and all of the above tests were within normal limits and the patient was not a chronic abuser, then I would proceed on an outpatient basis. I believe that the anesthetic of choice for routine outpatient inguinal herniorrhaphy is a field block that includes blockade of the ilioinguinal, iliohypogastric, and genitofemoral nerves. I usually supplement this with intravenous sedation. If the latter nerves are blocked with bupivacaine, then patients leave the facility with excellent analgesia and there is a low incidence of urinary retention with this technique. However, substance abusers are usually poor candidates for regional anesthesia, and general anesthesia supplemented with narcotics is most often what is best for all involved in the operating room. General anesthesia does not preclude the use of a supplemental ilioinguinal nerve block or infiltration of the wound with bupivacaine postinduction, which would lower postoperative narcotic requirements in the PACU. Anecdotally, these patients may require very high induction doses of barbiturates and high maintenance levels of anesthetics.

To summarize, as presented, I would not accept this patient for outpatient surgery in a hospital-based or freestanding ambulatory surgery center. He should be referred for detoxification and then rescheduled. Otherwise, in the case of the occasional cocaine user, surgery could be performed on an outpatient basis after an appropriate workup as outlined above.

REFERENCES

1. Coleman DL, Ross TF, Naughton JL: Myocardial ischemia and infarction related to recreational cocaine use. *West J Med* 136: 444, 1982
2. Isner JM, Estes NAM, Thompson PD, et al: Acute cardiac events temporally related to cocaine abuse. N Engl J Med 315: 1438, 1986
3. Alltieri PI, Toro JM, Banch H, Carron EH: Coronary artery spasm in patients with cocaine-induced acute myocardial infarction. J Am Coll Cardiol 9: 172A, 1987
4. Roth D, Alarcon FJ, Fernandez JA, et al: Acute rhabdomyolysis associated with cocaine intoxication. N Engl J Med 319: 673, 1989
5. Merrigan KS, Roberts JR: Cocaine intoxication: Hyperpyrexia, rhabdomyolysis and acute renal failure. J Toxicol Clin Toxicol 25: 135, 1987
6. Catravas JD, Waters IW: Acute cocaine intoxication in the conscious dog: Studies on the mechanism of lethality. J Pharmacol Exp Ther 217: 350, 1981

Response

Dr. Zahl has pointed out the very important point of unreliability in patients who are substance abusers. While the anesthesiologist can try to impress on these patients that for their welfare it is imperative to have honest answers to questions on substance use and abuse to provide the safest anesthesia care, I agree with Dr. Zahl that we must remain skeptical of the answers.

Although these patients usually are not good candidates for regional anesthesia, if the patient were willing to accept a regional technique such as a field block, epidural, or spinal anesthesia for his hernia repair, that would be my first choice. If general anesthesia were required, the wound field should be blocked with bupivacaine for a smoother recovery and postoperative course.

Toxic drug screens should be performed on such patients prior to surgery along with a detailed history of substance abuse. In addition, the usual care and precautions should be taken because of the possible risk of exposure to hepatitis or AIDS in substance abuse patients.[1] Unfortunately, substance abuse has infiltrated nearly all aspects of our society, and this type of problem patient is no longer isolated to the central urban city hospitals.

REFERENCE

1. Mathieu A, Dienstag JL: The hazard of viral hepatitis to anesthesiologists and other operating room personnel. In Orkin FK, Cooperman LH (eds): Complications in Anesthesiology. Philadelphia, JB Lippincott, 1983

◼ CASE REPORT NO. 18

A 10-year-old boy is scheduled for a cystoscopy under general anesthesia. The patient has clonic-tonic seizures of his upper extremities on almost a daily basis. In the preoperative interview, the mother stated that the child's pediatrician is aware that he is having this procedure but did not change his medications. He has been on the same dose of anticonvulsants for the past 6 months.

Discussion
L. Reuven Pasternak, M.D., M.P.H.
Assistant Professor, Anesthesiology and Critical Care Medicine, Director, Ambulatory Surgery Programs, The Johns Hopkins Hospital, Baltimore, Maryland

As the number and volume of ambulatory surgery procedures continues to grow at an accelerated pace, the anesthesiologist must often make clinical decisions without the guidance of definitive clinical studies. When faced with this circumstance, it is appropriate to apply a common-sense approach that requires several conditions to be met. The patient's medical problems, if any, must be appropriately evaluated and optimally managed. There should be no clear advantage to preoperative admission for further evaluation and preparation, and the nature of the procedure and associated anesthetic technique should be such that the patient can reasonably be expected to be discharged without subsequent adverse events. This last condition naturally includes the availability of appropriate post-discharge assistance.

The child with a persistent seizure disorder presents such a situation. While no definitive guidelines have emerged within the pediatric anesthesia community on this issue, we have been managing such children on an outpatient basis using the preceding guidelines. In evaluating this child, the etiology of the seizures must be known, especially with consideration of intracranial lesions or other pathologic processes that alter intracranial pressure. It also should be demonstrated that all reasonable efforts have been made to control the seizures; any recent change in severity or frequency of the seizures warrants a reevaluation by the pediatrician or neurologist before undertaking an elective procedure. It is not uncommon for children to experience a growth spurt with subsequent breakthrough of seizure activity due to insufficient anticonvulsant medication dosages. For this reason, and because of possible patient noncompliance with medication regimens, a serum anticonvulsant level should be determined within a week of the scheduled surgery for all patients on anticonvulsant drugs. Where the levels are subtherapeutic, the medication should be readjusted and a therapeutic level obtained regardless of the clinical presentation of the patient. Finally, any associated medical conditions also must be aggressively pursued, including a possible history of respiratory distress and aspiration associated with seizure activity. A radiograph of the chest may reveal findings consistent with chronic aspiration that is not evident from the history or physical examination.

Despite the persistence of seizure activity, a consistent and unchanging clinical presentation and satisfactory evaluation of the preceding issues reveal no significant advantage to preoperative admission to simply take medication that could be given as well at home in a less stressful environment. Special consideration should be given to scheduling the procedure so that the case is completed early in the day to allow for maximal observation before discharge. All anticonvulsant medications should be taken on schedule and brought to the surgery unit on the day of surgery. If doses are taken in the morning, their administration should be witnessed to ensure minimal fluid intake; similarly, if delays are encountered prior to discharge, the medications should be available to the patient later in the day. Any concern about compliance with medication administration warrants admission to prevent missing doses during the immediate preoperative and post-operative periods.

Choice of anesthetic and associated medication should be guided by the need to have the patient comfortable during the procedure and able to take fluids as soon as possible postoperatively. While spinal or epidural anesthesia enjoys con-siderable favor for cystoscopy in older patients, cooperation from a 10-year-old may be difficult and presents no distinct advantage. General anesthesia is the technique of choice, and fortunately, few of the commonly used agents are con-traindicated in patients with seizure disorders. Standard intravenous induction with thiopental is appropriate, with maintenance of anesthesia by a combination of nitrous oxide, oxygen, and halothane. Use of enflurane is not recommended because of its association with enhanced EEG activity. Similarly, ketamine is also contraindicated owing to its central nervous system interactions. Many alterna-tive techniques are also available, including a balanced technique utilizing 2 to 3 μg/kg fentanyl with low levels of halothane. While mask management is generally sufficient, any history of respiratory distress, especially aspiration, is an indica-tion for endotracheal intubation. Given the brief duration of the procedure and the limited postoperative pain when compared to such procedures as inguinal hernia repair, supplementation with caudal anesthetics is usually not indicated.

Everything having gone well in the operating room, discharge of the patient from the ambulatory surgery unit should only come after he regains full preop-erative medical status. Most important, the child must demonstrate the ability to take and retain oral fluids to ensure that he can resume his medications. As with all pediatric patients, there must be a responsible adult available to the child at all times and medical assistance readily available if necessary. Finally, any indi-cation of persistent altered mental status, whether irritability or lethargy, is an indication for overnight observation. While this phenomenon is not uncommon in postoperative pediatric patients, its presence in a child with preexisting neu-rologic deficit warrants conservative management for both clinical and medico-legal reasons.

Response

In order to ensure a safe perioperative course, there must be open communica-tion between the child, parents, pediatrician, and anesthesiologist. It must be documented that this child is taking a therapeutic level of anticonvulsants and that there has been no change in the frequency or duration of seizure activity. After the child has recovered from his anesthetic, I would observe this patient for 4 to 6 hours. It is during this time that the anesthesiologist and parent decide if all concerned are comfortable with sending the child home. I also would rec-ommend that at least *two* responsible adults be present to transport the child home. One adult would drive with the other sitting in the back seat with the child to provide comfort and support and to handle any emergencies.

To provide close follow-up for this child, a telephone call by the anesthesiol-ogist the evening of surgery would allow the parent to vent any special concerns as well as give the physician a chance to hear from the parent if there has been any change in the child's seizure activity since discharge from the ambulatory facility. When a patient has special needs, physicians and personnel involved in the ambulatory surgical experience should devote additional time to frequent follow-up calls to ensure a safe recovery period. This adds to the comfort level of the responsible parties providing home care.

■ CASE REPORT NO. 19

A 67-year-old woman is scheduled for a cataract procedure with a periorbital block. The patient takes the following medications: Cardiazem (30 mg TID), Diazide (1 q day), Lanoxin (0.125 mg q day), and Coumadin (2 mg q day). Preoperative laboratory testing on the morning of surgery reveals a prothrombin time of 16.5 (normal is 12). The patient's Coumadin was discontinued 2 days ago.

Discussion
Rebecca S. Twersky, M.D.
Medical Director, Ambulatory Surgery Unit, Assistant Professor of Anesthesiology, State University of New York, Health Science Center of Brooklyn, Brooklyn, New York

The factors in determining whether this patient is suitable for ambulatory surgery are physical status, anesthetic technique, and the surgical procedure. At our ambulatory surgery unit, all cataract patients and close to 95% of all other patients are seen preoperatively in our screening clinic. During this patient's preoperative screening, I would key in on her cardiac evaluation, in addition to the routine history, physical examination, and anesthesia assessment. Why is this patient taking these medications? Is there a history of myocardial infarction or angina? Are her symptoms controlled with calcium-channel blockers? What is her exercise tolerance? Is there a history of heart failure, atrial fibrillation, or syncope? Has she undergone specialized testing (*i.e.,* stress test, echo, Holter monitoring) to evaluate her condition? Why is she on the Coumadin? Has she ever been off Coumadin? Has she sustained a cerebral vascular event? Does she have any neurologic symptoms? Can she ambulate? I would need to consult with her internist and/or cardiologist to clarify any questions about her condition and to confirm that her medical status is well controlled and that she is in optimum condition to undergo this elective procedure. In our ambulatory surgery unit, I have given the ophthalmologists a form that they forward to the patient's internist to complete and return with the patient when scheduled for preoperative testing. This gives us a data base for comparison (including previous ECGs) and allows us to better evaluate the patient and decide whether he or she is indeed suitable for ambulatory surgery.

Natof analyzed the correlation of complications of ambulatory surgery with patients with preexisting medical problems and found that the incidence of major complications was the same in patients with or without preexisting disease.[1] This has been confirmed by a FASA survey of over 87,000 patients—there appeared to be little or no cause-and-effect relationship between preexisting disease and the incidence of complications.[2] The ASA physical status 3 patient and rarely physical status 4 patient are appropriate candidates for ambulatory surgery *if* their systemic diseases are *medically stable.*

Assuming that this woman is a stable physical status 3 patient and "medically cleared" to undergo the procedure, she presents with the additional problem of being on anticoagulants. Coumadin (warfarin sodium) interferes with the hepatic synthesis of vitamin K–dependent factors II, VII, IX, and X. It has a delayed onset of action of 8 to 12 hours and a half-life of 37 hours. The effect of Coumadin can be assessed by the prothrombin time, and the patient is considered anticoagulated if the prothrombin time is 25% of normal. The effect of the anticoagulation would normally be reversed within 5 days of discontinuance. The administration of parenteral vitamin K requires 3 to 6 hours to exert beneficial effect. Fresh frozen plasma is rapidly effective if active hemorrhage is present.

The key questions is: What risk, if any, is there to this patient of administering a periorbital block and performing surgery while the Coumadin effect is still present? The complication of concern from the regional block is retrobulbar hemorrhage. The etiology is considered to be puncture of an orbital vessel followed by either venous or arterial bleeding. Depending on the rapidity of the spread of blood, there can be minimal sequelae ranging from blood staining of the lids and conjunctiva to orbital swelling, proptosis, and increased intraocular pressure. Treatment is usually not necessary, but in extreme cases, blindness can follow unless it is appropriately managed.

This complication is virtually nonexistent with the periorbital block.[3] Utilizing a 25- or 27-gauge needle 1¼ inch in length with a rounded, short bevel, the needle can be inserted at an inferior temporal point no more than ½ to ¾ inch deep directed posteriorly. This eliminates nicking of any retrobulbar vessels. While periorbital hemorrhage may occur, it is of much less serious consequence.

Cataract surgery has undergone tremendous improvements that reduce bleeding potential. Ophthalmologists use smaller incisions, better sutures, cauterization under microscopic control, and improved anesthetics. Surgical technique can be modified to decrease the risk of bleeding (*i.e.,* a corneal incision that is avascular can be made rather than a limbal incision). The change from iris-supported to posterior chamber intraocular lenses as well as extracapsular extraction has further reduced the incidence of bleeding.

There is no clear agreement among ophthalmologists as to whether anticoagulants should be discontinued prior to cataract surgery. Stone and associates presented the summary of 135 Implant Society members and reported that 75% of the surgeons withheld Coumadin prior to cataract surgery.[4] Sequelae were not uncommon and were severe, including two deaths and other episodes of significant cardiovascular complications. In a review of over 2000 patients, 1% of whom were on anticoagulants, McMahan was unable to show an increase in sight-threatening complications when compared to the nonanticoagulated cataract patients.[5] Hall and coworkers reviewed a series of 49 cataract patients taking Coumadin and found no more than the usual amount of operative bleeding and no episodes of bleeding after the first postoperative day. Of the three patients who developed hyphemas, all cleared within 14 days with no loss of visual acuity.[6] It seems that the risks of serious life-threatening complications from stopping anticoagulation far outweigh the possibilities of sight-threatening complications from continued anticoagulation. Modern cataract surgery is so atraumatic that it can be accomplished without complications in patients on anticoagulant therapy. While good sight is important, the preservation of life takes precedence.

My answer is yes, this patient can have her surgery in an ambulatory facility (hospital or freestanding), but only after proper coordination between the internist, ophthalmologist, and anesthesiologist.

REFERENCES

1. Natof HE: Ambulatory surgery: Patients with preexisting medical problems. Ill Med J 166(2): 101, 1984
2. FASA Special Study I. Alexandra Va., Federated Ambulatory Surgery Association, 1987
3. Wang HS: Peribulbar anesthesia for ophthalmic procedures. J Cataract Refract Surg (14)4: 441, 1988
4. Stone LS, Kline OR, Sklar S: Intraocular lenses and anticoagulation and antiplatelet therapy. J Am Intraocular Implant Soc 11: 165, 1985
5. McMahan LB: Anticoagulants and cataract surgery. J Cataract Refract Surg (14)5: 569, 1988
6. Hall DL, Steen WH, Drummond JW: Anticoagulants and cataract surgery. Ophthalmic Surg (19)3: 221, 1988

Response

At Methodist Ambulatory SurgiCare, we do recommend that patients discontinue their Coumadin 5 days prior to their surgical procedure (standard of care in this community). In light of Dr. Twersky's presentation, there appears to be no sound medical reason for discontinuing Coumadin prior to surgery. In the face of severe underlying medical problems that require the patient to be anticoagulated, this can be more harmful than helpful. When faced with a patient taking Coumadin, communication between the internist, anesthesiologist, ophthalmologist, and patient is required before the anticoagulant is discontinued. The potential complication of retrobulbar hemorrhage should be thoroughly explained to the patient. This will allow the patient to have a voice in the decision to discontinue Coumadin prior to surgery. If the patient is medically stable and it is an absolute necessity that the anticoagulant be continued, a general anesthetic is also another option (albeit a weak one) for the patient.

■ CASE REPORT NO. 20

An 11-year-old boy with cystic fibrosis is scheduled for a nasal polypectomy. He has a remarkable past 5-year history of recurrent pneumonias and bronchitis. The patient receives occasional chest physiotherapy at the hospital but is poorly compliant for home physical therapy. The surgeon inquires about the appropriateness of ambulatory surgery for the procedure.

Discussion
Steven C. Hall, M.D.
Assistant Professor of Clinical Anesthesia, Northwestern University Medical School, Attending Anesthesiologist, Children's Memorial Hospital, Chicago, Illinois

Pathophysiology

Cystic fibrosis (CF) is the most frequent lethal genetic disease in childhood. Transmitted as an autosomal-recessive trait, CF is relatively common in Caucasians (1:2000 live births) and very uncommon in other racial groups. The primary defect is not understood, but the common problem is thick, viscid mucus that becomes inspissated in ductular structures, especially the pancreas, lungs, biliary tract, and intestine. In-utero bowel obstruction by thick mucus causes meconium ileus and peritonitis in 10% to 20% of newborns with cystic fibrosis, but most children present later in childhood with signs of pulmonary involvement.

Mucus obstruction of airways increases susceptibility to infection and subsequent destruction of the airway. Pneumonia, bronchitis, bronchiolitis, abscess formation, and empyema are among the frequent infectious complications. *Pseudomonas aeruginosa* and *Staphylococcus aureus* become the prevalent infectious organisms. Acute deterioration of pulmonary function can be precipitated by acute infection. Recurrent infections and plugging of the airway lead to irreversible fibrosis of the airways, emphysema, bronchiectasis, pneumothorax, and diffuse parenchymal fibrosis. Besides significant ventilation-perfusion mismatching, there are progressive signs of obstructive and restrictive disease. Expiratory flow rates are decreased, while airway resistance and residual volumes increase. The pulmonary manifestations of CF are the most debilitating, leading to chronic hypoxemia, cor pulmonale, and progressive respiratory and cardiac failure. Life expectancy is directly related to the success of management of the pulmonary aspects of CF.

All exocrine glands are involved in CF, although most are not of particular concern to the anesthesiologist. Obstruction of bile canaliculi may cause cholestatic jaundice in the neonate that resolves spontaneously. Later in childhood, the obstruction can lead to hepatic cirrhosis, portal hypertension, and gastrointestinal bleeding in a minority of patients, although liver failure is not a problem. Patients may, however, require vitamin K supplementation to improve production of coagulation factors. Abnormal glucose tolerance can develop later in childhood and will rarely require insulin therapy. Lastly, because of excessive salt excretion in sweat, hyponatremic, hypochloremic dehydration can occur in children stressed by hot weather.

Medical management of the child with CF includes a high-energy diet to compensate for malabsorption, vitamin and pancreatic enzyme supplements, and daily chest physiotherapy. Physiotherapy with postural drainage and mechanical percussion facilitates the expectoration of mucus from the respiratory tract.[1] Antibiotics, inhalation of mucolytic enzymes, and bronchodilators are added to the management as needed. There has been interest in the use of nocturnal oxygen therapy in CF patients with chronic hypoxemia to slow the increase in pulmonary vascular resistance and development of cor pulmonale. However, a recent long-term study has not demonstrated benefit from the technique.[2]

The prognosis of patients with CF has improved dramatically in recent years. Children who are diagnosed early and treated aggressively now usually live into their twenties, though a few with especially severe pulmonary disease die in early childhood.[3] As the average lifespan of children with CF increases, it is more likely that these patients will require surgery for lesions associated with the underlying disease (lobectomy, portocaval shunting, nasal polypectomy) or for unassociated lesions. The anesthesiologist must be prepared to adequately evaluate, prepare, and manage the perioperative course of these complicated patients.

Preoperative Evaluation

Because the primary concern in these patients is the pulmonary status, the degree of current respiratory impairment is the important determinant of suitability for anesthesia. The child without pulmonary signs needs no special attention. However, cough is usually present, and the amount of sputum is variable. The patient with foul-smelling or increasing sputum production, decreased exercise tolerance, cyanosis, hemoptysis, or fever is in poor control and at risk for significant morbidity with surgery. These children and their parents are often actively involved in the home management of the disease and are very astute in describing the child's clinical status. Because the family usually works closely with a pediatrician or pulmonologist, consultation with this physician is important to ensure adequate preparation.

Physical examination centers on the pulmonary system also. Signs of respiratory distress (tachypnea, accessory muscle use, cyanosis, wheezing) indicate a need to improve pulmonary status. In children, a strong cardiac system is an important part of compensation for the pulmonary disease. Signs such as a gallop rhythm, poor peripheral perfusion, or peripheral edema may suggest a decreased ability of the cardiac system to compensate for poor pulmonary function. If there is suspicion of cardiac decompensation, hospital admission is advisable.

Laboratory data depend on the need for further specific information. Chest x-rays are useful, especially in comparison with previous films, in evaluating changes in lung architecture. Pulmonary function tests are often abnormal, showing a decreased FEV_1 and vital capacity, increased residual volume, and normal or increased total lung capacity. However, unless there is suspicion of either a deterioration in lung function or a need for additional therapy (bronchodilators), pulmonary function tests and x-rays are not as important as the determination by history and physical examination of the current degree of cardiopulmonary compensation. Likewise, arterial blood gases are needed if there is suspicion of deterioration, but are not mandatory in all patients.

Because of the risk of anemia from both gastrointestinal bleeding and poor nutrition, a complete blood count is necessary. If there is a history of bleeding or easy bruisability, a coagulation profile is indicated. A blood glucose is obtained if there is a history of glucose intolerance, while electrolytes are drawn if there are signs or history of recent dehydration.

Preoperative Preparation

A great deal of attention must be directed to minimizing secretions, infection, and bronchospasm before surgery. With a cooperative patient and family, this can be done at home without admission to the hospital. Vigorous chest physiotherapy and adequate hydration are cornerstones of this management. Bronchodilators, mucolytic aerosols, and mist therapy are added as needed. If there is any indication of infection, sputum is cultured, and antibiotic therapy started. Fiberoptic bronchoscopy for bronchopulmonary lavage and direct antibiotic instillation has been advocated by some, but there is little evidence that there is significant benefit from this invasive therapy.

Premedication

These patients are chronically ill and have unique psychosocial problems. Their reactions to impending surgery may be more extreme than those of other children. Also, their parents may react differently than expected. Clear planning and discussions with the family are necessary to both provide support and guarantee cooperation.

Premedication, especially with narcotics, has often been avoided to prevent respiratory depression,[4] although there is no convincing evidence that any of the commonly used premedicants are detrimental. If anxiolysis is desired, premedication with a barbiturate or benzodiazepine, such as the short-acting midazolam, is a reasonable approach. If premedication is felt to be an important part of psychologically preparing a particular patient, it should be considered. It is often recommended to avoid atropine because of excessive drying of secretions. However, administration of atropine has not been associated with an overall increase in pulmonary complications.[5] Administration of a reasonable intramuscular dose or the smaller intravenous dose, coupled with vigorous attention to secretion control perioperatively, should be associated with minimal risk.

Anesthetic Management

Monitoring is especially useful in patients with CF. Pulse oximetry allows close monitoring of oxygenation, while capnography is an important trend monitor during general anesthesia. Arterial blood pressure and blood gas monitoring is not needed for most procedures but is especially useful for extensive surgeries (lobectomy, pleurectomy) and for patients with advanced disease and cor pulmonale.

Regional anesthesia has been advocated as a preferable technique for extremity and lower abdominal procedures.[6] The advantage of regional blockage, though, must be weighed against the potential of a depressed cough in the presence of a high spinal or epidural block.

General endotracheal anesthesia is commonly used. The largest endotracheal tube possible is used to both allow adequate suctioning and to minimize airway pressures when ventilating poorly compliant lungs. Volatile agents, with their advantage of high inspired $F_{I_{O_2}}$ and bronchodilation, are routinely used. Induction will often be slower than expected, however, because of extensive V/Q mismatching. A "balanced" technique with a narcotic and muscle relaxant can also be used.[7] Nitrous oxide is avoided in the presence of chronic hypoxemia (need for increased $F_{I_{O_2}}$), pneumothorax, or intestinal obstruction (possibility of gas trapping). At the end of the procedure, the patient is extubated "awake" after extensive suctioning.

Postoperative Management

Appropriate postoperative care starts during the operative procedure. Aggressive tracheobronchial toilet intraoperatively will help the first hours postoperatively, when the patient may not cough adequately. Vigorous hydration and gas humidification during the procedure will also help liquefy and remove secretions. Regional or local blockade with long-acting local anesthetics provides good pain relief for several hours after surgery without depressing the ability to cough.

In the postoperative period, the patient is at significant risk for atelectasis, pneumonia, and respiratory failure. Chest physiotherapy, hydration, humidification, and ambulation are encouraged at an early stage to minimize problems. Patients with severe preexisting disease and those who have had extensive surgery benefit from the increased resources and monitoring of postoperative hospitalization.

Conclusion

In the not so distant past, surgery was avoided when at all possible in children with cystic fibrosis. It was felt that the risks of morbidity and mortality were inordinate. With modern medical care, the child's pulmonary disability can be minimized with a variety of therapies. With an aggressive and resourceful family and medical staff, many patients can be properly prepared for surgery on an outpatient basis. With attention to the details of anesthetic care, these patients can then undergo a wide variety of procedures with minimal perioperative complications.

REFERENCES

1. Reisman JJ, Rivington-Law B, Corey M, et al: Role of conventional physiotherapy in cystic fibrosis. J Pediatr 113: 632, 1988
2. Zinman R, Corey M, Coates AL, et al: Nocturnal home oxygen in the treatment of hypoxemic cystic fibrosis patients. J Pediatr 114: 368, 1989
3. Dankert-Roelse JE, te Meerman GJ, Martijn A, et al: Survival and clinical outcome in patients with cystic fibrosis, with or without neonatal screening. J Pediatr 114: 362, 1989
4. Doershuk CF, Reyes AL, Regan AG, Matthews LW: Anesthesia and surgery in cystic fibrosis. Anesth Analg 51: 413, 1972
5. Salanitre E, Klonymus D, Rackow H: Anesthetic experience in children with cystic fibrosis of the pancreas. Anesthesiology 25: 801, 1964
6. Lamberty JM, Rubin, BK: The management of anaesthesia for patients with cystic fibrosis. Anaesthesia 40: 448, 1985
7. Todres ID: Cystic fibrosis. In Katz J, Steward DJ (eds): Anesthesia and Uncommon Pediatric Diseases, p 82–83. Philadelphia, WB Saunders, 1987

Response

Dr. Hall has presented a very thorough overview of the patient with cystic fibrosis. The patient with a significant disease problem must be evaluated by the anesthesiologist a minimum of several days in advance of scheduled surgery. A decision as to where this procedure can be safely performed (inpatient versus outpatient) should be made only after discussion involving the anesthesiologist, pulmonologist (or pediatrician), and parents. Ensuring a safe recovery from this child's anesthetic begins in the preoperative period with aggressive chest physiotherapy, secretion control, and medication administration; in the postoperative period, this child would require hydration, humidification, and continued chest physiotherapy. The genetic abnormality associated with cystic fibrosis has recently been recognized. Perhaps in the not too distant future cystic fibrosis will be diagnosed in utero and respiratory and cardiac abnormalities associated with the disease can be prevented.[1]

REFERENCE

1. National Institute of Diabetes and Digestive & Kidney Diseases: The CF Gene: A Fifty-Year Search, National Institute of Health, Bethesda, Maryland, August 1989.

A Successful Facility

A successful ambulatory surgery facility begins with sound planning. Planning encompasses all aspects of the program—from determining need, to understanding program functions, to marketing the program, to successfully operating the program. Development of an ambulatory surgery program without proper planning is similar to taking a long driving trip without a road map. You may go someplace, but is it the right direction?

A successful program influences the anesthesiologist's caseload and income. Hence our road map to a successful ambulatory surgery facility is a strategic planning route to our destination. The strategic planning process enables us to determine where we are today, where we want to be in the future, and how we will get there.

This chapter consists of three sections. The first section, which deals with facility planning, focuses on need and demand analysis; the functional/space programming process; and a step-by-step "how to" of planning and developing an ambulatory surgery program and facility. The second section discusses marketing as a responsibility of all managers. The last section considers fundamental operational and management issues.

Facility Planning

LESLIE K. LEIDER
PETER M. MANNIX

WHY IS PLANNING NECESSARY?

A well-designed and efficiently staffed surgery facility greatly contributes to the success of an ambulatory surgery program. A successful facility, however, doesn't happen by itself—it happens with planning. In any facility program, and specifically in planning ambulatory surgery facilities, we must first plan for the program's function and then determine the form that will permit this functioning. The cardinal rule of facility planning is *form follows function.*

Planning of the physical surgery facility is critical because its design affects so many aspects of the program. For example, staffing, operating costs, convenience, and often the success or failure of the ambulatory surgery program hinge on the physical facilities and design of the unit. Once constructed, the physical facility is the most difficult and expensive part of the ambulatory surgery program to change. Therefore, it is imperative that the facility be well planned in its early stages, so that its design conforms to the desired function.

WHAT IS THE STRATEGIC PLANNING PROCESS?

The strategic planning process is a structured approach used to determine the future direction of the organization. There are a number of steps in the process. Each step is based on the results of the previous step. The anesthesiologist who is involved in the strategic planning process should become familiar with these steps, since they will apply to most situations and specifically to ambulatory surgery program planning.

Need and Demand Analysis

Basic to the strategic plan is the need to know the role of the institution and the programs that fulfill this role. Therefore, you need to study a number of demographic factors, such as the following.

Service Area

An analysis must be done to determine where ambulatory surgery patients have come from in the past and where they might come from in the future. Is the geographic service area small and concentrated or large and spread out? If it is small and concentrated, what can we do to expand it? If it is large and spread out, how can we increase our market position?

Market Position

Market position identifies your share of the total ambulatory surgery market in your service area. As ambulatory surgery volume has grown over the years, market-position data for ambulatory surgery are becoming more available. State agencies or local health care associations may often collect and disseminate ambulatory surgery market-position data.

Your facility's ambulatory surgery market position should be carefully studied. What is it compared to that of your competitors and why? What is your market-position trend over the years and why? What actions are your competitors taking that affect market share. What can your facility do to enhance market position?

Population

Once the geographic service area and market position are defined, the character of the population should be analyzed. Perhaps the most important population variable is the age/sex specific breakdown of the service area. Although a high proportion of elderly patients (65 and over) historically indicated a heavy use of inpatient hospital services, shifting trends indicate that the elderly are now and will continue to be significant users of ambulatory surgery. Children, adolescents, and females aged 15 to 44 are frequently good candidates for ambulatory surgery. You should identify the population by age and sex categories and compare it with national figures to help determine ambulatory surgery use patterns.

Historical and projected population trends also should be analyzed. A geographic service area that has a growing population center bodes well for future use of ambulatory surgery services. In fact, a rapidly growing geographic area could potentially be a location for development of a freestanding ambulatory surgery facility, especially if it is conveniently near or adjacent to physician offices.

Physician Profile

Physicians have a great influence on the types of services offered in an ambulatory surgery program. A physician profile should focus on the following.

SPECIALTIES. Some specialties are geared more toward the use of ambulatory surgery facilities than others. Obstetric/gynecologic, otolaryngologic, orthopedic, plastic surgery, and ophthalmologic specialists are heavy supporters of ambulatory surgery. A successful program should include a strong component of physicians in these and other specialties.

AGE. A balance of younger and older physicians will contribute to the success of an ambulatory surgery program. It is particularly important to be aware of the numbers and specialties of elderly physicians. Physicians age 60 and over are likely to begin slowing their practices.

PRACTICE PATTERNS. It is important to have a reasonable understanding of the amount of work a given physician is likely to perform in your facility. You need to determine whether ambulatory surgery is conducive to his or her past practice patterns.

OFFICE LOCATION. Location often has a great effect on physician practice patterns. In planning your program, it is important to consider the location of existing physician offices, clinics, and services. A close location encourages use of the facility.

HUMAN RESOURCES, RECRUITMENT, AND RETENTION. Analysis of the factors listed above may indicate the need to recruit additional physician specialists to optimize use of your facility. If physician age, office location, or specialty representation is not ideal to support your program, the need to add physicians must be recognized early. Plans should be developed to fill gaps in patterns of health care delivery before they arise and adversely affect the ambulatory surgery program.

In some cases, a retention strategy is even better than a recruitment strategy, because it focuses on physicians who are already located in the area. Ask these physicians what you can do for them to increase their utilization of the ambulatory surgery facilities. Often physicians simply need to know they are wanted and important to the success of the facility.

Volumes of Service

HISTORICAL USE ANALYSIS. Volumes of surgery that historically have been handled in your facility should be carefully analyzed to determine trends. What percentage of the volume has been done on an outpatient basis? How does it compare to that of other surgical facilities in the area, across the state, and nationally? Why is it comparatively high or low? How can the relationship with health maintenance organizations (HMOs), preferred provider organizations (PPOs), or other alternative delivery systems (ADSs) affect your volume? In most instances, such relationships should be quite positive, since these organizations seek low-cost service delivery options such as ambulatory surgery.

PROJECTED USE ANALYSIS. Unfortunately, there is no totally reliable method to project future volumes of service. However, careful analysis and reasonable understanding of the factors listed above will give a high level of confidence in projecting future volumes. Projected volumes provide the base for the financial feasibility study. Hence projections should be carefully scrutinized because they will affect the bottom line.

Program Options

Ambulatory surgery programs can be developed in two locations: the hospital setting or a freestanding location. This section defines programs in these settings and discusses key features of each.

Hospital

Hospital-based ambulatory surgery units have two options for development. The program can be integrated or separated. In an integrated program, inpatient and outpatient surgery is combined in the same surgery suite. In a separated program, a self-contained ambulatory surgery suite located within the hospital is devoted to ambulatory surgery patients.

Integrated Unit

Advantages of an integrated hospital approach are

> Low startup costs, since the existing surgery suite is being used.
> Better utilization of existing and expensive facilities.
> Centralizes surgery in one location.
> Is convenient for staff and supply distribution and use.
> Is the most flexible, particularly if a hospital later decides to change to a separated or freestanding setting, based on the success of the integrated program. The integrated unit will still be used for inpatients.

Potential problems of the integrated setting are

> Scheduling can often result in the outpatient being "bumped" from the surgery schedule. Outpatients can be viewed as "second class citizens," which is perhaps the major single complaint of integrated units. On the other hand, some surgeons have a growing concern that ambulatory surgery is now a priority, leaving the inpatient schedule less convenient and flexible.
> An inpatient orientation is often focused on outpatients, whose needs are quite different. For example, participation of family members is an important feature of ambulatory surgery. Policies, procedures, and facilities must support this orientation, but often do not.
> Support space, location, and design are often an afterthought and may not functionally relate to the integrated surgery program.
> Physician-hospital joint ventures are difficult to structure in an integrated program.

Keys to success of an integrated ambulatory surgery unit are

> Adequate operating rooms and support space.
> Logical traffic flow between support spaces. This traffic flow is particularly critical for patients, visitors, staff, physicians, materials, and equipment.

The integrated program works best when the existing surgical suite has excess capacity, low outpatient volume is initially anticipated, travel patterns are clearly identified, and minimal dollars can be expended for the program. Many hospitals will find that the integrated approach is best for them. The reason is that the majority of hospitals are seeing a shift in surgery from the inpatient to the outpatient setting rather than significant increases in the total volume of surgery. Thus the existing operating room capacity is often adequate to support the numbers of surgeries. Renovating the unit to provide the appropriate support space is often a cost-effective solution to providing ambulatory surgery facilities.

One caveat should be noted here. That is, inadequate facilities will lead to poor ambulatory surgery utilization. If the appropriate support facilities for the ambulatory surgery program are not provided, physicians simply will not use the unit. The program will fail not because of lack of demand, but because of poor facility planning. Thus it is critical to provide the appropriate support spaces (family waiting room close to operating suite, second-phase recovery area to allow separation of ambulatory patients from more critically ill inpatients, space for family to be in attendance in phase-two recovery, and so on) in the proper location to facilitate traffic flows through the unit.

Separated Unit

Some hospitals prefer separated ambulatory surgery units. A hospital that has undergone a major renovation program that involved a new surgery suite might retain the old surgery suite and devote it to ambulatory surgery use. Other hospitals have converted labor and delivery units to ambulatory surgery use. Major advantages of the separated approach are

> Space is dedicated specifically for ambulatory surgery patients.
> There is no competition for inpatient operating rooms.

Potential problems that exist with a separated unit are duplication of staff and facilities, which can add to operating costs; ambulatory surgery facilities are expensive to develop and maintain; and travel distances for staff, patients, and supplies may be significant depending on location in the main hospital.

A separated ambulatory surgery program works best when the inpatient operating rooms are at maximum capacity and cannot easily be expanded or when a separate identity for the program within the hospital is desirable. In fact, the separated program offers a significant marketing advantage. A hospital can market the ambulatory surgery program as a freestanding unit with the convenience of hospital backup immediately available.

Freestanding Unit

Developers of freestanding ambulatory surgery units have two alternatives: freestanding on campus or freestanding off campus. Advantages of a freestanding on-campus facility are the following:

> Distinct identity for the program, yet still located on the main hospital campus.
> No competition for inpatient operating rooms.
> No competition for support space.
> Designed specifically for ambulatory surgery patients.
> Hospital backup immediately available.
> Joint ventures with physicians may be easier to arrange (although recent federal regulations and changes in tax laws result in greater scrutiny of such ventures).

Potential problems with a freestanding on-campus facility relate to expense. Many freestanding ambulatory surgery units begin with three or four operating rooms, which may result in a building from 8000 to 10,000 square feet. Thus the total project startup costs can easily exceed $2.5 million. Other potential problems are

> Waiting time for hospital backup.
> Location of the facility on the site. A common mistake is poor master-site planning and the incorrect location of an ambulatory surgery facility that prevents future growth of the ambulatory surgery unit or the hospital itself.

Keys to success of a freestanding ambulatory surgery facility on campus are design and access and backup procedures well organized. A freestanding on-campus facility works best when high ambulatory surgery volumes are projected that can justify the cost of the unit, a distinct identity on campus is desired, operating and capital dollars are available, and the site can adequately accommodate the new building.

For free-standing off-campus centers, many advantages are similar to the free-standing on-campus model:

> No competition for hospital operating rooms.
> No competition for support space.
> Designed specifically for ambulatory surgery patients.
> Physician linkages/joint ventures may be easier to arrange.

An additional advantage to freestanding off-campus facilities is that a distinct identity for the ambulatory surgery unit may be provided in an existing or new geographic area. A hospital or even a physician group will view this as a good opportunity to enter a new portion of their service area.

Potential problems are distance to the hospital for backup service, the costs associated with constructing the facility, and location of the facility on the site. Keys to success are similar to those for freestanding on-campus facilities: appropriate design and access and well-organized backup procedures. Proximity to a medical office building also will make the freestanding unit convenient to physicians and encourage their use.

Freestanding off-campus facilities work well when volume supports the new construction, when a geographic identity in a new location is desirable, when operational and capital dollars are available, and when the site can accommodate the building and parking.

Which Program Is Best for You?

The simple answer to this question depends on projected volume. Low-volume ambulatory surgery programs are probably best located in an integrated or perhaps a separated unit, because the existing overhead of the surgery unit can be shared. The high startup costs of a freestanding unit on campus or off campus will be prohibitive to a low-volume ambulatory surgery program. In fact, *the greatest danger for a hospital* in this instance is the risk that it will then be operating *two inefficient surgery suites,* one at the hospital and one at the freestanding site.

There are many advantages to the integrated program, particularly if surgery volume is mostly shifting from in to out and good physical facilities are available. However, if the volumes are increasing and existing operating rooms are at high capacity, then the freestanding program should be carefully considered. Obviously, this option offers the most alternatives for entrepreneurial physicians who want to develop a program on their own or a joint venture with the hospital.

Facility Analysis: Existing and Proposed

Existing buildings must be analyzed to determine what facilities are necessary to accommodate all the organization's programs (including ambulatory surgery). The sequence of events necessary to locate physical facilities on a site is called a *master site plan.* It is prepared in such a way as to identify major departmental zones and logical sequencing of construction and renovation. Together, the *role and program plan* and the *facility plan* form the organization's strategic plan.

Business Planning

To ensure consistency of thought regarding the proposed programmatic and facility components of ambulatory surgery, you should consider the development of a business plan. The business plan goes beyond strategic planning by incorporating the strategic planning, operational considerations, financing options, financial analysis, and other relevant information. To acquire outside capital, a business plan is usually needed.

Functional Programming

Once the master plan identifies a specific facility need for ambulatory surgery, that need must be described before architectural drawings are prepared. Functional/space programming is a planning process that clearly describes the need, function, and facilities required for an ambulatory surgery program. It contains a departmental description, workload analysis, staffing requirements, department organization, functional considerations, and space allocations. Simply stated, it delineates the number, size, and type of each room, together with the appropriate narrative to describe this information. This document is a *functional/space program* and, after revisions with staff input, is given to the architect to prepare drawings. It serves as the foundation for all further planning.

A *schematic design* is the architect's translation of the functional/space program into drawings. These first drawings roughly show the "scheme" of the departments, hence the title *schematics.* During this important stage of planning, basic layout and design are determined. If earlier planning steps have been completed properly, this step should proceed quickly and smoothly.

Certificate of Need (CON)

A *certificate of need (CON)* is a regulatory process a health care provider must go through to acquire approval of a particular project. You must check with your regulatory experts to determine whether a CON is needed for your project.

Once the schematics have been developed (at least in initial form), more accurate costing can be done. The cost estimates provide the basis, together with future volumes, to conduct a *financial feasibility study*. The long-range plan, schematic plans, financial feasibility study, and other related materials serve as the basis for the CON application.

Design Development

After the CON is submitted and the schematic design is finalized, the drawings are prepared in more detail, on a larger scale. In effect, the schematic design is developed further, and hence this step of planning is called *design development.*

In the course of design development, consideration is given to the details of the rooms. Major equipment items are identified (*equipment lists*); special mechanical systems (*e.g.,* ventilation needs and special lighting) are listed; specific door locations are noted. A *room detail summary* is prepared, identifying each room and its detail of equipment, finishes, and so forth.

Working Drawings and Specifications

Once the design development drawings and supporting narrative have been developed, very detailed drawings (called *working drawings* or *construction drawings*) are then prepared. These literally show every nut and bolt in the new facility with a narrative (specifications) to explain the drawings.

Bidding and Construction

Working drawings and specifications, when complete, are sent to several contractors who prepare bids. The project is awarded to the successful bidder, and the contractor begins to construct the facility.

WHAT IS THE ANESTHESIOLOGIST'S ROLE IN THE AMBULATORY SURGERY PLANNING PROCESS?

The anesthesiologist is a key player on the ambulatory surgery planning team. He or she generally participates in one of two roles: as a representative of the operating room in the hospital planning process or as an owner or representative of a group that is planning to build its own freestanding ambulatory surgery center (FASC). Each role is discussed below.

Hospital-Surgery Representative

The anesthesiologist has much to contribute regarding the hospital's role in, and design of, an ambulatory surgery program. His or her views should be collected in personal interviews with the planners, consultants, or whoever is conducting or coordinating the study. The anesthesiologist should discuss the volume of ambulatory surgery that is currently taking place, current and future anesthesia management practice, the potential for growth in volume, types of surgery programs that would be appropriate for the hospital to develop, need for additional physician specialties on staff, technology needs, and other topics. The anesthesiologist also should comment on the use of existing surgery facilities for ambulatory surgery, specifically the amount of space, department location, and department design. If new facilities are planned or existing facilities renovated, the anesthesiologist should participate in the planning process as it relates to the development of these facilities.

Owner

The anesthesiologist's role as an owner in the development of a freestanding ambulatory surgery facility is fairly commonplace. Under these circumstances the role of the anesthesiologist will be far greater than that of the hospital-surgery representative. Instead of relying on the hospital to coordinate the organizational planning process, the owners of the freestanding facility must be responsible for the planning function. A number of planning variables must be carefully analyzed to determine the freestanding facility's appropriate role and, just as importantly, its potential profitability. As discussed in the facilities planning portion of this chapter, construction of surgery facilities is very expensive. Construction of a new unit without thorough need and demand analysis could prove hazardous to the financial health of the facility owners.

WHO ELSE IS INVOLVED IN THE PLANNING PROCESS?

Generally speaking, the players in the planning process depend on the size of the project. In a major building program at a hospital, for example, the planning team often can be quite large. The planning team for construction of a freestanding ambulatory surgery facility, however, might be smaller. The following team members may be involved.

> *Planning or building committee:* This group represents the owners of the project. They do not need to be aware of the day-to-day events of the project. However, they should meet regularly, such as once a month, with planning team representative(s) to receive project updates. Major decisions and direction should be provided by this group.
>
> *Project manager:* The committee should select one individual in their employ to be the project manager. The project manager directs all of the other team members. He or she is responsible for the day-to-day activities of the project and should keep the building committee apprised of major events.
>
> *Planner/consultant:* This individual is responsible for conducting the market analysis of the study. Also, the planner/consultant provides objective input into the program's function and design. The planner/consultant also may provide financial analyses.

Architect/engineer: The architect takes the functional/space program and translates it into drawings. He or she also is responsible for coordinating the many disciplines (such as civil, mechanical, and electrical engineering) necessary to design the physical structure.

Construction manager or general contractor: In many large building projects, the owner employs a construction manager. This company serves as the owner's representative for the project, keeps close watch on materials used and project costs. For smaller projects, general contractors are usually used to coordinate the many construction disciplines.

This information is presented to give the anesthesiologist the basic background necessary to begin and participate in the ambulatory surgery planning process. The next section will describe in more detail some site selection considerations, the development and use of a functional/space program (F/SP), design criteria, and project budget estimate components.

SITE SELECTION: ON OR OFF CAMPUS?

As a primary participant in the planning process, you should become familiar with some of the basic concepts of site and facility planning. Your ability to translate concepts into architectural renderings and finally into an operational unit will aid in the eventual success (or failure) of the unit.

What are the important site-selection criteria for an ambulatory surgery facility? A real estate agent will tell you the three most important characteristics of purchasing and owning property are location, location, and location. Whether the ambulatory surgery unit is located inside or outside a hospital facility, its location must afford convenience, flexibility, and marketability.

Ambulatory surgery unit location must be convenient for the consumer, family, physician, and staff. It should be convenient to find, access, and circulate through. It should be reasonably accessible for support services (materials receipt and distribution, trash disposal, etc.) and amenable to operational systems (admitting, business, patient records, etc.). Physical constraints resulting from poor location will cause inconveniences and, most likely, create inefficiencies.

Location must promote flexibility in ambulatory surgery unit design, expansion, and, if necessary, alternative uses. Ideally, the unit's design should not be compromised by its location. Within an existing building, structural constraints or immediate "neighbors" may inhibit design. On a hospital campus or land with existing structures, the placement of the new ambulatory surgery unit may be dictated by predetermined site use plans (the master site plan) or situated in an area that limits design alternatives. Whatever the location, the building (and surrounding support zones, such as parking) should be expandable in such a way as to promote maximum integrity of the original or updated design. Also, the facility's location should not limit alternative uses of the site and buildings if the mix of services changes or if the ambulatory surgery program fails. You want to be sure that the site and buildings are attractive to other investors if you need to sell.

Finally, location should promote the marketability of the ambulatory surgery unit. Its visibility and image to the community, consumers, and physicians is important to its success. The concept of marketing is discussed in the second section of this chapter.

Site Selection

What are the key site characteristics to consider when evaluating site options? What type of professionals can assist you in the selection of a site? Once you've determined a general location for the ambulatory surgery facility through the use of marketing data or other sources, a real estate agent can point you in the direction of usable properties. However, you must be sure that the property is, or can be, zoned for use as an ambulatory surgery facility. In many cities and counties, an ambulatory surgery facility can be operated under zoning codes for health-related or medically related facilities. There are a number of areas, however, that do not have any zoning provisions for these facilities. Therefore, check with your real estate agent, lawyer, and local zoning authority for zoning provisions.

Next, you may want to conduct a general (nonscientific) survey of the "neighborhood." Who are your neighbors? Are they (or you) compatible with one another? Will they detract from the ambulatory surgery program's marketability? In other words, you don't want to locate your facility in a heavy industrial area or a "bad part of town."

As you select the site, visualize the access and egress to the site. Is it logical and convenient? Will it cause congestion off the main streets? Will it serve to enhance the visibility and image of the site and buildings? Usually, you will need the assistance of the architect and city planners to determine site access and egress patterns accurately.

The city authorities also can provide you with information regarding setbacks, rights of way, easements, and building height restrictions. *Setbacks* are the distances from streets or sidewalks that buildings are located; *rights of ways* and *easements* are portions of the property that are reserved for future use by city authorities or utility companies; and *building height restrictions* vary depending on local codes (although most freestanding ambulatory surgery facilities are single-story structures). Be sure to assess the impact of these items on both current building plans and plans for future site/building development.

Also, be sure the soil conditions of the site do not preclude desirable development or that it requires different and more costly foundations for the buildings. Your architect will inform you of soil implications following test borings by a soils sample specialist.

Site Development

Once you have selected the site, there are three major criteria to consider in developing it.

Location of Site Elements
Typically, you should master plan the total site before beginning specific drawings for the ambulatory surgery unit. *Master planning* describes the conceptual process one takes in considering all the potential programs, services, and facilities to be offered on the site for the next 5 to 10 years. Once these items are identified, the physical facilities required for them should be estimated (in terms of size) and situated on the site. This will provide you with a development plan for the future. It allows for orderly development of buildings and facilities.

Ideally, the site should be developed by using one-third for buildings, one-third for drives and parking, and one-third for landscaping. Following this general rule of thumb should result in an attractive and functional site.

Drives
On-site roadways should logically relate to the buildings and parking zones. Drives are planned to allow for easy and direct access to the site and buildings, especially by patients and visitors. Separation of service and staff traffic from patient and visitor traffic is desirable.

Parking/Entrances
Parking lots should be positioned to relate closely to various entrances. The key parking-entrance relationships include

> Patient and family parking to the main entrance of the building
> Physician parking to the physician entrance
> Staff parking to the staff entrance
> Service-related drives and parking to the receiving dock and service en
> trance

FUNCTIONAL/SPACE PROGRAMMING
A successful planning process begins with a concept. That concept is the foundation of the ultimate program and facility design. To define the concept (ambulatory surgery), a planning team needs to be assembled. Representatives from anesthesiology services, surgical nursing, medical staff (physician users), management, and marketing should be included. To successfully define the concept, different views must be considered and a consensus reached.

A functional/space program (F/SP) narratively describes the key considerations of the ambulatory surgery concept and program. Why is the F/SP important? It is the planning team's *plan* to coordinate all the different aspects of providing ambulatory surgery. It is the program for physical and operational development.

The F/SP comprises five major sections:

> *Description:* This section describes the proposed functions of the am
> bulatory surgery program. Obvious activities require only a brief
> description. Special activities or services require a more complete de

scription. Operational schedules also should be stated because they affect facility requirements. It is important that this section adequately describe the broad array of ambulatory surgery services to be provided, what types of patients will be served, and unique operational considerations that may affect volumes, staffing, space, and design.

Workload analysis: This section discusses historical and projected volumes of service. Specifically, the number of cases by specialty, average length of time per case, average recovery time, and other pertinent volume-related data should be presented here. These volumes will serve as the basis for projecting staffing requirements and space. Volumes should be projected for at least a 5-year period. Based on these projected volumes, the number of operating rooms, minor procedure rooms, primary postanesthesia care unit (PACU) stretchers, and secondary-stage PACU areas should be listed here.

Staffing levels: Based on workload analysis and the proposed hours of operation, staffing by job category should be provided here. Staffing levels should be projected for a 5-year period. It is also important to estimate the number of staff during the busiest time so that space requirements can be determined accordingly.

Program for design: This section lists the specific design criteria to be used for planning the facility. (Functional areas, relationships, and specific design criteria are discussed later in this section.) Design criteria generally fall into two categories: *Interdepartmental design* describes the proposed location of the ambulatory surgery unit and the major factors that influence its location. Such factors usually relate to vertical and horizontal patterns of public, patient, staff, physician, and materials traffic. For an ambulatory surgery unit within existing hospitals, this section usually describes the relationships between the unit and laboratory, radiology, admitting/business office areas, building entrances, and general circulation. For freestanding units, this section should describe the desirable site and building entrances and exits as well as locations for parking zones. *Intradepartmental design* describes the key factors affecting the layout/design of the ambulatory surgery unit. It discusses the flow of patients, family, staff, physicians, and materials within the area. It also describes the key locational relationships between major room elements. Also, unique design features of particular rooms (such as an operating room for cystoscopy or special ceiling lights) should be stated here.

Space allocation: In this section, ambulatory surgery facility rooms or areas are listed. Proposed net square feet on a room-by-room basis is also presented. Net square feet is defined as the usable space within a room and is usually calculated from the wall-to-wall dimension.

To move into master planning and other design activities, the architect relies heavily on the space allocation and program for design sections of the F/SP. These sections narratively describe the major design guidelines for the architect to follow. Therefore, these two sections require detailed consideration by the planning team.

GENERAL PLANNING GUIDELINES: OPERATING ROOMS AND PACUs

Ambulatory surgery programs should have at least two dedicated operating rooms. This allows for optimal patient throughput. Each ambulatory surgery operating room can accommodate 1300 to 2000 procedures per year, depending on average length of procedure, available hours of surgery per day, number of operating days per week, and the efficiency of operating room turnover. A "lean and mean" program and facility will have high throughput and high profitability.

In addition to the main operating rooms, minor operating rooms should also be considered. These rooms can be used for "lumps and bumps" and minimally time-consuming procedures. This also could be used for specialty services such as ophthalmology (YAG laser use) or endoscopy.

The preoperative holding area is used to prepare the ambulatory patient for surgery. Note the term *ambulatory*. The patient and family member should have easy access to this area, and it should have a nonclinical atmosphere. Because the majority of ambulatory surgery takes place in less than 30 to 40 minutes, there should be a minimum of 1.5 preoperative holding areas per operating room.

The primary recovery area is used for the immediate stage of postanesthesia recovery (regaining consciousness). Stretchers are used in this area. The number of primary recovery stretchers is usually a multiple of the number of operating rooms. Usually, 1.5 primary recovery stretchers to one operating room is sufficient. However, to determine the number of primary recovery stretchers appropriate to your particular situation, consideration must be given to the patient mix, volume per operating room, type of anesthesia used, and expected average length of immediate recovery time.

The second-stage recovery area is for patients who have regained consciousness, require less nursing care, and are being readied to go home. Second-stage recovery times vary between 1 and 6 hours, depending on the surgical procedure, the side-effects of anesthesia, and the patient's general physical and mental state. This area should be comfortably furnished for patients with recliners, chairs, couches, and, if necessary, a stretcher. This is a minimal care area, and hence a relative or friend of the patient should be allowed in this area.

ASSEMBLING THE FUNCTIONAL/SPACE PROGRAM

The ambulatory surgery planning team needs to carefully consider the major elements an ambulatory surgery program comprises. Not all the major issues can be addressed in this chapter. However, Exhibit 10-1 is provided to familiarize the anesthesiologist with the key issues. It is organized by the key sections of the F/SP. By responding to these issues and others pertinent to your situation, you will develop and refine the F/SP.

Once these issues are addressed, the F/SP can be assembled. Usually, four to

EXHIBIT 10-1. Functional Programming: Selected Issues in Ambulatory Surgery

DEPARTMENT DESCRIPTION

1. What are the goals and objectives of the ambulatory surgery program?
2. What types of surgical procedures and anesthetics will be allowed in the ambulatory surgery program?
3. What should be the maximum length of surgical procedures?
4. Will the ambulatory surgery unit be open 7 days a week?
5. What will be the hours of operation? At what time will the last general anesthesia case begin? The last local anesthesia case?
6. Should the ambulatory surgery program accept known contaminated cases?
7. What are our policies regarding ASA physical status 1 to 4 patients with respect to qualifications for ambulatory surgery?
8. Should an anesthesiologist be present at all times? If so, should the anesthesiologist or the attending physician be responsible for patient discharge?
9. Should non-M.D.s/D.O.s or others (podiatrists, oral surgeons, and so on) be allowed to use the facility?
10. Will students or residents of teaching or training programs participate in ambulatory surgery activities?
11. Should children under 12 years of age be operated on before 12 noon?
12. What laboratory and radiography diagnostic work will be needed for the patient? Will these services be provided in the ambulatory surgery facility?
13. Should all preregistration (admitting and financial) and preadmission testing (laboratory and radiographic tests as well as history and physical) occur prior to the date of surgery? If so, how many days in advance? Is it practical to have a preanesthesia screening clinic?
14. Will instrument cleanup, packaging, and processing occur in the ambulatory surgery department?
15. Is there need for an anesthesia induction room?
16. What is the function of the primary PACU? What is the function of the secondary stage PACU? At what time in the postanesthesia recovery process will the patient move from primary recovery to second-stage recovery?

WORKLOAD ANALYSIS

1. What are the projected annual volumes of service—by patient age, sex, and surgical specialty—for the next 5 years?
2. How many operating rooms, preoperative holding areas, and PACU beds (both primary and secondary) will be needed to support these projected volumes?

STAFFING

1. How will the ambulatory surgery operating room, preoperative holding areas, and PACUs be staffed?
2. How will the support departments/areas be staffed?

PROGRAM FOR DESIGN (FUNCTIONAL CONSIDERATIONS)

1. How will the internal design of the ambulatory surgery unit
   a. Maximize patient privacy?
   b. Minimize the mixing of inpatient and ambulatory surgery patients?
   c. Appropriately separate people, supply, and equipment flow?
   d. Maximize patient visibility?
   e. Provide for separation of functions?
   f. Allow for appropriate circulation linkage from waiting zone to preoperative holding and second-stage recovery zones (for family members)?
   g. *Provide for expansion?*
2. What external factors need to be considered in the location or design of the ambulatory surgery unit?

SPACE ALLOCATION

What physical facilities (including parking) should be made available to support the ambulatory surgery unit?

EXHIBIT 10-2. Ambulatory Surgery Functional Program
***

DEPARTMENT/PROGRAM DESCRIPTION

This hospital will provide facilities for scheduled ambulatory surgery. The *ambulatory surgery department* will be a separated unit—located within the hospital but not using inpatient surgical facilities. Existing hospital services will complement the ambulatory surgery department.

1. The ambulatory surgery program allows surgical patients to return home the same day as their surgery. No overnight hospital stay is required.
2. General, regional, and local anesthesia will be used.
3. It is anticipated that ambulatory surgery services will be available Monday through Friday between 7:00 A.M. and 5:00 P.M.
4. The surgery schedule will begin at approximately 7:30 A.M. and the last case will begin at approximately 2:00 P.M. for general anesthesia and 3:00 P.M. for local anesthesia.
5. Typically, surgical procedures of less than 2 hours will be permitted in the ambulatory surgery program. Depending on the surgery schedule, longer procedures may be scheduled if operating room time is available. There will be no time restrictions for local anesthesia as long as the patient can be discharged by 5:00 P.M.
6. Any type of surgical procedure will be allowed, providing
   a. It is not a known contaminated case
   b. Patients selected for surgery will be low risk as defined by ASA physical status 1 and 2 criteria. ASA physical status 3 patients will be accepted if their medical condition is under good control.
   c. It is safe on an ambulatory basis (recovery time less than 4 to 6 hours)
   d. Postoperative care does not require inpatient facilities
   e. A responsible person is available to take the patient home and appropriately monitor the patient's needs during the first postoperative day
   f. It is in accordance with the ambulatory surgical procedure list developed and approved by the medical staff's designated approval body
7. The anesthesiologist will have final authority for patient admission and discharge.
8. Patient scheduling, preoperative test results, history and physical examination, and registration will be completed in advance of surgery. Selected laboratory tests will be completed not more than 7 days before surgery.
9. Emergency inpatient admission protocols will be in effect should transfer to inpatient status be necessary.
10. All processing, packaging, and sterilization functions will be performed in the central service department. Flash sterilization equipment will be available in the ambulatory surgery department. A case cart system will not be used.

WORKLOAD ANALYSIS

1. Projected ambulatory surgery:
   a. First year: 3500 procedures
   b. Second year: 4100 procedures
   c. Third year: 4500 procedures
2. Four operating rooms, 6 preoperative holding beds, 6 primary PACU beds, and 10 secondary PACU beds will be needed to support projected volumes of service.
3. There should be 20 parking spaces allocated for ambulatory surgery unit patients and their families.

STAFFING AND ORGANIZATION

It is anticipated that

1. One anesthesiologist will be available and on site during normal hours of operation.
2. As volumes dictate, four to five anesthesiologists or certified registered nurse-anesthetists (CRNAs) will be available to staff the operating rooms.
3. As volumes dictate, four to five circulating nurses or surgery technicians will be available to staff the operating rooms. Scrub nurses will be used as necessary and in a cost-effective manner.
4. Five registered nurses will staff the PACU/holding area.

EXHIBIT 10-2. *Continued*

5. Total staffing, based on an approximate 9-hour working day:
   a. One to four anesthesiologists (or one anesthesiologist for every one to two CRNAs, if CRNAs are used).
   b. Four to five circulating nurses or surgery technicians.
   c. Five PACU/holding area nurses.
   d. Anesthesia aids or technicians, and so on.

FUNCTIONAL CONSIDERATIONS

1. Patient flow will be as follows: admission/reception → waiting → preoperative holding (change area/gowning) → operating room → primary PACU → second-stage PACU (change area) → discharge
2. Maximum nurse-patient visibility is desirable, allowing for reasonable patient privacy.
3. Family members will be allowed in the secondary recovery area.
4. There will be separate zones for waiting, preoperative and postoperative, and operating room areas.
5. Functions will be combined when feasible from a staffing, space, convenience, and economic viewpoint.
6. There will be minimum conflict of patient, family, staff, supply, and equipment traffic flow patterns.
7. Access to dedicated ambulatory surgery parking areas will be as convenient as possible.
8. Access to other hospital support departments will be as convenient as possible.

SPACE ALLOCATION BY DEPARTMENT AND SERVICE ELEMENT

Room Element	No.	Size	Total NSF	Comments
Operating room areas:				
General operating room	4	400	1600	
Scrub area	2	24	48	
Stretcher alcove	4	17	68	
Soiled utility room	1		80	
Equipment/laser storage	1		240	
Instrument storage	1		160	
Clean core:	1		340	
Flash sterilization				
Solution warmer				
Circulation				
Storage				
Medication				
Linen	—		——	
SUBTOTAL	14		2536	
Central staff support:				
Nursing/control station	1		120	
Anesthesiology workroom/ storage	1		140	
Supervisor office (1)/file (1)*	1		100	
Anesthesiology office (1)/ file (1)	1		100	
Waiting room—family (20)	1		300	
Staff lounge (8)	1		160	
Locker—male	1		100	
Toilet/shower	1		60	
Locker—female	1		140	
Toilet/shower	1		80	
Janitor closet	1		30	
SUBTOTAL	11		1330	

EXHIBIT 10-2. *Continued*

Room Element	No.	Size	Total NSF	Comments
Patient holding area:				
Children's playroom	1		80	
Preoperative holding room	6	70	420	
Primary PACU	6	80	480	
Second-stage PACU	10	70	700	
Clean supply/linen	1		120	
Soiled utility room	1		60	
Patient lounge	1		80	
Patient toilet	4	40	160	Disabled accessible
Storage	1		160	
Janitor closet	1		40	
SUBTOTAL	32		2300	
Total operating room NSF†	15		2616	
G/N @ 1.6 DGSF				4186
Total central staff support and patient holding areas	42		3550	
G/N @ 1.4 DGSF				4970
Total NSF	56		6086	
Total DGSF				9156

*Figures in parentheses refer to capacity of persons or items.

†NSF (net square feet) is usable space within rooms. DGSF is departmental gross square feet. DGSF is NSF plus circulation space, wall thickness, and other nonusable space within departments/areas. DGSF represents the total amount of space needed to support the ambulatory surgery program and is expressed as a multiple of net square feet. If a satellite or freestanding facility is planned, for cost estimating purposes you need to consider the building gross square feet (BGSF). BGSF considers all the space within the perimeter of the structure itself.

EXHIBIT 10-3. Typical Room Elements and Net Square Footage Range

Room Element	NSF Range*	
Operating room areas:		
General operating room	320–400	
Minor operating room	240–280	
Cystoscopic operating room	280–360	
Cysto control	30–50	
Cysto toilet	30–40	
Scrub area	15–40	
Flash sterilization area	20–40	
Medications/supply storage/linen	60–160	
Equipment storage	120–300	
Instrument storage	60–240	
Soiled utility room	60–140	
Stretcher alcove	17	Per stretcher
Substerile room	80–140	
Control desk	40–80	
Anesthesia workroom/storage	100–180	
Janitor closet	30–60	

EXHIBIT 10-3. *Continued*

Room Element	NSF Range*	
Central operating room staff support areas:		
Nursing/control station	80–140	
Physician office	80–120	
Supervisor office	80–120	
Anesthesiology office	80–120	
Male staff lounge/locker/toilet	160–300	
Female staff lounge/locker/toilet	180–400	
Staff lounge	140–220	
Scheduling office	60–80	
Patient holding area:		
Change/locker area	60–200	
Preoperative holding	60–100	Per patient
PACU (includes charting space)	80–120	Per patient
Second-stage postanesthesia care	70–120	Per patient
Induction room	80–100	Per patient
Examination room	80–100	
Patient toilet	40–60	
Supply/storage/linen	80–200	
Soiled utility room	60–120	
Children playroom	60–120	
Pantry	60–100	
Administrative support areas:		
Reception/switchboard/cashier/admitting	180–300	
Waiting room	120–500	
	or	
	12–15	Per person
Children's playroom	60–180	
Private consultation room	60–100	
Dining/vending area	100–300	
Public toilet	40–120	
Business office	60–80	Per work station
Medical records	60–80	Per work station
Administration	140–300	
Diagnostic services:		
Laboratory	100–300	
Radiology	340–580	
Supportive services:		
Central service	120–360	
Housekeeping	160–300	
Maintenance	160–400	
Pharmacy/gift shop	280–500	
Purchasing/storage	260–520	
Educational areas:		
Patient/community education	160 +	

*Depending on your particular situation, net square footage (NSF) by room element may fall outside of the NSF range.

five meetings are required to agree on a F/SP. You should provide ample time between meetings to allow for research and data collection, analysis, and consideration of major issues.

Exhibit 10-2 is an *example* of a completed F/SP. The space allocation is based on the functional requirements of this example program. It cannot be applied to individual situations. Your particular F/SP depends on functional programming requirements and budget considerations for your situation. This F/SP is presented for illustrative purposes only.

Exhibit 10-3 lists the common room elements (and their respective sizes) found in ambulatory surgery facilities. This list provides a range of room sizes. It should serve as a *guideline* when developing the space allocation section of the F/SP.

Room sizes and dimensions, when listed on paper or discussed in concept, are difficult to grasp for most people. When planning room spaces, measure a familiar area or room and use it as a guide for space comparisons. This will raise the comfort level of team members during this space planning phase.

Another important feature of Exhibit 10-3 is its obvious emphasis on including all the rooms needed to fit most ambulatory surgery programs. Most anesthesiologists and medical personnel are familiar only with the key areas used to support patient care or as individual work zones. It is important to recognize the different support-related rooms that allow patient care activities to occur (such as clean and soiled utility rooms, janitor closets, equipment storage, and offices).

WHAT ARE THE MAJOR AMBULATORY SURGERY FACILITY DESIGN FEATURES?

The space allocation section of the F/SP is organized into four major categories. The *zones* have differing purposes and design needs. They are discussed below.

> *Operating room (sterile) zone:* This zone includes the operating rooms, substerile area, scrub, and operating room support spaces.
> *Patient holding zone:* This area includes preoperative, primary PACU, second-stage PACU, induction room, nurse control, and support areas.
> *Central staff support zone:* This zone includes the offices, locker rooms, equipment/instrument clean-up, and sterilizing areas.
> *Reception/waiting zone:* This zone includes the reception, waiting, medical record, and business office areas.

The key functional relationships between these zones are as follows:

> The operating room zone should be in an isolated area, away from major traffic patterns.
> The holding areas should be situated between the reception/waiting zone and the operating room zone and should be conveniently accessible to the latter.
> The central staff support zone should be conveniently accessible to the holding areas and the operating room zone.

There should be two major entrances/exits from the ambulatory surgery unit. One is for the public—patients and families. The other is for staff, equipment, and supplies.

Within the individual zones, the following design criteria should be considered. In the operating room zone,

The substerile room should be situated between the operating rooms. This area provides access to a sterile work zone from the operating rooms.

Scrub areas should be adjacent to, and ideally have visibility into, the operating rooms.

The stretcher alcoves, equipment storage, clean supply room, and sterile instrument room should be situated across the hall from, or adjacent to, the operating rooms.

The soiled utility room should be situated between the operating room zone (relatively close to the operating rooms) and the central support area (to facilitate easy transport of soiled instruments, supplies, linen, and trash).

A janitor closet should be situated conveniently in the operating room zone.

In the patient holding zone,

The primary and secondary PACUs should each have access to a nurse control station and to clean and soiled utility rooms.

Patient toilets accessible to disabled persons should be located within the secondary recovery area.

Family members should be allowed in the preoperative holding and second stage PACU. Therefore, these areas should be conveniently accessible to the family waiting room to minimize family traffic flow throughout the unit. Public toilets should be located nearby.

The induction room, if used, should be adjacent to the operating room zone but accessible to family members.

In the central staff support zone,

Offices should be located near the staff entrance to minimize visitor travel through the unit.

The staff lounge should be conveniently accessible to the PACU and the operating room zone to facilitate breaks between cases.

The soiled utility room should have the following functional relationships: It should be situated between the operating room zone and the central support zone, and it should be adjacent to the pack makeup/sterilizer room (if part of the program).

The pack makeup/sterilizer room should be reasonably convenient to the sterile instrument room in the operating room zone.

In the reception/waiting zone,

> The reception office should be situated between the public entrance and the waiting room (to facilitate visual control).
> The waiting room should be situated near the reception office and the second-stage postanesthesia care unit (SSPACU).
> The private consultation room should be situated between the waiting room and SSPACU.

The most important design feature of all the areas, however, is that they be flexible and easily expandable. Don't let the unit's design limit the opportunity for expansion. Always plan a unit for possible expansion.

EXHIBIT 10-4. Major Zoning and Room Elements of an Ambulatory Surgery Facility by Functional Area

————————[**Service/Receiving Entrance**

Surgery
Operating room
Cysto/control room
Scrub area
Stretcher area
Soiled utility room
Equipment storage
Instrument storage
Flash sterilizer/substerile room
Control station
Clean utility room

Staff Support
Central sterilizing
Central stores
Anesthesia work areas

PACU/SSPACU
Primary- and second-stage recovery
Nursing station
Med room
Pantry
Supply room
Soiled utility room
Blanket warmer
Patient toilet
Child playroom (SSPACU)

Staff support
Lockers
Staff toilets
Staff lounge
Misc. staff offices

Physician & Staff Entrance }————————→

Patient
Change/locker area
Gowned waiting area
Children's playroom
Exam room
Preop holding room
Patient toilet
Supply room
Laboratory
Radiology

Public
Reception cashier
Switchboard
Admitting office
Business office
Waiting room
Private consultation
Dining, vending area
Public toilets
Patient records

Patient/Visitor Entrance }————————→

Ambulatory Surgery Facility Design (Exhibit 10-4 and Figure 10-1): Space program by Leslie K. Leider, Leider Planning Associates, Minneapolis, Minnesota; Schematic drawing by Hills Gilbertson Architects, Minneapolis, Minnesota.

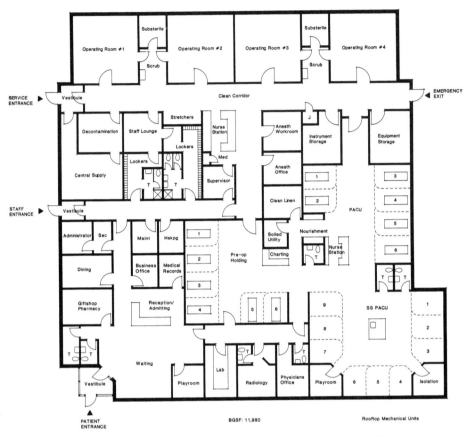

FIGURE 10-1. Prototype Floor Plan of a Freestanding Ambulatory Surgery Facility

Exhibit 10-4 and Figure 10-1 display the concepts and design of a freestanding unit. Each exhibit emphasizes a particular feature. Exhibit 10-4 diagrams the major zoning and access/egress patterns of the building. Figure 10-1 is a sample floor plan of a freestanding ambulatory surgery facility.

INTERIOR DESIGN

Only a qualified interior designer can help you make the best interior design decisions. All visual aspects of the ambulatory surgery facility must be pleasing and comfortable and present a nonclinical atmosphere. The colors and textures of floors, walls, and ceilings should exude a reasonable level of informality yet assure the patient that he or she is in a safe environment.

Colors are usually an important factor in soliciting a positive psychological response. Exhibit 10-5 lists general psychological responses by color. In planning your facility interiors, refer to this exhibit when working with your interior designer.

EXHIBIT 10-5. General Psychological Response by Color

Color	General Psychological Response
Black	Despondent, ominous, powerful, strong
Blue	Peaceful, comfortable, contemplative, restful
Green	Calm, serene, quiet, refreshing
Orange	Lively, energetic, exuberant
Pastel Colors	Neutral, nonrespondent, soothing
Purple	Dignified, mournful
Red	Stimulating, hot, active, happy
White	Cool, pure, clean
Yellow	Cheerful, inspiring, vital

EQUIPMENT PLANNING

In the latter part of schematic design and during design development, the planning team considers the type of equipment to be used in the facility. At first, a generic equipment list is prepared on a room-by-room basis. As the design process continues, specific equipment (by manufacturer and model) is selected.

Equipment is generally categorized into three groupings:

> *Group 1:* This equipment is often referred to as *fixed equipment.* Equipment in this category is permanently affixed to the structure; it is not "plugged in." Life expectancy is typically 10 years or more. Examples of group 1 items are sterilizers/washers, surgical lights, radiographic systems, communication systems, and built-in cabinetry.
>
> *Group 2:* This equipment is movable and is usually referred to as *movable equipment.* Life expectancy is typically 5 years or more. Examples of group 2 equipment are stretchers, wheelchairs, surgical tables, laboratory equipment, refrigerators, and furniture.
>
> *Group 3:* Equipment in this category consists typically of small, durable items, easily transported, and having a life expectancy of 3 years or more. Examples of items in this category are surgical instruments, diagnostic instruments, chart holders, reusable trays, and stainless steel jars and cannisters.

There are nine major steps in equipment planning. Each will be briefly discussed. Your consultant or architect can further detail each step.

> *Programming:* This is the assessment and documentation of equipment needs for the new facility.
>
> *Inventory and evaluation of existing equipment:* Existing equipment should be inventoried and evaluated for possible use in the new facility. Reusable equipment is documented, and a list of equipment to purchase is prepared (called a buy list).

Budget estimates: The buy list is priced out. This includes any costs associated with reinstallation of reusable equipment. Equipment budget estimates should be refined throughout the planning process.

Architectural planning and design: During the design development phase, equipment is laid out on the drawings on a room-by-room basis. At this stage, room function, workflow, and equipment use is carefully considered.

Purchased specifications: Buy-list equipment is categorized by who purchases and installs it (contractor or owner). Equipment specifications are developed to be used in asking for bids by vendors.

Bid evaluation and purchasing: Bids are received, reviewed, and awarded. A master equipment list is developed that includes the specific equipment, vendor, and final purchase price.

Coordination and scheduling of medical equipment delivery and installation: An equipment delivery and installation schedule is developed. Delays in equipment delivery and installation will adversely affect the opening and operation of the facility.

Coordination of staff orientation and training: Appropriate facility staff members need to be oriented and trained to use the equipment. This should occur 2 to 4 weeks before the opening of the facility to identify and resolve problem areas, if any exist.

Preventive maintenance programming: A preventive maintenance schedule of group 1 and 2 equipment should be developed. Improper, ill-timed, or avoided preventive equipment maintenance will result in unnecessary "down-time."

PROJECT COST COMPONENTS

Most major capital expenditures are long-term commitments and are accompanied by an element of risk. Decisions about capital expenditures are among the most difficult an organization must face, particularly for the renovation or new construction of physical facilities. The project cost budget aids facility planning through identification of capital needs. A well-planned expenditures budget provides assurance that the equipment and facilities needed are available at the proper time, helps to define the risk involved, and facilitates the establishment of priorities for asset acquisition.

Ambulatory surgery facility project costs consist of

Construction: Costs related to the physical structure ("bricks and mortar"), either new construction or renovation, as well as group 1 equipment

Site preparation: Costs related to physically preparing the site for construction, including the cost of roadways and parking areas

Equipment: Group 2 and 3 equipment costs

Professional fees: Fees associated with architectural, consulting, engineering, and other professional services.

Contingency: A sum of money dedicated to changes in the project scope or unexpected variations in costs

Financing: The cost of acquiring and using capital dollars during the planning and construction of a facility

Site acquisition: Costs associated with the purchase of land

Administrative: Costs for such items as soil tests, site survey, legal fees, and related expense that the owner is obliged to pay in connection with facility construction

Total project cost is typically 1.5 to 2 times the building cost. Hence, if the facility construction cost is estimated at $1 million, the total project cost may approximate $1.5 million to $2 million. Project costs can be controlled through reasonable and consistent review of all project phases.

Appropriately, most owners tend to concentrate on minimizing construction costs, since these costs constitute the greatest portion of the budget. However, the planning team needs to use a *life-cycle cost analysis* when evaluating building design, systems, and equipment. A life-cycle cost analysis considers the capital and *operating* costs of an item over its expected lifetime. Although an item may have a lower capital cost than another similar item, it may be more expensive to operate over its lifetime. Hence dollars may be saved initially, but greater operating expenses may significantly offset the initial capital cost savings.

The quality of the final ambulatory surgery facility design is directly related to the quality of time and effort given to the facility planning process. Each ambulatory surgery program is unique; an existing program cannot be simply transferred to a new situation.

The planning process presented here provides the anesthesiologist with an important concept and approach to planning ambulatory surgery facilities. The next two sections in this chapter discuss key marketing and operational considerations for the ambulatory surgery program.

SUGGESTED READINGS

Berkoff MJ: Planning and designing ambulatory surgery facilities for hospitals. J Ambulatory Care Management 4(3): 35–51, 1981

Breen PC: Circular patient flow highlights facility expansion program (interview). Same Day Surg 4(4): 49–50, 1981

Burn JM: Facility design for outpatient surgery and anesthesia. Int Anesthesiol Clin 20(1): 135, 1982

Hardy OB, Lammers LM: Hospitals: The Planning and Design Process. Boulder, Colo., Aspen Publishers, 1986

Leider LK: Business Planning Outline. American Hospital Association Seminar on Ambulatory Surgery, June 1987, Wash DC

Leider LK, Mannix PM: Facilities Planning Outline. American Hospital Association Seminar on Ambulatory Surgery, October 1984, Boston, MA

Medical Equipment Planning. Promotional brochure. Robert Douglass Associates, 1984

Reed WA, Dawson B: The ambulatory surgery facility. In Schultz RC (ed): Outpatient Surgery. Philadelphia, Lea & Febiger, 1979

Marketing the Ambulatory Surgery Center

A. BETH FROST
WILLIAM A. FLEXNER

BECOMING A MARKET-DRIVEN AMBULATORY SURGERY CENTER

Anyone with even a recessive marketing gene would be thrilled to be a health care David up against the Goliaths. And that is exactly the position you may well find yourself in operating a freestanding ambulatory surgery center among the well-established hospitals that may provide similar services. Even though your center may be fully or partially owned by the hospital, you still compete for the same customers. In the business of health care, just as in any competitive event, if you can't be bigger, you must be swifter, smarter, and smoother to succeed. From this point forward, that will be your marketing edge.

Whether they are owners, medical directors, or simply specialists involved in the delivery of ambulatory surgery services, anesthesiologists have a major impact on the way the service is delivered to customers. Producing customer satisfaction is the key to building demand in a growing and successful ambulatory surgery business. A *market* consists of two or more individuals, each having something the other wants and each wanting something the other has. A market transaction occurs when these individuals get together and make an exchange. Items that may be exchanged include, among others, goods, services, money, ideas, time, and attention. As long as both parties are satisfied with the transaction, each time they want to make an exchange of similar items, they will return to the marketplace and transact another piece of business.

We each do it hundreds of times every week, and even though many times unconsciously, there are always multiple factors that enter into our decision in choosing a provider of the goods and services. The days of the uncomplicated market structure in health care are largely over. In their place, organizations, professionals, and consumers are all changing in ways that require new knowledge and skills to manage a successful health care program.

MARKETING—THE USED AND ABUSED TERM

"We just need some marketing." This is an often said and simple phrase that can cause tachycardia in marketing professionals and can lead to severe economic depression in health care businesses when used without proper diagnosis, analysis, and treatment.

What is marketing? It is not just advertising, although that may be a part of it and that part is often assumed to be the whole. *Marketing*, by academic definition, is the performance of activities that direct the flow of services from the producer to the consumer based on market preferences. *Marketing*, by basic definition, is finding out what people want and giving it to them and finding out what people don't want and not giving it to them anymore.

This simple definition congeals when applied to our own experience as consumers. Think of your last purchase of services. What need of yours did it meet? Why did you purchase it from that particular provider? What was your perception of the company and the service before you made the decision to buy? The answers to all these questions are not merely happenstance, but the result of the company's detailed understanding and belief of your needs as you perceive them and the calculated development, communication, and delivery of the service according to those perceived needs.

As an anesthesiologist or medical director of an ambulatory center, you will be involved in the major decisions that affect the operations of your facility. Therefore, it is critical that you champion the perceived needs of your consumers to be the decision-making factor in all aspects of the business. Consumers only return if their needs continue to be met. Seeing that they are is the marketing approach to success in business.

In industry, marketing is the matching of a company's capabilities and resources with consumers' needs and wants. Needs and wants are the things that are important to consumers and that underlie their behavior. Because consumers' preferences and expectations vary, companies provide many different products and services. Through marketing, management can foster mutually beneficial exchanges between the organization and specified segments of the consumer population. To be successful, a business or any other organization must satisfy various consumer segments by providing appropriately designed products or services. Simultaneously, it must achieve its internal goals and objectives, whether these be profit, market share, health outcomes, or patient compliance. To reach these goals, a business or organization has to offer the right product or service at the right price and deliver it at the right time and place. When planning is market-based, effective and efficient exchanges are more likely to take place between the business or organization and its consumers. Such an orientation, however, requires an understanding on the part of management as to how and why consumers choose specific products or services in the marketplace.

HOW DO CONSUMERS IN A SERVICE INDUSTRY DETERMINE THAT THEIR NEEDS ARE BEING MET?

Quality seems to be the buzzword of the nineties that is interlinked with success for health care business survivors of the next decade. Physicians and managers have historically focused on the clinical perspectives of quality. Attention must now be focused on perceptual quality. "Beauty is in the eye of the beholder" can be adapted to "Quality is in the perception of the consumer."

Service organizations tend to be judged by the manner in which they provide services. The airline industry is a perfect analogy. When we purchase a ticket, what we really buy is transportation. If we travel safely from New York to Los Angeles, we should be satisfied consumers. But we *assume* technical competency of the pilots, because to think otherwise is too horrific. (Do we ever ask for a

pilot's flight record or if the navigator has been tested for alcohol or drug abuse?)
Our judgments are based on the peripherals: Was the flight on time? Were the
attendants pleasant? Did the luggage arrive at the same destination as the pas-
senger?

So it is with health care. Technical quality is assumed, and because health care
is such an intimate activity, even more emphasis is placed on the delivery mode.
Even though one of the key consumer groups is comprised of surgeons, they too
will often make utilization choices on whether or not their nonclinical needs are
being met.

WHO ARE THE CUSTOMERS?

The ambulatory surgery facility has two key consumer groups: surgeons and patients. It is a wise idea to establish from the very beginning the "corporate value"
that the surgery center exists *because and for* these two groups. How it affects
them should be a part of every decision that is made. This is critical in the attempt to continually satisfy their needs and maintain them as loyal customers.
Both surgeons and patients have many other choices, and you probably have a
competitor who is planning to take them away while you are reading this book.

The patient as customer is far more aware of his or her choices as a consumer
and rights as a patient. Participative care is becoming more of an expectation,
and the patient expects and should have a detailed explanation of what will take
place. More often than not, it is the surgery center staff that provides the information. The staff therefore becomes the primary agent for fulfilling the expectations of the patient consumer. A service-driven ambulatory facility makes it
everyone's responsibility to see that patient satisfaction is paramount.

The surgeon as customer finds that his or her satisfaction is more directly
related to those things which are controlled by the anesthesiologist. Equally important is the personal relationship that exists between the two. We most often
associate with those people and businesses with whom we feel most familiar and
accepted. The social relationship can be enhanced by activities as simple as operating room conversation and as structured as annual medical staff dinner
meetings. The critical part is to acknowledge the importance of the relationship
and to develop actions and activities to enhance it.

PRODUCT, PRICE, PLACE, AND PROMOTION—EVEN IF YOU'VE READ IT BEFORE, READ IT AGAIN

These well known "four P's" are the basics, and to ignore any one of them will
sabotage the other three. The creation and setting of the product, price, place,
and promotion is the strategic basis for all other activities in the marketing construct. The *marketing mix* must be carefully construed and balanced. The description and explanation of these critical components will not be extensive, but
they deserve some highlighting because of the crucial foundation that they lay.

Product

A simplistic view would identify *surgical services* as the main product. While this is an obvious component, it is the delivery of these services from all perspectives that is key. Let's divide this product into measurable units and consider how the sum of the parts equals the whole.

The product has significantly different components for the surgeon than for the patient. For the surgeon, it might consist of the following: ease of scheduling, available equipment, skills of the nursing staff, relationship with the anesthesiologist, time commitment for meetings, operating room turnover times, close and convenient parking, procedure cost for the patient, patient satisfaction, and general affability of the staff.

From the patient's perspective, although the product has some similarities, there are differences: care and compassion from the staff, physical environment, understanding and information from the business office on procedure and cost, education and consideration of the patient's family, close and convenient parking, safety and security, and very personalized care. It is challenging to simultaneously deliver the product to both consumer groups, but it is achievable when one commits to the service strategy that "it is a doctor's place and a patient's place" and when one uses this as a guidepost in decision making.

The benefits that consumers look for refer to the functional, social, and psychological utilities or values that are received. Health care organizations produce specific services, but people usually only purchase aspects of those services— things as tangible as a prescription for medicine or as intangible as the way the staff both talks and listens to them. Consumers look at health services in very different ways, because they are attempting to derive different benefits from the services. In ambulatory surgery, physicians may be seeking a competent, efficient staff, as well as a location and surgery schedule that are most compatible with their existing practices; patients may be seeking a less threatening environment along with the convenience of going home that day. It is incumbent on the manager (and particularly the anesthesiologist manager) to understand what aspects of the organization's services are being purchased, by whom, and why and then to translate these findings so that the producers of the services can maintain a high level of market responsiveness.

The range of services an organization produces is called the *product mix*. Most health care organizations have the capacity to offer a wide range of services. Whether they should do so is a different and strategically important question. In ambulatory surgery, the mix of specialties that will be invited to use the service should be based on the relative time and equipment needs of the surgeons, the compatibility of the specialties with each other, and the capacity of the facility to absorb the demand that each of the physicians in the specialties will generate.

In essence, the decision to include or eliminate a specialty should be made not only on the basis of what the center wants to do, but more importantly on what is feasible given a careful assessment of the potential market demand and the strength of existing ambulatory surgery services in the marketplace. The ambulatory surgery center, facility, unit, or program may not be capable physically or economically of being "all things to all people."

To control the organization's service offerings, a periodic review of the strengths and weaknesses of each service in relation to competitors should be carried out. The anesthesiologist, whether or not he or she has management responsibility, should be involved in the process; consumer input is essential if it is to be successful.

Place

We *Homo sapiens* are quite susceptible to taking a portion of what we see and applying it to the whole. This is why the place in which the service is delivered sets an image for the actual clinical service that is delivered, although in actuality they have the potential to be totally opposite. Have you ever ventured into a small neighborhood restaurant and, dismayed by its environment, chosen to eat elsewhere, even though the food was highly recommended? Or have you chosen not to try a new restaurant because it was unfamiliar or too distant? These factors may have overridden the fact that the restaurant prepared excellent food.

The *place* (or *distribution channel*) variable focuses attention on the problems, functions, and institutions involved in getting producers and consumers together. From the consumer's point of view, the place variable consists of three dimensions: time, location, and ability to obtain possession of the product or service. *Time* in this context refers to the ease or difficulty of getting to the site where services are obtained. *Location* refers to the physical and psychological environment in which the service is delivered. *Obtaining possession* refers to the number of service providers one might go through to obtain the needed service. The lay and professional referral chains are important components of the distribution segment. Ambulatory surgery managers should pay careful attention to where the demand for services will originate. The referral chain should be carefully assessed all the way back to primary care physicians and the employers or payors of the potential patients.

The location and physical attributes of the product, especially those which will form first impressions on the patient, deserve scrupulous review. Remember, the patient will consciously experience only the external structure, waiting room, preoperative areas, and postoperative areas. It is the first two that will set an expectation for what will happen during the actual surgery, and that mindset is unconsciously imprinted by the first impression of the physical environment. Historically, many assumptions about clinical excellence or lack thereof have been made about a hospital's operating suites as patients have walked through the front lobby. The physical environment must be clean, in good repair, up-to-date, and aesthetically pleasant. The location must be convenient and safe.

Price

Two things hold true: The glory years of the Green Bay Packers and the simple years of total reimbursement are both over. Ten years ago, price was an issue to neither the patient nor the physician. Very few patients now have carte blanche indemnity insurance, with most either having copayments or deductibles. Managed care plans are negotiating hard and swift to lock in prices. Government reimbursements are and will continue to decline for Medicare and Medicaid.

Price is now an issue, but this is not a recommendation to become the low-price leader. There is still a viable relationship between price and quality, and more and more third-party payors are asking for documentation of quality and outcome. However, ambulatory surgery facilities are positioned to take advantage of their singleness of mission and efficiency and can price their services to attract volume. Additionally, price is a particular issue for those services which are not covered by traditional plans, such as plastic surgery. (Package pricing of plastic surgery services can be used as a marketing tool to attract new patients for the plastic surgeons on staff.)

The *price variable* in marketing is what is exchanged for the satisfaction or benefits derived from the purchase—it is what is given up to get what has been purchased. In health care there are at least two conceptually different price variables that management can control. The first is the direct monetary price. From the organization's point of view, the price charged has typically been based on a formula that related total costs to total revenue requirements. With the advent of DRGs, HMOs, and PPOs, this is changing rapidly, ambulatory surgery services being a major tool to develop strongly competitive prices based on reduced costs.

The second concept of price in health care concerns the indirect costs to the consumer of getting into, through, and out of the health care setting. These costs include time, loss of control and dignity, hassle, opportunity costs, and actual loss of salary. Whenever possible, the ambulatory surgery center should be designed functionally to keep both types of costs to a minimum.

Promotion

Promotion is the final variable that management controls in its interactions with the marketplace. Special emphasis will be paid to promotion in this chapter. However, this is not an endorsement of its importance above the others. Now that your product, place, and price have been established, it is time to tell your consumers about it. This may sound simple, but choosing the right form of promotion and spending promotional dollars wisely can be compared to the very thin line between science and art that exists in medicine. There are many right ways. The key is to develop the right way that provides the most return for the investment of time and money. There are four different types of promotion that an organization can undertake: advertising, public relations, personal selling, and sales promotion.

Advertising

The most familiar is *advertising*, which is a paid form of nonpersonal communication. Advertising must be carefully chosen according to the target market group, and a misfire can be very expensive with little return. The target market must be chosen by demographic variables such as age, sex, income, geographic location, and so on. Once the target market has been identified, media can be chosen to reach them without wasted advertising dollars. All newspapers, television stations, and radio stations have readership or viewership information that will determine how to specifically reach your target group with the minimum investment. As an example, in advertising a cataract program, media information may show that radio is the key media for people over the age of 55 and that a particular station, because of its format, has a high listenership in that age group. It may not be the most popular station (and therefore not the most expensive) overall, but it clearly reaches the target market. The most common mistake made in advertising is choosing media placement in the media familiar to the business owner rather than the one that will best reach the target market.

Public Relations

The more commonly understood form of promotion in the health care industry is publicity, in which the organization actively seeks news stories and other public service announcements. This may be sought through varying types of activities.

COMMUNITY ACTIVITIES. Participation in community activities makes a statement that the organization gives as well as receives. Participation may be the contribution of funds, staff time, or professional services when appropriate. The benefits of your contribution, in whatever form, are many: media coverage, relationships with community business and government leaders, and a positive image with your potential patient population. A side benefit is the morale boost and good will often experienced by the staff when participating in such activities.

MEDIA CONTACTS. The media connection is initially made through a press release, sent in proper format and with ample time for response. The topic of the news release may be a medical procedure that is new in the marketplace for ambulatory surgery, new technological capabilities, a new physician who will be joining the staff, or any honors or achievements that are awarded to the organization. The media is bombarded with news releases, and they will be judicious in their selection. It is important to send a news release only when the item is newsworthy and significant.

Once a relationship is made with a media source, it is important to cultivate that relationship so that the ambulatory facility becomes a first-choice source for media inquiries. This is accomplished through a quick response to media pursuits and through courteous and honest responses to questions.

SPECIAL EVENTS. A *special event* is any activity that gathers your consumers together for a purpose other than the provision of services. This would include an open house to tour your facility; educational seminars for the public, physicians, or physicians' office staffs; health screening (*i.e.,* cholesterol, glaucoma, blood pressure, and so on); an athletic event such as a run; or a health fair. The purpose of special events is to once again expose your presence to the community (consumers and potential consumers) to provide name recognition, so that when the choice of a surgery facility is at hand, your hospital or freestanding center is the first called to mind.

INTERNSHIPS/MENTOR PROGRAMS. Many colleges and universities offer programs that allow technical, medical, and clinical students an opportunity to participate in their field of study before receiving their degree. This is an excellent opportunity for increased exposure in the marketplace and often provides additional high-caliber staff support at little or no cost.

Personal Selling

A third form of promotion that is typically not recognized for its importance is personal selling. This form represents all the interpersonal communication that occurs between members of the organization and consumers. Each employee is a salesperson for the organization. Almost all staff members work in close association with both consumer groups and have opportunities on a daily basis to meet the consumer's needs and expectations. Each of the staff members involved in an ambulatory surgery facility (e.g., aides, receptionists, nurses, physicians) should be aware of and practice effective communications skills with customers at all times. This starts with simple courtesy with patients, family and friends, and physicians and their office staffs, whether in personal or telephone interactions. Simple courtesies are not forgotten by customers and can make a difference in whether the patients or physicians use the facility on a repeat basis.

In addition to the day-to-day personal sales responsibilities, a formal sales program may be initiated. This would involve sending out staff (i.e., a nurse, a receptionist, or a scheduler) to meet with a physician and his or her office staff. This activity accomplishes several goals. It shows the physician that the ambulatory surgery center is personally interested in him or her and in his or her practice. It also builds a relationship between the office staff and the ambulatory surgery staff that may have an impact on facility selection in the future. In addition, that relationship may help to make smooth clerical transactions and accurate charging of fees because of the ease of working with a familiar person. Sales calls to physician offices should be made at least semiannually, and office staffs should be invited to the surgery facility for an annual event, such as a breakfast seminar.

Sales Promotion

The final type of promotion is sales promotion, which consists of the booklets, brochures, stationery, newsletters, signs, office displays, and direct mailings that are used to enhance the relationship between the organization and consumers. These may be utilized to provide basic information about the procedures and systems of utilizing the facility, such as a patient handbook; may be used as a direct-mail marketing piece, such as a physician recruiting brochure; or may be used to announce a special event, such as an open house invitation. It is imperative that the piece be produced professionally, since it will unconsciously indicate to the receiver the clinical professionalism of your program. The consistent use of a logo, format, design, and colors will solidify your image in the mind of the consumer and will help to separate and clarify your identity from your competitor's.

MARKET RESEARCH: HOW TO MARKET-DRIVE THE FOUR P'S

It is an expensive and dangerous thing to assume that you know what your consumers are thinking. What happens if you use your perceptions as a base for decision making and your perceptions are different from those of your consumers? Generally, failure follows. Formal and informal methodologies exist to gather the thoughts of those who will decide to utilize your facility. The most important and critical factor is the acceptance of those perceptions as truth. Market research is a management tool, not a report card, and objectivity in accepting the perceptions of the consumer groups as truth must be maintained.

Market research gathers quantitative and qualitative information from consumers that forms a basis for decision making. Formal collection of data may be obtained through use of primary research, which may include written or telephone surveys, personal interviews, or focus groups. Secondary research may be available from government agencies, libraries, or health care organizations. Informal collection is often the result of one-on-one conversations with surgeons or patients. Statistical reliability of anecdotal information is limited but still should be at least considered in the decision-making process.

TYING IT ALL TOGETHER: THE MARKETING PLAN

If you were to take an automobile trip from Chicago to New York without driving on the major freeways, one of the first things you would do would be to outline your highway itinerary. If you got halfway there and discovered that one of the roads you had planned on taking was closed, you could look at your plan and, knowing what your goal was, select another road that would still take you to New York. This application is true of facility and program marketing. If you know what your goals are and you have them mapped out in detail, when a change in your marketplace takes place, you can alter your plan and still reach your goals. In addition, having a written marketing plan helps to clarify to all involved what the strategic marketing direction will be, and also serves as a calendar guideline to ensure that activities are accomplished. It is important to note that the marketing plan is a key part of the strategic business plan. That plan includes all the operational decisions regarding product, place, and promotion as described in the prior sections of this chapter.

The following outline is a general marketing plan format that has been adapted for ambulatory surgery facility use:

I. Executive summary
II. Situation analysis
III. Strengths, weaknesses, opportunities, and threats
IV. Mission statement
V. Target consumer groups
VI. Goals
VII. Action plan
   A. Research
   B. Public relation activities
   C. Advertising
   D. Promotional publications
   E. Internal communications
   F. Budget

Program Packaging

Product-line marketing is a term that is used to describe a particular way in which generic products or services are packaged so as to separate them in the minds of consumers by their particular attributes. For instance, Ford Motor Company makes cars but packages them in product lines that we know as Ford, Mercury, Lincoln, and so on. Each of these is known for its distinct attributes, generally related to price and quality. Product-line marketing for the ambulatory surgery center can mean the packaging of services according to their attributes, generally related to specialty and target market. Cataract surgery, plastic surgery, and others can be effectively packaged and marketed to key consumer groups. This is often a more effective use of promotional expenditures that general image advertising because it specifically asks the consumer to take an action to purchase the service.

COMPETING IN THE AMBULATORY SURGERY MARKET

The key to competing in the ambulatory surgery market is to follow a three-step process: (1) understand your consumers' (physicians, patients, third-party payors) needs and wants and how they go about deciding where to go for specific services, (2) design your services to respond to the consumers who represent the market segments most likely to use your type of service in the volume that you will need to successfully run the service, and (3) locate, price, and promote the services in such a way as to provide maximum attractiveness to targeted market segments.

If these steps are not followed, either formally or at least intuitively, market failures may occur. These failures are likely to be caused by one of four different actions:

1. Treating the market as undifferentiated and assuming that all consumers behave basically the same. All consumers are not the same, and they do not want the same things. The task of the ambulatory surgery manager is to understand how consumers differ and then to respond effectively to these differences.

2. Developing programs that competitors have without understanding the potential demand remaining in the market. For any product or service, demand is limited. Clearly, there is growth in the ambulatory surgery area, but this does not mean that every organization can successfully enter that marketplace and grow. One must carefully assess the strength of competitors and the potential demand remaining in the market before going head to head with them.

3. Designing programs as you think they should be designed rather than the way the consumer wants them. Because demand has exceeded supply for many years in the health care system, professionals have become accustomed to determining how and what the consumer will get from the organization. With the excess supply in the current marketplace, this will no longer work effectively.

4. Thinking that public relations, communications, and marketing will create demand. If the demand is not there, no amount of communications will get people to come and use your services. The demand has to be there in one form or another, and it is essential for the ambulatory surgery manager to understand where the demand is and how best to attract it.

SUGGESTED READINGS

Leebov, W: Service Excellence: The Customer Relations Strategy for Health Care. American Hospital Publishing, 1988.

Ries, A, Trout J: Bottom-Up Marketing. New York, McGraw-Hill, 1989

Zemke, R: The Service Edge. New York, New American Library Books, 1989

Fundamentals for Success

ANNE FREY DEAN

ORGANIZATION

Lack of communication is the root of all (or at least most) evil. Poor communication can be the cause of a failed relationship or business venture. An ambulatory surgery facility is not immune to this problem.

Effective communication among team members takes on even more importance in an ambulatory surgery facility than in a traditional hospital setting. The facility is smaller in size, all patients are there for surgery (resulting in higher stress levels), and almost all the staff makes contact with the patient. Patients of the 1990s want information about their treatment; communicating information effectively among patients, staff, and physician is good practice from the standpoints of health care and marketing.[1]

When interviewed, physician owners of surgery centers cited many different reasons for leaving the hospital environment. But all these reasons referred back to communications problems. Lack of control over their patients; too much bureaucracy, red tape, and paperwork; lack of follow-through on problems; and lack of interest in the physicians' or ambulatory patients' problems are all complaints centering on defects in communication channels. The hospital's organizational chart must be designed not only to identify but also to simplify channels of communication. Flexibility and quick response is essential to the ambulatory surgery facility if it is to retain satisfied patients and physicians.

Organizational Structure

In most hospital-oriented health care facilities, the traditional organizational structure is a pyramid with five levels of management hierarchy (Fig. 10-2). The top three levels set policies and goals, plan strategy to effect the policies and obtain the goals, and assume the responsibility for implementing the plans. The department director serves as the middle manager who has direct responsibility

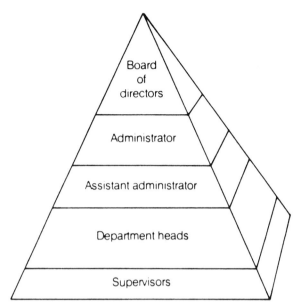

FIGURE 10-2. The traditional management pyramid.

for the functioning of the unit. Reporting to the department directors are area chiefs (charge nurses) who are responsible for the day-to-day functioning of their areas.[2] Reporting and communication channels assume an upward-downward configuration, as weighty as the pyramid design in Figure 10-2, and as cumbersome. In examining this design, one cannot help but notice the distinct divisions depicted much like fences dividing lines of authority. Such fences defeat the team concept of health care delivery, and as they relate to a hospital-affiliated ambulatory surgery facility depict a common but weighty problem.

Regardless of the format used by a facility, the organization's structure should be easy to implement, simple to use, understood by the staff, and able to facilitate the team concept.

Ambulatory surgery organizational charts that duplicate the structure found in hospitals will reflect many of their problems, such as "poor morale, decreased productivity, poor communication, lack of concern, and, ultimately, a lack of progress in creative thinking."[3] In the ambulatory surgery center, it is essential to promote the concept of team management. Organizational charts must be simplified to incorporate this concept. The fewer persons involved, the less cumbersome are communication channels. Don't become management heavy. A football team composed of all captains is not a team.

The Team Concept

Let's look at the ambulatory surgery health care team. The patient would be the captain. He or she has called the plays by electing to have ambulatory surgery and keeping his or her surgical appointment. The anesthesiologist (coach) evaluates the patient and procedure and decides on appropriate anesthesia. The surgeon (quarterback) picks up the ball and runs with it (quickly, we hope) to the

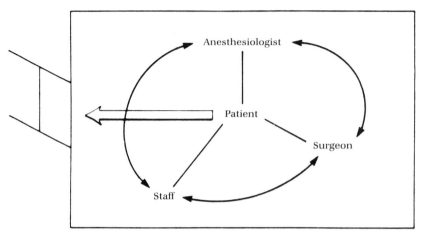

FIGURE 10-3. The team concept for ambulatory health care.

goal. The surgery center staff (blocking backs) lead the way by preventing problems (regarding scheduling, interviewing and data collection, equipment and supplies, or staffing) that might interfere with attaining the goal. The field of play is the surgery center. The configuration this team assumes in planning, implementing, and evaluating patient care is the circle of the team huddle. All team members go toward one goal—a satisfactory ambulatory surgery experience.

The area of most concern in a physician-owned or -managed facility is the question of where the duties and responsibilities of the administration and those of the physician owner or director merge, separate, or diversify? Identifying these roles may be a more difficult political task. Separating them may be an even greater challenge. Enforcing and adhering to the separate role descriptions and responsibilities is essential if the members are to work as a team. To do otherwise creates confusion, reduces morale, and decreases the quality of health care services provided. Ultimately, fewer goals are attained. Frequently, the temptation to call individual plays becomes too much for many physician-owners or medical directors who may attempt to assume the administrator or nurse's role. This temptation may manifest itself in many forms, from counseling a staff nurse, arbitrarily changing policies, or rearranging furniture and equipment. Operational functions such as staffing, counseling, patient flow, and nursing procedures should be left to the persons hired to manage those functions. Problems in these areas should be noted for discussion in future management meetings. Management must appear as a unified team if the facility is to be successful. Theodore Roosevelt once said that the "best executive is one who has sense enough to pick good men for the job and self-restraint enough to keep from meddling while they do it."

The Medical Director
Regardless of any problems the administrator and medical director may discover in defining their relationship, the advantages of having an on-site medical director far outweigh the disadvantages. In a hospital-affiliated program, the medical

director is frequently the chief of anesthesiology services. Since the medical director conducts or supervises the preanesthesia assessment, his or her knowledge and expertise are invaluable in determining the surgeon's compliance to patient selection criteria (an essential component in the utilization review process). He or she frequently will uncover valuable information pertinent to the anesthetic-surgical plan.

As an impartial member of the team, the medical director's professional input is most valuable in such areas as meeting selection criteria, rescheduling a patient, or even cancelling the case altogether. The medical director's knowledge of the philosophy and the daily functioning of the facility is valuable in this role as he or she assumes the capacity of advisor over front-line manager.

Who is going to be the medical director of the unit? This person will have the responsibility for

1. Preoperative risk evaluation, both surgical and anesthetic
2. Dealing with all of the surgical specialties fairly, without being accused of favoring his or her own specialty
3. Examining and signing patients out of the facility
4. Providing continuity of care for patients by being available in the facility until the last patient has been discharged[4]
5. Reviewing all quality assurance activities.

The medical director's assumption of these duties relieves the executive director from the role of "policing" physicians and permits physicians to consult together. An anesthesiologist would easily qualify in all areas. Having an anesthesiologist as medical director is a special bonus; it guarantees the availability of this important specialist. As part of the team, the anesthesiologist will be most eager to identify educational deficiencies and provide inservice education programs. His or her knowledge and experience are immeasurable in assessing patient problems and in performing discharge assessments.

Nursing Staff
The nursing staff selected for the ambulatory surgery center must have a different orientation from that of traditional hospital-oriented nurses. Staff members must be selected for their people orientation. The person applying for a position in a patient-centered, family-oriented unit who never mentions the patient during the interview would probably be incompatible with the ambulatory work setting.

Frequently, nurses coming from an inpatient hospital background have not been indoctrinated to the special requirements of ambulatory surgical care. The imbalance between attention given to inpatients and that given to outpatients has forced many surgeons to admit potential ambulatory surgery patients in order for them to receive first-class operating room treatment. In hospitals that are established for inpatient care, staff members tend to place greater emphasis on the sick patient.[5] As a result, the ambulatory surgery patient may suffer from skillful neglect as the staff rushes to meet the acute needs of the sick. In comparison, the needs of a well patient may not seem as important. There has been so much emphasis placed on care of the sick that few staff members are truly knowledgeable about the special needs to be met in caring for the well patient.

The Patient

The ambulatory surgery patient has health range needs that are different from the acutely or chronically ill patient; he or she

1. Is independent, maintains himself or herself well within the community setting, and wishes to do so
2. Desires to return to a social environment in as short a period of time as possible with the least disruption as can be attained
3. Does not view himself or herself as being sick
4. Suffers ambivalence, for by coming to the hospital, the ambulatory surgery patient is inclined to assume the sick role arbitrarily

The hospital environment may create ambivalence on the part of the patient in that it tends to validate the patient's reason for being there as an illness. Sick people do not care for themselves; rather, they assume a *passive* role. The ambulatory surgery patient is more desirous of maintaining an *active* role in his or her own health care, and thereby maintain control over therapy. These are very basic—but essential—needs.

When planning the care of the sick hospitalized patient, it seems fairly simple to identify needs, for they center on the illness. Even when applying biopsychosocial delineations, the focus remains primarily on the illness. In the ambulatory surgery environment, wellness is promoted. The patient enters as a normal person with a temporary problem. As such, he or she ambulates into and out of the facility (in some facilities even walking to the operating room). The whole philosophy of ambulatory care promotes the patient's self-image as an otherwise healthy, intact, socially active person with special needs. Care is designed around promoting individualized attention, and, as such, flexibility in standing procedures is the rule.

Health care professionals, like all people, tend to develop routines that become carved in stone. These, then, become rigid rituals irrespective of the needs of the individual patients. There seems to be no impetus to change approaches used for years by both physicians and patients. If the approach to patients that was taught in nursing or medical schools has worked, there seems to be a resistance to changing it. The problem, however, is that the approach taught in the last three decades has centered on the sick patient; as a result, when hospital oriented medical persons enter the ambulatory environment, they take the same approach with the patients, to the potential detriment of all concerned. This standard approach can be clearly recognized in the following example:

> Patients enter the ambulatory surgery facility for their surgical appointments as scheduled, and are greeted warmly by the preop nurse. After advising the responsible persons accompanying the patients to remain in the waiting room, the nurse accompanies the *patients* to their assigned changing areas and has them change into a *patient* hospital

gown. The nurse has the patient get in bed, starts appropriate intravenous lines, and puts up the side rails on the *stretchers*. Skin preps may be performed at this time, followed by preoperative medication. The patients' responsible persons enter, visit, and *leave* to remain in the *waiting room*. The patients are pushed to the operating room on their stretchers. After surgery, they may be given ice chips before leaving the facility in a wheelchair.

With this approach, the only difference separating the inpatient preoperative routine from the outpatient is that the patient comes into the facility on the morning of surgery and hopefully goes home the same day.

Examine the words used in the example above:

Patients
Waiting room
Hospital gown
Put to bed
Stretcher

They are all connected with and identified with hospitals and sick people. They hardly promote an image of the surgical guest as a well person. Yet, in just a few hours this person will be returned to home and be responsible for effecting his or her own transition back to full activity.

Now, examine the approach used when the staff has internalized the ambulatory health care philosophy of promoting wellness:

The surgical *guests* enter the ambulatory surgery facility and are warmly greeted by the staff. After collecting the necessary last-minute information, the guests and their responsible persons are escorted to the preoperative dressing area where the nurse shows them the *scrub suit or pajamas*, located in the cubicle, that will need to be put on. The nurse remains nearby if assistance in changing is needed. Family members frequently enjoy being of help in this activity. In some instances, changing clothes may not be necessary. This is depending on the type of procedure and location of the incision site. After determining the guest's readiness, the nurse returns and determines the need for venous access. If such a need is indicated, a prn adapter is started in the hand, covered with a clear plastic adhesive strip (tape covers wounds). The guest's responsible person may stay in attendance. This option is offered prior to the procedure. Since no premedication will be given, the surgical guest relaxes in a comfortable recliner. Skin preps or marking can be accomplished quite comfortably here. With appropriate equipment this area can be used for regional block induction. With no premedication, the guest will ambulate to the operating room accompanied by the circulating nurse. After surgery (depending on type of anesthesia), the guest may ambulate or be transported to the postanesthesia care unit (PACU). At an appropriate time light nourishment will be given while the patient is seated in another recliner. Upon discharge, the nurse will escort the guest and responsible person to their car.

In both models, the patients received "good care." In the second example, however, the nurse promoted the guest's image of wellness while recognizing the role of the responsible person in the guest's health care. In assessing the otherwise healthy patient, the nurse must be able to determine the patient's level of self-sufficiency accurately. This skill comes from learned knowledge and experience.

The temptation to rotate staff from other hospital areas to the ambulatory surgery area is great. Such practices may seem cost-effective and efficient initially; however, rotating staff members often do not possess the necessary philosophy, knowledge, or skills to provide quality ambulatory care. Ambulatory surgery nursing is a specialty in which the nurse is committed to promoting individualized, quality health care at a reduced cost with the least emotional, psychological, and physical trauma possible. The ambulatory nurse team member must be aware of the cost of health care, and stringent cost-containment measures should be enforced among staff members without compromising the quality of the care delivered.

Ambulatory surgery nurses must be aware of their role in marketing to both the physician and the patient. They promote the image of themselves and their fellow staff members as people pleasers. These members are especially interested in cooperating and assisting at each step of the plan to attain the common goal of a satisfactory ambulatory surgery experience for all involved parties. As such, these nurses approach their jobs as eager agents in data collection, assessment, preparation, and planning. As team members, the ambulatory surgery nurse specialist erases any adversarial role in relating to physicians and administrators while recognizing the importance of their functions being accomplished promptly in providing consumer satisfaction. Tact and diplomacy are innate characteristics. Surgeons should find their visits to the facility productive and satisfying. Highly skilled, productive staff members should exhibit motivation, initiative, and enthusiasm in a positively spirited environment. Such enthusiasm and positive interest filters down from the top (*i.e.*, the nursing director).

The Nursing Director

In choosing a nursing director, physicians and administrators frequently choose a "good nurse" from among the staff nurses with whom they have worked. In these instances, an injustice may be done to the physician, the nurse, and the facility, since being a good nurse implies skill in the technical field and not, necessarily, in management. Often, the director may not be a nurse at all, but a person especially skilled in business, finance, or office management. Whatever the person's background, it should reflect a mixture of all the above as well as a strong ability and interest in marketing. This skill should cover not only developing advertising copy, brochures, physician letters, flyers, and newsletters, but also the ability to call on doctors' offices and communicate effectively with them and their staffs.

The director must exhibit enthusiasm, for the enthusiasm generated can be felt and appreciated by those fortunate enough to enter its bright circle. It is contagious and may well be among the most positive attributes a manager possesses. Enthusiasm springs from enjoyment. That enjoyment springs from gaining pleasure from one's commitments. The manager who is able to emit enthusiasm for the ambulatory surgery facility as well as the concept of ambulatory health care will find staff and physicians alike responding to that enthusiasm, basking in its pleasure and passing it on to other patients, physicians, staff members, and community representatives.

It is a wise manager who includes staff members in the management of the facility and who becomes involved in it also. This may mean digging in side by side with the staff, working together to set up materials management programs, develop policies and staffing patterns, or on a particular day even make coffee, escort patients, or provide staff relief. Such occasional involvement "in the trenches" will do much to promote a strong sense of camaraderie while serving to identify rough spots in the system to the manager. While delegating is important, shared responsibility is a must. However, managers must be aware that their primary function is to manage the facility overall—not to staff it. Sharing staff duties should be reserved for occasional shortages; as a steady diet, it affects the manager's primary responsibility, and by so doing leaves the manager position temporarily vacant.

The key to good management will always lie in effective communication, both overt and covert. The effective manager makes it a point to visit each area of the facility frequently, even if it means donning scrubs to mingle with staff and physicians. Being interested in individual staff members is essential. Remembering particular aspects of each member's life reflects this concern and interest. Developing thorough orientation and evaluation programs is a part of effective management. Holding frequent staff meetings, promoting open discussion, soliciting opinions and concerns, responding with appropriate explanations or changes, sharing budget restrictions and plans, and soliciting staff participation in every phase of operation promotes mutual interest and satisfaction. Being involved with the staff is essential to the promotion of harmony and participation; however, the wise manager also knows it is essential to keep a certain distance in order to maintain objectivity in evaluating staff and in assessing the large picture. Becoming close friends with individual staff members will cause problems detrimental to the overall functioning of the facility. Wise managers will seek their own counsel while maintaining the confidentiality of those who confide in them. The temptation to become a pal is great, but will lead to graying of the lines of authority. It's essential for management to maintain a professional image in order to be a role model for the staff.

POLICIES AND PROCEDURES
Developing policies and procedures seems to be one of the most overwhelming tasks facing the management team. These written guidelines must be clear, concise, practical, and applicable to the day-to-day functioning of the facility. Do not establish policies you do not or cannot follow. Rewrite them when needed, to reflect what you are doing. Policies must be established for all operational aspects, while goals, objectives, and philosophies must be written in such a manner as to reflect the true spirit desired by the governing body. Policies must cover

> Medical staff credentialing
> Committees required

Quality assurance programs, safety, and risk management plans
Infection control practices
Fire and disaster procedures
General personnel policies
Staffing
Emergency transfer or admission arrangements
Consultant use and criteria for selection
Job descriptions
Medical/surgical staff privileges
Anesthesia services
Pathology services
Radiology services
Medical direction
Hours of operation
Scheduling procedures
Preadmission criteria
Preoperative and postoperative contact with patients
Distribution of clothing and valuables
Responsible person requirements
Acceptable procedures and anesthetic agents
Laboratory requirements
Inservice education plans

The explicit guidelines provided by credentialing bodies as well as organizations responsible for developing recommended standards and codes aid greatly in developing policies and procedures for accreditation and daily operations. Such guidelines issue from the

Accreditation Association for Ambulatory Health Care
Joint Commission on Accreditation of Healthcare Organizations
Association of Operating Room Nurses
Centers for Disease Control
Environmental Protection Agency
Department of Labor Relations
Medicare Certification Guidelines
Occupational Safety and Health Authority
American Society of Anesthesiologists
American Society of Post Anesthesia Nurses

These groups set optimal, achievable standards designed to provide quality patient care. Developing policies designed to identify and implement these standards of recommended practices will prevent last-minute rewrites prior to credentialing visits. Additional policies designed to meet standards would include

A statement on patients' rights
Governance/organizational structure

Medical records practice and administration
Facility environmental control
A survey process for evaluation of services

Combined with the standards required to meet state licensure codes and certification, these policies do much to ensure that the quality of care rendered at the facility will be optimal, thus providing a safe environment for patients, physicians, and staff members alike.

It is not enough merely to develop an impressive-looking policy and procedure manual. Each staff member, including the medical director, should read the manual prior to assuming active duty and should document that they have read it. This responsibility should be a routine part of the basic orientation program. Additions or changes should be announced at regular staff meetings. Typewritten copy should be hung on the communication board for at least 2 weeks in order for everyone to sign it and to become familiar with the new policy. Updating should be an ongoing process. Time should be set aside on a regular basis to review sections of the manual for accuracy and applicability (are you following it? can you follow it?). This will ensure that the manual is an active part of the functioning of the facility and is realistic in reflecting actual practices. Such a practice also keeps persons knowledgeable about the governing policies while eliminating the formidable task of last-minute review prior to credentialing visits.

Any policy should be expansive enough to permit growth and individual flexibility in carrying it out while strict enough to provide the necessary governance. Do not try to establish a policy for everything.

FORMS AND RECORDS

The basic concept of ambulatory health care incorporates the KISS principle ("Keep it simple, stupid"). Implementation of this principle can be easily accomplished through consolidation and streamlining of existing forms. In the hospital environment, this requires educating the medical records committee to the need for redesigning existing forms and omitting others that are specific to inpatients. In the hospital outpatient department it is not uncommon to find at least 22 forms on the patient's chart. This number can effectively be reduced to a reasonable number (5–9) by

Consolidating and streamlining existing forms
Eliminating unnecessary forms
Using preprinted orders and instructions designed with space for additional, individualized notes
Using both the front and back of forms
Using dictation stations to replace written records

Nurses may complain of not having enough space to write, but if the forms are well designed, a mere check in the appropriate space will adequately document care while providing the added bonus of an easier chart review process.

Physicians enjoy the streamlined chart, since its efficiency saves valuable time. The physician's signature may be required on only a few of the forms. Preprinted instructions and orders can be individually checked for appropriateness and signed.[6] Physicians' preference cards should always be used and should include the preference of individual anesthesiologists on cards stating use of intravenous access and other preferences. An ambulatory surgery facility should reduce paperwork and bureaucratic red tape while promoting nurse initiative.

EQUIPMENT

Purchasing equipment can be somewhat like purchasing a surprise gift—unless selected carefully, the equipment can end up in the back of the closet just like last year's Christmas tie.

Equipment lists should be developed from the accepted procedures to be performed at the facility, but individualized to the personal requirements of the physicians in the area. Do not try to second-guess the items that will be needed, the style, or the manufacturer. If the manager or director of nursing is from one of the area hospitals, a common mistake is to assume that the same equipment will be acceptable at the ambulatory facility to all the physicians. Whether this is true or not depends on the scope of the physician draw area. Will the facilities physician staff be composed only of physicians with privileges at that particular hospital, or will other physicians in the area also be using the facility? This must be determined in order to ensure acceptability of selected equipment.

In order to provide knowledgeable data for the physician, collect information about styles, sizes, costs, probable discounts, and service and maintenance agreements. All this information should be considered in selecting equipment as well as the return on investment determined by use and overhead. Solicit a commitment from physicians prior to the purchase. Will the item keep you abreast of hospital activity, or maybe even provide a competitive edge over the other facilities in town? Is it state of the art or is it about to be replaced by something newer and better (and maybe less expensive)?

Before the facility opens, make use of an ad hoc or advisory committee composed of physicians representing all specialties planning to use the facility. This group can assist in effectively choosing between similar items, thus taking the burden of selecting controversial items away from the management—a wise political move.

As equipment comes in, it should be checked, inventoried, and inserviced. Maintenance programs should be planned in the initial phase. Warranties and instruction manuals should be filed in a handy manual accessible to all. One person should assume responsibility for this.

The astute manager will scurry to stay abreast of changing trends in order to determine possible future equipment needs. Being receptive enough to a physician's request for a new item to explore and study the feasibility of procurement will gain many friends for the facility. This means faithful scanning of equipment ads and articles in professional journals and a keen interest in progressive new trends—another basic concept of ambulatory surgery centers.

MATERIALS MANAGEMENT

Materials management refers to the overall use and control of supplies and equipment within the facility. An active materials management and inventory control program is the financial backbone of a successful ambulatory surgery program and should be approached with determination and forceful consistency. A lack of understanding results from a lack of education in the financial process of materials management. Cost containment and cost reduction are essential for the financial survival of ambulatory care. It will work if staff members assume an active role in the budgeting process and are cognizant of line item costs, overhead expenses, profit margins, and procedure fees. Share this information with physician users.

Monthly budget and inventory review meetings enhance compliance and promote enthusiasm for the program among staff members who recognize their important role in making the program financially successful.

Staff members should always be actively involved in the inventory control program, providing valuable input about specific items needed and those best suited to meet the objectives of the facility. One of the staff members should be recognized as the official materials manager. This person would be responsible for all the ordering and organization of supplies in order to provide a smooth flow of materials.

Determine a specific ordering day. Identify the primary receiving day (and clerk). Use purchase orders, batch receiving slips, packing slips, and invoice copies (hold these separate); do not pay incomplete orders until complete; identify back orders. Keep shelves stocked, but not overstocked. The phrase "A place for everything, and everything in its place" can effectively be fulfilled with spacesaver shelves on tracks, wall-hung bins, and even rectangular laundry baskets to store loose supplies in bulk. Each shelf and bin should be labeled with the item, vendor, and quantity stocked. Frequent stock reviews will identify little-used items that may be omitted in order to add a new one. Keeping inventory low but adequate keeps costs down.

In order to curtail costs, inventory and overhead must be determined. Set realistic goals. Analyze procedure costs at least every 6 months on high-volume procedures. Determine the break-even point and push for it, keeping the original goals in mind. With staff members especially cognizant of these factors, promote cost-containment and reduction ideas—even the smallest. Turn lights and suction off when not in use. Monitor environmental temperatures. Practice stringent use of physician preference cards. Do not overstock rooms or oversupply cases. Do not hoard supplies. Do not open supplies unless you are certain of their being used.

ASSESS STAFFING NEEDS. Do not overstaff or understaff. Develop a PRN pool and an active volunteer program to assist professional staff members. These persons will be of great assistance on especially busy days. Each area should be concisely planned and staffed for the most efficient use. Such organization and planning of duties will go far to decrease overtime and staffing budgets. Part-time pool staff should be selected by the same stringent criteria used for full-time employees. Volunteer and PRN services should reflect the personalized, people-oriented philosophy of the facility. These persons must also be motivated enough to stay abreast of policy changes or additions and interested enough to participate in pertinent inservice programs.

Budgeting should, of course, reflect facility use and growth for staffing purposes. The initial budget may be difficult to determine; however, knowledge of area health patterns will provide a guide to facility use. For example, in the Sun Belt, January, February, and March are heavy tourist months for retired persons who may choose to have surgical procedures performed during this time. Hence, use may increase during this period. On the other hand, school vacations usually result in increases in pediatric and adolescent surgery.

Plan your growth rate realistically. Can you add 10 cases per month or 1 to 3 new physicians per month? What methods will you use to solicit their participation? Will they be effective? To what extent? Is the growth rate dependent on service expansion requiring major or minor equipment purchases? Have these been included in the annual budget? For example, are there plans to expand orthopedics to include arthroscopy and radiology services?

SCHEDULING

One of the primary advantages of a separated or freestanding ambulatory surgery facility is the flexibility afforded in scheduling procedures. This is a prime asset, especially when it comes to marketing, since most physicians list "problems with scheduling" as one of their primary problems with hospital operating rooms. The ambulatory surgery facility scheduling staff should exhibit an eagerness to please, cooperate, and accommodate when scheduling procedures (they must be knowledgeable as to type of procedures performed, equipment needs, and availability of equipment) through the physician or his or her office staff. Block scheduling should be promoted in the initial phase of the marketing and development program. Such a service becomes highly feasible and profitable if the facility is designed efficiently to incorporate alternate treatment or procedure rooms, and if equipment is designed to be movable. Developing minor procedure rooms for local lumps and bumps frees up valuable sterile operating room space and increases flexibility. In developing block scheduling policies, determine how this service can be most effective and, especially, how long a block of time will be held for a specific surgeon or group. Resistance in the medical community to the idea may be high initially, if the concept is not currently being practiced in other facilities. Many surgeons feel it is more efficient for them to use two rooms in a hospital operating suite on their surgery day. They perform major procedures in one room and minor in the other, alternating between the two. However, grouping all their outpatient cases on one day in a block at the ambulatory surgery unit will enable them more time for major inpatient procedures while increasing patient satisfaction. The ambulatory surgery staff recognizes a time savings, since changing surgeons increases room turnover time. Surgeons using this concept find they can better schedule their time knowing they have a definite block each week for their ambulatory surgery cases.[7,8]

Equipment and instrument needs also benefit from block scheduling. Instead of having several physicians arguing over the use of a microscope, the facility can stagger the schedule so that on any given day only one physician would be working with a microscope. Block scheduling not only helps to project staffing needs, but also helps staff to project supplies, equipment, and instrument needs.

Keep equipment and staff mobile. Put locking wheels on everything. This practice enhances flexibility and will prove invaluable in handling "add-ons" as well as scheduled blocks. Many physicians prefer using ambulatory surgery centers for minor emergencies presenting to their office (e.g., a child with a dog bite that needs attention or a young woman suffering a spontaneous abortion). Facilities with limited space can optimize space use by combining examination and procedure rooms and having movable furniture and equipment. Developing treatment facilities in ancillary areas such as a pain clinic in postanesthesia care or preoperative holding capitalizes on space. Mobility should be promoted even in a dedicated room such as cystoscopy. Tables can be mobile, enabling this specialty space to be used for other radiographic purposes as well as routine procedures.

QUALITY ASSURANCE

Quality assurance is a term heard repeatedly in all industries. It encompasses all the goals, objectives, standards, and plans formulated to deliver a quality product to the consumer. It involves staff, physician, and management representatives participating together in defining the components of quality care, methods for implementation, and tools for evaluating or measuring the process. Quality assurance is the identification of potential problem areas, the development of policies and procedures to prevent their occurrence, studying compliance, and reassessing problem-solving solutions to determine if there has been a successful outcome or if there is a need to restudy.

The development of an active quality assurance program can readily be achieved by organizing a defined committee, consisting of no less than the medical director, the nursing director, a medical records statistician, and a member of the nursing staff.[9]

The committee will

Identify all activities concerned with the delivery of quality care
Recommend additional activities or modification of existing activities
Establish outcome, process, and structure standards and criteria
Develop assessment and evaluation tools designed to identify discrepancies between practices and standards
Recommend corrective action and monitor the results of the change in behavior or performance as it applies to the delivery of quality care

Natof lists six basic components of a quality assurance program:[10]

1. *Identify* problems.
2. *Develop* solutions.
3. *Disseminate* information.
4. *Reassess* at a later date.

5. *Correlate* with educational activities.
6. *Report* activities to responsible parties.

In order to appraise the quality of care as well as the process, periodic formal assessments must be performed with a measuring tool or audit. The audit tool should be developed to reflect the standards of practice. The audit process involves review of documentation such as the operating room or anesthesia records.[11] There are two methods that can be used to identify substantive problems. A *problem-oriented* audit involves a review of a number of charts to look for substantive problems (deviation from the norm); a problem we would be embarrassed to defend with our peers. A *topic-oriented* audit establishes a particular topic for review (e.g., postoperative instructions). There must be a problem-oriented question (e.g., are patients obtaining instructions and do they understand them?). Charts are also reviewed to see if instructions were received and patients can additionally be called to see if they understood them.

Quality assurance is an ongoing, cyclic, nonpunitive process designed to promote excellence in the health care delivery system.

HAPPINESS

Happiness is an essential component of any successful ambulatory surgery program and refers to the happiness of the persons concerned—physicians, guests (patient and responsible person), and staff.

The primary consumer for any surgery center remains the physician. Surveys reveal 98% of patients contacted used a given facility on the recommendation of their physician. With that fact in mind, it is imperative to keep the physician happy by

>   Being pleasant, obliging, and cooperative
>   Anticipating needs and problems
>   Practicing effective problem solving and follow-through
>   Using updated preference cards
>   Keeping instrument trays and equipment neat and in good working
>   order
>   Minimizing room turnover time
>   Maximizing efficiency
>   Soliciting ideas

The surgery center guests assume the facility has state-of-the-art technology. The guests' happiness (assuming a satisfactory outcome) will stem from the staff providing psychosocial gratification by

>   Being pleasant and sincere
>   Displaying warmth and empathy
>   Exhibiting a genuine interest in the patients, their problems, and their
>   responsible persons

Providing personalized care to meet their needs

Maintaining a professional attitude, providing patients with a sense of security as to the staff's skills

Holding preoperative and postoperative conferences to impart information and answer questions

Providing extras such as teaching tools or special touches such as toys or extra blankets

Providing written instructions for ready reference by the patient or family member

Promoting the image of wellness

Practicing patient-centered, family-oriented care

Providing follow-up contact

The happiness of staff members is essential to maintain the high morale that will provide an ambiance of warmth and relaxation. Flexibility and communication remain at the core of happiness. This is achieved by

Allowing free days and time off when the facility is not busy

Flexibility with hours and breaks

Providing rotation and cross-training within the facility

Distribution of praise and recognition

Open group discussions and participation in the management circle

Development of continuing education

Profit sharing and incentive plans

CONCLUSION

Physicians, managers, staff, and patients need to be aware of the advantages of ambulatory surgical care. As each group participates in a satisfactory ambulatory surgery experience, each will in its own way promote the advantages to colleagues, friends, coworkers and the community at large—all potential users.

Although providing quality care is an essential ingredient of success, it alone will not ensure a successful facility. In addition to making the facility easily accessible to both physician and patient, Wetchler feels the following are essential components that every facility must incorporate as part of its game plan in order to become or remain successful.[4]

1. *The team concept:* Continually interacting within the facility are three different groups. The physician, the patient, and the staff must work toward a common goal of providing a successful, satisfying ambulatory surgery experience for all involved parties. Each of the three groups are equal in importance, and one group should not attempt to gain importance at the expense of either of the other groups. Professional turf battles must be minimized.

2. *Simplified medical records:* Develop medical records that are easy for

You and your doctor chose the METHODIST AMBULATORY SURGERY CENTER for your surgical care and treatment. We have tried to make your Ambulatory Surgery experience as comfortable and convenient as possible. We are interested in your assessment of our services, personnel, and facilities. Please take a moment to complete this postage paid comment card and return it to us. Your comments and suggestions help us to evaluate our services. Your cooperation is appreciated. Thank you.

CIRCLE ONE:

1. If you came to the hospital for testing several days prior to your surgery:

   (a) Were you treated in a courteous, pleasant and professional manner? Yes No

   (b) Did you have laboratory tests? Yes No

   (c) Did you have a chest X-ray? Yes No

   (d) Did you have an EKG? Yes No

   (e) Were your tests carried out smoothly and efficiently? Yes No

   (f) Do you feel your visit to the Ambulatory Surgery Center (prior to surgery) was beneficial? Yes No

   (g) How long did it take for your testing to be completed?_____(hours)

2. Do you feel your instructions prior to surgery were adequate? Yes No

3. Were your personal and informational needs met? Yes No

4. Do you feel the Ambulatory Surgery Center personnel were interested in you as a person? Yes No

5. Were you comfortable in our facilities regarding lighting, temperature control, and furniture? Yes No

6. Were the facilities convenient to use? Yes No

7. Do you feel your separation from your family member or friend was minimal? Yes No

8. If your child had surgery, as a parent, do you feel you were reunited with your child as soon as possible? Yes No

9. Do you feel you have been given adequate post-operative instructions? Yes No

10. Were the waiting room facilities adequate for whoever accompanied you the day of your surgery? Yes No

11. If you would have this surgery again, would you prefer to be an Ambulatory Surgery Patient? Yes No

12. How would you rate your overall surgery experience at the Methodist Ambulatory Surgery Center?

    ☐ Excellent   ☐ Good   ☐ Fair   ☐ Poor

Please list any general comments, suggestions, or employees who provided exceptional service:

_____

_____

_____

_____

DATE OF SURGERY:_____

NAME: (Optional)_____

FIGURE 10-4. Patient satisfaction questionnaire used at the Methodist Medical Center of Illinois. This form is given to the patient at the time of discharge from the facility.

the physician and staff to use and are specific for the ambulatory surgery patient and procedure.

3. *Physician convenience:* Develop channels of communication so that information flows freely from the facility to the physician's office in scheduling procedures. Work out block scheduling time. Involve the physician's office in problem solving. Develop standing preoperative and postoperative orders and discharge instructions. Regularly monitor the physicians and their office staff's level of satisfaction with the facility.

4. *VIP (very important patient):* Let the patients know how important they are by preoperative and postoperative phone calls, priority registration, patient education through brochures, an attractive environment, and limited waiting time. Regularly monitor patient satisfaction levels (Fig. 10-4). Keep family members or responsible persons informed about the patient's progress. "The secret of the care of the patient is in caring for the patient."[12]

5. *Careful selection criteria:* Selection involves not only the patient, but also the surgical procedure, as well as physicians and staff who will work in the facility.

6. *Careful discharge criteria:* Discharge criteria should be practical. A responsible person should monitor the patient's care at home. Both the patient and the responsible person should have all discharge information explained and provided to them in writing.

7. *Separate outpatients from inpatients:* Breen feels "patients just entering the in and out surgery unit should never be exposed to post-anesthesia patients returning from the operating or recovery rooms. The psychology of ambulatory surgery is very important in all aspects ... even the registration and scheduling should be separate, it should be located in the same area as the outpatient surgery."[13] Every effort should be made to have a separate ambulatory surgery PACU.

8. *Medical director:* The medical director must be available, impartial, and knowledgeable in the complete selection process. Direction fairly administered makes it easier for all physicians who wish to schedule procedures in the facility.

9. *Be competitive:* As we continue to have constraints placed on the way we practice and as competition springs up around us, it is essential that we evaluate the way we deliver health care and make every effort to do it
   a. Better
   b. At greater convenience
   c. At a lower price

10. *Market appropriately—everybody sells:* Every member of the staff must be aware of the facility's philosophy, policies, goals, and objectives. We are our own best salespeople when it comes to providing physician, patient, and staff satisfaction.

Ambulatory surgery is a concept whose time has come. However, merely constructing a facility and opening its doors will not guarantee success. This will require the active participation of all parties who are involved in working in the ambulatory surgery facility. Success is multifaceted and depends directly on any and all the factors mentioned in the preceding pages.

REFERENCES

1. Winston WJ: Proven marketing strategies. Fifth National Conference on Same-Day Surgery. Dallas, 1984
2. Herkimer AG, Jr: Understanding Hospital Financial Management. Germantown, Md., Aspen Systems, 1978
3. Skagg RL: Programming and design of ambulatory care facilities: Hospitals. J Am Hosp Assoc 00: 42, 1977
4. Wetchler BV: Development of a successful ambulatory surgery program. In Jackson J, Roach C, Myers M, Norins LC (eds): Development of a Successful Ambulatory Surgery Program, p 67. Atlanta, American Health Consultants, 1981
5. Ford JL: Outpatient surgery: Present status and future projections. South Med J 5(7): 311, 1978
6. Perks M: Preprinted discharge instructions save time and trouble. Same Day Surg 5(7): 81, 1981
7. Battaglia CJ: New block approach smooths OR scheduling. Same Day Surg 7(7): 61, 1983
8. Drier CA, VanWinkle RN, Wetchler BV: Block scheduling contributes to ambulatory surgery center success. AORN J 39(4): 673, 1984
9. Batalden PB, O'Conner JP: Quality Assurance in Ambulatory Health Care. Germantown, Md., Aspen Systems, 1980
10. Natof H: Managing a successful quality assurance program. Fourth Conference on Same-Day Surgery, Atlanta, 1983
11. Kneedler J: Nursing audit: Challenge to the operating room nurse. University of Texas Health Science Center Teleconference Network Program, San Antonio, Texas, June–August 1978
12. Peabody FW: Care of the patient: JAMA 88: 877, 1927
13. Breen P: Facility design. Same Day Surg 5(4): 50, 1981

SUGGESTED READINGS

Burn J: Facility design for outpatient surgery and anesthesia, In Developing and Managing An Ambulatory Surgery Program, p 135. Boston, Little, Brown, 1981

Davis JE: Developing the ambulatory surgery unit: The physician's responsibility. J Ambulatory Care Management 4(3): 27, 1981

Davis JE: Major Ambulatory Surgery. Baltimore, Md., Williams & Wilkins, 1986

Kirkpatrick KW, Flasck ED: How to implement a quality assurance program, Today's OR Nurse 3:(12): 26, 1982

Forms and Policies

■ ■

COMPILED BY BERNARD V. WETCHLER

INTRODUCTION

As ambulatory surgery is becoming a popular alternative to inpatient care, more hospital facilities are following the example of the independent, freestanding facilities by consolidating and streamlining existing forms and making them applicable to the needs of their ambulatory surgical population. In Chapter 10, Anne Dean addresses the need to have forms specific for ambulatory surgery; in this section, I have gathered forms from a variety of ambulatory surgical facilities so that the reader may evaluate and compare forms and records used elsewhere. I wish to thank the medical directors who provided these forms for review:

Willis A. McGill, M.D.
Director, Department of Anesthesia and Short Stay Unit
Children's National Medical Center
Washington, D.C.
(pages 595–607)

Carolyn Greenberg, M.D.
Medical Director, Ambulatory Surgery Unit
Columbia-Presbyterian Medical Center
The Presbyterian Hospital in the City of New York
New York, New York
(pages 608–624)

Jean M. Millar, M.B., Ch B, FFARCS
Consultant in Administrative Charge, Day Surgery Unit
Nuffield Department of Anaesthetics
Oxford, United Kingdom
(pages 625–631)

Thomas J. Conahan, M.D.
Medical Director, Day Surgery Unit
Hospital of the University of Pennsylvania
Philadelphia, Pennsylvania
(pages 632–642)

Martin S. Bogetz, M.D.
Medical Director, UCSF Surgery Center
Medical Center at the University of California, San Francisco
San Francisco, California
(pages 643–646)

Bernard V. Wetchler, M.D.
Medical Director, Ambulatory SurgiCare
Methodist Medical Center of Illinois
Peoria, Illinois
(pages 647–656)

Carl J. Battaglia, M.D.
Medical Director
Texas Outpatient Surgicare Center
Houston, Texas
(pages 657–661)

Michael F. Roizen, M.D.
Professor and Chairperson, Department of Anesthesia and
Critical Care, Professor of Medicine, University of Chicago,
Pritzker School of Medicine, Chicago, Illinois
(pages 662–665)

CHILDREN'S HOSPITAL NATIONAL MEDICAL CENTER
AMSAC
PRE-OPERATIVE TELEPHONE SCREENING   Patient's Name: _____

DATE SCHEDULED FOR SURGERY:	HOME PHONE:	WORK PHONE:
SURGEON/DENTIST:	DATE AND TIME OF CALL:	DISPOSITION:
CHIEF COMPLAINT: *(TYPE OF SURGERY):*		AGE:
RESPONDANT:	RELATIONSHIP	

SUBJECTIVE FINDINGS:

Does your child have or ever had:

CHECK (✓) BOX
YES   NO   **COMMENTS**

	YES	NO	COMMENTS
Asthma	☐	☐	
Breath-holding spells *(apnea)*	☐	☐	
Croup/Bronchitis/Pneumonia	☐	☐	
Heart problems, heart murmurs *(Rheumatic)*	☐	☐	
Hepatitis *(Hepatitis B Carrier/liver disease)*	☐	☐	
Kidney Disease	☐	☐	
Bleeding disorders *(bruises easily)*	☐	☐	
Diabetes	☐	☐	
Sickle Cell Disease or Trait	☐	☐	
Seizures or convulsions	☐	☐	
Allergies to medicines, food, environmental factors	☐	☐	
Prematurity	☐	☐	
Was O_2 or ventilator required	☐	☐	
History of Apnea/Bradycardia	☐	☐	
Is your child currently on any medications	☐	☐	

Has your child ever had:

	YES	NO	
Previous hospitalization/surgery	☐	☐	

If the child had previous surgery:

	YES	NO	
Problems with anesthesia	☐	☐	
(delayed awakening, unexplained fever, MH, jaundice/vomiting/difficult intubation)	☐	☐	

Does anyone in your family have a history of

	YES	NO	
Bleeding disorders	☐	☐	
Muscle disease	☐	☐	
Trouble with anesthesia/M.H.	☐	☐	
Does your child wear any prosthesis	☐	☐	
Glasses/Braces/Bridges/Hearing aid/Trach/ Wheelchair/Crutches	☐	☐	

Does your child have:

	YES	NO	
Any developmental delays/learning disabilities	☐	☐	
Is your child prepared for surgery	☐	☐	
Will you bring your child in on the day of surgery? If NO, who will?	☐	☐	
Does your child have any problems I have not mentioned?	☐	☐	

Adolescents:

	YES	NO	
History of smoking	☐	☐	
Drug/alcohol use	☐	☐	
Chance of being pregnant	☐	☐	

PAGE 1

CHILDREN'S HOSPITAL NATIONAL MEDICAL CENTER

PLANS: (1) Counsel:

	CHECK (✓) BOX		
	YES	NO	COMMENTS
Phone call from Admissions Counselor, RN will call day before with food instructions, time of surgery, time to arrive	☐	☐	_____
Puppet show and why prepare	☐	☐	_____
Explain NPO and why	☐	☐	_____
Any questions parent has	☐	☐	_____
Rules of SSRU/Surgical Unit	☐	☐	_____

AMSAC/SSRU
DAY BEFORE SURGERY TELEPHONE CALL

Signature: _____

DATE AND TIME OF CALL:	DISPOSITION:	RESPONDANT:	RELATIONSHIP:
DATE OF SURGERY:		ARRIVAL TIME TO AMSAC:	
TIME OF SURGERY:	NPO TIME:FULL		CLEAR:

SUBJECTIVE FINDINGS:

Does your child now have:

	CHECK (✓) BOX		
	YES	NO	COMMENTS
Cold symptoms/sore throat/cough	☐	☐	_____
GI symptoms *(diarrhea)*	☐	☐	_____
Fever	☐	☐	_____
Rashes/cold sores	☐	☐	_____
Loose teeth, tooth aches, dental problems	☐	☐	_____
Has your child been exposed to: Chicken pox, German measles, measles, mumps in the past 3 weeks	☐	☐	_____
Is your child now taking any medications?	☐	☐	_____
Did you and your child attend the Puppet Show or Is your child prepared for surgery?	☐	☐	_____
Are there any other medical problems not discussed?	☐	☐	_____
Does your child have any nicknames	☐	☐	_____

ASSESSMENT: _____

PLANS: (1) Counsel:

	CHECK (✓) BOX		
	YES	NO	COMMENTS
Times as above	☐	☐	_____
Reinforce What and Why NPO *(No tooth-brushing, gum)*	☐	☐	_____
Review rules of SSRU/Surgical Unit	☐	☐	_____
Other *(Trach protocol, crutches, etc.)*	☐	☐	_____
Any questions parents have?	☐	☐	_____

Signature: _____

ASSESSMENT: _____

CHNMC 144.1/144.2

CHILDREN'S HOSPITAL NATIONAL MEDICAL CENTER
DEPARTMENT OF ANESTHESIOLOGY

Instructions For Not Eating or Feeding Before Surgery
(Nothing By Mouth - N.P.O.)

In order to shorten the length of your child's stay in the hospital, your child has been scheduled for surgery as an outpatient. It is most important that your child have an empty stomach when given an anesthetic. This will reduce the danger of vomiting and inhaling stomach contents into the lungs while asleep. You must follow these instructions or your child's surgery may be cancelled.

I. If your child is under 1 year of age:

A. A day before surgery call your surgeon or Children's Hospital after 5:00 P.M. at 745-3317 to find out the time surgery is scheduled (not the time you are asked to arrive at the hospital).

B. Your child must not be fed any solid food after midnight the evening before the day of surgery no matter what time the surgery is scheduled.

C. Your child may be fed milk or formula up to six hours before the time surgery is scheduled.

D. Four hours before surgery your child should be offered up to 4 ounces of clear liquids (sugar water, kool-aid, ginger ale, apple juice, but NOT milk, food or formula) then your child should have nothing else by mouth.

E. If your child is being breast fed, you may continue to breast feed your child up to four hours before surgery is scheduled.

F. If your child must take medicine by mouth for a medical condition during the period when no food or drink is allowed before surgery, please give the medicine at its scheduled time with a sip of water (no more than 2 teaspoons).

G. If you have any questions about these directions or about what your child should eat or drink before surgery, please call 745-3317 after 5:00 P.M. weekdays. We will be happy to answer your questions and discuss any special problems your child may have. You may also discuss any questions you have about feeding your child with the nurse who will telephone you a day or two before your child is scheduled for admission.

Form #1

CHILDREN'S HOSPITAL NATIONAL MEDICAL CENTER
DEPARTMENT OF ANESTHESIOLOGY

Instructions For Not Eating or Feeding Before Surgery
(Nothing By Mouth - N.P.O.)

    In order to shorten the length of your child's stay in the hospital, your child has been scheduled for surgery as an outpatient. It is most important that your child have an empty stomach when given an anesthetic. This will reduce the danger of vomiting and inhaling stomach contents into the lungs while asleep. You must follow these instructions or your child's surgery may be cancelled.

II. If your child is 1 to 6 years old:

   A.   A day before surgery call your surgeon or Children's Hospital after 5:00 P.M. at 745-3317 to find out the time surgery is scheduled (not the time you are asked to arrive at the hospital).

   B.   If surgery is scheduled between 7:30 a.m. and 12 noon your child must not eat or drink anything after midnight the evening before the day surgery is scheduled.

   C.   If surgery is scheduled at 12 noon or later, your child must not have any solid food, milk or milk products after midnight the evening before surgery is scheduled. Before 6:00 a.m. the morning of surgery your child may have up to 8 ounces of clear liquid only (kool-aid, apple juice, ginger ale but NOT milk or food). After 6:00 A.M. your child must have nothing else to eat or drink before surgery.

   D.   If your child must take medicine by mouth for a medical condition during the period when no food or drink is allowed before surgery, please give the medicine at its scheduled time with a sip of water (no more than 2 teaspoons).

   E.   If you have any questions about these directions or about what your child should eat or drink before surgery, please call 745-3317 after 5:00 P.M. weekdays. We will be happy to answer your questions and discuss any special problems your child may have. You may also discuss any questions you have about feeding your child with the nurse who will telephone you a day or two before your child is scheduled for admission.

CHILDREN'S HOSPITAL NATIONAL MEDICAL CENTER
DEPARTMENT OF ANESTHESIOLOGY

Instructions For Not Eating or Feeding Before Surgery
(Nothing By Mouth - N.P.O.)

In order to shorten the length of your child's stay in the hospital, your child has been scheduled for surgery as an outpatient. It is most important that your child have an empty stomach when given an anesthetic. This will reduce the danger of vomiting and inhaling stomach contents into the lungs while asleep. You must follow these instructions or your child's surgery must be cancelled.

III. If your child is older than 6 years:

A. Your child must not eat or drink anything at all after midnight the evening before surgery is scheduled.

B. If your child must take medicine by mouth for a medical condition during the period when no food or drink is allowed before surgery, please give the medication at its scheduled time with a sip of water (no more than 2 teaspoons).

C. If you have any questions about these directions or about what your child should eat or drink before surgery, please call 745-3317 after 5:00 P.M. weekdays. We will be happy to answer your questions and discuss any special problems your child may have. You may also discuss any questions you have about feeding your child with the nurse who will telephone you a day or two before your child is scheduled for admission.

Dear Parents,

Your opinions and comments about the Short Stay Recovery Unit help us to meet the needs of our patients. We would appreciate your cooperation in filling out this questionnaire. Feel free to comment as well as answer the questions. Your name is not required on the questionnaire, but you may write it if you wish.

Thank you for your cooperation.

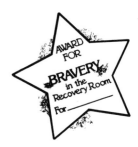

1. What was your overall impression of the Short Stay Recovery Unit (SSRU)?

   ☐ Favorable
   ☐ Unfavorable
   ☐ Indifferent

   Comments: _____
   _____

2. Did the unit meet you and your child's needs?

   ☐ Yes
   ☐ No

   Comments: _____
   _____

3. Did you receive a call the night before surgery from a nurse from the SSRU?

   ☐ Yes
   ☐ No

4. If yes, did you find the information helpful?

   ☐ Yes
   ☐ No

   Comments: _____
   _____

5. Were you informed that —

   - no siblings allowed?   ☐ Yes   ☐ No
   - only two (2) adults allowed?   ☐ Yes   ☐ No
   - no food or drinks allowed?   ☐ Yes   ☐ No
   - one (1) adult must stay with child at all times?   ☐ Yes   ☐ No

6. Were you satisfied with the discharge instructions given by the nurse?

   ☐ Yes
   ☐ No

   Comments: _____
   _____

7. Did you feel comfortable taking your child home at the time of discharge?

   ☐ Yes
   ☐ No

   Comments: _____
   _____

CHNMC FORM (Rev 1/84) Disk 1601

Parent's Instructions for SSRU

Short Stay Recovery Unit
Children's Hospital National Medical Center
111 Michigan Avenue, N.W.
Washington, DC 20010

SHORT STAY WELCOMES YOU

Our unit is designed to care for children who have undergone surgery requiring a minimum of 1 hour of short-stay recovery time. Your child's stay in our unit will vary usually from 1 to 4 hours or longer, depending on the type of surgical procedure done and your child's individual recovery rate.

We realize that the surgical experience is stressful for both you and your child. We hope this introduction to our unit will help minimize anxiety by providing you with some important and helpful information. Feel free to let us know your specific needs, concerns, or questions so that we may work together to make your child's stay here a pleasant one.

RULES AND REGULATIONS

In order for your child to receive safe, comprehensive care, let us review a few regulations designed to promote recovery.

Visiting: For safety reasons, we require one parent or visitor to stay with your child at all times. No siblings under 12 years old, and no more than two visitors per patient are allowed on this unit.

Smoking, Eating or Drinking: These activities are not permitted on any hospital unit. You are welcome to use the cafeteria or snack bar located on the 2nd floor.

Breakfast	6:30 A.M.–9:30 A.M.
Lunch	11:00 A.M.–2:00 P.M.
Dinner	4:30 P.M.–7:00 P.M.
Fast Foods	10:00 A.M.–4:00 P.M.

WHILE YOU'RE HERE

We encourage your participation in your child's care to the point at which you feel comfortable. You and your child may watch the television located in the play room, or use the telephones provided in each room.

AFTER SURGERY

When your child returns from surgery, you may notice that an IV (intravenous fluid) bottle will be regulating fluids through an attachment to the child's arm or foot. This IV will be removed when your child can tolerate fluids without vomiting.

GOING HOME

Before being discharged from the unit to go home, your child must meet certain criteria by the medical team for the type of procedure that was performed. Your nurse will discuss these criteria with you.

Before leaving, you will receive discharge instructions and will be requested to sign your child's chart. In addition, we ask that you please answer the questionnaire to help us evaluate and improve our unit.

Thank you.

SHORT STAY STAFF

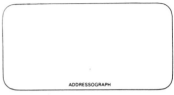

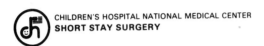

CHILDREN'S HOSPITAL NATIONAL MEDICAL CENTER
SHORT STAY SURGERY

ADDRESSOGRAPH

POST-OPERATIVE INSTRUCTIONS REGARDING ANESTHESIA

(LAST NAME)	(FIRST)	(MIDDLE INITIAL)	OPERATION SCHEDULED

IF YOUR CHILD HAD GENERAL ANESTHESIA or LOCAL ANESTHESIA WITH SEDATION, PLEASE PAY ATTENTION TO THE FOLLOWING INSTRUCTIONS:

1. The child may experience lightheadedness, dizziness or sleepiness following surgery. Please do not leave the child alone.

2. Let the child rest at home with moderate activity as tolerated. It may not be necessary to keep your child in bed, but it is important to rest until the next morning following general anesthesia. Do not let the child ride bikes, skate boards, etc.

3. Progress slowly to a light regular diet unless otherwise instructed. Start with liquids, then semi-solids and if appropriate for age, gradually work up to solid foods.

4. If your child should experience difficulty in breathing or persistant nausea and vomiting, please call short stay unit at **745-5122** or the anesthesiologist-on-call. An anesthesiologist can be reached 24 hours a day through the hospital operator at **745-3060**.

IF THE PATIENT IS LEGALLY AN ADULT:

5. Do not drink alcoholic beverages for 24 hours. Alcohol increases the effects of anesthesia and sedation.

6. Do not drive a motor vehicle, operate machinery or power tools for 24 hours.

7. Do not make any important decisions or sign important papers for 24 hours. You may be forgetful due to the medications administered.

OTHER INSTRUCTIONS:

Nurse Signature: _____

I HAVE RECEIVED and UNDERSTAND THE POST-OPERATIVE INSTRUCTIONS GIVEN TO ME:

Date: _____   *Parent's Signature:* _____

CHNMC FORM 129 (4/85) Disk 1 7N2   **MR**

CHILDREN'S HOSPITAL NATIONAL MEDICAL CENTER
NURSING DEPARTMENT
NURSING DISCHARGE SUMMARY

Patient's Primary Diagnosis: _____

Primary Nurse _____

ADDRESSOGRAPH

PART I - HOME CARE INSTRUCTIONS: INGUINAL HERNIORRHAPHY and/or HYDROCELLECTOMY and/or ORCHIDOPEXY

NOTE:
If you have printed instructions from your private physician, please follow those and use this as a supplement.
ACTIVITY:
May begin normal activities, but no strenous activities such as running, skating, jumping or playing hard for two weeks. *(Children over 8 years should stay home from school for 1 week.)* Other children may return to school in 2 - 4 days, when child is comfortable, but no playground or gym activities for 1 week. Infants may lie on their tummies.
DIET:
Progress slowly to a regular diet. We have given your child clear liquids in the Short Stay Unit. Continue with clear liquids at home with the addition of milk products, soups, eggs and soft cereal. Include and increase solid intake as tolerated.
Babies: ½ strength formula for the first feeding and advance to full strength as tolerated.
VOMITING:
If vomiting occurs, do not feed for 1 hour, and start over with ice chips or clear liquids, building up to regular food.
CARE OF INCISION:
Some children have a "clear coating" over the incision, this type of dressing peels off by itself in 3 - 5 days. It does not require any special care other than keeping the area clean and dry. Other children have a gauze pad dressing that should not get wet and should be kept clean and dry; if the tapes become loose, they can be trimmed or replaced. It may be difficult, but try to keep your child from scratching the incision. Please do not use baby powder or creams for diaper rash for two weeks. Loose clothing will be more comfortable for your child.
BATHING:
May have a sponge bath. But may not take a bath for _____ days.
MEDICATIONS:
Give Tylenol *(Acetaminophen)* _____ mg every _____ hours for discomfort. *(Generally, do not give more than four times daily.)*
WHEN TO CALL A DOCTOR:
- Any obvious bleeding. Some dried blood may be over the incision, *this is normal!*
- Redness or swelling around the incision.
- Fever over 101° F. or 38.4° C.
- Drainage *(pus)* from the wound.
- Persistent pain in the incision that is not relieved by Tylenol.
ADDITIONAL INSTRUCTIONS: _____

WHERE TO CALL WITH QUESTIONS:
- SHORT STAY UNIT—745-5122; open 8:00 a.m. to 11:00 p.m., Monday through Friday.
- Clinic/Private Doctor: _____
- *IN AN EMERGENCY,* call _____
FOLLOW-UP APPOINTMENT: _____ Make an appointment with _____
I have received and understand the above instructions:

_____
(PARENT SIGNATURE)

PART II

DISCHARGED: ☐ Home   ☐ Extended Care Facility   Other: _____
VIA: ☐ Ambulatory   ☐ Wheelchair   ☐ Stretcher   ☐ Carried

ACCOMPANIED BY: ☐ Parent: _____   ☐ Other: _____

Patient's physical/emotional condition at discharge: _____

Summary of patient/family understanding of discharge instruction *(i.e., by verbalization or demonstration):* _____

Date of Discharge: _____

Time of Discharge: _____
_____
(DISCHARGING NURSE'S SIGNATURE)

(TO DOCUMENT ANY ADDITIONAL INFORMATION ON ANY ITEM ABOVE, PLEASE INDICATE DATE OF CORRESPONDING PROGRESS NOTE.)

COPY DISTRIBUTION: WHITE - Chart   PINK - Parent   CHNMC FORM 113A (Rev 11/85) Disk 18E2 **MR**

CHILDREN'S HOSPITAL NATIONAL MEDICAL CENTER
NURSING DEPARTMENT
NURSING DISCHARGE SUMMARY

Patient's Primary Diagnosis: _____

_____

Primary Nurse: _____

ADDRESSOGRAPH

PART I - HOME CARE INSTRUCTIONS: EYE SURGERY

(SPECIFICALLY: _____)

NOTE:
If you have printed instructions from your private physician, please follow those and use this as a supplement.

DIET:
We have given your child clear liquids in the Short Stay Unit. Continue with a light diet at home, of cracked ice, sip carbonated beverages and juices for approximately 6 hours. As recovery progresses, you may include milk products and solid intake as tolerated.
     Babies: Breast feed immediately on ½ strength formula for the first feeding, and regular strength thereafter.

VOMITING:
If vomiting occurs, do not feed for one hour and start over with ice chips or clear liquids, building up to a regular diet.

MEDICATIONS: _____

_____

ACTIVITY:
Quiet play, preferably indoors for 2 - 3 days. School is normally resumed on third to fourth post-operative day, but no playground or gym activities for 10 days. Guard against getting filth into the eyes *(i.e., sandbox, playground, wading pool, basement.)* Swimming is not allowed for 2 weeks. No showers for 5 days.

SPECIAL INSTRUCTIONS:
Eyes may be uncomfortable—but should not be painful. Discourage rubbing eyes as much as possible. Child may be unusually sensitive to sunlight for several days. Use sunglasses. No restrictions are imposed on using the eyes immediately after surgery, including television and reading. Expect reddened eyes for about 2 weeks. Do not be surprised if your child prefers to keep both eyes closed or squints excessively for the first few days. Expect bloody eye drainage for about 5 days. This should lessen every day. Double vision may occur after surgery but this usually disappears in several days. Please do not try to evaluate the outcome of the surgery during the first few days following surgery. Frequently, there is a good deal of change in eye position during the first few days.

WHEN TO CALL THE DOCTOR:
- Increased swelling of the eyes
- Yellow eye drainage
- Fever over 101°
- "Runny nose" secretions *(may possibly be wiped into freshly operated eye, antibiotic thereapy may be needed).*

WHERE TO CALL WITH QUESTIONS:
- SHORT STAY UNIT—745-5122; open 8:00 a.m. to 11:00 p.m., Monday through Friday.
- Clinic/Private Doctor _____
- *IN AN EMERGENCY,* call _____

FOLLOW-UP APPOINTMENT: Make an appointment with _____

I have received and understand the above instructions:

_____
(PARENT SIGNATURE)

PART II

DISCHARGED: ☐ Home   ☐ Extended Care Facility   Other: _____
VIA: ☐ Ambulatory   ☐ Wheelchair   ☐ Stretcher   ☐ Carried

ACCOMPANIED BY: ☐ Parent: _____ ☐ Other: _____

Patient's physical/emotional condition at discharge: _____

_____

Summary of patient/family understanding of discharge instruction *(i.e., by verbalization or demonstration)*: _____

_____

Date of Discharge: _____

Time of Discharge: _____   _____
                                                  (DISCHARGING NURSE'S SIGNATURE)

(TO DOCUMENT ANY ADDITIONAL INFORMATION ON ANY ITEM ABOVE, PLEASE INDICATE DATE OF CORRESPONDING PROGRESS NOTE.)

COPY DISTRIBUTION: WHITE - Chart   PINK - Parent   CHNMC FORM 1130 (Rev 11/85) Disk 18F2 **MR**

CHILDREN'S HOSPITAL NATIONAL MEDICAL CENTER
NURSING DEPARTMENT
NURSING DISCHARGE SUMMARY

Patient's Primary Diagnosis: _____

_____

Primary Nurse: _____

ADDRESSOGRAPH

PART I - HOME CARE INSTRUCTIONS: CIRCUMCISION

NOTE:
If you have printed instructions from your private physician, please follow those and use this as a supplement.

ACTIVITY:
Begin normal activity. May return to school in 2 - 4 days, when child is comfortable.

DIET:
Progress slowly to a regular diet. We have given you child clear liquids in the Short Stay Unit. Continue with liquids at home with the addition of milk products, soups, eggs, and soft cereal. Include and increase solid intake as tolerated.

        Babies: ½ strength formula for the first feeding. Advance to full strength as tolerated.

VOMITING:
If vomiting occurs, do not feed for 1 hour and start over with ice chips or clear liquids, building up to regular food.

MEDICATIONS:
Give Tylenol *(Acetaminophen)* _____ mg every _____ hours for discomfort. *(Generally, do not give more than four times a day.)*

SPECIAL INSTRUCTIONS:
- If there is a gauze dressing on the penis, it should be removed in the morning.
- Begin giving a warm tub bath _____ days after surgery and every day thereafter, rinse well. Do not scrub the penis, just wash gently. May go without wearing pants for a day or so for more comfort. Loose diapers and loose fitting clothes may be more comfortable for several days.
- Baby may sleep on his stomach.
- *Stitches* - Don't worry if the stitches fall out, this is normal. The stitches are not removed, they dissolve.
- Some redness and swelling is expected, but be sure to have the nurse show you what the penis looks like before you go home.
- Do not use any medications, ointments, vaseline, powder, etc., on the penis, unless specifically instructed to do so.
- If the skin slips over the head of the penis during the first week after surgery, gently pull the skin back down with your fingers. If the skin cannot be brought back, *please call your doctor.*

WHEN TO CALL THE DOCTOR:
- Swelling that does not gradually lessen. *(Swelling should be gone by 1 week.)*
- A fever over 101° F. or 38.4° C., not relieved by Acetaminophen, *(Tylenol, Tempra, etc.)*
- Any bright red bleeding that does not stop after applying pressure for 10 continuous minutes; take your child to the Emergency Room. *(This is most unlikely to occur.)*

WHERE TO CALL WITH QUESTIONS:
- SHORT STAY UNIT—745-5122. Open 8:00 a.m. to 11:00 p.m., Monday through Friday.
- Clinic/Private Doctor _____
- *IN AN EMERGENCY,* call _____

FOLLOW-UP APPOINTMENT: Make an appointment with _____

I have received and understand the above instructions:

_____
(PARENT SIGNATURE)

PART II

DISCHARGED: ☐ Home   ☐ Extended Care Facility   Other: _____

VIA: ☐ Ambulatory   ☐ Wheelchair   ☐ Stretcher   ☐ Carried

ACCOMPANIED BY: ☐ Parent: _____ ☐ Other: _____

Patient's physical/emotional condition at discharge: _____

_____

Summary of patient/family understanding of discharge instruction *(i.e., by verbalization or demonstration):* _____

_____

Date of Discharge: _____

Time of Discharge: _____

_____
(DISCHARGING NURSE'S SIGNATURE)

(TO DOCUMENT ANY ADDITIONAL INFORMATION ON ANY ITEM ABOVE, PLEASE INDICATE DATE OF CORRESPONDING PROGRESS NOTE.)

COPY DISTRIBUTION: WHITE - Chart   PINK - Parent   CHNMC FORM 113C (Rev 11/85) Disk 18F1 **MR**

CHILDREN'S HOSPITAL NATIONAL MEDICAL CENTER
NURSING DEPARTMENT
NURSING DISCHARGE SUMMARY

Patient's Primary Diagnosis: _____

_____

Primary Nurse: _____

ADDRESSOGRAPH

PART I - HOME CARE INSTRUCTIONS: ORAL EXTRACTION PROCEDURES

NOTE:
If you have printed instructions from your private physician, please follow those and use this as a supplement.

ACTIVITY:
Quiet activity for the first 24 hours. This helps reduce bleeding and permits formation of a clot in area which is necessary for healing.

DIET:
Liquid diet for the first 24 hours: Then soft foods high in vitamins and protein; *examples*—eggs, soups, milk shakes, mashed potatoes, chopped meats. Increased fluid intake is recommended. Gradually add solid foods. Temperature of foods will not affect site.

MEDICTIONS:
Give Tylenol *(Acetaminophen)* _____ mg every _____ hours for discomfort. *(Generally, do not give more than four times daily.)*

SPECIAL INSTRUCTIONS:
The operated area will swell. May place an ice pack on cheek for swelling. Other teeth may ache temporarily. A sore throat or slight ear ache may develop. There will be a cavity where the tooth was removed. *Do not rinse or brush teeth the day of surgery.* The day following surgery the area should be gently rinsed after meals and at bedtime with warm salt water. The cavity will gradually fill-in with new tissue. Slight bleeding is expected and may persist until the next day. Avoid spitting, it may cause bleeding.

WHEN TO CALL THE DOCTOR:
- Bleeding—which persists after applying pressure with a gauze pad or wet tea bag for 30 minutes twice.
- Fever over 101° which persists 24-48° past surgery.
- Pain not relieved by Tylenol and/or prescription given.

WHERE TO CALL WITH QUESTIONS:
- Short Stay Unit - **745-5122**; open 8:00 a.m. to 11:00 p.m., Monday through Friday.
- Clinic/Private Doctor: _____
- In an Emergency; call: _____

FOLLOW-UP APPOINTMENT: Make an appointment with _____

I have received and understand the above instructions:

_____
(PARENT SIGNATURE)

PART II

DISCHARGED: ☐ Home   ☐ Extended Care Facility   Other: _____
VIA: ☐ Ambulatory   ☐ Wheelchair   ☐ Stretcher   ☐ Carried

ACCOMPANIED BY: ☐ Parent: _____ ☐ Other: _____

Patient's physical/emotional condition at discharge: _____

_____

Summary of patient/family understanding of discharge instruction *(i.e., by verbalization or demonstration)*: _____

_____

Date of Discharge: _____

Time of Discharge: _____   _____
                                                          (DISCHARGING NURSE'S SIGNATURE)

*(TO DOCUMENT ANY ADDITIONAL INFORMATION ON ANY ITEM ABOVE, PLEASE INDICATE DATE OF CORRESPONDING **PROGRESS NOTE**.)*

COPY DISTRIBUTION: WHITE - Chart   PINK - Parent   CHNMC FORM 113E (12/86) Disk 18F3   **MR**

CHILDREN'S HOSPITAL NATIONAL MEDICAL CENTER
NURSING DEPARTMENT
NURSING DISCHARGE SUMMARY

Patient's Primary Diagnosis: _____

ADDRESSOGRAPH

Primary Nurse _____

PART I - HOME CARE INSTRUCTIONS: ADENOIDECTOMY

NOTE:
If you have printed instructions from your private physician, please follow those and use this as a supplement.

ACTIVITY:
Limited activity for the first 2 - 3 days. May return to school after _____ days.

DIET:
Progress slowly to a regular diet. We have given your child clear liquids in the Short Stay Unit. Continue with clear liquids at home with the addition of milk products, soups, eggs, and soft cereal. Avoid hot, spicy, very acid *(example: orange juice)* and rough *(example: chips, crusted bread)* foods for the first _____ days. As recovery progresses, you may include and increase solid intake as tolerated. If vomiting occurs, do not feed for one hour and start over with ice chips or clear liquids, building up slowly to soft, then regular food.

MEDICATIONS:
Tylenol *(Acetaminophen)* _____ mg every _____ hours, if needed for discomfort. Generally do not give more than four times a day. Since aspirin, and products containing aspirin interfere with blood clotting, avoid these preparations.

SPECIAL INSTRUCTIONS:
- Coughing, gargling, straining, shouting, clearing the throat, or blowing the nose should be kept at a minimum.
- Expect some bleeding or brown mucous from the nose for the first 24 hours.
- You may notice that your child's voice is changed. If it persists by your office visit—bring this to the attention of your doctor.

WHEN TO CALL THE DOCTOR:
- Any bleeding of bright red blood from the nose or throat that does not stop in 5 minutes.
- Persistent pain that is not relieved by Acetaminophen *(i.e., Tylenol, Tempra).*
- Fever over 102⁰ F. *(not relieved by Acetaminophen)*
- Persistent Cough

WHERE TO CALL WITH QUESTIONS:
- Short Stay Unit—745-5122; open 8:00 a.m. to 11:00 p.m., Monday through Friday.
- Clinic/Private Doctor.
- *IN AN EMERGENCY,* call _____

FOLLOW-UP APPOINTMENT:
Make an appointment with _____

I have received and understand the above instructions:

_____
(PARENT SIGNATURE)

PART II

DISCHARGED: ☐ Home   ☐ Extended Care Facility   Other: _____
VIA: ☐ Ambulatory   ☐ Wheelchair   ☐ Stretcher   ☐ Carried

ACCOMPANIED BY: ☐ Parent: _____   ☐ Other: _____

Patient's physical/emotional condition at discharge: _____

Summary of patient/family understanding of discharge instruction *(i.e., by verbalization or demonstration):* _____

Date of Discharge: _____

Time of Discharge: _____   _____
(DISCHARGING NURSE'S SIGNATURE)

(TO DOCUMENT ANY ADDITIONAL INFORMATION ON ANY ITEM ABOVE, PLEASE INDICATE DATE OF CORRESPONDING PROGRESS NOTE.)

COPY DISTRIBUTION: WHITE - Chart   PINK - Parent

CHNMC FORM 113 (Rev 11/85) Disk 18E1   **MR**

THE PRESBYTERIAN HOSPITAL
in the City of New York
at
Columbia-Presbyterian Medical Center

NAME:

DATE OF
BIRTH/SEX:

LOCATION CODE:

UNIT NO.:

AMBULATORY SURGERY UNIT ADMISSION CHECKLIST

Date _____   Arrival time _____

DIAGNOSIS_____ SURGERY_____

( )   NPO
( )   No URI or acute illness
( )   Contact lenses and glasses removed
( )   Dentures and bridges removed
( )   Makeup and jewelry removed
( )   Medical questionnaire completed
( )   Physical exam completed
( )   Lab reports complete
( )   Surgical consent signed
( )   Anesthesia consent signed
( )   Identification bracelet
( )   Mental status clear
( )   Surgical prep
( )   Voided on call

Where will the patient be staying tonight? Telephone number?

_____

With whom?

_____

How will they get there?

_____
_____

VITAL SIGNS
B.P. _____
P. _____
R. _____
Temp. _____

MEDICATIONS

Name	Dose	Route	Time	R.N.

Additional information

_____
_____
_____

To O.R.   Time _____

_____ R.N.

Babies Hospital • Dana W. Atchley Pavilion • The Edward S. Harkness Eye Institute • Harkness Pavilion • Neurological Institute
New York Orthopaedic Hospital • Presbyterian Hospital • Sloane Hospital • Squier Urological Clinic • Vanderbilt Clinic

AMBULATORY SURGERY UNIT ADMISSION CERTIFICATION

I am aware of the danger of food or liquid in my stomach during anesthesia and surgery.

I certify that I have had nothing to eat or drink since midnight.

Exceptions:_____

I certify that I have an escort home.

Name of escort: _____

Patient's signature _____

Witness_____

Date _____

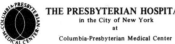

THE PRESBYTERIAN HOSPITAL
in the City of New York
at
Columbia-Presbyterian Medical Center

UNIT NO.:

NAME:

DATE OF
BIRTH/SEX:

LOCATION CODE:

AMBULATORY SURGERY PREOPERATIVE TELEPHONE INSTRUCTIONS

( ) NPO after midnight. Nothing to eat or drink the day of surgery. No candy, gum, smoking.
     Exceptions: _____
( ) Patient informed when to arrive in unit 1 hr. prior to surgery.   Time: _____
( ) Location of unit
( ) Parking facilities
( ) Patient should wear loose fitting clothing, flat shoes, no makeup, no contact lenses
( ) Leave money, jewelry, valuables at home
( ) Health survey reviewed with patient
     Does patient have a URI? _____
     Has patient had a illness since they last saw the surgeon? _____
( ) Anesthesia questions _____
     _____
( ) Surgery questions _____
     _____
( ) Medications _____
     _____
( ) Recommend shower or bath the evening before or morning of surgery
( ) Recommend brushing teeth the morning of surgery
( ) Has patient made arrangements for an escort?   YES   NO
     Escort must accompany patient to and from unit
     Responsible adult must be with patient the evening of surgery
     Inform patient about waiting facilities for escort
     Inform patient of expected length of stay

Special Instructions _____
_____

Patient questions or concerns _____
_____

Impression _____
_____

RN/MD_____

Date/Time _____

Babies Hospital • Dana W. Atchley Pavilion • The Edward S. Harkness Eye Institute • Harkness Pavilion • Neurological Institute
New York Orthopaedic Hospital • Presbyterian Hospital • Sloane Hospital • Squier Urological Clinic • Vanderbilt Clinic

AMBULATORY SURGERY POSTOPERATIVE TELEPHONE FOLLOWUP

( ) ACTIVITIES
Has patient resumed normal activities?   YES   NO

( ) DIET
Is patient tolerating liquids/solids/normal diet?   YES   NO
Any nausea or vomiting?   YES   NO

( ) PAIN
Does patient have pain?   YES   NO   If so, describe

Was pain medication prescribed?   YES   NO
What medication? How effective?

( ) BATHING
Is patient bathing normally?   YES   NO

( ) WOUND
Is dressing/cast dry and intact?   YES   NO

Is there any swelling, redness, or drainage?   YES   NO
Describe

Neurovascular check, if applicable

( ) MISCELLANEOUS
Did patient experience:
Muscle discomfort? YES   NO   Sore throat?   YES   NO
Headache?   YES   NO   Voiding difficulties? YES   NO
Pain at i.v. site? YES   NO   Fever?   YES   NO

( ) Review of postoperative instructions?   YES   NO
( ) Review of special instructions?   YES   NO

( ) Did patient need to contact their doctor, the Ambulatory Unit or
the Emergency Room?   YES   NO

( ) Patient's comments or concerns

( ) Surgeon/anesthesiologist contacted regarding above?   YES   NO

( ) Additional followup necessary?   YES   NO

RN/MD_____   Date/Time_____

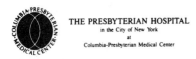

THE PRESBYTERIAN HOSPITAL
in the City of New York
at
Columbia-Presbyterian Medical Center

UNIT NO.:

NAME:

DATE OF
BIRTH/SEX:

LOCATION CODE:

PEDIATRIC MEDICAL QUESTIONNAIRE
AMBULATORY SURGERY UNIT

Please take a few minutes to complete this health questionnaire. Accurate information will help us in evaluating your child's medical status and taking care of your child's medical needs.

Child's name _____ Name of Parent/Guardian _____

Address _____

Home telephone (area code) _____ (number) _____   (if none – how can you be reached?) _____

Parent's work telephone (area code) _____ (number) _____

Reason for surgery _____

Age _____ Occupation _____ If student, what grade _____

Has your child had any serious illnesses?   YES   NO   List
_____
_____

Has your child been hospitalized?   YES   NO   List hospital, date, reason
_____
_____

Did your child have any problems with previous surgery or anesthesia?   YES   NO   Describe
_____
_____

Has anyone in your family had problems with anesthesia?   YES   NO   Describe
_____
_____

Does your child take any medicines regularly?   YES   NO   List
_____
_____

Does your child have any general allergies or allergies to medicine?   YES   NO
List and describe reaction
_____
_____

Has your child had any problems with his/her HEART or CIRCULATION?
Heart murmur   YES   NO
Irregular heartbeat   YES   NO
Rheumatic fever   YES   NO

Explanation or additional problems _____
_____

Babies Hospital • Dana W. Atchley Pavilion • The Edward S. Harkness Eye Institute • Harkness Pavilion • Neurological Institute
New York Orthopaedic Hospital • Presbyterian Hospital • Sloane Hospital • Squier Urological Clinic • Vanderbilt Clinic

– 2 –

Has your child had any problems with his/her LUNGS or BREATHING?

Asthma	YES	NO
Pneumonia	YES	NO
Bronchitis/Bronchiolitis	YES	NO
Cough	YES	NO
Shortness of breath	YES	NO

Explanation or additional problems _____

Has your child had any problems with his/her KIDNEYS or BLADDER?

Infections	YES	NO
Difficulty with urination	YES	NO

Explanation or additional problems _____

Has your child had any problems with his/her BLOOD?

Anemia	YES	NO
Prolonged bleeding or easy bruising	YES	NO
Sickle cell disease	YES	NO
Blood transfusions	YES	NO

Explanation or additional problems _____

Has your child had any problems with his/her NERVES, MUSCLES, or BONES?

Seizures	YES	NO
Fainting spells or dizziness	YES	NO
Head, neck, or facial injury	YES	NO
Scoliosis	YES	NO
Muscle weakness	YES	NO
Dislocated joint(s)	YES	NO

Explanation or additional problems _____

Does your child smoke? YES NO How much? _____

Does your child drink alcohol? YES NO How much? _____ How often? _____

Does your child use marijuana or similar drugs? YES NO

Type of drug _____. How much? _____ How often? _____

– 3 –

Has your child had any of the following?

Thyroid disease	YES	NO
Glasses or contact lenses	YES	NO
Problems with hearing	YES	NO
Physical disabilities	YES	NO
Loose, capped, missing or chipped teeth	YES	NO
Dentures, bridges (permanent or removable), braces	YES	NO

Explanation or additional information _____

_____

Has your child had chicken pox?   YES   NO

   If No, has your child been exposed to chicken pox recently?   YES   NO

   If Yes, what date? _____

If not immunized for measles or mumps, has your child been exposed to either measles or mumps in the past 2 weeks?   YES   NO

   If Yes, what date? _____

Does your child menstruate?   YES   NO   Date of last menstrual period _____

YOUR CHILD MUST BE ESCORTED BY A PARENT OR LEGAL GUARDIAN
who will stay with them during the day and take them home from the hospital.

Only two adults can accompany a child to the pediatric ambulatory surgery unit. Children who are not having surgery cannot come to the unit.

I will be accompanying my child to ambulatory surgery:

Name _____ Relationship _____

Address _____

Telephone (area code)   (number) _____

Hospital Emergency Room nearest your home _____

I understand that my child should not have anything to eat or drink after TIME_____ DATE _____
Failure to follow this instruction will result in cancellation of my child's surgery.

                                   _____

                                   Parent/Guardian Signature

                                   _____

                                   Date

– 4 –

PHYSICIAN HISTORY

Diagnosis _____

Surgical procedure _____

History of present illness _____

_____

_____

PHYSICAL EXAMINATION

Ht _____ Wt _____ BP _____ P _____ R _____

HEENT _____

Heart _____

Lungs _____

Abdomen _____

Extremities _____

Neurologic _____

LABORATORY TESTS

Required for patients having local anesthesia with sedation, regional, or general anesthesia. To be obtained within 2 weeks of surgery.

TEST	RESULTS	DATE
( ) CBC	RBC _____ Hgb _____	_____
	WBC _____ Hct _____	_____
( ) Urinalysis	_____	_____
( ) Other	_____	_____
_____	_____	_____
_____	_____	_____

If tests are obtained from an outside laboratory, the surgeon is responsible for reporting the results to the Unit at least 48 hours prior to surgery.

Physician's signature _____ Date _____

THE PRESBYTERIAN HOSPITAL
in the City of New York
at
Columbia-Presbyterian Medical Center

UNIT NO.:

NAME:

DATE OF
BIRTH/SEX:

LOCATION CODE:

ADULT MEDICAL QUESTIONNAIRE
AMBULATORY SURGERY UNIT

Please take a few minutes to complete this health questionnaire. Accurate information will help us in evaluating your medical status and taking care of your medical needs.

Name _____

Address_____

Home telephone (area code) _____ (number) _____

Work telephone (area code) _____ (number) _____

Reason for surgery_____

Date of surgery _____ Unit Number _____

Age_____ Height_____ Weight_____ Sex M   F

Marital status S M D W   Occupation _____

Have you had any serious illnesses?   YES   NO   List
_____
_____

Have you been hospitalized?   YES   NO   List hospital, date, reason
_____

Did you have any problems with previous surgery or anesthesia?   YES NO   Describe
_____

Has anyone in your family had problems with anesthesia?   YES NO   Describe
_____

Do you take any medicines regularly?   YES   NO   List
_____

Have you taken any other medicines in the past 2 years?   YES NO   List
_____

Do you have any general allergies or allergies to medicine?   YES NO
List and describe reaction
_____
_____

Have you had any problems with your HEART or CIRCULATION?

Heart murmur	YES	NO
Irregular heartbeat	YES	NO
Rheumatic fever	YES	NO
Mitral valve prolapse	YES	NO
Heart failure	YES	NO
Shortness of breath	YES	NO
Chest pain or pressure (angina)	YES	NO
High blood pressure	YES	NO
Difficulty climbing stairs	YES	NO
Chest pain or shortness of breath with exercise	YES	NO
Waking up at night short of breath	YES	NO
Sleeping on more than one pillow	YES	NO
Ankle swelling	YES	NO
Heart attack	YES	NO
Abnormal EKG	YES	NO

Explanation _____

Babies Hospital • Dana W. Atchley Pavilion • The Edward S. Harkness Eye Institute • Harkness Pavilion • Neurological Institute
New York Orthopaedic Hospital • Presbyterian Hospital • Sloane Hospital • Squier Urological Clinic • Vanderbilt Clinic

– 2 –

Have you had any problems with your LUNGS or BREATHING?

Asthma	YES	NO
Pneumonia	YES	NO
Bronchitis	YES	NO
Emphysema	YES	NO
Cough	YES	NO
Do you cough up anything?	YES	NO
Shortness of breath	YES	NO
Abnormal chest x-ray	YES	NO

Explanation _____

Have you had any problems with your KIDNEYS or BLADDER?

Infections	YES	NO
Stones	YES	NO
Difficulty with urination	YES	NO
Kidney failure	YES	NO

Explanation _____

Have you had any problems with your BLOOD?

Anemia	YES	NO
Prolonged bleeding or easy bruising	YES	NO
Sickle cell disease	YES	NO
Abnormal blood tests	YES	NO
Blood transfusions	YES	NO

Explanation _____

Have you had any problems with your NERVES, MUSCLES, or BONES?

Seizures	YES	NO
Strokes	YES	NO
Fainting spells or dizziness	YES	NO
Head, neck, or facial injury	YES	NO
Back injury	YES	NO
Muscle weakness	YES	NO
Numbness of arms or legs	YES	NO
Extreme nervousness or anxiety	YES	NO
Psychiatric illness	YES	NO

Explanation _____

Do you smoke? YES NO   How much? _____
Do you drink alcohol? YES NO   How much? _____ How often? _____
Do you use marijuana or similar drugs?   YES NO
Type of drug _____ How much? _____ How often? _____

– 3 –

Have you had any of the following?

Diabetes	YES	NO
Thyroid disease	YES	NO
Hepatitis or jaundice	YES	NO
Frequent vomiting or diarrhea	YES	NO
Weight loss or gain	YES	NO
Hiatus hernia	YES	NO
Frequent fevers	YES	NO
Problems with vision	YES	NO
Glaucoma	YES	NO
Glasses or contact lenses	YES	NO
Problems with hearing	YES	NO
Physical disabilities	YES	NO
Loose, capped, missing or chipped teeth	YES	NO
Dentures, bridges (permanent or removable), braces	YES	NO

Explanation _____

Are you pregnant?   YES   NO   Date of last menstrual period _____

YOU MUST HAVE AN ESCORT
Person who will take you home from the hospital

Name _____
Address_____
Telephone number (area code)   (number) _____
Relationship_____

Hospital Emergency Room nearest your home
_____

Patient's signature _____
Date _____

– 4 –

HISTORY

Diagnosis _____
Surgical procedure _____
History of present illness _____   _____
_____
_____

PHYSICAL EXAMINATION

Ht_____ Wt _____ BP_____ P _____ R _____
HEENT_____
Heart_____
Lungs _____
Abdomen _____
Extremities _____
Neurologic _____

LABORATORY TESTS

Required for patients having local anesthesia with sedation, regional, or general anesthesia. To be obtained within 30 days of surgery.

TEST	RESULTS	DATE
( ) Hemoglobin or hematocrit (all patients)	_____	_____
( ) Urinalysis (all patients)	_____	_____
( ) EKG (over age 40 or cardiovascular disease)	_____	_____
( ) Chest x-ray (over age 50 or pulmonary or cardiovascular disease unless obtained within previous 6 months)	_____	_____
( ) Chem 7 (diabetes, cardiovascular or renal disease or taking antihypertensive medications or diuretics)	_____	_____
( ) Sickle cell test (required by law in black patients unless previous results available)	_____	_____
( ) Other (as indicated by medical status of patient)	_____	_____
	_____	_____
	_____	_____

If test are obtained from an outside laboratory, the surgeon is responsible for reporting the results to the Unit at least 48 hours prior surgery.

Physician's signature _____ Date _____

The Presbyterian Hospital in the City of New York

Columbia-Presbyterian Medical Center, New York, NY 10032-3784

PEDIATRIC AMBULATORY SURGERY
HOME CARE INSTRUCTIONS

1. After general anesthesia, children may develop nausea or vomiting. The symptoms are usually mild and will disappear by the next day. Nausea may be managed at home with sips of juice or soft drinks which are not too fizzy. Do **not** give solid food until nausea or vomiting have disappeared for three hours.

2. On the night following the child's surgery there may be a slight fever (100°F) or some discomfort; these can be managed nicely with Tylenol. Give as directed on the bottle.

3. If during your first week at home your child has a fever of 101°F or above, call Pediatric Ambulatory Surgery (-   ) between 8am and 5pm or your surgeon's office. If your child has a fever of 101°F or above, continues to vomit or has any other problems and you are unable to reach your doctor, contact the emergency room nearest to your home at _____ hospital.

4. Medications: Mild pain is not unusual and may be relieved by Tylenol or a similar non-aspirin pain medication. A prescription for other medications may be given to you by your doctor.

   MEDICATION   DOSE   INSTRUCTION

   _____

   _____

5. Your child's followup visit is: Date: _____ Time: _____

   Place: _____ If you are unable to keep this appointment, please

   call: _____ .

A ☐   Additional Discharge instructions provided in a separate handout

B ☐   Additional Discharge instructions:

   _____

   _____

   _____

   _____

I have read and understand the above Discharge instructions.

Parent/Guardian signature _____

        Instructed by _____ RN

        Discharged by _____ MD   Date _____

( ) **Discharge Instructions given in Spanish**

Babies Hospital   •   Dana W. Atchley Pavilion   •   The Edward S. Harkness Eye Institute   •   Harkness Pavilion   •   Neurological Institute
New York Orthopaedic Hospital   •   Presbyterian Hospital   •   Sloane Hospital   •   Squier Urological Clinic   •   Vanderbilt Clinic

The Presbyterian Hospital in the City of New York

Columbia-Presbyterian Medical Center, New York, NY 10032-3784

AMBULATORY SURGERY UNIT

To our patients:

Please take a few minutes to share your impressions of the Ambulatory Surgery Unit. This information will help us in our continuing effort to improve services to all patients and to make the experience as comfortable and convenient as possible. Thank you for your cooperation.

Did you find the admitting procedure satisfactory?	YES	NO
Were the personnel pleasant and attentive to your individual needs?	YES	NO
Were you taken care of promptly?	YES	NO
Were the preoperative and postoperative telephone calls helpful?	YES	NO
Were the discharge instructions presented clearly and completely?	YES	NO
Was the facility convenient to use?	YES	NO
Did everything go as smoothly as expected?	YES	NO
If you were to need one day surgery in the future, would you return to this Ambulatory Surgery Unit?	YES	NO
If your laboratory tests were done at Presbyterian Hospital, were the arrangements satisfactory?	YES	NO
Did you encounter any problems with parking?	YES	NO

Do you have any comments or suggestions?

_____

_____

_____

_____

Date of surgery _____

Name (optional) _____

Babies Hospital • Dana W. Atchley Pavilion • The Edward S. Harkness Eye Institute • Harkness Pavilion • Neurological Institute
New York Orthopaedic Hospital • Presbyterian Hospital • Sloane Hospital • Squier Urological Clinic • Vanderbilt Clinic

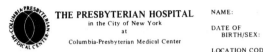

THE PRESBYTERIAN HOSPITAL
in the City of New York
at
Columbia-Presbyterian Medical Center

NAME: UNIT NO.:

DATE OF
BIRTH/SEX:

LOCATION CODE:

AMBULATORY SURGERY UNIT POSTOPERATIVE INSTRUCTIONS

1. ACTIVITIES

    Rest today. It is normal to experience some dizziness or drowsiness following surgery or treatment. Do not consume alcohol, drive, operate machinery, or make important personal or business decisions for 24 hours.

    Activity level
    ( ) Full
    ( ) Work
    ( ) Exercise
    ( ) Other:

2. DIET

    Progress as tolerated without nausea or vomiting.
    ( ) Liquids
    ( ) Light meals
    ( ) Normal
    ( ) Other:

3. MEDICATIONS

    Mild aches, pains, or cramps are not unusual, and may be relieved by tylenol or similar non-aspirin pain medication. A prescription for other pain medication may be given by your doctor.

    ( ) Prescription given

    Medication   Dose   Instructions
    _____
    _____
    _____

4. BATHING

    ( ) Sponge
    ( ) Shower
    ( ) Tub
    ( ) Normal

5. WOUND CARE

    A small amount of bright red blood is to be expected. If you feel the amount is excessive, call your doctor.

    ( ) Keep dressings dry
    ( ) Change dressings as necessary
    ( ) Do not change your dressing until you see your doctor
    ( ) Other:

Babies Hospital • Dana W. Atchley Pavilion • The Edward S. Harkness Eye Institute • Harkness Pavilion • Neurological Institute
New York Orthopaedic Hospital • Presbyterian Hospital • Sloane Hospital • Squier Urological Clinic • Vanderbilt Clinic

6. EMERGENCIES

    Call your doctor if problems arise such as bladder difficulties, persistent nausea or vomiting, bleeding that does not stop, unusual pain, fever, redness, swelling, or drainage of pus. If you are unable to reach your doctor, you may contact the Ambulatory Surgery Unit, the Presbyterian Hospital Emergency Room, or the hospital emergency room nearest your home.

7. SPECIAL INSTRUCTIONS

    _____
    _____
    _____
    _____

8. FOLLOW-UP CARE

    ( ) Call your doctor's office to schedule an appointment
    ( ) Call the clinic to schedule an appointment
    ( ) An appointment has been scheduled
        Date: Time:

    You will receive a call from the Ambulatory Surgery Unit staff in a day or so to find out how you are feeling.

    I have read and understand the above discharge instructions.

    Patient's signature_____

    Instructed by _____ R.N.

    Orders by _____ M.D.   Date _____

    Ambulatory Surgery Unit telephone number: (212) 305-2574
    Hours of operation: Monday-Friday 7 a.m. to 6 p.m.

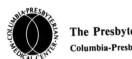

The Presbyterian Hospital in the City of New York
Columbia-Presbyterian Medical Center, New York, NY 10032-3784

AMBULATORY SURGERY
POSTOPERATIVE FOLLOWUP FORM

To maintain the quality of patient care, as well as to comply with
State regulations, a review of the post operative course is required.
This form should be completed during the postoperative period and
returned to the Ambulatory Surgery Unit - PH16W.

Patient's name: Unit number:
Name of surgeon:
        Service: Date of Surgery:

Procedure(s):

_____ Uneventful postoperative course.
           (If you check this blank, please stop here,
            sign the form and return it. Thank you)

           Did patient return for emergency treatment to the:
_____ Office
_____ Clinic
_____ Emergency Room

           Did patient require hospital admission:
_____ from the Recovery Room
_____ after discharge from the ambulatory surgery unit

           Postoperative problem list:

_____ Bleeding   _____ Pain
_____ Infection   _____ Respiratory complications
_____ Persistent nausea or vomiting _____ Cardiac complications
_____ Bladder or bowel dysfunction _____ Other

Description of problem:
_____
_____
_____

Brief description of therapy and followup plan:
_____
_____
_____

_____ M.D.   Date_____

Babies Hospital • Dana W. Atchley Pavilion • The Edward S. Harkness Eye Institute • Harkness Pavilion • Neurological Institute
New York Orthopaedic Hospital • Presbyterian Hospital • Sloane Hospital • Squier Urological Clinic • Vanderbilt Clinic

OXFORDSHIRE HEALTH AUTHORITY

The Churchill Hospital   Day Surgery Unit
Old Road   Consultant in Administrative Charge: Dr J. Millar
Headington   **NEW TELEPHONE NUMBER**
Oxford   Telephone: As from 3rd DECEMBER 1988 ext 679
                                                              The Churchill Hospital
                                                              Telephone number
                                                              will be
                                                              OXFORD (0865) 741841

Dear

Your admission to the Churchill Day Surgery Unit has been arranged for:

_____

If this is unsuitable please ring the Admissions Officer on Oxford 64841, Extension 653.

You should also notify ext 653 by telephone as soon as possible if you cannot keep the appointment because of acute illness, including the common cold or sore throat.

A map showing the way to the Day Surgery Unit is enclosed. Parking is provided in the Visitors' Car Park, which is signposted.

The Day Surgery Unit has been established to allow patients to come in for surgical treatment and go home on the same day. It is very important that the following conditions are fulfilled or it will not be possible to carry out your treatment:

1. No food or drink must be taken after midnight the night before your operation.

2. If you normally take tablets or medicines or use inhalers, these should be taken as usual, with only a sip of water if this is necessary. Bring them with you.

3. You must arrive at the Day Surgery Unit at 8.00 a.m.

4. If you are under 16 years, you must be brought by your parent or guardian.

5. You must arrange for a responsible adult to take you home by car or taxi before 5 p.m. He or she should telephone the Churchill Hospital, Oxford 64841, extension 679 between 12.30 and 1.30 to find out when to collect you.

6. There must be a responsible adult at home to look after your overnight.

7. You must not drive a car or any other vehicle, or operate machinery, or use a cooker or kettle for 24 hours after your anaesthetic. Alcohol should be avoided. It is inadvisable to sign documents or take important decisions.

8. Do not work if this is strenuous or involves machinery, or take strenuous exercise the day after your operation.

OAH 3313

PLEASE:

Have a bath before coming.

Make a note of your weight.

Remove makeup and nail varnish.

Leave money and valuables at home.

Bring your medical card, if possible.

Bring a wash bag, dressing gown and slippers or soft indoor shoes.

Bring sanitary towels, if having a gynaecological operation.

Bring reading material/knitting etc. to occupy waiting time.

The Staff of the Day Surgery Unit wish to make your treatment as pleasant as possible. Please telephone the Unit if you have any problems.

Yours sincerely,

Dr J. Millar
Consultant in Administrative Charge
Day Surgery Unit

OXFORDSHIRE HEALTH AUTHORITY

Tel: Oxford 64841
ext. 679

The Churchill Hospital,
Headington,
Oxford.

DAY SURGERY UNIT

TO BE GIVEN TO THE ESCORT OF:

Name ....

Please telephone between 12.30 and 13.30 hours to see when your friend or relative will be ready for collection, and be available to come when requested to do so. You should ask which car park to use.

PLEASE READ THE FOLLOWING INSTRUCTIONS CAREFULLY

The patient must be taken home by you in a private car or taxi and kept under observation for at least 12 hours.

You are reminded that the patient must not be allowed to drive a car or any other vehicle or to operate apparatus or machinery (including cookers) for 24 hours after discharge from the Day Surgery Unit.

You may be handed pain-killing tablets (and for some patients, anti-sickness tablets) to be given to the patient. Please keep them safe. You may also be given special written instructions for the patient, and a letter to be delivered to the General Practitioner.

Dr J. Millar
Consultant in Administrative Charge

If post-operative problems: Telephone Oxford 64841
Gynaecology Patients: ask for duty Gynaecological S.H.O.
Urology Patients; ask for Staff Nurse or Sister, Ward 15.
Others:

OAH 3314

DAY SURGERY UNIT

TO BE HANDED TO PATIENTS' ATTENDING OUT PATIENTS' <u>BEFORE</u> SEEING DOCTOR.

ASSESSMENT QUESTIONNAIRE

<u>NAME</u>:   <u>DATE</u>:

<u>RECORD NO</u>:

It is possible that you may need to come into hospital for an operation. It would be greatly appreciated if you could help by answering the following questions:

1. Do you suffer or have you suffered from any of the following:

		YES	NO
1.	Heart disease	☐	☐
2.	Palpitations	☐	☐
3.	High blood pressure	☐	☐
4.	Chest pains	☐	☐
5.	Swelling of ankles	☐	☐
6.	Shortness of breath	☐	☐
7.	Asthma	☐	☐
8.	Chronic cough	☐	☐
9.	Diabetes	☐	☐
10.	Epilepsy	☐	☐
11.	Heartburn	☐	☐
12.	Jaundice	☐	☐

Other diseases (Please list) ....

2. Are you taking any tablets, pills, inhalers,
    or medicine — for any reason?   ☐   ☐

If yes, please list ....

Please turn over . . .

	YES	NO
3. Have you any allergies?	☐	☐

If yes, please list ....

4. Do you smoke?	☐	☐

If yes, what and how many ....

5. Have you had any operations or anaesthetics before?	☐	☐

If yes, please list ....

Were there any complications? If so please give details ....

6. Do you have false, capped or loose teeth?	☐	☐
7. Is there anything about yourself or your family's medical history you think we should know?	☐	☐

If yes, please give details ....

It is possible you may be suitable for Day Case Surgery which would mean you would not have to spend the night in hospital. This will normally only be the case if you can answer "yes" to the following:

1. Would you like the opportunity to have your surgery done and be sent home all on the same day?	☐	☐
2. Would it be acceptable to you to have no premedication (premed) before surgery?	☐	☐
3. Can you make your own way to the Churchill Hospital by 8.00 a.m.?	☐	☐
4. Can someone collect you from the Churchill Hospital between 4 p.m. and 5 p.m. on a weekday?	☐	☐
5. Will there be a responsible and physically fit person available to look after you for the first night?	☐	☐

Thank you for your help.

O H 3315

INSTRUCTIONS FOR PATIENTS WHO HAVE HAD A GENERAL ANAESTHETIC

Anaesthetic drugs remain in the body for 24 hours, and gradually wear off over this time. During the 24 hours following your anaesthetic you are under the influence of drugs, and it is important to obey the following instructions:

1. Do not drive a car, or any other vehicle, including bicycles.

2. Do not operate machinery or appliances such as cookers or kettles.

3. Avoid alcohol.

4. Do not lock the bathroom or toilet door, or make yourself inaccessible to the person looking after you.

5. Drink plenty of fluids and eat a light diet, avoiding heavy or greasy foods.

6. Take things easy the day after your operation and do not work with machinery or take strenuous exercise.

7. Do not make important decisions, or sign important documents for 24 hours after your anaesthetic.

8. If there are any problems after your return home, please telephone the Churchill Hospital on Oxford (0865) 64841.
   Gynaecology Patients: ask for duty Gynaecological S.H.O.
   Urology Patients: ask for Staff Nurse or Sister, Ward 15, extension 418.
   Others:

O H 3316

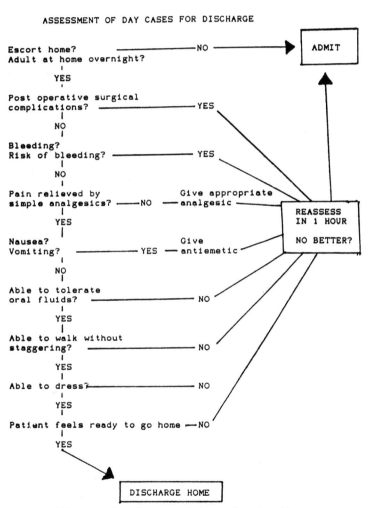

OXFORDSHIRE HEALTH AUTHORITY

ASSESSMENT OF DAY CASES FOR DISCHARGE

Escort home? ———————————NO ——————→ ADMIT
Adult at home overnight?
          |
        YES
          |
Post operative surgical
complications? ———————————— YES
          |
         NO
          |
Bleeding?
Risk of bleeding? ————————— YES
          |
         NO
          |
Pain relieved by   Give appropriate
simple analgesics? ———NO —analgesic
          |
        YES
          |
Nausea?   Give
Vomiting?   ———— YES — antiemetic
          |
         NO
          |
Able to tolerate
oral fluids?   ———————————— NO
          |
        YES
          |
Able to walk without
staggering?   ———————————— NO
          |
        YES
          |
Able to dress?————————————— NO
          |
        YES
          |
Patient feels ready to go home ——NO
          |
        YES

REASSESS
IN 1 HOUR

NO BETTER?

DISCHARGE HOME

- with a supply of appropriate analgesics if necessary
+ instructions not to drive, operate machinery, cook or
  drink alcohol for 24 hours postoperatively

MARFORMS

☑ CHECK PATIENT UNIT – PRESS FIRMLY

☐ **DAY SURGERY UNIT** (Yellow)

☐ **AM ADMIT UNIT** (Pink)

☐ **SHORT STAY UNIT** (Blue)

IMPORTANT

1. CHECK PATIENT UNIT AT LEFT.

2. REMOVE THE 2 INFORMATION
   SHEETS THAT DO NOT APPLY.

BRING THIS WITH YOU ON THE DAY OF YOUR PROCEDURE

HOSPITAL OF THE UNIVERSITY OF PENNSYLVANIA
3400 Spruce Street   Philadelphia, PA 19104-4283

DAY SURGERY UNIT PATIENT INFORMATION
662-3529 or 662-2312

You are to have surgery on _____ , 19 _____ , at _____ o'clock.

We ask that tests ordered by your surgeon be completed AT LEAST FIVE WORKING DAYS BEFORE you are scheduled for surgery so that they can be reviewed by the Day Surgery Unit's nurses and physicians. A member of the Day Surgery Unit staff will call you the day before your operation to tell you about our Unit and to answer any questions you may have. Occasionally we experience difficulty in reaching patients. If you have not been contacted by 3:00 P.M. the day before your surgery, please call the Unit (662-2312 or 662-2313) between 3:00 and 4:30 P.M.

To reach the Day Surgery Unit, take the Silverstein elevators to the 4th floor. PLEASE PLAN TO ARRIVE AT THE DAY SURGERY UNIT RECEPTION DESK AT _____ AM/PM (ONE HOUR BEFORE YOUR OPERATION). Once you arrive, you will be taken to the dressing area to await surgery and to see your anesthesiologist if you are to receive anesthesia care.

A member of our Unit will also call you the day after your operation to see how you are recovering.

Thank you for your help and cooperation. We look forward to caring for you in our Unit and will do our best to ensure that your experience with us is as safe and pleasant as possible.

Thomas J. Conahan, M.D.
Medical Director, Day Surgery Unit

YOUR COMPLIANCE WITH THE FOLLOWING PREREQUISITES IS MANDATORY TO AVOID DELAYS OR CANCELLATION OF YOUR OPERATION:

1) DO NOT SMOKE AND DO NOT EAT OR DRINK ANYTHING (NOT EVEN COFFEE, TEA, MINTS, GUM OR WATER) AFTER MIDNIGHT THE EVENING BEFORE SURGERY. (This is important to prevent vomiting during surgery which could have serious consequences for you.) TAKE NO MEDICATIONS UNLESS SO INSTRUCTED.

2) IF YOU ARE GOING TO HAVE GENERAL ANESTHESIA OR ARE GOING TO RECEIVE ANY SEDATIVE MEDICATIONS, YOU **MUST** HAVE AN ADULT TO ESCORT YOU HOME. YOU SHOULD HAVE A COMPANION AVAILABLE TO YOU AT HOME AFTER YOUR SURGERY.

3) SHOULD YOU HAVE A COLD OR OTHER ILLNESS THE DAY BEFORE SURGERY, OR SHOULD YOU BE UNABLE TO KEEP YOUR DAY SURGERY UNIT APPOINTMENT FOR ANY REASON, PLEASE CALL THE UNIT IMMEDIATELY SO THAT YOU MAY BE RESCHEDULED OR EVALUATED FURTHER.

4) IF YOU ARE NOT HOME THE DAY PRIOR TO SURGERY, PLEASE CALL THE UNIT (662-2312 or 662-2313) BETWEEN 3:00 and 4:30 P.M. FOR INSTRUCTIONS.

5) PLEASE ARRIVE AT LEAST ONE (1) HOUR BEFORE YOUR OPERATION IS SCHEDULED.

DAY SURGERY UNIT

☑ CHECK PATIENT UNIT – PRESS FIRMLY

IMPORTANT

☐ **DAY SURGERY UNIT** (Yellow)

1. CHECK PATIENT UNIT AT LEFT.

☐ **AM ADMIT UNIT** (Pink)

2. REMOVE THE 2 INFORMATION SHEETS THAT DO NOT APPLY.

☐ **SHORT STAY UNIT** (Blue)

BRING THIS WITH YOU ON THE DAY OF YOUR PROCEDURE

HOSPITAL OF THE UNIVERSITY OF PENNSYLVANIA
3400 Spruce Street   Philadelphia, PA 19104-4283

AM ADMIT PATIENT INFORMATION
662-6450

You are to have surgery on _____ , 19 ____ and are to be admitted to the Hospital of the University of Pennsylvania after your surgery.

Your blood tests and any other tests that have been ordered <u>MUST</u> be completed <u>FIVE DAYS BEFORE</u> your procedure is scheduled.

You will be contacted by the AM Admit nurse coordinator the day prior to your scheduled surgery. Occasionally we experience difficulty in reaching patients. If you have not been contacted the day before your operation or if there are any questions, please call the nurse coordinator (662-6450) between the hours of 3:00 p.m. and 6:00 p.m. On the day of operation, please plan to arrive at the <u>ADMISSIONS OFFICE.</u> From there, you will be escorted to the AM Admit - Short Stay Unit on 1 Dulles to await surgery and to see an anesthesiologist if you are to receive anesthesia care. Clothing, dentures, valuables, etc., will either be sent with you to the operating room in a patient belonging bag, or be given to a friend or family member for safe keeping.

Should you have a cold or other illness the day before surgery, or should you be unable to keep your appointment for any reason, call both your doctor's office and the AM Admit nurse coordinator immediately so that you may be rescheduled or evaluated further.

If you are to receive anesthesia (other than local), an anesthesiologist will also call you the day prior to your operation to familiarize you with our procedures and to answer any questions you may have.

DO NOT SMOKE AND DO NOT EAT OR DRINK ANYTHING INCLUDING WATER, MINTS OR GUM AFTER MIDNIGHT, THE EVENING BEFORE SURGERY. This is important to prevent vomiting during surgery which could have serious consequences for you. Take no medications or water unless so instructed.

Thank you for your help and we look forward to caring for you.

Operating Room Team
Hospital of the University of Pennsylvania

AM ADMIT UNIT

☑ CHECK PATIENT UNIT — PRESS FIRMLY

☐ **DAY SURGERY UNIT** (Yellow)

☐ **AM ADMIT UNIT** (Pink)

☐ **SHORT STAY UNIT** (Blue)

IMPORTANT

1. CHECK PATIENT UNIT AT LEFT.

2. REMOVE THE 2 INFORMATION SHEETS THAT DO NOT APPLY.

BRING THIS WITH YOU ON THE DAY OF YOUR PROCEDURE

HOSPITAL OF THE UNIVERSITY OF PENNSYLVANIA
3400 Spruce Street   Philadelphia, PA 19104-4283

SHORT STAY PATIENT INFORMATION
662-6450

You are to have a procedure on _____ , 19 _____ .

Your blood tests and any other tests that have been ordered <u>MUST</u> be completed <u>FIVE DAYS</u> <u>BEFORE</u> your procedure is scheduled.

You will be contacted by the nurse coordinator the day prior to your scheduled procedure. Occasionally we experience difficulty reaching patients. If you have not been contacted or if there are any questions, please call the nurse coordinator (662-6450) between the hours of 3:00 p.m. and 6:00 p.m. the day before your procedure. On the day of your procedure, please plan to arrive at the <u>SHORT STAY UNIT ON</u> <u>THE FIRST FLOOR OF THE DULLES BUILDING</u> at the appointed time. You will await your procedure there and see an anesthesiologist if you are to receive anesthesia care. Clothing, dentures, valuables, etc., will be placed in a locked closet.

Should you have a cold or other illness the day before your procedure, or should you be unable to keep your appointment for any reason, call both your doctor's office and the nurse coordinator immediately so that you may be rescheduled or evaluated further.

If you are to receive anesthesia (other than local), an anesthesiologist will also call you the day prior to your procedure to familiarize you with our Unit and to answer any questions you may have.

DO NOT SMOKE AND DO NOT EAT OR DRINK ANYTHING, INCLUDING WATER, MINTS OR GUM AFTER MIDNIGHT, THE EVENING BEFORE YOUR PROCEDURE. This is important to prevent vomiting which could have serious consequences for you. Take no medications or water unless so instructed.

Following your procedure you may spend about an hour in the recovery room before returning to the Short Stay Unit. You will remain in the Unit until you are ready for discharge home.

YOU MUST HAVE AN ADULT TO ACCOMPANY YOU HOME OR YOUR PROCEDURE MAY BE CANCELLED. You should also have a companion available to you at home after your procedure.

Thank you for your help and we look forward to caring for you.

Short Stay Unit
Hospital of the University of Pennsylvania

132068 6-88 Copyright ©HUP   **SHORT STAY UNIT**

☐ **DAY SURGERY UNIT** (Yellow)

☐ **AM ADMIT UNIT** (Pink)

☐ **SHORT STAY UNIT** (Blue)

HISTORY NO.

NAME

RACE

AGE

SEX

Imprint with Name Plate or Print Patient's Name, Hosp. No. & Physician

TO BE COMPLETED BY SURGEON

MINIMUM STUDIES FOR PHYSICAL STATUS I & II PATIENTS.

(When in doubt about need for a study, contact one of the designated anesthesia consultants)

	Under Age 40	Over Age 40	Over Age 60	Diuretic or Antihypertensive Use
☐ CBC	YES	YES	YES	YES
☐ EKG	NO	YES	YES	YES
☐ Chest X-Ray	NO	NO	YES	YES
☐ SMA-6	NO	NO	YES	YES
☐ OTHER				

OPERATIVE
PROCEDURE: _____

_____
Requesting Physician's Signature
(Must be present to obtain studies)

SURGEON TO COMPLETE FOR AM ADMIT AND SHORT STAY PATIENTS ONLY

PATIENT'S OLD RECORDS REQUESTED	☐ YES ☐ NO	INITIALS/DATE _____
OLD RECORD FORWARDED TO AM ADMIT-SHORT STAY UNIT	☐ YES ☐ NO	INITIALS/DATE _____

HISTORY AND PHYSICAL EXAM:

SENT TO ADMISSIONS WITH PATIENT	☐ YES ☐ NO	INITIALS/DATE _____
TO BE FORWARDED BY SURGEON'S OFFICE	☐ YES ☐ NO	INITIALS/DATE _____

HEALTH SURVEY QUESTIONNAIRE — TO BE COMPLETED BY ALL PATIENTS

Dear Patient:

We welcome the opportunity to participate in your medical care. To save you an extra trip to the hospital, we depend on your surgeon to evaluate your health and to order appropriate studies. We depend on you to provide accurate health screening information on this form.

To help us, please complete the following survey.

Thank you for your help and we look forward to caring for you.

Hospital of the University of Pennsylvania

NAME	DATE SURVEY FILLED OUT

STREET ADDRESS	CITY	STATE	ZIP CODE

AGE	HEIGHT	WEIGHT	HOME TELEPHONE	OTHER TELEPHONE

HOSPITAL OF THE UNIVERSITY OF PENNSYLVANIA

List All Allergies
(including medication allergies)

_____

_____

_____

_____

List All Medicines You Now Take

_____

_____

_____

_____

List All Medications You Have Taken In The Past
Five Years.

_____

_____

_____

_____

List All Medical Illnesses You Have Had

_____

_____

_____

_____

List All Operations You Have Had

OPERATION	DATE
_____	_____
_____	_____
_____	_____
_____	_____

	NO	YES	
1. Have you ever had a problem with anesthesia other than nausea or vomiting?	☐	☐	_____
2. Has anyone related to you ever had a problem with anesthesia other than nausea or vomiting?	☐	☐	_____
3. Could you be pregnant?	☐	☐	_____
4. Do you smoke? If so, how many packs per day?	☐	☐	_____
5. Do you have a cough?	☐	☐	_____
6. Do you bring anything up when you cough?	☐	☐	_____
7. Have you had asthma?	☐	☐	_____
8. Do you have a cold?	☐	☐	_____
9. Can you walk up two flights of stairs without getting short of breath?	☐	☐	_____
10. Have you had any difficulties with breathing?	☐	☐	_____
11. Do you have any bleeding tendencies?	☐	☐	_____
12. Have you ever been anemic?	☐	☐	_____

	NO	YES	
13. Do you have a heart murmur?	☐	☐	_____
14. Have you ever had a heart attack?	☐	☐	_____
15. Have you ever had angina or pain in the chest related to your heart?	☐	☐	_____
16. Have you ever had high blood pressure?	☐	☐	_____
17. Do you ever wake up short of breath at night?	☐	☐	_____
18. Do you have diabetes?	☐	☐	_____
19. Have you had significant weight loss in the past 4 months without trying to diet?	☐	☐	_____
20. Have you ever had thyroid problems?	☐	☐	_____
21. Have you ever had an abnormal chest x-ray?	☐	☐	_____
22. Have you ever had a stroke?	☐	☐	_____
23. Have you ever had epilepsy, seizures or falling out?	☐	☐	_____
24. Do you have frequent headaches?	☐	☐	_____
25. Have you ever had eye problems?	☐	☐	_____
26. Have you ever had kidney disease?	☐	☐	_____
27. Have you ever been jaundiced?	☐	☐	_____
28. Have you ever had hepatitis?	☐	☐	_____
29. Have you ever had an arm or leg become numb or weak?	☐	☐	_____
30. Do you have any physical disabilities?	☐	☐	_____
31. Do you have any chipped or loose teeth, dentures, caps, bridgework or braces?	☐	☐	_____
32. Would you describe yourself as being extremely anxious about your pending procedure?	☐	☐	_____
33. Have you ever been under the care of a psychiatrist?	☐	☐	_____

STATEMENT OF PATIENT COMPLIANCE

1) I AM AWARE OF THE DANGER TO ME OF FOOD OR LIQUID (INCLUDING WATER, COFFEE, OR TEA) IN MY STOMACH DURING ANESTHESIA AND I <u>CERTIFY</u> THAT I HAVE HAD NOTHING TO EAT OR DRINK SINCE MIDNIGHT.

NOTE EXCEPTIONS: _____

_____
(Local anesthesia, water with prescribed morning medication, etc.)

2) **FOR PATIENTS BEING DISCHARGED ON THE DAY OF SURGERY:**
I CERTIFY THAT I HAVE AN ESCORT HOME WHOSE NAME IS:

_____

PATIENT SIGNATURE _____

WITNESS _____

DATE _____

PRE-OP CHECKLIST

CIRCLE ONE:

1. FALSE TEETH: None/Removed

      If Removed: _____ Given to family member/friend

      _____ Other

2. PROSTHESES: (Wig, Contact lenses, Eyeglasses, Artificial limb, etc.)

      Describe _____

      None/Removed

      If removed: _____ Given to family member/friend

      _____ Other

3. VALUABLES: None/Removed

      If Removed _____ Given to family member/friend

      _____ Locker No. _____ Other

4. ID BRACELET VERIFICATION

      L Wrist / R Wrist   (circle one)

RN SIGNATURE _____ DATE _____

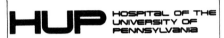

HUP HOSPITAL OF THE
UNIVERSITY OF
PENNSYLVANIA

DAY SURGERY UNIT
662-3529
662-2312

HISTORY NO.

NAME

RACE

AGE

SEX

Imprint with Name Plate or Print Patient's Name, Hosp. No. & Phys'n

DAY SURGERY UNIT POST OPERATIVE INSTRUCTIONS

1. Do not drive or operate hazardous machinery for 24 hours.
2. Do not make important personal or business decisions for 24 hours.
3. Do not drink alcoholic beverages for 24 hours.
4. Eat light foods (jello, soups, etc.) as you can tolerate them without feeling sick to your stomach.
5. Drink as much water or carbonated beverages (cola, 7-up, etc.) as you can tolerate, up to eight glasses a day.
6. If your bandages become soaked with bright red blood, place another dressing pad over your bandages. (Do not remove the original bandage.) Call your surgeon for further instructions. A small amount of bright red blood is to be expected.
7. Limit your activities for 24 hours. Do not engage in heavy-work until your surgeon gives you permission.
8. Report the following signs or any questions regarding your physical condition to your surgeon immediately:
   * Excessive swelling of or around the wound area.
   * Redness
   * Temperature of 100° F or above.
   * Excessive pain.

SPECIAL INSTRUCTIONS AND MEDICATIONS

1. _____
2. _____
3. _____
4. _____
5. _____
6. _____

FOLLOW UP APPOINTMENT

DATE _____ TIME _____

CALL _____ FOR APPOINTMENT TIME

_____ M.D.
Physician Signature

INSTRUCTIONS GIVEN BY:

_____ M.D./R.N.

PATIENT ACKNOWLEDGEMENT:

_____
Patient Signature

_____
Date

Rev. 9/82

WHITE — MEDICAL RECORDS   YELLOW — PATIENT COPY

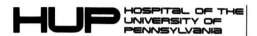

DAY SURGERY

PATIENT FLOW SHEET

(IMPRINT WITH PATIENT PLATE)

PREOPERATIVE INSTRUCTIONS	POSTOPERATIVE FOLLOW UP

PREOPERATIVE INSTRUCTIONS

Date/Time called _____

Nurse/MD _____

Patient informed NPO after midnight _____

   No food after 8PM _____

   May have clear liquids from 8PM to 12M _____

   After 12M nothing to eat or drink _____

   In AM nothing to eat or drink (no mints, gum, smoking) _____

Patient informed when to arrive in unit (one hour prior

   to surgery) _____ Hr.

Location of unit (fourth floor Dulles) _____

Parking facilities (Hilton, Civic Center, etc.) _____

Attire—suggest loose fitting clothing, flat shoes, no makeup,

   no jewelry, glasses vs. contact lenses _____

Instruct patient not to bring money, jewelry, valuables, etc.

   with them _____

Health survey reviewed with patient   Yes/No

   Does patient have a cold _____

Has patient had an illness since they last saw their

    surgeon _____

Anesthesia questions _____

_____

_____

   Use of medications _____

_____ MD

Recommend a shower or bath the evening before or morning

   of surgery _____

Has patient made arrangements for someone to take them

   home? _____

    Inform patient that individual must accompany patient to

      and from unit _____

    Inform patient that they must have a responsible adult with

      them the evening of surgery _____

    Inform patient that there are waiting facilities for visitors _____

    Inform patient of the expected length of stay _____

Special instructions_____

Patient comments or concerns_____

_____

_____

Instructor's impression _____

_____

POSTOPERATIVE FOLLOW UP

Date/Time called_____

Nurse/MD_____

Has patient resumed ADL's (Activities of Daily Living)?   Yes/No

   If not why not?_____

_____

_____

Is patient tolerating liquids/solids/normal diet?   Yes/No

Any nausea or vomiting?   Yes/No   If so when?   Number of

   episodes? _____

_____

   What did patient do for relief? _____

Does patient have pain?   Yes/No   If so describe? (duration, location

   etc.)_____

_____

   State factors which alleviated pain._____

   Was pain medication prescribed?   Yes/No   Was pain

     medication effective?

Is dressing/cast dry and intact?   Yes/No _____

Is there any drainage?   Yes/No   If so describe? _____

_____

Is there swelling, redness at operative site?   Yes/No   If so explain

_____

Neurovascular check if applicable _____

_____

Did patient exhibit any of the following?

   Muscular discomfort?   Yes/No   Sore throat?   Yes/No

   Headache?   Yes/No   Elevated temp.?   Yes/No

   Pain at IV site?   Yes/No   Voiding difficulties?   Yes/No

Review of postoperative instructions.   Yes/No

What are patient's concerns/comments about experience?_____

_____

Was surgeon/anesthesiologist contacted regarding any of the above?

   Yes/No _____

_____

Additional follow up necessary?   Yes/No_____

UCSF SURGERY CENTER

Preoperative Health Questionnaire

Patient's Name_____ Age_____ Sex_____ Today's date_____

Planned operation_____ Date of Surgery_____ Surgeon_____

Home phone_____ Work phone_____ Best time to call_____

Questions answered by_____ Relation to patient_____

	Yes	No	?	Comments
General Health				
1. Do you excercise regularly? (Describe)	❑	❑	❑	_____
2. Are you limited in your activity? (Describe daily activity)	❑	❑	❑	_____
3. Are you ill now or were you recently ill? (cold, fever, chills or flu)	❑	❑	❑	_____
4. Are you **ALLERGIC** to any medicines? (List)	❑	❑	❑	_____
5. Women: Could you be pregnant?	❑	❑	❑	_____
6. Do you or did you ever smoke? (Quantify in packs/day for ? years)	❑	❑	❑	_____
7. Do you drink alcohol? (How much?)	❑	❑	❑	_____
8. Do you have a productive cough? (Describe recent changes.)	❑	❑	❑	_____
9. LIST ALL MEDICINES YOU NOW TAKE (INCLUDE "OVER-THE-COUNTER" DRUGS)				_____ _____ _____
Medical History				
10. Do you have or have you had any problems with your heart? (Describe nature of problem, e.g., chest pain, high blood pressure, heart attack, abnormal ECG, skipped beats.)	❑	❑	❑	_____
11. Do you have or have you had any problems with your lungs or chest? (Describe nature of problem, e.g.,shortness of breath, chest pain, emphysema, bronchitis, asthma, TB, abnormal chest x-ray.)	❑	❑	❑	_____
12. Have you or anyone in your family had a serious bleeding problem? (Prolonged bleeding from nosebleed, teeth and gums, tooth extractions, surgery?)	❑	❑	❑	_____
13. Have you ever been anemic? (Have you ever had black/tarry stools, heavy periods, coffee ground emesis?)	❑	❑	❑	_____
14. Do you have diabetes? (Do you wake up at night to urinate; have excessive thirst?)	❑	❑	❑	_____
15. Have you ever been treated for cancer with chemo- or radiation therapy?	❑	❑	❑	_____

	Yes	No	?	Comments

16. Have you ever had any problem with your:

Liver (cirrhosis, hepatitis, jaundice, malaria)? ❑ ❑ ❑ _____

Kidney (stones, infection, failure, dialysis)? ❑ ❑ ❑ _____

Blood (anemia, leukemia, sickle cell disease)? ❑ ❑ ❑ _____

Thyroid gland? ❑ ❑ ❑ _____

Back or neck? ❑ ❑ ❑ _____

Muscle cramps or spasms? ❑ ❑ ❑ _____

Digestive system (heartburn, hiatal hernia, ulcer)? ❑ ❑ ❑ _____

17. Have you ever had:

Frequent and/or severe headaches? ❑ ❑ ❑ _____

Epilepsy, fits, or seizures? ❑ ❑ ❑ _____

Stroke, leg or arm weakness? ❑ ❑ ❑ _____

18. **LIST ALL MEDICAL ILLNESSES** _____

_____

_____

19. **LIST ALL OPERATIONS** _____

_____

_____

Anesthesia and Surgery

20. Have you or any blood relative ever had problems with anesthesia or surgery? (nausea, vomiting, hyperthermia, prolonged drowsiness, anxiety) ❑ ❑ ❑ _____

21. Do you have a problem with motion sickness? ❑ ❑ ❑ _____

22. Do you have any particular concerns about your anesthesia? (anxiety, fears, questions) ❑ ❑ ❑ _____

23. Do you have any particular concerns about your surgery? (anxiety, fears, questions) ❑ ❑ ❑ _____

24. Do you have any chipped or loose teeth, dentures, caps, bridgework or braces? ❑ ❑ ❑ _____

25. **ADDITIONAL COMMENTS**_____

END OF QUESTIONNAIRE, THANK YOU.
Adapted from the SKR Preoperative Patient Questionnaire and HUP Day Surgery Unit Health Survey

R.N. Review: ❑ Phone ❑ In-Person Date_____ Time_____ RN_____

Vital signs: BP_____P_____ RR_____ T°_____ WEIGHT (KG)_____

Comments_____

1/31/89

UCSF SURGERY CENTER
Preoperative Evaluation for Anesthesia

Proposed Operation _____

Age _____   Male   Female   **Scheduled date** _____

Pertinent History

_____

_____

Past Medical History	date	procedure	anesthetic	complications

no ❑   Previous surgery   _____   _____   _____   _____

no ❑   Anesthetic problems in past or in family   _____

no ❑   **Medical problems** _____

no ❑   Cardiac   _____

no ❑   Respiratory   _____

no ❑   **Pregnant?**   ❑ yes or uncertain **(note below in special considerations)**

no ❑   **Allergies** _____

no ❑   **Present medications**_____

no ❑   Other drugs   _____

	no	yes	comments
Smoking	❑	❑	_____
Alcohol	❑	❑	_____
Dentures	❑	❑	_____
Contact lens	❑	❑	_____
Other	❑	❑	_____

Physical Exam   Wt _____kg   T° _____   BP _____/_____   P _____   RR _____   Height _____

normal	abnormal findings	normal		abnormal findings
❑ Airway _____		❑ Dental	_____	
❑ Neck _____		❑ Chest	_____	
❑ Cardiac_____		❑ Neurologic	_____	
❑ Musculoskeletal _____		Other	_____	

Laboratory Data   Hct _____   ECG_____   CXR_____

Other lab _____

Special Considerations_____

Evaluated by _____ M.D.__ __ __ __   _____   _____

Signature   Date   Time

Day of Surgery NPO for _____ hours   **ASA Physical Status**_____   **Anesthetic Plan:** General   Regional   MAC

Consent ❑ Anesthetic procedures and risks explained to patient; all questions answered.   ❑ Above history and physical reviewed.

Comments_____

Evaluated by _____ M.D.__ __ __ __   _____   _____

Date   Time

Attending Anesthesiologist_____ M.D.__ __ __ __   _____   _____

Date   Time

UCSF Surgery Center
Post Anesthesia Care Unit
STANDING ORDERS

1. Admit to PAR.

2. Vital Signs
   Phase I: On admission and every 15 minutes until transfer to Phase II Recovery Area.
   Phase II: On transfer and every 30 minutes until discharge.
   Temperature every hour.

3. Oxygen Therapy
   Adults: 3 l/min O_2 via nasal prongs until awake and responsive, then discontinue.
   Children: 40% O_2/air mixture via face tent or cup until awake and responsive, then discontinue.

4. IV Fluid
   ☐ 2 ml/kg/hour of fluid given intraoperatively. Discontinue i.v. just before discharge.

   _____

5. PAR Medications
   Pain: ☐ Fentanyl 0.2 µg/kg iv q 3 min prn pain. Contact anesthesiologist after 8 doses.

   _____

   Nausea: ☐ Droperidol 10 µg/kg iv q 10 min prn nausea. Contact anesthesiologist after 4 doses.

   _____

6. Activity: Gradual progression as tolerated. Increase head of bed as tolerated.

7. Call anesthesiologist for:
   • systolic blood pressure < 90 mmHg or > 180 mmHg; diastolic blood pressure > 110 mmHg.
   • heart rate < 50 bpm or > 120 bpm.
   • respiratory rate < 8/min or > 30/min.
   • urine output < 0.5 ml/kg/hour if a catheter is present.
   • any cardiac dysrhythmia.

8. Discharge: May occur when discharge criteria are met and on the written order of a physician. Discharge
   instructions are to be reviewed with the patient and acknowledgement of these instructions documented.
   Patients given general anesthesia, regional anesthesia or sedative drugs will be discharged with a
   responsible person. Discharge medications per surgeon (below).

9. Other_____

   _____

_____M.D.___ ___ ___ ___ Date_____Time_____
Anesthesiologist/Surgeon

LOCAL ANESTHETIC ONLY: Discharge when discharge criteria are met. Review discharge instructions.

DISCHARGE MEDICATIONS: ☐ Tylenol #3,_tabs orally every___hours prn pain. DISP_____

_____

_____

_____M.D.___ ___ ___ ___ Date_____Time_____
Surgeon

Version 2/24/89

Surgery Center
(415) 476-8384
Home Care Instructions
Child

Your child was given an anesthetic for surgery today.

You may expect your child to:
- be sleepy during the day, but he/she should arouse easily.
- have some nausea or vomiting, but this should not persist.
- have some discomfort depending on the type of surgery, but this should not be excessive.
- have a sore throat.

We recommend you:
- return directly home with your child so that he/she may rest for the remainder of the day.
- **not** expose your child to situations that require quick reflexes such as using stairs or riding a bicycle.
- allow your child to eat as he/she desires. Begin with a light diet (**clear** juice, soup, jello) then progress to more solid food as tolerated. Babies may be fed as soon as they are awake and hungry.
- telephone your surgeon if you notice any unusual redness, drainage, bleeding, pain or fever.

Special Instructions for _____
Surgical procedure

Activity
resume normal activity	as tolerated	in _____ days
resume strenuous/playground activity	as tolerated	in _____ days
return to school	as tolerated	in _____ days

Care of the Incision
keep the area clean and dry; trim or replace any loose dressing material;
keep your child from scratching the incision as much as possible

Bathing
You may bathe your child: anytime   wait _____ days

For Pain
Give_____every_____ hours if needed for discomfort.

Other medications and instructions:

_____

If your child has any peculiar behavior (excessive sleepiness, vomiting, excessive pain) or if anything concerns you, call your surgeon, Dr. _____at_____ .

If you are unable to reach your surgeon, call UCSF at 476-1000 and ask the operator to connect you with the surgical resident on-call for the_____ surgery service.

In an emergency, contact your local hospital's Emergency Room.

688-04 2/88

Return Appointment Date_____	**Instructions given by:**
Day_____Time_____ a.m. p.m.	_____R.N.
Phone_____ for an appointment	**Instructions received by:**
Dr._____	
	parent or guardian date

SURGERY CENTER HOME CARE INSTRUCTIONS - CHILD

Surgery Center
(415) 476-8384
Home Care Instructions
Adult

You were given an anesthetic for surgery today.

You may expect to:
- be sleepy during the day, but not excessively so.
- have some nausea or vomiting, but this should not persist.
- have some discomfort depending on the type of surgery, but this should not be excessive.
- have a sore throat.

We recommend you:
- return directly home so that you can rest for the remainder of the day.
- begin with a light diet (**clear** juice, soup, jello) then progress to more solid food as tolerated.
- drink as much water or carbonated beverages as you can.

Do not drive a car or operate hazardous machinery for at least 24 hours.
Do not make important personal or business decisions for at least 24 hours.
Do not drink alcoholic beverages for 24 hours.
Call your surgeon if you notice any unusual redness, drainage, bleeding, pain, or fever.

Special Instructions for _____
                                        Surgical procedure

Activity
     resume normal activity   as tolerated   in_____days
     resume strenuous activity   as tolerated   in_____days

Care of the Incision
     keep the area clean and dry; trim or replace any loose dressing material; avoid scratching the incision

Bathing
     You may bathe: anytime   wait_____days

For Pain
       Take   (circle)   **Tylenol #3**   (or write in drug)_____
       _____ **tablets by mouth every** _____ **hours as needed for discomfort.**

Other medications and instructions:

If anything concerns you, call your surgeon, Dr. _____at_____.
If you are unable to reach your surgeon, call UCSF at 476-1000 and ask the operator to
connect you with the surgical resident on-call for the_____surgery service.
        In an emergency, contact your local hospital's emergency room.

688-03 2/88

Return Appointment Date_____	**Instructions given by:**
Day_____Time_____ a.m. p.m.	_____R.N.
Phone_____ for an appointment	**Instructions received by:**
Dr._____	patient or guardian date

UCSF
The Medical Center
at the University of California, San Francisco
San Francisco, California 94143

SURGERY CENTER HOME CARE INSTRUCTIONS - ADULT

The Methodist Medical Center of Illinois
Ambulatory SurgiCare

Preoperative Instructions

Arrive at _____ □ AM □ PM on Day: _____ Date: _____ Your surgery is
scheduled for _____ , however, unforeseen circumstances may result in
delays. Our staff will attempt to keep you informed, but feel free to make inquiries at the
Reception Desk.

- Do not have anything to eat or drink (no water, gum, mints, coffee, juice) after midnight the
  night before your surgery. **This may not apply to medications prescribed by your
  physician. Please note special instructions.**

- Do not drink any alcoholic beverages for 24 hours before or after your surgery.

- Park your car in parking deck I on level 2A or 2B and bring your parking ticket to the unit to
  be validated.

- You must have someone with you to drive you home. You must have a responsible person with
  you the rest of the day of surgery and also during the night. You should not drive a car for 24
  hours following your surgery.

- You should wear comfortable clothes. Do not bring a large amount of money or jewelry. Do not
  wear make-up, particularly mascara, the morning of your surgery. You should wear your
  glasses instead of contacts. You should shower or bathe the evening before or morning of surgery.

- You have received a Patient Information Booklet regarding Ambulatory SurgiCare from your
  doctor or from the unit. Please read the information and instructions prior to the day of surgery.

- You understand if you do not follow the instructions or if your physical condition changes your
  surgery may be canceled.

You have had the following done today:

    □ Blood   □ Urine   □ EKG   □ Chest x-ray   □ Other_____

Special Instructions: _____

_____

□ by telephone   □ in person
□ Patient verbalized understanding of all indicated instructions.
□ Needs Reinforcement

I have read above statements. These statements have verbally been communicated to me. I
understand these instructions and my questions have been answered.

    Patient Stamp   _____

                                     Patient Signature

                                     _____

                                     MASC Personnel Signature

                                     _____ _____

                                     Time   Date

MASC   The Methodist Medical Center
Phase II   of Illinois

Date_____ Time in_____ Time out_____

Operation_____

Anesthesia   General   ☐
             Regional   ☐
             Local with
             sedation   ☐
             Local   ☐
             ET   ☐

Time		
BP V A	240	
	220	
	200	
	180	
	160	
Pulse ●	140	
	120	
	100	
	80	
Resp. ○	60	
	40	
	20	
	0	
Temp		

Discharge Criteria

☐ Vital signs stable

☐ Swallow, cough **present**

☐ Able to ambulate

☐ Dressings checked   ☐ Take home medication   ☐ Nausea, vomiting, dizziness minimal

☐ Voided   ☐ Authorization signed   ☐ Absence of respiratory distress

☐ Patient given discharge instruction sheet   ☐ Alert and oriented

☐ Responsible adult present to escort patient home   ☐ Postanesthesia recovery score 10

Medications	Nurses Notes

_____ **R.N.**
      Signature of RN discharging patient

_____ **M.D.**
         Responsible Physician

Discharge criteria, Methodist Ambulatory SurgiCare

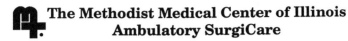

The Methodist Medical Center of Illinois
Ambulatory SurgiCare

Home Care Instructions
Local Anesthesia

Activity
You may resume activities of daily living as your doctor directs you.

Medications
You may have some pain. A prescription for pain may be given by the doctor. This should be taken as directed. If it does not help the pain, contact your doctor. If your doctor does not prescribe anything for pain, then you may take a non-prescription, non-aspirin pain medication such as, Tylenol or Advil. Please be sure to follow directions on the label. Take all pain medication with some food to prevent upset stomach.

Diet
Progress slowly to a regular diet. Start by taking liquids such as water or carbonated soft drinks. If you have no nausea try soup and crackers and, finally solid foods.

When to Call the Doctor
If you develop:
- A fever over 101° orally.
- Pain not relieved by pain medication.
- Any bleeding or unexpected drainage from the wound.
- Extreme redness or swelling around the incision.

Where to Call with Questions
- Your doctor. If unable to reach your doctor, then call:
  - Ambulatory SurgiCare - **672-5935** open 7:00 a.m. to 5:00 p.m., Monday through Friday
  - At night and on weekends, phone the Emergency Room - 672-5500.

Follow-Up Appointment _____

Additional Instructions _____
_____
_____

I have received and understand the above instructions.

_____   _____
(Patient Signature)   (Nurse's Signature)

                                           _____
                                                       (Date)

The Methodist Medical Center of Illinois
Ambulatory SurgiCare

Patient Acknowledgment and Agreement

☐ **This Applies To All Patients**

1. To the best of my knowledge the information on the Patient Questionnaire is correct.

2. I understand if a condition develops during my surgery or during my recovery and my doctor feels that it is necessary to admit me to the medical center to aid in my recovery, my doctor will admit me as an inpatient.

3. I will call my doctor if I have any unusual bleeding, respiratory problems or severe pain after my release from Ambulatory Surgery to home.

☐ **In Addition To Items 1, 2, and 3 Above, This Applies to Patients Receiving General/Regional Anesthesia Or Sedation.**

1. I have read and I understand the Patient Instructions I have been given. I have a responsible person to accompany me home after I leave the medical center and I understand that it would be best to have a person remain with me through the first night after my surgery.

2. I did not drink any liquid or eat any food after the time listed in my instructions. I have taken my medicine as I was told to do.

3. I understand that for twenty-four (24) hours following my surgery, I should not:
   • Drive a car
   • Operate any machinery or power tools
   • Drink any alcoholic beverages
   • Make any important decisions

_____	_____
Witness	Patient
_____	_____
Date	Responsible Person for the Patient
	_____
	Relationship

Consent 24-AS 1-Rev. 8/89

The Methodist Medical Center of Illinois
Ambulatory SurgiCare

Patient Preanesthesia/Surgery Questionnaire

Name————————————— Age ————— Weight ————— Height —————

Date/Time of Operation ————————————————— Arrival Time —————————

Person to drive you home_____ Phone# _____

1. Please tell us if you have or have had any of the following; if you check yes, please explain.
   Blood pressure problems: □Yes □ No_____
   Heart problems/chest pain: □Yes □ No_____
   Hepatitis/jaundice: □Yes □ No _____
   Bleeding problems: □Yes □ No_____
   Diabetes: □Yes □ No _____
   Epilepsy/seizures/severe headache: □Yes □ No _____
   Asthma/breathing problem: □Yes □ No_____
   Loose, false or capped teeth: □Yes □ No _____

2. List any major illnesses other than usual childhood illnesses: _____
   _____
   _____

3. List any operations you have had: _____
   _____
   _____

4. List any medicines, steroids, inhalers or drugs you take now or have taken in the past year.
   _____

	Yes	No
5. Have you or a blood relative ever had a problem with an anesthetic?	□	□
6. Are you allergic to local anesthesia, any medicines, iodine or tape?	□	□
7. Date of last period: ————— Could you possibly be pregnant?	□	□
8. Do you smoke? _____	□	□

(Please check if you take any medicine, injections or pills for:)
    □ Heart   □ Lungs   □ Diabetes   □ Kidney   □ Blood Pressure

Patients, please do not write below the double line - for use of Anesthesia Department.

Anesthesia Note

    □ NPO   □ Chart Reviewed   □ Lab Data Reviewed

    □ Anesthesia management and risk explained to patient/responsible party

    □ Patient's condition satisfactory to proceed with anesthesia as planned

    □ General   □ Regional   □ Local with Sedation

Date_____ Time_____ Signature _____

The Methodist Medical Center of Illinois
Ambulatory SurgiCare

Home Care Instructions   ☐ Local With Sedation
                              ☐ General Anesthesia

Activity
You might feel a little sleepy for the next 24 hours. This is due to the medicine you received to relax you. For the next 24 hours you should not:
- Drive a car, operate machinery or power tools.
- Drink any alcoholic beverages, including beer.
- Make any important decisions or sign important papers.

You should have a responsible adult with you for the rest of the day and during the night. This is for your own safety and protection. You may be up and about according to doctor's instructions.

Medications
You may have some pain. A prescription for pain may be given by the doctor. This should be taken as directed. If it does not help the pain, contact your doctor. If your doctor does not prescribe anything for pain, then you may take a non-prescription, non-aspirin pain medication such as, Tylenol or Advil. Please be sure to follow directions on the label. Take all pain medication with some food to prevent upset stomach.

Diet
Progress slowly to a regular diet. Start by taking liquids such as water or carbonated soft drinks. If you have no nausea try soup and crackers and, finally solid foods.

When to Call the Doctor
If you develop:
- A fever over 101° orally.
- Pain not relieved by pain medication.
- Any bleeding or unexpected drainage from the wound.
- Extreme redness or swelling around the incision.

Where to Call with Questions
- Your doctor. If unable to reach your doctor, then call:
  - Ambulatory SurgiCare - **672-5935** open 7:00 a.m. to 5:00 p.m., Monday through Friday
  - At night and on weekends, phone the Emergency Room at - 672-5500.

Follow-Up Appointment _____

Additional Instructions _____

_____

_____

I have received and understand the above instructions.

_____   _____
    (Patient Signature)   (Nurse's Signature)

_____   _____
 (Responsible Party's Signature)   (Date)

**The Methodist Medical Center of Illinois
Ambulatory SurgiCare**

Home Care Instructions
Epidural Anesthesia

Activity:
- Rest at home; no strenuous activity is recommended for the rest of the day and during the night unless otherwise instructed by your physician.
- You may have a pillow under your head and can sit to eat.
- You should have a responsible adult with you for the rest of the day and during the night. This adult must accompany you to the bathroom and be with you until the following morning.

Diet:
Progress slowly to a regular diet. Start by giving liquids such as water or carbonated soft drinks. If you have no nausea try soup and crackers and, finally solid foods. You should drink fluids frequently.

When to Call the Doctor:
If you develop:
- A headache that is not relieved by Tylenol.
- A stiff neck.
- A fever over 101° orally.
- Pain not relieved by pain medication.
- Any bleeding or unexpected drainage from the wound.
- Extreme redness or swelling around the incision.

Where to Call with Questions:
- Your doctor. If unable to reach your doctor, then call:
  - Ambulatory SurgiCare - **672-5935**; open 7:00 a.m. to 5:00 p.m., Monday through Friday
  - At night and on weekends, phone the Emergency Room - 672-5500.

Follow-Up Appointment: _____

Additional Instructions: _____

_____

_____

_____

_____

I have received and understand the above instructions.

_____   _____
(Patient Signature)   (Nurse's Signature)

_____   _____
(Responsible Party Signature)   (Date)

The Methodist Medical Center of Illinois
Ambulatory SurgiCare

Home Care Instructions
Spinal Anesthesia

Activity:
- Bed rest is recommended for the rest of the day and during the night unless otherwise instructed by your physician.
- You may have a pillow under your head and can sit to eat.
- You should have a responsible adult with you for the rest of the day and during the night. This adult must accompany you when you get up to go to the bathroom.

Diet:
Progress slowly to a regular diet. Start by giving liquids such as water or carbonated soft drinks. If you have no nausea try soup and crackers and, finally solid foods. You should drink fluids frequently.

When to Call the Doctor:
If you develop:
- A headache that is not relieved by Tylenol.
- A stiff neck.
- A fever over 101° orally.
- Pain not relieved by pain medication.
- Any bleeding or unexpected drainage from the wound.
- Extreme redness or swelling around the incision.

Where to Call with Questions:
- Your doctor. If unable to reach your doctor, then call:
  - Ambulatory SurgiCare - **672-5935**; open 7:00 a.m. to 5:00 p.m., Monday through Friday
  - At night and on weekends, phone the Emergency Room - 672-5500.

Follow-Up Appointment: _____

Additional Instructions: _____
_____
_____
_____
_____

I have received and understand the above instructions.

_____   _____
(Patient Signature)   (Nurse's Signature)

_____   _____
(Responsible Party Signature)   (Date)

The Methodist Medical Center of Illinois
Ambulatory SurgiCare

Pediatric Home Care Instructions
General Anesthesia

Activity

Your child might feel a little sleepy for the next 24 hours. This is due to the medicine your child received. Please do not leave the child alone. Children should rest at home, but may be up and about according to doctor's instruction. Do not let the child ride bikes, skateboards, etc., for 24 hours.

Medications

Your child may have some pain. A prescription for pain may be given by the doctor. This should be taken as directed. If it does not help the pain, contact your doctor. If your doctor does not prescribe anything for pain, then you may give your child a non-prescription, non-aspirin pain medication such as, Tylenol. Please be sure to follow directions on the label. Take all pain medication with some food to prevent upset stomach.

Diet

Progress slowly to a regular diet. Start by giving liquids such as water or carbonated soft drinks. If your child has no nausea try soup and crackers and, finally solid foods.

When to Call the Doctor:

If your child develops:
* A fever over 101° orally.
* Pain not relieved by pain medication.
* Any bleeding or unexpected drainage from the wound.
* Extreme redness or swelling around the incision.
* Croupy cough.
* Nausea and vomiting that is not getting better.

Where to Call With Questions

* Your doctor. If unable to reach your doctor then call:
  * Ambulatory SurgiCare - **672-5935** open 7:00 a.m. to 5:00 p.m., Monday through Friday
  * At night and on weekends, phone the Emergency Room - 672-5500.

Follow-Up Appointment:_____

Additional Instructions: _____

_____

_____

_____

I have received and understand the above instructions.

_____   _____
(Responsible Party Signature)   (Nurse's Signature)

                                         _____
                                                    (Date)

The Methodist Medical Center of Illinois
Ambulatory SurgiCare

Postoperative Follow Up

Phone#: _____ Age: _____ Date/Time called: _____

Date of Surgery: _____ MD: _____

Procedure: _____

Anesthesia: ☐ Intubation ☐ General ☐ Sedation ☐ Regional

Has patient resumed ADL'S (Activities of Daily Living)? ☐ Yes ☐ No If not, why? _____

_____

Is patient tolerating liquids/solids/normal diet? ☐ Yes ☐ No

Any nausea or vomiting? ☐ Yes ☐ No If so when? Number of episodes? _____

What did patient do for relief? _____

_____

Does patient have pain? ☐ Yes ☐ No If so describe? (duration, location, etc.) _____

_____

Was pain medication effective? ☐ Yes ☐ No ☐ N/A. _____

_____

Is dressing/cast dry and intact? ☐ Yes ☐ No ☐ N/A _____

Is there any drainage? ☐ Yes ☐ No If so describe. _____

_____

Is there swelling, redness at operative site? ☐ Yes ☐ No If so explain. _____

_____

_____

Did patient exhibit any of the following?

Muscular discomfort?   ☐ Yes ☐ No _____

Sore throat?   ☐ Yes ☐ No _____

Elevated temp.?   ☐ Yes ☐ No _____

What are patients concerns/comments about experience? _____

_____

_____

Additional follow up necessary? ☐ Yes ☐ No _____

_____

Physician Notified ☐ Yes ☐ No. Name: _____ Time: _____

        Patient Stamp   Nurse Signature: _____

Texas Outpatient Surgicare Center

An Affiliate of Medical Care International, Inc

17080 Red Oak Drive
Houston, Texas 77090
713/444-0065

SPECIAL INFORMATION FOR PEDIATRIC OUTPATIENT SURGERY

Because hospital admissions may have profound emotional consequences in children, physicians who perform surgery on children are turning more to outpatient surgery in an attempt to avoid separating the child from its parents, while performing needed surgical procedures in a safe but unthreatening atmosphere.

Children are rewarding patients. They will amaze you by bouncing back quickly from surgical procedures. As a parent, your attention to a few details before you bring your child to the outpatient surgery unit will help to make your child's surgery as pleasant an experience as possible.

In general, it's best for you, the parent, to discuss the upcoming procedure honestly with your child before the day of surgery. During this discussion, be sure to emphasize why the surgery is necessary. Use simple language, but try to insure that your child knows that the planned procedure is being done to improve his well-being. Tangible results such as better hearing, fewer colds and "runny noses", and things of that nature should be stressed.

On the day of surgery, encourage your child to bring with him to the Surgery Center a favorite toy, doll, blanket or other object which provides a sense of security. The Surgery Center personnel will be sure that this object accompanies your child to the operating room and is with him or in the recovery room upon awakening from anesthesia.

You will be encouraged to stay with your child right up until the time he or she goes to surgery, and you will be present when your child is emerging from the anesthetic. Emergence from anesthesia, when the child may be in some pain and is disoriented, can be a frightening experience. You should assure your child that you will be there to comfort, console, and care for him or her.

Although a parent is not present during the induction of anesthesia, this is generally not an unpleasant experience for the child. For most types of outpatient surgery, no pre-anesthetic drugs are employed, so your child will not be given any "shots". It is important for your child to know that - emphasize this positive aspect of the experience to your child during your discussion.

Most often, anesthesia is induced by having the child breathe an anesthetic gas mixture out of a small mask attached to a balloon containing the gas. The Surgery Center personnel try to make a game out of this procedure, so you might explain to your child that he will fall into a pleasant sleep while blowing up a balloon.

Ether is no longer used in modern anesthesia, having been replaced by several other agents which are not unpleasant smelling, and result in a much quicker induction. In fact, if your child has a favorite flavor such as strawberry, cherry, or watermelon, tell the Surgery Center personnel since the anesthetic gas can be altered to smell like any of these or several other fruits.

A word about PREOPERATIVE FEEDING: Although adults are asked not to have anything to eat or drink after midnight before surgery, it is difficult to withhold nourishment from a child. If your child is scheduled for early morning surgery, it is generally easier to adhere to the nothing after midnight rule. However, if surgery is scheduled for late morning or afternoon, it may be possible for the child to have clear liquids up to SIX hours before surgery (depending on the age of the child and the nature of the surgery). Please ask your Doctor or the Surgery Center office staff to check with the Anesthesiologist for specific instructions.

One final word about anesthesia for children. Many children have had pets "put to sleep" by the veterinarian and have never seen them again. Although adults understand the distinction between being "put to sleep" as a form of euthanasia and being "put to sleep" for anesthesia, make sure that if your child has had a pet "put to sleep" that you either make the distinction very clear to him or avoid using the term "put to sleep".

TEXAS OUTPATIENT SURGICARE CENTER
17080 RED OAK • HOUSTON, TEXAS 77090 • 713/444-0065

For Office Use Only	
TIPS	Date Injured
PSIC	2nd Opinion YES NO
Old Chart	Pre Cert YES NO
Student YES NO Where	Lab

Texas Driver's License # of responsible adult   Date this surgery

Patient Name   Last - First - Middle   Address   City   State   Zip

Insured address if different from above.

Date of Birth   Age   Sex M F   Ht.   Wt.   Home Phone

INSURED PERSON - PRIMARY	Social Security #	INSURED PERSON - SECONDARY	Social Security #
	— —		— —
Relationship to Patient		Relationship to Patient	
Employer	Work Phone	Employer	Work Phone
Address		Address	
#1 Insurance		#2 Insurance	
Address		Address	
Group #	Telephone #	Group #	Telephone #

Workman's Comp.   Address   Claim #   Telephone #

Nearest Relative (Other than Spouse)   Address   Telephone #

Past Hospitalizations (last 5 years) - Use back if necessary   Previous Surgeries

Previous Anesthetic Complications	Drug Allergies	Type of Surgery	by Dr.

Social History
Smoke YES NO   How Much   Drink YES NO   What   How Much

| Past Medical Illness | | | If yes explain or list |
Have you ever had or do you have:	NO	YES	below, except number 11:
1. A PROBLEM WITH YOUR NERVES			
2. A PROBLEM WITH YOUR MUSCLES			
3. CHRONIC HEADACHES, NECK, BACK, LEG PAIN, FAINTING			
4. HEART TROUBLE			
5. ASTHMA, TB, PNEUMONIA LUNG PROBLEM			
6. DIABETES, GLAUCOMA			
7. HIGH BLOOD PRESSURE			
8. STEROID THERAPY			
9. JAUNDICE, HEPATITIS OR LIVER PROBLEMS			
10. BLEEDING DISORDERS			
11. DENTURES			
12. CONTACT LENSES (Must be removed)			
13. ARE YOU PRESENTLY TAKING ANY MEDICATIONS			Kind and amount
14. DO YOU CONSIDER YOURSELF TO BE IN GOOD HEALTH			
15. ANY HISTORY OF SEIZURES			
16. ASPRIN USE			

TOPS - 14 Rev. 5/88

Texas Outpatient Surgicare Center   17080 Red Oak Drive
An Affiliate of Medical Care International, Inc   Houston, Texas 77090
                                                        713/444-0065

PRE-OP POINTERS

1. Please bring a gown or robe, or something appropriate to wear after your surgery. (For example, shorts or warm-up suit after surgery on your knee.)

2. Have pillows or blankets in your car to elevate the operative site, if necessary, during the ride home.

3. DO NOT WEAR MAKE UP or NAIL POLISH to the center the day your surgery is scheduled.

4. Please DO NOT bring jewelry or valuables to the center with you.

5. Comfortable, loose-fitting shoes or slippers (no high heels) are safer and easier to dress into after your procedure.

6. All contact lenses INCLUDING EXTENDED WEAR LENSES should be removed. We are not responsible if they are lost or damaged. Should you remove your lenses at the Center, bring your container for storing them.

7. Warm socks for leg warmers may be worn in surgery unless your surgery is on your knee, leg, or foot.

8. If you are to have general anesthesia, or local with sedation, or Monitored Anesthesia Care (MAC), nothing to eat or drink after midnight – NOT EVEN CHEWING GUM OR ICE CHIPS. If you are having a local anesthesia or an epidural procedure, there are no restrictions.

POST ANESTHESIA INSTRUCTION SHEET

These instructions MUST be read carefully and followed!!!!!!!!

1. You must arrange for a responsible adult to accompany you home.

2. Do not take a public conveyance without the presence of another adult.

3. Some of the anesthesia drugs you may receive can take up to 24 hours to leave your system completely. For this reason, you should not ingest any alcoholic beverages, drive a car, operate any dangerous machinery, or make any important decisions for 24 hours after your surgery.

4. Please contact or have your responsible adult contact your surgeon anytime following discharge from the center, if you have any problems or questions regarding your surgery.

5. Please follow all post surgery instructions your surgeon has given you.

6. Please discuss these instructions with the adult to be responsible for you and leave them in his/her possession prior to your surgery.

Accredited By Accreditation Association for Ambulatory Health Care, Inc.

Texas Outpatient Surgicare Center

An Affiliate of Medical Care International, Inc

17080 Red Oak Drive
Houston, Texas 77090
713/444-0065

POST-OPERATIVE INSTRUCTIONS
THESE INSTRUCTIONS MUST BE READ CAREFULLY AND FOLLOWED FOR YOUR CARE.

DIET--------------------------CLEAR LIQUIDS SHOULD BE TAKEN INITIALLY, IF YOU ARE NOT NAUSEATED. SOLID FOOD OR MILK SHOULD NOT BE TAKEN UNTIL CLEAR LIQUIDS ARE TOLERATED.

ACTIVITY----------------------REST IS RECOMMENDED FOR THE FIRST 24 HOURS. SOME OF THE ANESTHESIA DRUGS YOU MAY RECEIVE CAN TAKE UP TO 24 HOURS TO LEAVE YOUR SYSTEM COMPLETELY. FOR THIS REASON, YOU SHOULD NOT INGEST ANY ALCOHOLIC BEVERAGES, DRIVE A CAR, OPERATE ANY DANGEROUS MACHINERY, OR MAKE ANY IMPORTANT DECISIONS FOR 24 HOURS AFTER YOUR SURGERY OR WHILE TAKING PAIN MEDICATION.

MEDICATION--------------------YOUR PHYSICIAN HAS PRESCRIBED THE FOLLOWING:

_____

_____

_____

_____

SPECIAL
INSTRUCTIONS------------------NOTIFY YOUR DOCTOR OF TEMPERATURE OF 101 OR ABOVE (OR AS SPECIFIED BY YOUR DOCTOR), OR EXCESSIVE BLEEDING FROM OPERATIVE SITE.

PLEASE CALL YOUR DOCTOR'S OFFICE WITHIN THE NEXT 2-3 DAYS AND MAKE AN APPOINTMENT FOR A POSTOPERATIVE CHECKUP UNLESS ALREADY SCHEDULED.

SHOULD YOU DEVELOP A PROBLEM AND CANNOT REACH YOUR DOCTOR, GO TO THE NEAREST EMERGENCY ROOM.

_____

_____

_____

_____

_____

_____
PATIENT'S NAME

_____
SIGNATURE OF PERSON RECEIVING INSTRUCTIONS   DATE

_____
SIGNATURE OF NURSE GIVING INSTRUCTIONS

YOU MAY EXPECT A CALL FROM ONE OF THE RECOVERY ROOM NURSES IN THE NEXT FEW DAYS. THIS WILL BE A ROUTINE CHECK ON YOUR PROGRESS.

TOPS - 20

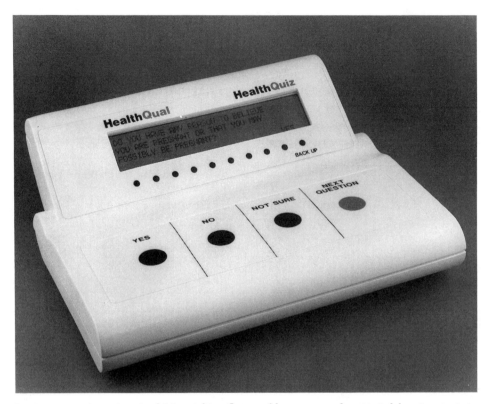

Lap top computer automates history taking, flags problem areas and suggests laboratory tests to be ordered. (SOURCE: Developed at The University of Chicago by Michael F. Roizen, M.D. Used with permission).

HEALTH QUIZ

Michael F. Roizen, M.D. has invented a computerized machine that automates the taking of patient histories. Health Quiz is a simple lightweight lap top computer with four buttons—*yes, no, not sure,* and *next question.* Dr. Roizen has shown that his machine can save time and expense lost on unnecessary laboratory testing. When used in an initial multicenter evaluation, average savings of $68.70 were realized by more efficient use of laboratory testing.

The questions appear in a simple format on a liquid crystal display screen and can be understood by anyone who is functionally literate. The patient answers up to 134 questions on a small video display. The number of questions varies because they are based on a "decision tree" whereby positive answers to particular questions generate additional questions. Although it may take upwards of 30 minutes for the patient to complete the Health Quiz (depending on patient age and physical status), the mean time for completion is approximately 8 minutes.

The machine's software is written on a "smart card," a credit card-size disk that fits into the back of the machine. Another "smart card" records answers to questions. For recordkeeping, the machine's data on an individual patient can be directly transferred to a larger desk top or mainframe computer. In this fashion, the need to store paper can be eliminated; if a physician already has a computerized recordkeeping system, the direct data transfer eliminates the need to hire a clerk to input data.

Health Quiz may alternatively be connected to a printer. In addition to answers to questions, physicians may obtain a printout of important facts (such as allergies, the presence of dentures, or difficulty with a previous anesthetic), a list of patient's symptoms, and suggestions for laboratory testing. Because Health Quiz analyzes the answers to questions as the test is being given, the recommendations to the physicians for preoperative testing are available as soon as Health Quiz is connected to a printer. See examples of symptom summary forms for alleged ASA physical status 1 and ASA physical status 3 patients on the following two pages.

```
HEALTHQUAL SYMPTOM SUMMARY FORM        PREOP-R.1          Page   1
COPYRIGHT 1988                                       NOV 27, 1989
IDENTIFICATION NUMBER : 1111111111

PATIENT NAME: _____

PHYSICIAN: _____

PRESENT COMPLAINT: _____

The patient's answers to the HealthQuiz may suggest disease in
the following systems as indicated by the following symptoms:

SYSTEM          SYMPTOMS

HEMATOL         ASA INTAKE




SOME ITEMS PERTINENT TO ANESTHESIA CARE ARE:

Patient has capped teeth.
Patient wears contact lenses.
Patient has loose, cracked, or chipped teeth.
Patient has previously had Anesthesia.
Patient or a family member had problems with Anesthesia.
Patient has restrictions in opening mouth.
Patient has clicking, popping or pain in jaw joints.
Patient has taken ASA or similar medication in the last week.

               SUGGESTED LABORATORY TESTS

HCT

Consider stool for occult blood


If operation involves insertion of a prosthesis or foreign material,
you might obtain a URINALYSIS to rule out a urinary tract infection.
```

```
HEALTHQUAL SYMPTOM SUMMARY FORM        PREOP-R.1          Page   1
COPYRIGHT 1988                                      DEC  3, 1989
IDENTIFICATION NUMBER : 2222222222

PATIENT NAME:  _____

PHYSICIAN:  _____

PRESENT COMPLAINT:  _____

The patient's answers to the HealthQuiz may suggest disease in
the following systems as indicated by the following symptoms:

SYSTEM          SYMPTOMS

CV              SOB
CV              ? MI
CV              ANGINA OR SKIPPED HEART BEATS
CV              CV MEDS
CV              DOE
CV              SLEEPS WITH MORE THAN ONE PILLOW

PULM            ? COPD




SOME ITEMS PERTINENT TO ANESTHESIA CARE ARE:

Patient has previously had Anesthesia.
Patient gets SOB with minor exertion.
Patient takes heart active drugs (see question 115).
Patient takes heart active drugs (see question 116).

                SUGGESTED LABORATORY TESTS

POTASSIUM                          BUN AND/OR CREAT
CHEST XRAY PA/LAT                   EKG


Consider stool for occult blood


If operation is associated with significant blood loss, you might
obtain Hgb or HCT.


If operation involves insertion of a prosthesis or foreign material,
you might obtain a URINALYSIS to rule out a urinary tract infection.
```

Index

■ ■